TEXTBOOK OF VETERINARY DIAGNOSTIC RADIOLOGY

DONALD E. THRALL, DVM, PhD

Professor of Radiology, North Carolina State University, School of Veterinary Medicine, Raleigh, North Carolina

W.B. SAUNDERS COMPANY

Philadelphia   London   Toronto   Mexico City
Rio de Janeiro   Sydney   Tokyo   Hong Kong

W. B. Saunders Company: West Washington Square
                          Philadelphia, PA 19105

Library of Congress Cataloging in Publication Data
Main entry under title:

Veterinary diagnostic radiology.

1. Veterinary radiology.   2. Veterinary medicine—Diagnosis.   I. Thrall, Donald E. [DNLM: 1. Radiography—veterinary.   SF 757.8 V586]

SF757.8.V48 1986   636.089′607572   85–8386

ISBN 0–7216–1199–0

Editor: Darlene Pedersen
Designer: Bill Donnelly
Production Manager: Laura Tarves
Illustration Coordinator: Walt Verbitski
Page Layout Artist: Patti Maddaloni

Veterinary Diagnostic Radiology   ISBN   0–7216–1199–0

Last digit is the print number: 9   8   7   6   5   4   3   2

This book is dedicated to Drs. W. C. Banks (deceased), W. D. Carlson, M. A. Emmerson, W. H. Rhodes, and G. B. Schnelle (deceasced), who, as members of the organizing committee for the American Board of Veterinary Radiology, now the American College of Veterinary Radiology, were instrumental in the establishment of veterinary radiology as a recognized specialty.

CONTRIBUTORS

Graeme S. Allan, B.V.Sc., M.V.Sc., F.A.C.V.Sc.; Diplomate, American College of Veterinary Radiology
Specialist Veterinary Radiologist; Attending Veterinary Radiologist, Sydney University Veterinary Hospital and Clinic, Sydney University, Sydney, Australia.
Radiographic Signs of Joint Disease—Companion Animals

Robert J. Bahr, D.V.M.
Associate Professor of Veterinary Radiology, College of Veterinary Medicine, Oklahoma State University; Section Chief, Boren Veterinary Medical Teaching Hospital, Stillwater, Oklahoma.
The Thoracic Wall—Companion Animals
The Heart and Great Vessels—Companion Animals

Don L. Barber, D.V.M., M.S.
Professor of Veterinary Radiology; Coordinator of Radiologic Services, Veterinary Teaching Hospital, Virginia-Maryland Regional College of Veterinary Medicine, Blacksburg, Virginia.
The Peritoneal Space—Companion Animals
Abdominal Lymph Nodes
The Adrenal Glands
The Stomach—Companion Animals

Jan E. Bartels, D.V.M., M.S.; Diplomate, American College of Veterinary Radiology
Professor and Head of Department of Radiology, School of Veterinary Medicine, Auburn University, Auburn, Alabama.
Intervertebral Disc Disease—Companion Animals

Darryl N. Biery, D.V.M.
Professor of Radiology, University of Pennsylvania School of Veterinary Medicine, Philadelphia, Pennsylvania.
The Large Bowel—Companion Animals

J. Gregg Boring, D.V.M., M.S.
Professor and Chief of Radiology Services, College of Veterinary Medicine, Mississippi State University, Mississippi State, Mississippi.
The Carpus—Equidae

Sydney M. Evans, V.M.D.
Instructor in Radiology, Veterinary Hospital, University of Pennsylvania, Philadelphia, Pennsylvania.
Avian Radiography

Charles S. Farrow, D.V.M.
Professor of Radiology, University of Saskatchewan, Western College of Veterinary Medicine; Chief, Special Clinical Services, Veterinary

Teaching Hospital, Western College of Veterinary Medicine, University of Saskatchewan, Saskatoon, Saskatchewan, Canada.
The Larynx, Pharynx, and Trachea—Equidae
Neck and Thorax—Equidae

Daniel A. Feeney, D.V.M., M.S.
Associate Professor of Radiology, College of Veterinary Medicine, University of Minnesota; Radiologist, University of Minnesota Veterinary Teaching Hospitals, St. Paul, Minnesota.
The Kidneys and Ureters—Companion
*   Animals*
The Uterus—Companion Animals
The Ovaries and Testes—Companion Animals

Patrick R. Gavin, D.V.M., Ph.D.
Associate Professor of Radiology, College of Veterinary Medicine, Washington State University, Pullman, Washington.
The Equine Spine

Gary R. Johnston, D.V.M., M.S.
Associated Professor of Radiology, College of Veterinary Medicine, University of Minnesota; Radiologist, University of Minnesota Veterinary Teaching Hospitals, St. Paul, Minnesota.
The Kidneys and Ureters—Companion
*   Animals*
The Uterus—Companion Animals
The Ovaries and Testes—Companion Animals

Stephen K. Kneller, D.V.M., M.S.
Associate Professor, Department of Clinical Veterinary Medicine; Chief of Radiology Section, Veterinary Medicine Teaching Hospital, College of Veterinary Medicine, University of Illinois, Urbana, Illinois.
The Metacarpus and Metatarsus—Equidae
The Larynx, Pharynx, and
*   Trachea—Companion Animals*

Jimmy C. Lattimer, D.V.M., M.S.;
Diplomate, American College of Veterinary Radiology
Assistant Professor of Radiology, College of Veterinary Medicine, University of Missouri—Columbia, Columbia, Missouri.
Equine Nasal Passages, Sinuses, and Guttural
*   Pouches*
The Prostate—Companion Animals

John M. Losonsky, D.V.M., M.S.
Associate Professor, Department of Veterinary Clinical Medicine, College of Veterinary Medicine, Staff Radiologist, Veterinary Medical Teaching Hospital, University of Illinois, Urbana, Illinois.
The Pulmonary Vasculature—Companion
*   Animals*

Mary B. Mahaffey, D.V.M., M.S.;
Diplomate, American College of Veterinary Radiology
Assistant Professor of Radiology, College of Veterinary Medicine, The University of Georgia, Athens, Georgia.
The Stifle and Tarsus—Equidae
The Peritoneal Spaces—Companion Animals
Abdominal Lymph Nodes
The Adrenal Glands
The Stomach—Companion Animals

Sandra V. McNeel, D.V.M.; Diplomate, American College of Veterinary Radiology
Associate Professor, Radiology Section, Department of Veterinary Clinical Sciences, College of Veterinary Medicine, Iowa State University, Ames, Iowa.
The Phalanges—Equidae
The Small Bowel—Companion Animals

Michael R. Metcalf, D.V.M., M.S.
Assistant Professor of Radiology, School of Veterinary Medicine, North Carolina State University, Raleigh, North Carolina.
Diseases of the Immature
*   Skeleton—Companion Animals*

Wendy Myer, D.V.M., M.S.
Associate Professor of Veterinary Radiology, The Ohio State University College of Veterinary Medicine; Veterinary Radiologist, The Ohio State University Veterinary Teaching Hospital, Columbus, Ohio.
The Cranial Vault and Associated
*   Structures—Companion Animals*
The Nasal Cavity and Paranasal
*   Sinuses—Companion Animals*

Richard D. Park, D.V.M., Ph.D.; Diplomate, American College of Veterinary Radiology
Professor, Department of Radiology and Radiation Biology, College of Veterinary Medicine and Biomedical Sciences, Colorado State University; Head, Section of Radiology, Veterinary Teaching Hospital, Colorado State University, Fort Collins, Colorado.
The Diaphragm—Companion Animals
The Urinary Bladder—Companion Animals

Robert D. Pechman, Jr., D.V.M.
Associate Professor of Veterinary Radiology, Louisiana State University, School of Veterinary Medicine, Baton Rouge, Louisiana.
The Liver and Spleen—Companion Animals
The Urethra—Companion Animals

Norman W. Rantanen, D.V.M., M.S.
Lexington, Kentucky.
Alternate Imaging

Charles R. Root, D.V.M., M.S.; Diplomate, American College of Veterinary Radiology
Animal Radiology and Radiography Service, Bothell, Washington.
The Thoracic Wall—Companion Animals
The Heart and Great Vessels—Companion Animals
Abdominal Masses

Ronald D. Sande, D.V.M., M.S., Ph.D.
Professor of Veterinary Radiology, Washington State University; Services Division Head, Washington State University Teaching Hospital, Pullman, Washington.
The Metacarpo-(Metatarso-) Phalangeal Articulation—Equidae
The Pleural Space—Equidae

Russ Stickle, D.V.M.
Assistant Professor, Michigan State University, College of Veterinary Medicine, East Lansing, Michigan.
The Equine Skull

Jon Stowater, D.V.M., M.S.
Assistant Professor of Radiology, Tufts University, School of Veterinary Medicine, North Grafton, Massachusetts.
Aggressive vs Nonaggressive Bone Lesions

Donald E. Thrall, D.V.M., Ph.D.
Professor of Radiology, North Carolina State University, School of Veterinary Medicine, Raleigh, North Carolina.
Introduction to Radiographic Interpretation
Neoplasia—Companion Animals
The Stifle and Tarsus—Equidae
The Mediastinum—Companion Animals
The Pleural Space—Companion Animals

Robert L. Toal, D.V.M., M.S.
Assistant Professor of Radiology, Department of Rural Practice, College of Veterinary Medicine, The University of Tennessee, Knoxville, Tennessee.
Fracture Healing and Complications—Companion Animals
The Navicular Bone—Equidae

Michael A. Walker, D.V.M.; Diplomate, American College of Veterinary Radiology
Associate Professor, College of Veterinary Medicine, The University of Tennessee, Knoxville, Tennessee.
The Vertebrae—Companion Animals

Barbara J. Watrous, D.V.M.; Diplomate, American College of Veterinary Radiology
Assistant Professor, Oregon State University, College of Veterinary Medicine, Corvallis, Oregon.
The Esophagus—Companion Animals

John W. Watters, D.V.M., M.S.; Diplomate, American College of Veterinary Radiology
Professor of Veterinary Radiology, School of Veterinary Medicine; Assistant Director of the Veterinary Teaching Hospital and Clinics—Ancillary Services, Louisiana State University, Baton Rouge, Louisiana.
The Lungs—Companion Animals

Jeffrey A. Wortman, V.M.D., Ph.D.
Assistant Professor of Radiology; Chief, Section of Radiology, University of Pennsylvania, School of Veterinary Medicine, Philadelphia, Pennsylvania.
Alternate Imaging

PREFACE

The level of sophistication of veterinary radiology has increased considerably in the past 15 years. So has the number of books dealing with the subject. Yet a need remains for a comprehensive general veterinary radiology book to be used as a text by students of veterinary medicine and as a reference by practitioners of companion animal or equine medicine and surgery. This need prompted the writing of this book.

It is my opinion that it is impossible for any one person to produce a comprehensive, accurate textbook of veterinary diagnostic radiology. Thus, the genesis of the multiple-author format contained herein. I am honored that so many distinguished radiologists agreed to take time from their busy schedules to contribute chapters. Without their cooperation and expertise this book would not have been possible.

The method of radiographic interpretation recommended by and utilized in this text is the roentgen sign method. The basis of this method is recognition of radiographic abnormalities and correlation of those abnormalities with the signalment, history, and clinical and laboratory data in order to formulate a differential diagnosis.

We hope that the book we have produced is a useful one. It is conceptually a basic information source that we hope will make interpretation of radiographs easier for students of radiology.

DONALD E. THRALL

CONTENTS

SECTION 1

PRINCIPLES OF INTERPRETATION

CHAPTER 1

INTRODUCTION TO RADIOGRAPHIC INTERPRETATION

DONALD E. THRALL

X RAYS AND RADIOGRAPHS

X rays are a type of electromagnetic radiation, similar to visible light. The wavelength of x rays, however, is shorter than that of visible light, making them more energetic. The higher energy of x rays allows them to penetrate many types of matter that light rays cannot. The science of radiology is based upon the property of x rays being able to penetrate matter. For example, the intricate internal spiraling of a conch shell is impossible to perceive from its exterior because the shell cannot be penetrated by light. By using x rays to "see through" the shell, the internal spiraling pattern becomes apparent (Fig. 1–1). Thus, x rays provide a means to visualize the internal structures of objects or patients.

A radiograph is a picture of the number of x rays passing through an object. The radiographic image is recorded on photographic film consisting of a silver-containing photographic emulsion bound to a transparent base. X rays interacting directly with the emulsion result in precipitation of metallic silver (black) when the film is processed. In clinical practice, however, silver precipitation is usually produced by light

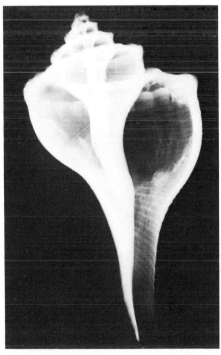

Figure 1–1. Radiograph of a conch shell illustrates the ability of x rays to provide images of the internal structure of nontransparent objects. The intricate internal spiraling pattern is not apparent when viewing the exterior of the shell. Radiology is based on the ability to "see" internal structures of patients by using x rays and a photographic emulsion recording system.

1

emitted from an intensifying screen, which fluoresces when struck by x rays. Intensifying screens are used because the x ray film emulsion is more sensitive to light than to x rays. Some individuals use the term "x ray," "film," "plate," and "picture" as jargon for the term radiograph; this is incorrect practice and should be avoided.

The degree of blackness of a radiograph is directly related to the number of x rays that reach the film or intensifying screen. Thus, areas of the film emulsion struck by a large number of x rays or a large amount of light from the intensifying screen are black after film processing. Conversely, areas struck by no light or radiation are transparent. Between these two extremes is a range of gray film tones, the blackness of which is directly related to the number of x rays that reach the film or the intensifying screen (Fig. 1–2).

The degree of blackening of the x ray film is

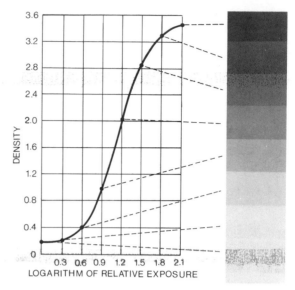

Figure 1–3. Relationship between relative radiation exposure (x-axis) and resulting optical film density (y-axis). As radiation exposure increases, so does optical film density, i.e., blackness. (From Fundamentals of Radiography, 12th ed. Eastman Kodak Comapny, 1980, with permission.)

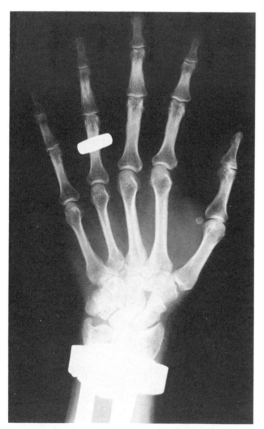

Figure 1–2. Radiograph of a human hand. Black regions represent areas of the film over which no x rays were absorbed from the x-ray beam before reaching the cassette. Homogeneously white areas, such as the watch and ring, are those over which *all* x rays were absorbed before the beam reached the cassette. Between these two extremes are many shades of gray resulting from various degree of x-ray absorption from the primary beam. It should be obvious that bones absorbed more x rays than fleshy parts of the hand.

measured in terms of optical density. Optical density and film blackness are directly related (Fig. 1–3). The term density is also often used to describe the degree to which the patient or object radiographed absorbs incident x rays. For example, in Figure 1–2, some would refer to the ring, watch, and bones as more dense than the adjacent soft tissue. This usage is confusing because the degree of the *optical* density of the film in these areas is low, whereas that of the *object* density is high. Further confusion arises when the added variable of physical density (g/cm^3) of the patient or object is considered. As the physical density of the patient or object increases, the optical film density decreases, whereas the object or radiographic density increases. This confusing terminology can be avoided by using the term density as it refers to the radiograph only in relation to the measurable optical density of the film. The degree of blackness or whiteness of the patient or object being radiographed should be referred to in terms of radiolucency or radiopacity, respectively. For example, in Figure 1–2, soft tissues of the hand are more radiolucent than the bones; both are more radiolucent than the watch and the ring. It may also be said that the watch and the ring are more radiopaque than the remainder of the hand. Describing radiographic appearance in terms of radiolucency (lucency) and radiopacity (opacity) avoids the confusion associated with the use of the term density for such purposes.

IMAGE FORMATION AND DIFFERENTIAL ABSORPTION

It is possible to use x rays to produce an image of a patient or object on film because some x rays are absorbed by the patient or object and some pass through unchanged, producing film blackening. Of particular importance in patient radiography is the fact that x rays are not absorbed homogeneously by the body; some tissues absorb x rays more efficiently than others. This phenomenon is called differential absorption. If absorption of x rays by the patient were uniform (no differential absorption), the resulting radiographic image would be gray or white. On the other hand, if no absorption occurred, the resulting radiograph would be homogeneously black. The effect of differential absorption is illustrated in Figure 1–2 wherein the areas between the fingers and adjacent to the hand are black because no x rays from the incident beam were absorbed before reaching the intensifying screen. Soft tissues of the hand are visible because they have absorbed some x rays from the primary beam. Bones of the hand are more radiopaque than soft tissues; the bones have absorbed more x rays and thus that part of the intensifying screen under the bones was struck by fewer x rays than the part under the fleshy parts of the hand. The watch and ring appear totally radiopaque because no x rays were able to pass through them. The degree of differential absorption of x rays by a patient or object depends on the energy of the x rays and the composition of the patient or object.

A detailed discussion of radiographic technique is beyond the scope of this book, but it is important to recognize that the degree of differential absorption of x rays by the patient is a function of x-ray energy. As the energy of x rays increases, so does their penetrability. Thus, when higher energy x rays are used, the lesser is the degree of differential absorption by the patient. When lower energy x rays are used there is more difference between the radiopacity of bone and soft tissue.

IMPORTANCE OF TISSUE COMPOSITION

Although the effect of x-ray energy on differential absorption is important, it is the dependence of x-ray absorption on tissue or object composition that allows radiographic images of patients to be produced. X-ray absorption by a substance is affected by the effective atomic number of its elements and the physical density of the substance. Consider the physical density and effective atomic number of the substances listed in Table 1–1. By recognizing the direct relationship between the absorption of x rays,

TABLE 1–1. PHYSICAL DENSITY AND EFFECTIVE ATOMIC NUMBER OF VARIOUS SUBSTANCES

Substance	Physical Density (g/cm^3)	Effective Atomic Number
Air	0.001	7.8
Fat	0.92	6.5
Water	1.00	7.5
Muscle	1.04	7.6
Bone	1.65	12.3

physical density, and effective atomic number, the substances in Table 1–1 may be ranked in order of increasing radiopacity. If your calculations are correct, air would be listed as the most radiolucent substance. The radiolucency of air and other gases results from their low physical density. Even though the effective atomic number of air is higher than that of fat, air is more radiolucent because of its lower physical density, i.e., there are many fewer molecules per unit area to absorb x rays. If air could be compressed until its physical density equaled that of fat, it would be more radiopaque than fat because of its greater atomic number.

The next more radiopaque substance in Table 1–1 is fat. Although the effective atomic number of fat is less than that of air, its physical density is greater, making fat more radiopaque than air. Next, consider the physical density and effective atomic number of water and muscle. It may be theorized that muscle would be more radiopaque than water because of its higher physical density and effective atomic number. The sensitivity of the radiographic imaging system, however, is not great enough to allow detection of differences in the radiopacity of substances with such small differences in physical density and effective atomic number. Thus, the radiopacity of most fluids (blood, urine, transudates, exudates, bile, and cerebrospinal fluid) and nonmineralized, nonadipose tissues (cartilage, muscle, fascia, tendons, ligaments, and parenchymal organs) is essentially the same. The radiopacity of these fluids and tissues is referred to as soft-tissue radiopacity. The most radiopaque substance in Table 1–1 is bone; its physical density and effective atomic number are higher than those of the other substances listed. Thus, there are five perceivable degrees of inherent tissue radiopacity: air, fat, soft tissue, bone, and metal (Fig. 1–4). Most metals have a high physical density and atomic number and absorb diagnostic x rays efficiently, thereby being rendered totally radiopaque.

In the discussion of relative inherent radiopacities, thickness was not mentioned. Thickness of the object radiographed and "total" resulting radiopacity are interrelated; as thick-

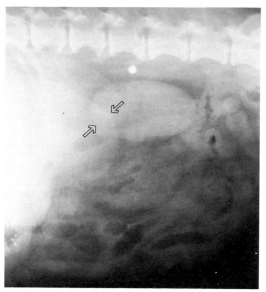

Figure 1–4. Lateral view of abdomen in which the five different radiopacities are represented. Air radiopacity: gas in the bowel. Fat radiopacity: adipose tissue in the retroperitoneal space, which is more radiopaque than gas, but less radiopaque than the kidneys themselves. Soft tissue radiopacity: the kidneys; note the summation shadow created by overlapping of the caudal pole of the right kidney and the cranial pole of the left kidney *(arrows)*. Bone radiopacity: the vertebrae. Metal radiopacity: the shotgun pellet. The exact location of the pellet cannot be determined from this lateral view alone. It could be in the skin, intraperitoneal space, or retroperitoneal space, or lying on top of the x-ray table, under the dog. Two views, at 90 degrees from each other, are necessary to identify the location of such foreign bodies. The ventrodorsal abdominal radiograph of this dog is shown in Figure 1–14. By evaluating these views, the location of the pellet may be determined.

the same magnitude. For example, although we state that fat is inherently more radiolucent than bone, if a block of fat measuring 24 cm × 24 cm × 24 cm is placed on a cassette next to a slice of bone of a thickness of 1 mm, the fat would appear more radiopaque; i.e., its total radiopacity would be greater. It is critical to remember that radiopacity depends on thickness and inherent radiopacity.

RADIOGRAPHIC GEOMETRY

Now that the basic principles of image formation and differential absorption are understood, it is important to recognize that certain geometric factors can affect the quality of the resultant image. Two important factors are magnification and distortion.

Magnification refers to the enlargement of the image relative to the actual object size. Magnification depends on the subject-film distance and tube-film distance. In clinical practice, subject-film distance affects magnification more than does tube-film distance. When subject-film distance increases, magnification increases. In the magnified image, each piece of visual information is spread over a larger area of the film, which makes the image less sharp. It must be appreciated that some parts of the patient are always farther from the film than other parts (Fig. 1–6). Thus, whenever possible, the area of primary interest should be placed in the closest proximity to the cassette.

Distortion is present when the image misrepresents the true shape or position of the object. Distortion results from unequal magnification of different parts of the same object; it can be minimized by keeping the object and the film planes parallel. Some distortion occurs in every radiograph because there are always parts of the patient that are not parallel to the film plane. Severe distortion, however, may limit the diagnostic quality of the radiograph (Fig. 1–7).

ness increases, radiopacity increases (Fig. 1–5). Thus, the different radiopacities discussed previously (air, fat, soft tissue, bone, and metal) are relative inherent radiopacities, assuming that the substance thickness is of approximately

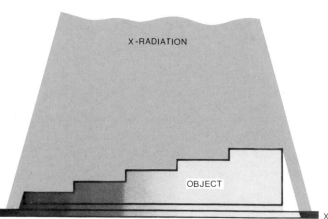

X-RADIATION

OBJECT

X-RAY FILM

Figure 1–5. Effect of object or patient thickness on radiopacity. Areas of the film under thicker parts of the patient or object are more radiolucent than those under the thinner parts. Therefore, radiopacity is directly proportional to patient thickness. (From Fundamentals of Radiography, 12th ed. Eastman Kodak Company, 1980, with permission.)

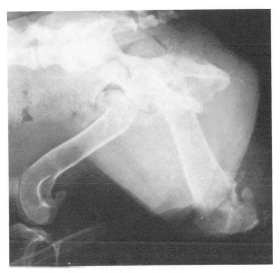

Figure 1–6. Lateral view of the pelvis of a dog in right lateral recumbency. The right pelvic limb was pulled cranially, the left pelvic limb caudally. Notice the increased diameter of the left femur in comparison with the right because of magnification—the left femur is farther from the cassette. Margins of the magnified left femur are less sharp than those of the right.

Thinking in Three Dimensions. It must be remembered that a radiograph is a two-dimensional image of a three-dimensional object. Thus, the radiographic image of the object depends on its orientation with respect to the primary x-ray beam. In some instances, the image may not resemble the object to the degree that it cannot be identified (Fig. 1–8). Therefore, patient positioning for radiography is important and must be standardized. Another result of the two-dimensional radiographic image is the loss of depth perception. To evaluate depth radiographically, it is necessary to make two radiographs of the object, with one view at

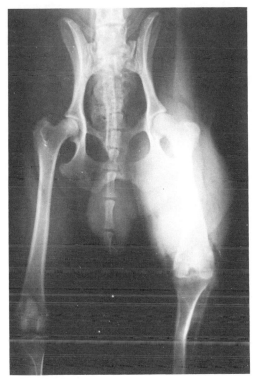

Figure 1–7. Ventrodorsal view of the pelvis. The right femur was held parallel to table top; the left femur was positioned with the stifle farther away from the table top. The left femur appears shorter than the right and is asymmetrically magnified because of distortion, i.e., it was not struck perpendicularly by the x-ray beam. The left thigh also appears more radiopaque than the right because the thickness of tissue traversed by the x-ray beam was greater on the left owing to the leg angulation.

a 90 degree angle from the other. Depth can then be mentally reconstructed (Fig. 1–4). In addition, some lesions are apparent in only one radiographic projection (Fig. 1–9). Thus, for

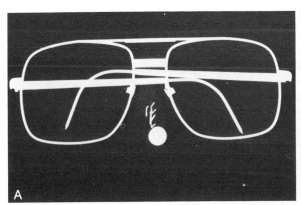
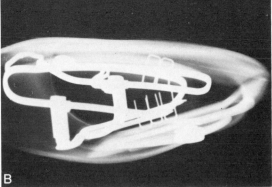

Figure 1–8. How recognizable an object, or body part, is from its radiograph depends on its relationship to the primary x-ray beam. The object in *A* is easily recognizable. The object in *B* is difficult to recognize as the same pair of eyeglasses, unless one knew the identity of the object before radiography and that the glasses case was viewed on end (parallel to the primary beam).

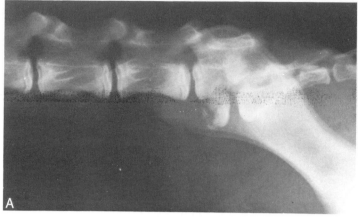

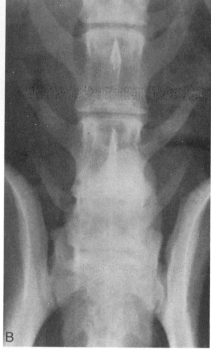

Figure 1–9. Lateral (A) and ventrodorsal (B) radiographs of a canine lumbar spine. A, There is a displaced fracture of L7. B, The fracture itself canot be seen; L7, however, appears decreased in length. Some lesions are more apparent on one radiographic projection than on others. Thus, at least two projections of a body part should be made routinely.

each patient, a minimum of two views at 90 degrees from each other, should be obtained; other oblique views may be necessary.

A final consequence of the radiograph being a two-dimensional image of a three-dimensional object is the summation effect. When parts of a patient or object in different planes are superimposed, the result is a summation image representing the degree of x-ray absorption by all superimposed objects. For example, consider the structure of a block of Swiss cheese. There are holes apparent on the exterior of the block; cuts have been made through cavities formed by gas accumulation as the cheese was processed. Inside the block are more cavities, some of which are superimposed. When a radiograph of the block is made, fewer x rays are absorbed by the cheese in areas where cavities overlap; the more cavities that overlap, the greater the number of x rays that reach the film

(Fig. 1–10). Thus, in the instance of Swiss cheese, the resulting summation shadows are radiolucent because they represent summation of radiolucent images. Summation shadows can also be radiopaque (Fig. 1–4). One must remember that radiographs are summation shadowgrams. When a suspicious radiopacity or radiolucency is identified, consideration must be given to the possibility that it represents a summation shadow produced by the overlapping of normal structures.

RADIOGRAPHIC NOMENCLATURE

Radiographic projections are named according to the direction in which the central ray of the primary x-ray beam penetrates the body part of interest, from *point of entrance* to *point of exit*. Directional terms used to describe radiographic views should be those listed in the *Nomina*

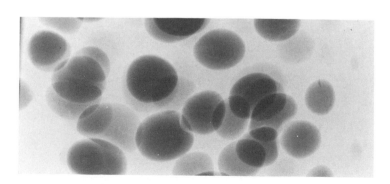

Figure 1–10. Radiograph of a block of Swiss cheese illustrates the principle of summation shadows. Gas-filled cavities in the cheese are apparent. Areas in which gas cavities overlap are more radiolucent than areas in which no overlapping has occurred. Increased radiolucency is due to decreased x-ray absorption in areas where cavities overlap. There are areas where none, two, three, and four cavities have overlapped. Can you identify them? These summation shadows are negative, because they result in increased radiolucency. See Figure 1–4 for an example of a positive summation shadow.

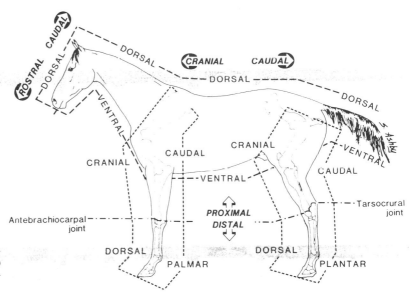

Figure 1–11. Proper anatomic directional terms as they apply to various parts of the body. (Courtesy of Dr. J. E. Smallwood.)

Anatomica Veterinaria. An abdominal radiograph made with the dog in dorsal recumbency and the use of an overhead, vertically directed x-ray beam is called a ventrodorsal view; with the dog in ventral recumbency, it would be called a dorsoventral view. The same method is used for other body parts, with the appropriate directional term applied (Fig. 1–11). In some instances, it is customary to specify only the point of entrance of the x-ray beam. For example, lateromedial projections of extremities are commonly referred to as laterals. Mediolateral radiographs of extremities are also usually referred to as laterals. It is impossible to determine from the radiographic anatomy alone whether extremity radiographs were of lateromedial or mediolateral projection; some external marking system is necessary for such distinction.

Oblique projections should be named by using the same method as standard views, i.e., by designating anatomically the points of entrance and exit (Fig. 1–12). Angles of obliquity can also be designated by inserting the number of degrees of obliquity between the directional terms involved. If the dorsolateral-palmaromedial oblique (DL-PaMO) projection in Figure 1–12 were made by positioning the x-ray tube 60 degrees laterally with respect to dorsal, the designation could be D60L-PaMO. This term implies that, beginning dorsally, one proceeds 60 degrees to the lateral side to locate the point of entrance of the x-ray beam. This same view could also be called either a dorsolateral oblique or a dorsal 60 degree lateral oblique, because the point of exit is obvious once the point of entrance is known.

RADIOGRAPH VIEWING

To assist in developing a mental picture of normal radiographic anatomy, radiographs should always be placed on the illuminator in a standard manner. Lateral views of any part, i.e., anatomy viewed in a sagittal plane, should be viewed with the cranial (rostral) aspect of the animal to the viewer's left. Ventrodorsal or dorsoventral radiographs of the head, neck, or trunk, i.e., anatomy viewed in a dorsal plane, should be placed with the cranial (rostral) part of the animal pointing up and with the left side of the animal on the right side of the image.

Figure 1–12. Description of radiographic projections by direction of penetration of the x-ray beam, from point of entrance to point of exit (proximal view of equine proximal carpal bones). (Courtesy of Dr. J. E. Smallwood.)

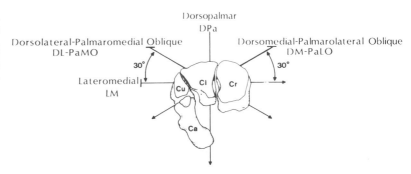

Caudocranial (plantarodorsal, palmarodorsal) or craniocaudal (dorsopalmar, dorsoplantar) radiographs of the extremities should be placed on the illuminator with the proximal end of the extremity at the top; there is no convention regarding whether the medial or lateral side of the extremity should be to the viewer's left. Random positioning of radiographs on the illuminator increases the difficulty in establishing a mental picture of normal radiographic anatomy.

When interpreting radiographs, an isolated, quiet environment should be sought; distractions cause one's diagnostic accuracy to decrease. Adequate illumination, such as a good quality, evenly illuminated viewbox, is essential for accurate film interpretation. At least two illuminators are desirable so that at least two views can be evaluated simultaneously. At all costs, avoid interpreting radiographs by holding them toward a room light. A valuable aid in interpreting radiographs, particularly of large animals, is a spotlight, sometimes referred to as a hot light. A spotlight is an intense light source that allows observation of overexposed areas on a radiograph, such as soft tissues adjacent to bone. Minimal new bone growth, which may be easily overlooked under normal illumination, can become apparent when the radiograph is viewed with a spotlight.

Radiographs should be examined with the viewer positioned at an appropriate distance from the viewbox. Often an abnormality is missed if the viewer is too close to the illuminator; it may only be apparent when the examiner moves back and looks at the entire radiograph from a distance of 4 to 6 feet.

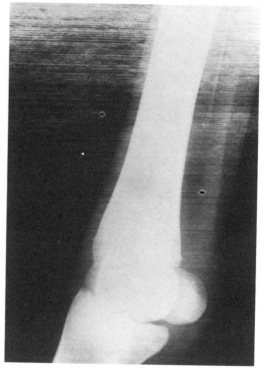

Figure 1–13. Inappropriate alignment between the primary x-ray beam and the grid resulted in grid "cut-off" and underexposure. Visible structures cannot be evaluated sufficiently from this radiograph.

PRINCIPLES OF INTERPRETATION

Radiographic interpretation is neither mysterious nor difficult if certain basic procedures are followed. Reading a radiograph is a matter of compiling all of the evidence, analyzing it, and arriving at reasonable conclusions. There are a number of important steps to this process.

Step 1: The Signalment and Case History. As in any phase of clinical diagnosis, the breed, sex, and age, as well as complete knowledge of the medical history of the animal, must be known for accurate radiographic assessment. As an example, previous trauma may have resulted in appreciable alteration of the normal anatomy. If the existence of such previous trauma was unknown, the radiographic manifestations of the altered anatomy could be misinterpreted with significant consequences.

Step 2: The Physical Examination. A radiographic examination is performed only afer a clinical opinion of the possible abnormality has been formed. Generally, the purpose of a radiographic examination is to confirm a clinical diagnosis or impression, not to make the diagnosis. A detailed and complete physical examination is necessary to establish a reason for radiographic evaluation and to determine the part or parts of the animal to be examined radiographically.

Step 3: The Correct Radiographic Procedure. As stated previously, a discussion of the technical aspects of radiography is beyond the scope of this book. Nevertheless, its importance cannot be overlooked. No matter how astute the clinician becomes at radiographic interpretation, if a radiographic examination is technically inadequate because of an insufficient number of views, improper exposure factors, inadequate axillary equipment such as cassettes and screens or poor darkroom technique, important information may be overlooked and the correct diagnosis may be missed (Fig. 1–13). A poor quality radiograph is at best inconclusive and at worst totally misleading.

Step 4: Evaluating the Radiograph. Evaluating a radiograph consists of determining whether an abnormality exists, defining the anatomic location of the lesion, classifying the lesion according to its roentgen signs, and making a differential diagnosis.

In the process of trying to determine whether

or not an abnormality exists, the entire radiograph must be evaluated. The organ approach or the area approach may be used. In the organ approach, the evaluator makes a conscious effort to evaluate every organ on the radiograph. In the area approach, the evaluator approaches the radiograph by starting the analysis centrally and working peripherally or vice versa. Whether to use the organ or area approach is an individual decision. Nevertheless, whichever approach is adopted, the entire radiograph should be interpreted in a systematic manner.

Determining whether or not an abnormality exists is often the most difficult part of radiographic interpretation. One reason for this difficulty is that the range of normal anatomic variation is broad. It is virtually impossible to remember, or even see in a lifetime, all of the anatomic variations present in domestic animals. This does not mean, however, that anatomic variation will always be misinterpreted as abnormal. There are published radiographic anatomy references available for comparison. In addition, if the suspected abnormality involves an extremity, the contralateral limb can be used for comparison.

The value of experience in deciding if a

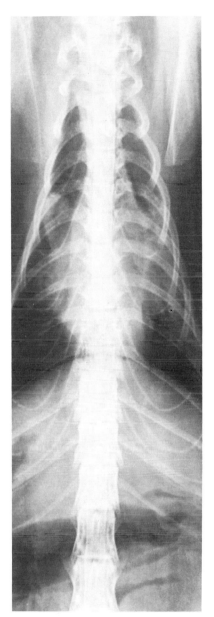

Figure 1–15. Roentgen sign example: number. There are 14 pairs of ribs.

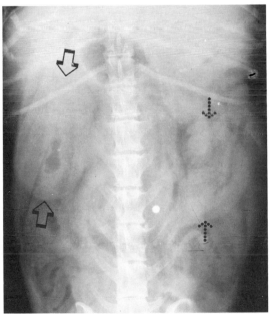

Figure 1–14. Roentgen sign example: size and position. The size of the right kidney is increased *(open arrows)*; compare it with the normal left kidney *(dotted arrows)*. The position of the caudal pole of the right kidney is abnormal; it is displaced laterally. This is the ventrodorsal view of the abdomen of the dog in Figure 1–4. Note the location of the shotgun pellet. By mentally reconstructing the third dimension after viewing both radiographs, one can deduce that the shotgun pellet is lodged in the retroperitoneal space medial to the caudal pole of the left kidney.

radiographic abnormality is present cannot be underestimated. Those individuals just beginning to evaluate radiographs should not be discouraged by the relative ease with which more experienced persons discover radiographic abnormalities. The more radiographs one systematically analyzes, the easier is the detection of lesions.

Once a lesion has been identified, the next step is to determine its anatomic location. In certain instances, such as an abnormality involving a long bone, determination of lesion location is easier than when a more complex anatomic area is involved. Difficulty in identi-

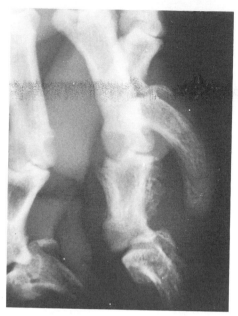

Figure 1–16. Roentgen sign example: margination. There is periosteal proliferation on the middle phalanx of the fourth digit.

fying the location of an abnormality is compounded by the fact, as noted previously, that the radiograph is a two-dimensional image of a three-dimensional object. Thus, a minimum of two radiographic projections, at a 90 degree angle from each other, are needed of any body part. Without two such views, the third dimension of depth cannot be mentally reconstructed, and it is therefore impossible to locate accurately the lesion in question (Fig. 1–4). Oblique projections may also be required. It is also necessary, of course, to have a thorough knowledge of gross anatomy. A skeletal model, particularly of complex areas such as the carpus and tarsus, is often helpful.

Once a lesion has been identified and located, the next step is to describe the lesion according to its roentgen signs. Roentgen signs have been defined as changes in size, shape, number, location, margination, and radiopacity. By describing the lesion according to its roentgen signs, the error-prone method of immediately jumping to a diagnosis because the lesion "looks like something you may have seen or heard about before" (the so-called Aunt Minny approach) can be avoided. The Aunt Minny approach to radiographic diagnosis can be quite impressive and attractive to those individuals who are beginning to learn how to evaluate radiographs; users of the Aunt Minny approach appear to have *supernatural* ability. Aunt Minny is a *charlatan,* however, and proponents of this method soon learn there is more than one possible cause for most radiographically detectable lesions. Thus, the roentgen sign approach is more reliable. By first describing a

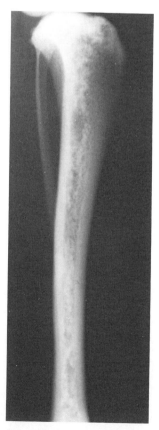

Figure 1–17. Roentgen sign example: radiopacity. There are multifocal areas of increased radiopacity in the medullary cavity of the tibia.

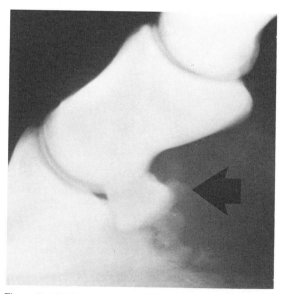

Figure 1–18. Roentgen sign example: shape. There is an osteophyte on the proximal aspect of the navicular bone *(arrow).*

TABLE 1–2. GAMUTS FOR TWO COMMONLY OBSERVED ROENTGEN SIGNS

Increased Bronchial Wall Thickness	Increased Pulmonary Radiopacity—Alveolar, Patchy Distribution
Allergy	Pneumonia
Chronic inflammation	Hemorrhage
	Edema
	Allergy
	Thromboembolism
	Primary tumor
	Secondary tumor
	Toxicosis

lesion according to its roentgen signs rather than immediately attempting to designate the cause for the detected abnormality, diagnostic accuracy increases considerably. Examples of roentgen signs are given in Figures 1–14 to 1–18.

Once roentgen signs have been defined, the next step is to consider what diseases can result in the production of these roentgen signs; this is called the *gamut* approach. A gamut is a list of diseases that may result in the production of a certain roentgen sign. Some gamuts are more extensive than other gamuts (Table 1–2). For patients in whom more than one roentgen sign is present, gamuts for all such signs should be considered collectively with the signalment, history, clinical signs, physical findings, and laboratory data so as to formulate a list of differential clinical diagnoses.

PITFALLS IN INTERPRETATION

There are a few circumstances in which the accuracy of radiographic interpretation decreases considerably: (1) The presence of an obvious lesion that distracts the evaluator, preventing the systematic evaluation of the remainder of the radiograph; (2) Discovery of a lesion that answers the clinical question that prompted the radiographic examination, thereby distracting the evaluator from further analysis of the radiograph; (3) Tunnel vision, which is a preconception of what will be found on the radiograph so that when the preconception is confirmed, the viewing of the radiograph ends.

Radiographic interpretation is both art and science. It is a skill that can be learned by most individuals. The more organized and analytic the approach to evaluating a radiograph, the more astute the individual becomes in diagnostic radiology.

CHAPTER 2

AGGRESSIVE VS. NONAGGRESSIVE BONE LESIONS

JON STOWATER

The area of orthopedics affords the veterinarian perhaps the greatest opportunity to use radiology as a diagnostic and prognostic tool. Most of these instances involve acute orthopedic trauma, and the radiographic interpretation of such trauma is rather straightforward. There are, however, many other causes of orthopedic disease, and radiographic interpretation in these cases can be more difficult. Bone is limited to either lysis, production, or a combination of both in response to any insult or disease; therefore, different lesions can have similar radiographic patterns. It should also be remembered that many lesions commonly associated with a characteristic radiographic feature may have an atypical appearance. Rather than memorize the characteristic radiographic features for each orthopedic disease, it is more beneficial to understand the pathophysiologic significance of each roentgen sign, to integrate all changes seen, and to characterize the lesion according to its aggressiveness. Once that evaluation is made, the task of making a specific diagnosis is greatly simplified.

Bone is dynamic, living tissue undergoing constant change. It is a supportive structure that adapts to mechanical loads and stresses by remodeling itself to be functionally competent while using the minimal appropriate amount of bone tissue.[1] This process of functional adaptation is widely referred to as Wolff's law.[1, 2] The remodeling process occurs through the activity of osteoblasts, osteoclasts, and osteocytes. Osteoblasts are situated on bone surfaces (periosteal, endosteal, and within haversian canals) and produce new bone by laying down a collagenous matrix, which in a normal metabolic state becomes mineralized. The osteoblast is trapped within the bone and becomes an osteocyte. Osteoclasts are also on the bone surface but remove or resorb bone. Osteocytes also resorb bone by enlargement of their lacunae in a process referred to as bone flow; older osteocytes die and are replaced by younger osteocytes that move inward from the surface.[3] Under certain conditions of local inflammation, macrophages may also participate in focal bone resorption.[2]

In normal (nonpathologic) circumstances, bone undergoes the remodeling and turnover process continuously from the embryologic state until death. These changes come about not only due to the stress of weightbearing, but also the intermittent pressure of active muscles on the periosteum cause bone resorption and result in alterations in shape.[1] This change is also observed in pathologic conditions in which pressure is applied to the periosteum over time by expanding masses adjacent to the bone (soft-tissue neoplasm or chronically distended joint capsule).[4] The protuberances that exist at the sites of muscle attachment become more evident with increased muscle function. Osteoblastic new bone formation is stimulated at these sites by forces mediated through Sharpey's fibers, which are enmeshed in the periosteum.[1]

Bone remodeling is also subject to many influences that have little or nothing to do with mechanical factors. The skeleton represents a readily mobilized store of calcium and phosphate upon which the body may call in times of increased need (pregnancy, lactation, and egg laying) or dietary insufficiency.[1] The parathyroid glands maintain calcium homeostasis by secreting parathormone, which accelerates bone resorption (osteoclastic and osteocytic) and allows the release of calcium from bone.[1, 3, 5, 6] Parathyroid function is affected by any alteration in calcium homeostasis, including chronic renal disease, dietary deficiencies, and neoplasms secreting parathormone-like substances.[5] Other nonmechanical causes of bone remodeling may include excessive circulating adrenal glucocorticoids or diminished gonadal secretion of anabolic steroids.[6] The reader is encouraged to consult appropriate texts for an explanation of the pathophysiologic mechanisms involved in these processes.

BONE RESPONSE TO DISEASE OR INJURY

There are a multitude of pathologic conditions that affect bone, but there are only two avenues of response: bone destruction (osteolysis) and bone production (osteogenesis). Osteolysis usually precedes osteogenesis, although the amount of either seen radiographically and the specific pattern of lysis, production, or both is a function of the pathophysiology of the injury.[4, 7, 8] After radiographic examination the lesion may be classified and the differential diagnosis formulated. The radiographic appearance of the lesion can be related to the aggressiveness and duration of the offending agent or injury; the variability of the reparative response of the animal; and the influences of other factors, such as medical or surgical intervention or the preexistence or superimposition of other pathologic processes.

The initial step in interpreting a bone lesion radiographically is to categorize it according to its aggressiveness. This process simplifies the task of diagnosis by ruling out those lesions inappropriate to the category selected. Specific discussions of individual orthopedic diseases are presented elsewhere in this text and should be used as a reference once this initial evaluation is made. After describing the aggressiveness of the lesion, the clinician can select the appropriate philosophy of treatment, e.g., an aggressive bone lesion requires aggressive therapy, whereas no therapy is needed for a nonaggressive lesion.

An *aggressive* bone lesion is active and is usually acute or subacute at first presentation. The disease process rapidly expands into the normal bone, and there is usually minimal to no evidence of an effective reparative and counteractive process by the host bone. Aggressive is not synonymous with but includes malignant neoplasia. A *semiaggressive* bone lesion is subacute to chronic and implies a moderate rate of activity. A reparative response by the host bone is evident, but it has not confined the disease completely. The lesion may be expanding slowly and the outcome is still uncertain. A nonaggressive lesion is usually chronic and has minimal to no activity. There is a well-defined host-bone response that has confined the disease, and the process has been or continues to be resolved successfully.

These terms represent a continuum of events in a pathologic process. A lesion may change from aggressive to semiaggressive and may ultimately become nonaggressive as the host bone responds. Other lesions may never change. An osteosarcoma by virtue of its malignant nature is always an aggressive lesion, whereas a congenital bone cyst may be nonaggressive for the lifetime of the animal. Because the aggressiveness of a bone lesion can change, radiographic re-evaluation is essential, especially regarding aggressive lesions for which an assessment of the response to therapy may be critical.

The radiographic assessment of aggressiveness in bone lesions is based on the degree of activity and the presence and effectiveness of a reparative response by the host bone. Activity and reparative response are recognized radiographically by the degree and pattern of osteolysis and osteogenesis; the margination of the lesion, the zone of transition between diseased and normal bone, and the rate of change seen on follow-up radiographs must also be considered.

Bone Lysis

Osteolysis is usually the first response of a bone to injury or disease. The radiographic detection of osteolysis is dependent on several factors, such as the opacity of the surrounding bone, the ability to define the margin of the radiolucent area, and the amount of superimposed periosteal new bone.[4, 7, 8] Lysis is more easily seen in cortical than in cancellous bone by virtue of greater contrast. The lesion with a well-defined margin is easier to see than one with a poorly defined margin. If new bone production is also present, which is common, the lytic component may be less visible or may not be seen at all. Osteolysis is a reactive phenomenon; it is not directly caused by pathogenic bacteria, tumor cells, or other pathologic agents, but rather is due to stimulation of osteoclastic and osteocytic resorption.[8] By virtue of their secretory activity, osteoclasts lyse both the mineral and organic matrix of bone. Halisteresis or the decalcification of bone with a residual normal matrix is not considered a valid concept, except perhaps on a minor scale.[4] The earliest radiographic signs of bone lysis are a subtle alteration of bone texture as a result of resorption of small trabeculae and a loss of bone opacity due to the removal of mineral. Under the most favorable circumstances, there is a latent period of about 10 days between histologic and radiographic evidence of osteolysis;[4, 8] this period is longer with less aggressive processes and in rarified bone.[4]

Generalized Bone Lysis. Bone lysis can be classified as generalized or localized. Generalized lysis involves an entire bone, several bones in a limb, or perhaps the entire skeleton in uniform fashion. This pattern is attributed to a generalized disturbance in normal bone turnover, which could be caused by disuse of a limb, dietary deficiency or imbalances, or endocrine disturbances. The radiographic changes associated with generalized osteolysis are often subtle and require familiarity with normal skeletal appearance at different stages of life to avoid misinterpretation. If only one limb is affected, it can be compared radiographically to the opposite normal limb. The radiographic changes associated with generalized osteolysis are an overall decrease in skeletal radiopacity, a coarse trabecular pattern, thinning of the cortices, and loss of distinction of endosteal margins.[4] As a general rule, a 30 to 50 percent loss of bone substance is required before radiographic detection is possible.[4, 9] Thus, radiography is not a sensitive indicator of generalized osteolysis until the process is fairly advanced.

Localized Lysis. Localized bone lysis usually indicates an aggressive process and may be divided into three major patterns: geographic, moth-eaten, and permeative (Fig. 2–1).[8] *Geographic* lysis is characterized by a single, fairly large-sized hole that in its pure form has a sharp line of transition from the lysed to the intact bone. The margin of the lesion, however, may be irregular, scalloped, or ragged. The overlying cortex may be destroyed or remodeled by periosteal proliferation, creating a new cortex that slowly expands to contain the lesion. Cortical destruction implies an aggressive lesion. An expanded yet intact cortex overlying an area of geographic lysis indicates a semiaggressive to nonaggressive lesion, such as a congenital bone cyst, benign tumor, focal area of resolving osteomyelitis, or bone sequestrum.

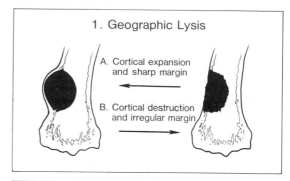

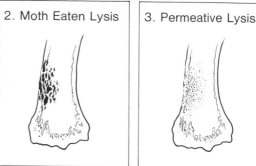

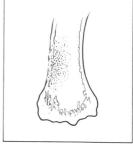

Figure 2–1. Localized bone lysis may be divided into categories of geographic, moth-eaten, and permeative. Geographic lysis is subdivided into those that expand the cortex and are sharply marginated (IA) and those that destroy the cortex and may have an irregular margin (IB). An expanded, yet intact cortex indicates a less aggressive lesion than one that destroys the cortex. Moth-eaten lysis (2) is more aggressive than geographic lysis, and permeative lysis (3) is the most aggressive.

Moth-eaten lysis is characterized by multiple medium- to small-sized holes that are often confluent. The margins are irregular and poorly defined. The overlying cortex may be totally destroyed or may have multiple areas of discontinuity.

Permeative lysis has numerous small, nearly imperceptible holes that are reasonably uniform in size but tend to be smaller and more scattered toward the periphery of the lesion. Thus, the margin of a permeative lesion is broad and indefinable. The cortex may be extensively involved, but distinct areas of destruction may not be identified. The multiple, small lytic foci give the appearance of a generalized reduction in radiopacity of the cortex.

The degree of aggressiveness increases from geographic to moth-eaten to permeative forms of lysis. Moth-eaten and permeative lysis imply penetration of the cortex. A sharp distinction between these two patterns may be impossible at times as they often occur together. In fact, mixed patterns of lysis occur frequently, with the more aggressive form being evident at the periphery of the lesion; a central area of geographic lysis may have a surrounding zone of moth-eaten lysis. In instances of mixed patterns, the more aggressive form should be utilized as the true indicator of the nature of the lesion. Also, the clarity of the margin of the lytic process indicates aggressiveness; a well-defined margin suggests a well-organized, slower process, whereas a poorly defined margin implies a less-organized, more aggressive lesion. Complete absence of bone lysis is not characteristic of an aggressive lesion. Osteolysis may be difficult or impossible to visualize, however, if significant, new bone production has occurred. In these instances, other criteria, such as the pattern of new bone production and the rate of change on follow-up radiographs, must be used to assess aggressiveness.

New Bone Production

The second response of host bone to insult is new bone production. Radiographically, there is roughly a 2-week lag between the initial stimulus and the detection of new bone.[4, 8] The periosteum is a specialized connective tissue membrane that surrounds the bone, except at the intracapsular portions of joints; it is composed of a dense, fibrous outer layer and a looser inner layer of osteoblasts and their precursor cells. The inner layer, often referred to as the cambium layer, has an osteogenic potential that is activated after injury (Fig. 2–2).

Periosteal new bone forms when the periosteum is elevated from the cortex by any disease process or agent.[10, 11] Histologically, numerous fine connective tissue strands (Sharpey's fibers) and small blood vessels maintain a connection between the periosteum and the cortex, extending in a perpendicular manner from the elevated periosteal membrane to the cortex. If the cambium layer has not been destroyed, it forms osteoid, which follows the fibers and blood vessels downward. This osteoid then becomes mineralized, forming tiny bone spicules or rays that are visible on the radiograph as periosteal new bone. If the lesion is benign and is allowed to resolve, the formation of new bone continues and fills the spaces between the bone spicules until a solid layer of new bone is formed.

The process just described is the first type of periosteal reaction, which is called the *solid* pattern. It may be thin or thick, straight or undulating, variable in opacity, and with distinct or indistinct margins. These features signify only the progress and age of the process and perhaps the aggressiveness of the initial irritant.[7] A smooth, solid, distinctly marginated periosteal reaction usually signifies a benign or nonaggressive process of minimal or no activity. The less distinct and more irregular the margin is, the more active and aggressive the lesion. A thin, indistinct, focal periosteal reaction may

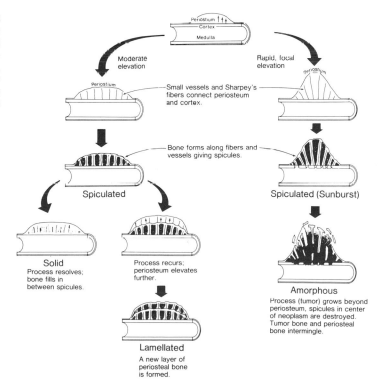

Figure 2–2. Periosteal new bone forms as a result of elevation of the periosteum by any process. Small blood vessels and Sharpey's fibers may maintain a connection between the periosteum and cortex, providing a framework on which new bone may form. The various patterns may be related to the pathophysiologic events that are occurring.

appear solid, yet may be the earliest visible sign of an aggressive or semiaggressive lesion if the lytic component is of insufficient magnitude to be recognized. Follow-up radiographs reveal the true nature of this type of lesion.

The second pattern of periosteal reaction is the *interrupted* type, which is subdivided into lamellated, spiculated, and amorphous forms.[7] The *lamellated* form has a layered or onion-skin appearance. It is thought to represent intermittent elevations of the periosteum by an expansile process, which has cycles of rapid and slow growth.[7, 8, 11] After each cycle of periosteal elevation is complete, a layer of new bone is formed subperiosteally. This pattern is not common, but it may be found at the edge of an expanding bone tumor in the area known as Codman's triangle or in instances of bacterial osteomyelitis.

The *spiculated* variety is seen in early semiaggressive to aggressive lesions and may persist, becoming more prominent if the lesion fails to resolve. With clearing of the offending agent or tissue from the spaces between the spicules, new bone continues to form, converting the spiculated pattern into a solid one. This filling process may occur rapidly or slowly, depending on the nature of the inciting agent. During this period, the spicules become thicker as new bone formation progresses; this is typical of chronic bacterial or fungal osteomyelitis.[12] In nonresolving (aggressive) lesions, such as malig-

nant bone tumors, the spicules are frequently thin and may become quite long as the periosteum is elevated a considerable distance from the cortex. Eventually, many malignant bone tumors grow through and beyond the periosteum in the central part of the neoplasm, and the spicules may be destroyed.[8] Tumors or expansile lesions that penetrate the cortex from a focal point on the bone and rapidly elevate the periosteum produce a radiating pattern of bony spicules; the fine fibers and vessels connecting the periosteum and the cortex radiate from the point of cortical penetration to the stretched periosteum with which they maintain a perpendicular relationship.[10] This pattern, often referred to as a "sunburst," is commonly associated with osteosarcoma.[7, 8, 12] It is identified, however, in less than one half of patients with this type of tumor.[13] Osteomyelitis and focal trauma may also produce a sunburst pattern of spicules. Therefore, the length and thickness of the spicules, the pattern of bone lysis if present, and the rate of change noted on follow-up radiographs must be considered to differentiate these processes.

The third subtype of interrupted periosteal reaction is referred to as an amorphous pattern.[7] As the name implies, it has no particular form The new bone may appear in clumps, clouds, or wispy strands, and may intermingle with the spiculated pattern. Its margins are poorly defined, with the new bone fading into the soft

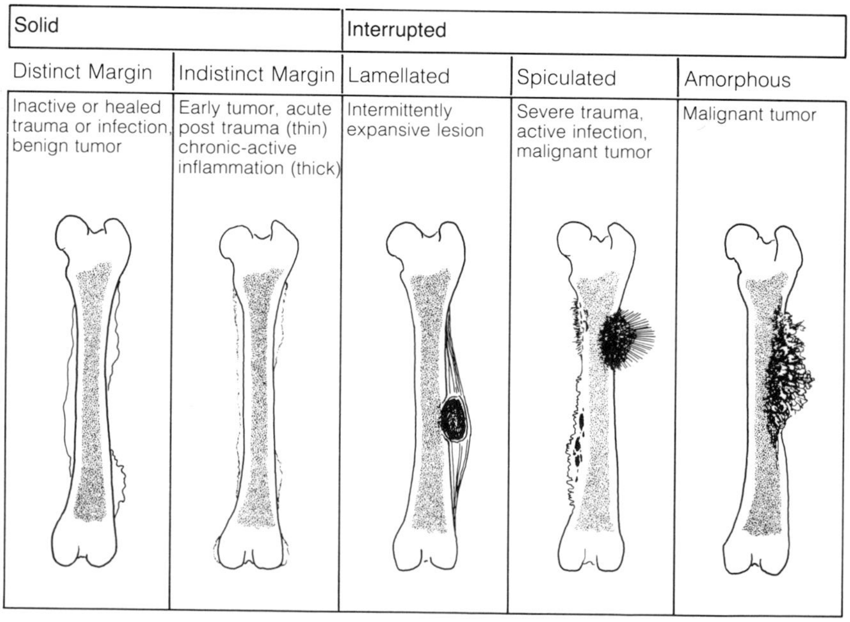

Solid		Interrupted		
Distinct Margin	Indistinct Margin	Lamellated	Spiculated	Amorphous
Inactive or healed trauma or infection, benign tumor	Early tumor, acute post trauma (thin) chronic-active inflammation (thick)	Intermittently expansive lesion	Severe trauma, active infection, malignant tumor	Malignant tumor

Figure 2–3. A differential diagnosis of periosteal reactions may be formulated once a pattern has been selected. In general, the lesions become more aggressive when the spectrum of solid to interrupted patterns is considered. Note, however, that a focal solid, indistinctly marginated reaction may be seen with early neoplasia or osteomyelitis. Follow-up radiographs 7 to 10 days later should disclose the aggressive nature of this kind of lesion.

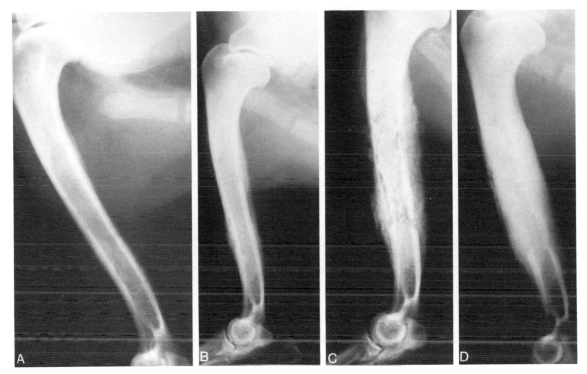

Figure 2–4. Lateral radiographs of the humerus of an 11-year-old miniature greyhound demonstrate the dynamic nature of bone disease and the importance of follow-up radiographs. The dog had surgery for correction of pyometritis. Febrile episodes occurred during the first post-surgical week. Two weeks after ovariohysterectomy, a shifting lameness developed. Three weeks after surgery, radiographs of the long bones were obtained. *A*, 21 days after surgery. A faint, irregular yet solid, periosteal reaction is seen on the caudal cortex of the proximal humeral diaphysis. This finding can be an early change associated with an aggressive or semiaggressive lesion preceding the appearance of lysis. *B*, 33 days after surgery. A definite moth-eaten pattern of lysis and an irregular yet solid pattern of periosteal new bone are seen along the entire caudal diaphyseal cortex and in focal areas of the cranial diaphyseal cortex. This lesion would best be described as semiaggressive (see Table 2–1). *C*, 49 days after surgery. There is progression of both the moth-eaten lysis and the periosteal reaction, which is now thick and irregular yet with definable margins. More periosteal new bone is visible on the cranial cortex, and it too is irregular as well as somewhat interrupted. The patterns indicate continued aggression by the disease process and continued reparative response by the host bone. The lesion would still be classified as semiaggressive. *D*, 117 days after surgery. There is resolution of the process by the host bone. The lytic process has been replaced by smooth, solid, new bone along the cranial and caudal cortices. The lesion would now be classified as nonaggressive.

tissues. The amorphous pattern represents the least organized type of periosteal reaction and is associated with the most aggressive lesions, primary malignant bone tumors. Radiographically, it may be difficult to distinguish this type of periosteal new bone from the actual tumor bone of osteosarcoma. Initially, early mineralization of a hematoma or other forms of dystrophic soft-tissue mineralization adjacent to a bone may appear similar to an amorphous periosteal pattern.[12] Other criteria, such as the presence or absence of bone lysis, should then be considered (see Fig. 2–3 for differential diagnosis of periosteal reactions). The absence of new bone production in the presence of an aggressive form of lysis indicates the lack of a reparative response and is thus associated with aggressive bone lesions.

OTHER CRITERIA

In the evaluation of the aggressiveness of bone lesions, the type of margin of the osteolytic component, the breadth of the zone of transition between the osteolytic margin and the normal bone, and the rate of change noted on follow-up radiographic studies are important factors to consider. The margin of a destructive lesion is an indication of its aggressiveness and the reparative response by the host bone.[4] A clearly defined or distinct margin of the area of osteolysis indicates a less aggressive lesion than one with a poorly defined margin. A dense zone of sclerotic bone at the margin of an osteolytic lesion indicates a reparative process and thus suggests a less aggressive lesion than one in which there is no sclerosis.[8] The zone of transition is the area between the margin of the osteolytic lesion and the normal-appearing bone.[14] The length of this zone is determined by the rate of expansion of the lesion (aggressiveness) and the ability of the host bone to produce a reparative response.[12, 14] A relatively long zone of transition implies an aggressive lesion, whereas a short zone suggests a less aggressive lesion. Follow-up radiographs are made days, weeks, or even months after the initial examination to assess rate of change. The appropriate time interval between radiographic examinations is based on how aggressive the lesion appears initially and, therefore, how soon significant change may be anticipated. A primary malignant bone tumor may show dramatic changes in 7 to 10 days; benign lesions may change slowly over a period of weeks to months (Fig. 2–4).

The aforementioned radiographic changes should be carefully evaluated individually and then integrated to form an impression of the aggressiveness of an orthopedic lesion (Fig. 2–5). Generally, lesions should be classified according to the most aggressive changes, with the results of follow-up radiographs used for further clarification. Very aggressive lesions may also have nonaggressive components, such as primary malignant bone tumors that have a solid periosteal reaction at the periphery of the lesion in the area of Codman's triangle.[4, 11] This occurrence is due to the physical lifting of the periosteum beyond the confines of the actual neoplasm. The importance of integrating the radiographic changes and using follow-up studies for evaluating aggressiveness cannot be overemphasized, because radiographs, like any diagnostic test, are subject to misinterpretation. By using these criteria, it should be possible to classify most osseous lesions into one of three major categories: aggressive, semiaggressive, or nonaggressive. This classification then provides a means to limit the list of differential diagnoses and to determine a plan for therapy or further diagnostic testing.

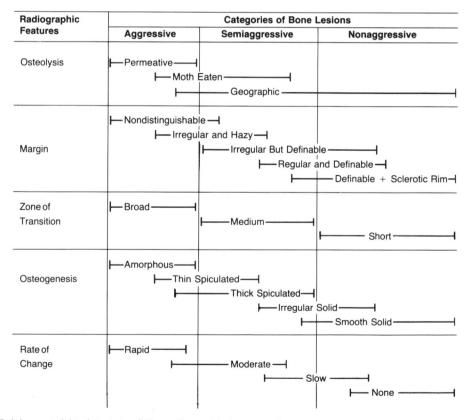

Guidelines for Classification of Bone Lesions

Figure 2–5. It is essential to integrate all the radiographic features of a bone lesion to arrive at the proper classification of aggressiveness. Many of the patterns listed overlap, emphasizing the need to carefully evaluate the radiograph for all possible changes that may be related to the disease process. Follow-up radiographs should be compared with originals to determine the progress of the disease and the reparative response.

References

1. Lanyon LE: Mechanical function and bone remodeling. *In* Sumner-Smith G (Ed): Bone in Clinical Orthopaedics. A Study in Comparative Osteology. Philadelphia, WB Saunders, 1982, pp. 273–304.
2. Matthews JL: Bone structure and ultrastructure. *In* Urist MR (Ed): Fundamental and Clinical Bone Physiology. Philadelphia, WB Saunders, 1980, pp. 4–44.
3. Whalen JP: The resorption of bone and its control. Radiology 113:257, 1974.
4. Greenfield GB: Radiology of Bone Diseases. Philadelphia, JB Lippincott, 1969.
5. Capen CC, Belshaw BE, and Martin SL: Endocrine disorders. *In* Ettinger SJ (Ed): Textbook of Veterinary Internal Medicine. Diseases of the Dog and Cat. Philadelphia, WB Saunders, 1974, pp. 1351–1452.
6. Ganong WF: Review of Medical Physiology. Los Altos, CA, Lange Medical Publications, 1967, p. 324.
7. Edeiken J, and Hodes PJ: Roentgen Diagnosis of Diseases of Bone. Baltimore, Williams & Wilkins, 1967.
8. Lodwick GS: Solitary malignant tumors of bone: The application of predictor variables in diagnosis. Semin Roentgenol 1:293, 1966.
9. Lodwick GS: Reactive response to local injury in bone. Radiol Clin North Am 2:209, 1964.
10. Grunow OH: Radiating spicules, a nonspecific sign of bone disease. Radiology 65:200, 1955.
11. Brunschwig A, and Harmon PH: Studies in bone sarcoma. III. An experimental and pathological study of the role of the periosteum in the formation of bone in various primary bone tumors. Surg Gynecol Obstet 60:30, 1935.
12. Hanlon GF: Radiologic approach to bone neoplasms. Vet Clin North Am [Small Anim Pract] 12:2, 1982.
13. Morgan JP: Radiology in Veterinary Orthopedics. Philadelphia, Lea & Febiger, 1972.
14. Morgan JP: Radiographic diagnosis of bone lesions in the appendicular skeleton of the dog. Comp Contin Ed 1:395, 1979.

SECTION 2

AXIAL SKELETON—COMPANION ANIMALS

CHAPTER 3

THE CRANIAL VAULT AND ASSOCIATED STRUCTURES

WENDY MYER

RADIOGRAPHIC EVALUATION

Normal Anatomy

The skull is one of the most complex and specialized parts of the skeleton. It houses the brain as well as the sense organs for hearing, equilibrium, sight, smell, and taste. Radiography is commonly used to evaluate abnormalities of these organs. This evaluation is difficult, however, because the shape and size of the skull in domestic dogs vary more than in any other mammalian species.

Three head shapes have been described in the dog: dolichocephalic, mesaticephalic, and brachycephalic. This classification is based upon the relative proportions of the facial bones and the cranial vault. Dolichocephalic breeds, such as collies, have long, narrow skulls with longer facial components than those of the cranial vault. Mesaticephalic breeds, such as the beagle and setter, have heads of medium proportions, whereas brachycephalic breeds, such as the Boston terrier and Pekingese, have short, wide heads with shorter facial than cranial vault components.[1] Examples of these normal breed variations are shown in Figure 3–1.

In addition to these differences, marked changes also occur during miniaturization of the dog; these changes are illustrated in Figure 3–2. Notice that decreases in body size are accompanied by decreasing prominence of the occipital protuberance and frontal sinuses and by progressive doming and cortical thinning of the calvarium. The more a breed digresses from the ancestral German shepherd type, the more pronounced are the changes in the shape and relative size of the calvarium.

Differences in skull shape are also evident between the dog and the cat. The normal cat skull is illustrated in Figure 3–3. Notice especially the alteration in the shape of the nasal passages with doming of the frontal and nasal bones, the more complete bony orbits due to large postorbital processes, the increased width of the skull through the zygomatic arches, and the large occipital fossa and tentorium osseum surrounding the cerebellum.[2] Although there are some breed differences in the shape of the cat skull, these differences are slight when compared to those of the dog.

Because of the complexity of the skull, good radiographic positioning is essential for adequate evaluation. Optimal positioning usually requires general anesthesia or heavy sedation. When proper positioning is achieved, the bilateral symmetry of the skull allows comparison between a unilateral abnormality and the corresponding normal structure on the opposite side. Even minor obliquity during positioning causes considerable anatomic distortion and su-

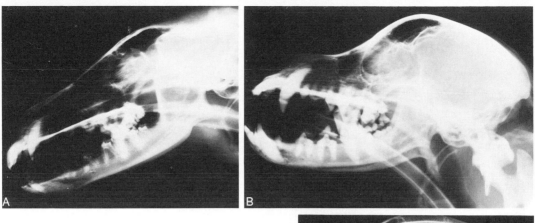

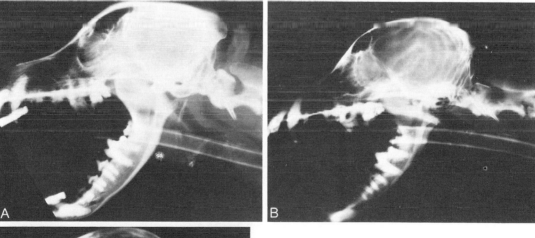

Figure 3-1. Lateral views of the skull illustrate breed variations in canine head shape. *A*, a collie (dolichocephalic breed); *B*, a terrier (mesaticephalic breed); *C*, a Boston terrier (brachycephalic breed).

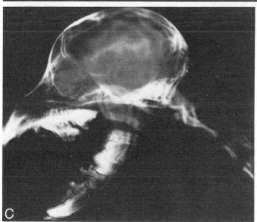

Figure 3-2. Lateral views of the canine skull illustrate differences in shape due to miniaturization. Note the progressive decrease in the prominence of the occipital protuberance and increased prominence of the calvarial component of the skull. *A*, a setter; *B*, a beagle; *C*, a toy poodle.

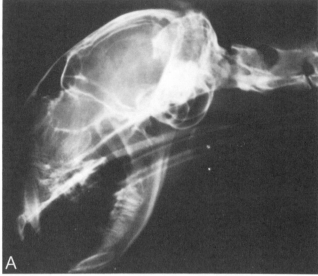
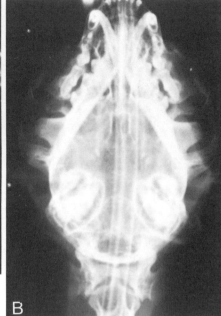

Figure 3–3. Lateral *(A)* and ventrodorsal *(B)* radiographs of the skull of a normal domestic shorthair cat.

perimposition. Routine positions include the lateral and dorsoventral, or ventrodorsal, views. In addition, oblique, rostrocaudal, and open mouth views are often used, depending on the area to be evaluated.[3] Detailed descriptions of these special views have been reported.[4]

Alterations in Size, Shape, and Margination

Alterations in brain size are frequently reflected in the calvarium. Microcephaly (decrease in the size of the brain) and anencephaly (absence of the brain) are usually accompanied by decreased calvarial size. These congenital anomalies are uncommon and are incompatible with life.

Internal hydrocephalus is excess fluid accumulation in the cerebral ventricles. The degree of resultant calvarial distortion depends on the rate at which fluid accumulates, the severity of ventricular enlargement, and the stage of ossification of the cranial sutures at the onset of the disease.[5] The most severe changes occur in

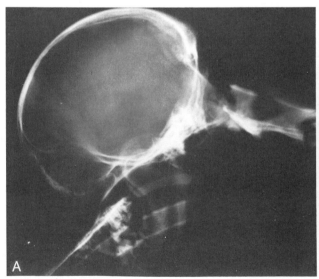
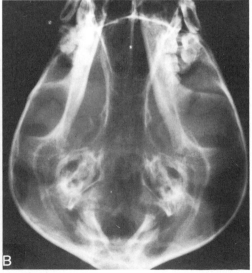

Figure 3–4. Lateral *(A)* and ventrodorsal *(B)* radiographs of a 7-month-old mixed-breed dog with severe hydrocephalus. Note especially the loss of the normal convolutional skull markings and the resulting homogeneous appearance of the calvarium.

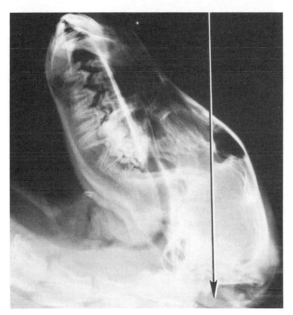

Figure 3–5. Position used for evaluation of the foramen magnum. *Arrow*, direction of the central x-ray beam.

congenital hydrocephalus, with less severe alterations in those animals that acquired hydrocephalus after calvarial ossification.[6] Hydrocephalus is most often described in the small breeds of dogs, such as the Yorkshire terrier and Chihuahua. Only rarely has this condition been described in the cat.[7]

Radiographic signs suggestive of hydrocephalus are enlargement of the calvarium with cortical thinning, decreased prominence of the normal calvarial convolutional markings, open fontanelles and cranial sutures, and a brain that appears homogeneous (Fig. 3–4).[8] Ventricular size and shape can be assessed with pneumoventriculography.[9]

Occipital dysplasia, an abnormal dorsal extension of the foramen magnum, is another common congenital anomaly in the smaller breeds of dogs. This condition was first described in 1965 and usually occurs in toy and miniature poodles, Yorkshire terriers, and Chihuahuas.[10] It is impossible to estimate the prevalence of occipital dysplasia. Two studies suggest that the condition is relatively common in smaller dogs. In 1979, Wright found a 100 per cent rate of incidence in 15 asymptomatic small breed dogs.[11] In another study, Watson found a 50 per cent incidence rate in 45 normal beagles.[12] Most of these animals had only a minor dorsal extension of the foramen magnum, and it is unlikely that the anomaly alone was clinically significant. This condition, however, is often accompanied by other abnormalities, such as hydrocephalus or atlantoaxial malformation, which may result in signs of neural dysfunction.

The size of the foramen magnum is best evaluated by using a rostrodorsal-caudoventral skull radiograph. The anesthetized animal is placed on its back with its neck flexed so the nose moves toward the sternum. The central x-ray beam passes between the eyes and exits through the foramen magnum (Fig. 3–5).[13] The angle of the beam from the vertical axis varies from 25 to 40 degrees, depending on the shape of the calvarium. Figure 3–6 illustrates the normal and abnormal appearance of the foramen magnum.

Several congenital calvarial malformations have been described in the cat. Mucopolysaccharidoses have been described in Siamese and domestic shorthair cats. These diseases are caused by inborn errors in glycosaminoglycan metabolism. Although the metabolic error in these two breeds is not identical, the clinical appearance of the cats is similar. Characteristically, the cats have a broad, short maxilla with

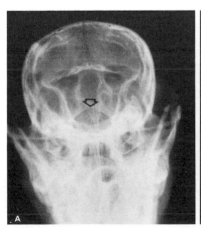
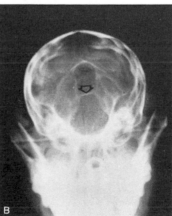
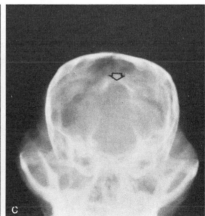

Figure 3–6. Rostrodorsal-caudoventral oblique views of the skull illustrate the foramen magnum in three small-breed dogs. *Arrows*, the dorsal extent of the foramen. *A*, a normal foramen; *B*, moderate occipital dysplasia; *C*, severe occipital dysplasia.

depression of the nasal bridge. Concurrent dysplasias of other areas of the skeleton are often present. In people and in the Siamese cat, this condition appears to be inherited as an autosomal recessive trait. Inheritance in the domestic shorthair cat has not been determined.[14]

Another congenital abnormality is craniofacial malformation in the Burmese cat. This lethal, inherited defect is characterized by cerebral exencaphaly in which the forebrain protrudes through an opening in the front of the skull at the level of the frontoparietal suture. The frontal and nasal bones are greatly reduced, the eyes are small, and there is shortening of the upper jaw (superior brachygnathia). There is duplication of the maxilla with four upper canine teeth and absence of the incisive, nasal, and ethmoidal bones and cartilages. The condition appears to be an example of incomplete conjoined twinning.[15]

Trauma is the most common cause of acquired alterations in skull shape and margination in the dog and cat. Skull injuries may occur from a number of different causes, including automobile accidents, falls, animal interactions, weapons, and crushing forces. Automobile accidents, animal interactions, and injuries of unknown causes accounted for approximately 75 percent of traumatic lesions in one report.[16] The exposed portion of the calvarium is more prone to injury than is the more protected base of the skull. Fractures of the calvarium are not as common in dogs as in people, suggesting that some protection from the thick calvarium and heavy calvarial musculature is present in the medium-sized dog. Smaller dogs have a greater risk of injury due to their domed and relatively thin calvarium.[17]

Severely displaced fractures of the calvarium are likely to result in immediate death. In surviving animals, skull fractures are either hairline (nondisplaced) or minimally displaced depression fractures, both of which may be difficult to detect. They may appear as radiolucent linear or curvilinear fissure lines or, if there is overlapping of the fracture edges, as radiopaque lines (Figure 3–7). Good positioning and the use of oblique views facilitate the radiographic evaluation of suspected fractures. Comparison with normal radiographs of an animal of similar skull type may be useful. Anesthesia is helpful but is not always possible if the cardiovascular status of the animal is impaired. It must be realized that damage to the brain, such as concussion and subdural or intracranial hemorrhage, cannot be accurately evaluated using conventional radiographic techniques. Brain damage may be considerably more serious than would be estimated from the severity of the skeletal damage. Therefore, a complete neurologic evaluation of the animal should be performed before the radiographic examination.

Maxillary and mandibular fractures are more common than fractures of the calvarium (Fig. 3–8).[18] Oblique and open mouth views are especially helpful when evaluating these fractures. Fractures of the facial bones are often accompanied by soft-tissue swelling and are generally enough displaced to be readily evident on routine views. If the nasal passages or frontal sinuses are invaded, subcutaneous air accumulation is a frequent finding; this appears as a radiolucent area between the skin and facial bones.

Perhaps the most common mandibular injury is symphyseal separation in the cat.[19] These fractures may result from automobile accidents, animal interactions, or falls. In urban areas, where multiple story housing is common, cats may sustain severe injuries after falls from great

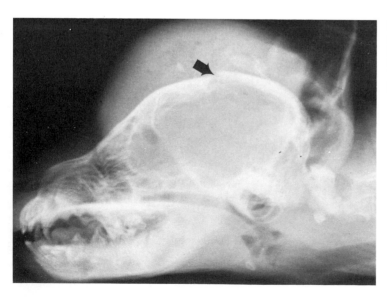

Figure 3–7. Lateral skull radiograph of an 8-week-old mixed-breed dog that was hit by a car. *Arrow*, a minimally displaced fracture of the calvarium. There is marked soft-tissue swelling due to a large subcutaneous hematoma.

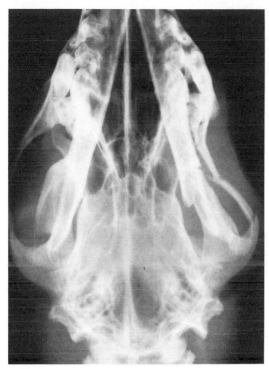

Figure 3–8. Ventrodorsal view of the skull of a 2-year-old male German shepherd with comminuted fractures of the left zygomatic arch and mandible after the dog was hit by a car. Note the marked depression of the zygomatic arch fragments.

ease. Age also affects the relative severity of skull changes compared to those in long bones. Skull demineralization tends to predominate in secondary renal hyperparathyroidism, whereas cortical thinning of the long bones is most marked in the secondary nutritional form of the disease. This difference may be because the nutritional disease occurs more often in young animals in whom there is rapid skeletal turnover. The nutritional form of the disease now occurs less frequently with the increased use of balanced commercial rations.

One of the first radiographic signs of hyperparathyroidism in the skull is the loss of the lamina dura, the bone that forms the dental alveolus. The normal appearance of the teeth is shown in Figure 3–15. The disappearance of the bony socket causes the teeth to appear as if they are "floating" (Fig. 3–9). Concomitant fibrous osteodystrophy may result in thickening of the maxilla and filling of the nasal cavity with soft tissue (Fig. 3–10). The teeth may become displaced, and, in the young animal, eruption of the permanent teeth may be impaired. This impairment is especially common in the subhuman primate.[22]

Increases in bone opacity may result from a number of factors. One acquired cause of in-

heights. Because cats usually land on all four feet, these falls result in a uniform pattern of fractures. The force of the landing results in the cat hitting its nose, with resultant fracture of the mandibular symphysis and splitting of the hard palate. Femoral fractures and carpal dislocations with or without forelimb fractures also frequently occur.[20] This pattern of injuries is called the high-rise syndrome.

Alterations in Radiographic Opacity

These alterations may be focal or diffuse. Generalized loss of radiographic opacity is most often due to primary or secondary hyperparathyroidism. Primary hyperparathyroidism results from hyperplasia or neoplasia of the parathyroid gland, whereas secondary hyperparathyroidism is due to a dietary imbalance (low calcium and high phosphorus levels) or to renal disease with abnormal phosphorus retention. In small animals, secondary hyperparathyroidism occurs more often than the primary type. The bone response in hyperparathyrodism from any cause is similar.[21]

The degree of cortical thinning and decreased bone opacity depends on the severity of the mineral imbalance and the duration of the dis-

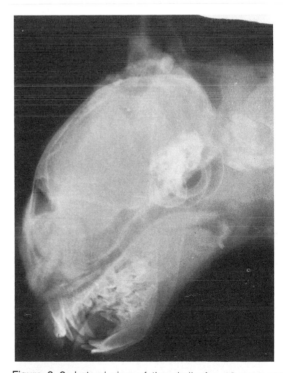

Figure 3–9. Lateral view of the skull of a 12-week-old kitten with severe secondary nutritional hyperparathyroidism. Note the overall loss of bone opacity, the loss of the lamina dura, and the marked cortical thinning of all of the bones of the skull.

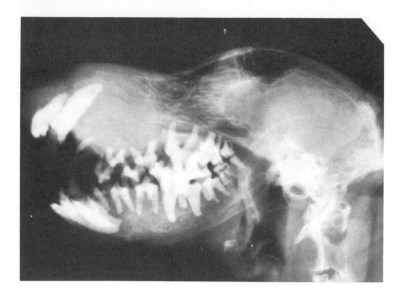

Figure 3–10. Lateral skull radiograph of a 12-year-old female Scottish terrier with primary hyperparathyroidism and severe fibrous dysplasia with thickening of the maxilla and displacement of the teeth. Note the absence of the lamina dura around the teeth.

creased bone opacity in the dog is craniomandibular osteopathy. The etiology of this non-infectious, non-neoplastic proliferative bone disease is unknown. It occurs most often in West Highland White, Scottish, and Cairn terriers, but isolated instances in other breeds have been reported.[23] The disease affects young, growing animals between 4 and 11 months of age. Affected animals have fever, anorexia, atrophy of the temporal and masseter muscles, and mandibular pain, especially during mastication.[24]

Craniomandibular osteopathy usually involves the occipital, parietal, and temporal portions of the calvarium, especially the tympanic bullae and the mandibular rami. One or more of these bones may be affected and the involve-

ment is often symmetric. Bony proliferation near the temporomandibular joints may result in bridging and ankylosis of these joints, thus interfering with the ability of the dog to open its mouth (Fig. 3–11). Proliferative changes on the long bones, which resemble those seen in hypertrophic osteodystrophy (HOD), have also been reported. Bony proliferation ceases when the animal reaches skeletal maturity.

Focal areas of increased opacity in the skull may occur with radiopaque foreign bodies and calcified brain tumors. Most brain tumors do not produce bony changes in the calvarium, although cerebral meningiomas may calcify and therefore are seen on survey radiographs. Bone destruction or proliferation involving the calvarium usually results from primary bone neo-

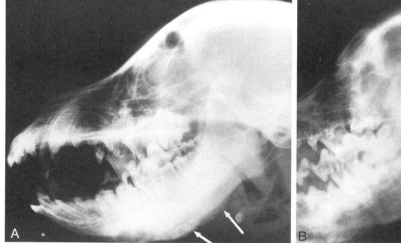
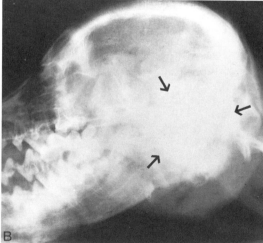

Figure 3–11. Lateral skull radiographs of two West Highland white terriers with craniomandibular osteopathy. *A,* the dog has proliferation primarily on the mandibular ramus *(arrows). B,* the second dog has proliferation involving the tympanic bullae and temporomandibular joints *(arrows).*

plasms or from neoplasia of the surrounding soft tissues.

Malignant bone neoplasms occur more frequently in the dog than in the cat.[25] The most common neoplasm of bone in both species is osteosarcoma.[26] Between 10 and 15 percent of all osteosarcomas are found in the skull. In one report concerning the distribution of osteosarcomas in the dog skull, 36 percent of neoplasms arose from the cranial vault, 36 percent from the facial bones, and 27 percent from the mandible.[27]

Radiographically, osteosarcomas arising from the cranial vault do not resemble those arising from the appendicular skeleton or from other areas of the skull. These neoplasms of the cranial vault tend to appear osteoblastic, have well-defined borders, and contain granular areas of calcification. Facial and mandibular osteosarcomas more closely resemble neoplasms of the extremities, and are characterized by osteolysis, cortical destruction, and new bone formation in the surrounding soft tissues.

When compared with osteosarcomas, other primary bone neoplasms of the skull are rare. Those types that occur more commonly include chondrosarcomas, osteomas, and osteochondromas.

Osteomas and osteochondromas are benign lesions. Osteomas are composed of dense homogeneous bone; they have a smooth, well-defined margin and a slow growth rate (Fig. 3–12). Osteomas may arise from the mandible, the cranial vault, or the sinuses, do not cause bone destruction at their attachment site, and often are amenable to surgical removal. Those lesions that arise from the cranial vault may predispose to neurologic signs. Osteochondromas resemble osteomas radiographically, but characteristically occur in immature dogs and usually involve multiple areas of the skeleton, especially the spine and ribs.

Another neoplasm, which has been infrequently described in the dog, is the multilobular osteoma and chondroma. Synonyms for this lesion include chondroma rodens, juvenile aponeurotic fibroma, and calcifying aponeurotic fibroma. Lesions in the dog most often involve the temporo-occipital area of the skull, although involvement of the orbit has been reported.[28] The neoplasm occurs most frequently in medium to large-breed dogs, at an average age of 7 years (range: 15 months to 12 years); no sex predilection has been reported. This neoplasm appears as a multilobular soft-tissue mass that contains nodular to stippled areas of mineralization with lysis of the underlying bone. Histologically, the neoplasm consists of a lobulated mass with islands of partially calcified or ossified cartilage, or both, surrounded by dense fibrous tissue. The neoplasm is locally invasive but can

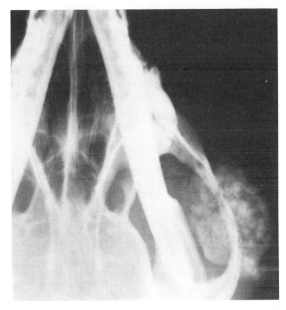

Figure 3–12. Ventrodorsal radiograph of a 9-year-old female mixed-breed dog with an osteoma of the left zygomatic arch. Note the opaque, well-ossified appearance of this neoplasm.

undergo malignant transformation with rare distant metastasis.[29] Surgical excision, with or without radiation therapy, appears to be the treatment of choice.[30]

Malignant soft-tissue neoplasms of the skull frequently invade adjacent bone with varying amounts of destruction and proliferation, i.e., an aggressive lesion; rarely are these lesions purely osteoblastic. Malignant melanomas, squamous cell carcinomas, hemangiosarcomas, reticulum cell sarcomas, fibrosarcomas, and adenocarcinomas are examples of this type of neoplasia.[31] Bone destruction of the nasal region is especially common and is discussed in Chapter 4. Metastatic neoplasms of the skull and mandible occur rarely.

Alterations in bone opacity may also occur with osteomyelitis. Bacterial and fungal infections of the skull in the dog and cat usually involve the teeth, sinuses, or tympanic bullae. Radiographic signs related to these areas are described elsewhere. Bacterial osteomyelitis may occur after fractures of the facial bones or surgical repair of mandibular fractures. Osteomyelitis generally causes a combination of bone destruction and proliferation. The presence and degree of proliferation depend on the virulence of the infectious organism; thus, low-grade infections tend to produce a sclerotic bone reaction. *Cryptococcus neoformans* is a saphrophytic fungus that usually involves the respiratory or central nervous systems, although ulcerated skin lesions on the head with lysis of the underlying bone may also result.[32]

Abnormalities of the Middle and Inner Ear

Radiography is useful in the evaluation of otitis media. Oblique and open mouth projections of the skull usually require the use of general anesthesia, but these views are necessary for adequate radiographic evaluation of the tympanic bullae. Although the anatomy of the petrous temporal bone is complex, most animals have unilateral involvement, allowing comparison of the affected and unaffected sides.

Otitis media is generally a sequela to chronic otitis externa, and thus narrowing of the external ear canal may be seen on the ventrodorsal radiograph. Ossification of the annular cartilages may also result from chronic otitis externa. Radiographic signs of otitis media include thickening and sclerosis of the wall of one or both tympanic bullae and filling of these normally well-aerated structures with soft-tissue material (Fig. 3–13). In advanced disease, bony prolif-

eration may involve the remaining petrous temporal bone, the temporomandibular joint, or both. Although sclerosis of the petrous temporal bone may be seen, otitis interna does not produce readily apparent radiographic signs in most animals, and diagnosis of this condition must be based on clinical signs.[33]

Other conditions that affect the middle ear include neoplasms and craniomandibular osteopathy. Malignant soft-tissue neoplasms, most notably squamous cell carcinoma of the ear canal, may result in extensive bone destruction, proliferation, or both and involves the petrous temporal bone, with occasional extension to the temporomandibular joint. This occurrence is more common in cats than in dogs (Fig. 3–14).

As previously mentioned, craniomandibular osteopathy may also result in marked bony proliferation affecting the tympanic bullae. Differential diagnosis is based on the age and breed

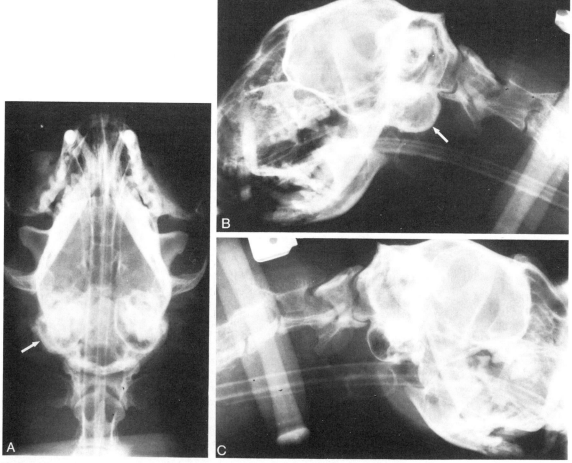

Figure 3–13. Ventrodorsal *(A)* and oblique views *(B* and *C)* of the skull of a 5-year-old domestic shorthair cat with chronic otitis externa of the right ear. *B,* oblique view of the left bulla. Compare the markedly thickened, fluid-filled right tympanic bulla *(arrows)* with the normal left side. Changes in the right bulla indicate secondary otitis media.

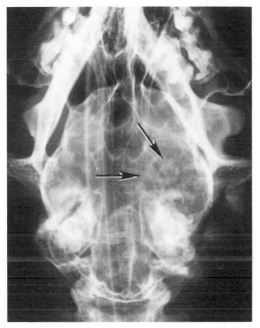

Figure 3–14. Ventrodorsal radiograph of the skull of a 12-year-old domestic shorthair cat with a squamous cell carcinoma of the left ear canal. There is lysis of the base of the skull *(arrows)* as well as of the lateral aspect of the left tympanic bulla.

of the animal as well as the absence of otitis. In addition, involvement with craniomandibular osteopathy is frequently bilateral with concurrent mandibular periostitis.

Evaluation of the Teeth

A tooth is composed of two parts: the root, which is embedded in the cancellous bone of the skull, and the crown, that part within the oral cavity. The bone between adjacent teeth is called the alveolar crest. The dentin, enamel,

TABLE 3–1. DENTAL FORMULAS

Species	Deciduous	Permanent
Dog	$2 \times \dfrac{3\ \ 1\ \ 3}{3\ \ 1\ \ 3} = 28$	$2 \times \dfrac{3\ \ 1\ \ 4\ \ 2}{3\ \ 1\ \ 4\ \ 3} = 42$
Cat	$2 \times \dfrac{3\ \ 1\ \ 3}{3\ \ 1\ \ 2} = 26$	$2 \times \dfrac{3\ \ 1\ \ 3\ \ 1}{3\ \ 1\ \ 2\ \ 1} = 30$

and lamina dura are radiopaque, whereas the pulp cavity and periodontal membrane are radiolucent. Figure 3–15 shows the normal anatomy of a tooth. The dental formulas for the dog and cat are provided in Table 3–1. Special radiographic positions and film types are recommended for optimal evaluation of teeth.[34]

Changes in the appearance of the teeth may occur owing to age, trauma, infection, or neoplasia. Congenital adontia (complete absence of the teeth) is rare, whereas oligodontia (partial absence of the teeth) is common, especially in the brachycephalic breeds of dogs. Supernumerary teeth also occur. Rarely are congenital alterations in the number of teeth clinically significant.[35]

The appearance of the teeth changes markedly during normal development and maturation.[36] The apical foramina of the teeth in the young animal are open (Fig. 3–15). The permanent teeth develop beneath or to one side of their deciduous precursors. All of the permanent teeth usually erupt by 7 months of age. Shortly after this eruption, the apical foramina close and the size of the pulp cavity gradually decreases. Regression of the alveolar crest, decreased prominence of the lamina dura, and coarsening of the bony trabeculation surrounding the teeth are normal changes that occur with age.[37]

Periodontal disease is a frequent form of

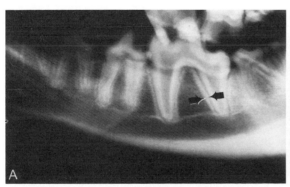

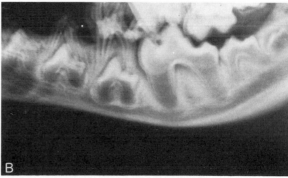

Figure 3–15. *A,* close-up lateral view of the mandible of a mature dog. Notice the well-defined lamina dura *(arrows)* marking the dental alveoli. *B,* close-up lateral view of the mandible of a 4-month-old dog. Notice the open apical foramina of the teeth and the location of the permanent premolars under their deciduous precursors.

dental disease in dogs and cats. Radiographic signs include resorption of the alveolar crest, rounding of the amelocemental junction, widening of the periodontal space with loss of the lamina dura, and lysis of the bone surrounding the teeth. Loss of bone opacity around the teeth also occurs with primary or secondary hyperparathyroidism. Bone lysis in hyperparathyroidism is more genralized and is not restricted to the periodontal area.

Periapical infections are common in older animals and may be secondary to periodontal disease. Other causes include fracture of the tooth or of the adjacent bone, neoplasia, and hematogenous infections. Periapical abscesses may arise in more than one tooth concurrently and may be found incidentally in asymptomatic aging dogs and cats that are examined radiographically for other reasons. In the dog, infection of the fourth upper premolar (carnassial tooth) frequently results in an externally draining fistulous tract just below the eye. Open mouth oblique views of the teeth are necessary for full evaluation of this condition. Radiographic signs of periapical disease include widening of the periodontal space surrounding the apex, bone lysis or sclerosis adjacent to the apex, resorption of the tooth root, and osteomyelitis of the adjacent bone (Fig. 3–16). Complications such as delayed gingival healing and nasal discharge after dental extractions may occur due to retained roots or the presence of sequestered fragments of alveolar bone.[38]

Focal destruction of bone adjacent to teeth may also occur with neoplasia (Fig. 3–14), which may arise from the dental elements themselves or from the adjacent bone or soft tissues. Malignant neoplasms tend to be more lytic, whereas benign processes tend to have a more sclerotic, well-demarcated border, reflecting their slower growth rate.

Periodontal epulides are the most common type of benign oral neoplasm in the dog. The nomenclature of these neoplasms was recently changed to alleviate the confusion resulting from previous classifications. All epulides arise from the periodontal membrane. Under the revised classification, there are three types of epulis: fibromatous, ossifying, and acanthomatous. Only the acanthomatous epulis has the potential to infiltrate locally into the bone.[39] Aggressive surgical excision or radiation therapy is the treatment of choice for these neoplasms.

Odontogenic neoplasms in dogs are rare.[40] These neoplasms arise from the dental laminar epithelium and usually contain enamel inclusions, dental pulp stroma, or organized dental structures, which distinguish them from the epulides. One classification scheme outlines the odontogenic neoplasms as ameloblastomas, keratinizing ameloblastomas, ameloblastic fibroodontomas, compound odontomas, and complex odontomas.[41] Ameloblastomas occur most frequently in the dog. These lesions often cause osteolysis around involved tooth roots, but may also be accompanied by an osteoblastic reaction. A rare odontogenic neoplasm that was described in young cats (less than 14 months of age) is the fibroameloblastoma. This neoplasm contains ameloblastic epithelial tissue and dental pulp–like stroma, and causes bone lysis and proliferation of the maxilla. Wide surgical excision is the most successful form of treatment in that these neoplasms are not radioresponsive.[42]

Disorders of the Temporomandibular Joints

The temporomandibular joint is a condylar joint that allows considerable lateral sliding movement. The transversely elongated mandibular condyle does not correspond exactly with the articular surface of the temporal bone. In addition, the synchondrosis at the mandibular symphysis allows independent motion between the mandibular rami, which in turn permits congenital or traumatic luxations of the temporomandibular joints to occur without fracture.[43]

Disorders of the TM joints in the dog and cat include congenital dysplasias, traumatic luxations, fractures, and osteoarthritis. Involvement of this joint in craniomandibular osteopathy has been discussed. Radiographic examination is often the only method of reaching a definitive diagnosis of temporomandibular region abnor-

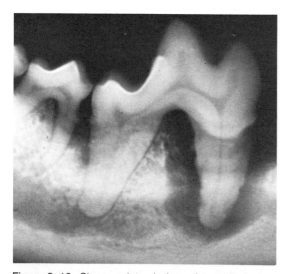

Figure 3–16. Close-up lateral view of a periapical abscess around the rostral root of the first mandibular molar. Note the marked lysis of the alveolus with loss of the normal lamina dura. There is also erosion of the dental enamel.

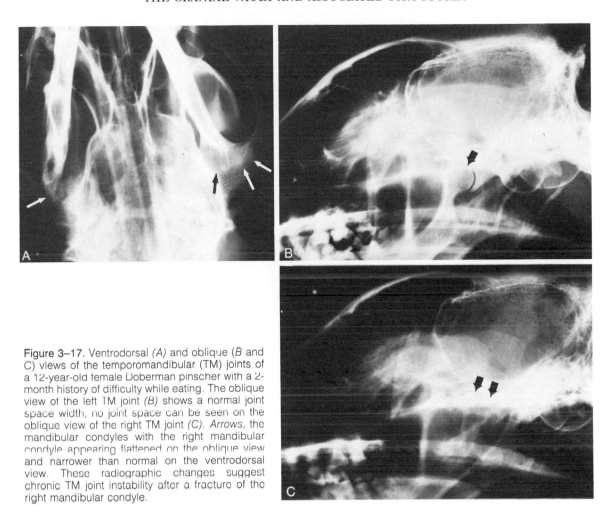

Figure 3–17. Ventrodorsal *(A)* and oblique *(B* and *C)* views of the temporomandibular (TM) joints of a 12-year-old female Doberman pinscher with a 2-month history of difficulty while eating. The oblique view of the left TM joint *(B)* shows a normal joint space width; no joint space can be seen on the oblique view of the right TM joint *(C)*. *Arrows,* the mandibular condyles with the right mandibular condyle appearing flattened on the oblique view and narrower than normal on the ventrodorsal view. These radiographic changes suggest chronic TM joint instability after a fracture of the right mandibular condyle.

malities. In addition to the standard ventrodorsal and lateral views, oblique views with the animal under anesthesia or heavy sedation are generally required for adequate evaluation of these joints. These views are described elsewhere.[44]

Open-mouth jaw locking is a prominent clinical sign of congenital dysplasia of the temporomandibular joints. Jaw locking is precipitated by yawning or excessive opening of the mouth. The condition is uncommon but is most frequently reported in the Bassett hound.[45] In this breed, the condition appears to be due to abnormal angulation of the condyloid processes with resulting subluxation. Stretching of the lateral ligament of the affected joint and excessive lateral movement of the condyloid process allows the coronoid process to become entrapped lateral to the zygomatic arch. Jaw locking usually occurs on the contralateral side from the joint with the most severe dysplastic changes. This condition has been treated successfully by removal of the ventral portion of the zygomatic arch.[46] A similar problem with jaw locking may result from callus formation after fracture of the zygomatic arch.[47]

Traumatic injuries that affect the temporomandibular region are especially common in the cat, perhaps due to the relative frequency of mandibular symphyseal injury as well as the lack of structural suport for the mandibular fossa. Traumatic dislocations generally result in rostrodorsal displacement of the mandibular condyle. Dislocations may be unilateral or bilateral and may occur alone or in combination with a variety of fractures, including fractures of the condylar portion of the joint (Fig. 3–17), the base of the condylar portion, the mandibular fossa or retroarticular process, and the zygomatic process.[48] Oblique and ventrodorsal views are especially helpful in the characterization of these lesions. Malocclusion is a prominent feature of temporomandibular joint injuries (Fig. 3–18). Radiography is helpful in eliminating a diagnosis of rostral mandibular fractures as the cause of the malocclusion.

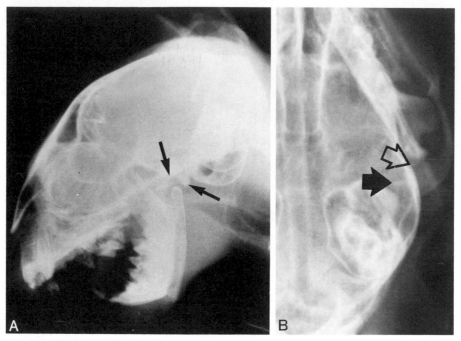

Figure 3–18. *A,* lateral skull radiograph of a 4-year-old domestic shorthair cat with bilateral temporomandibular luxations, mandibular symphyseal fracture, and some fractured teeth. The mandible has dropped in a rostroventral direction with marked malocclusion. *Arrows,* the temporal portion of one of the joints. *B,* dorsoventral radiograph of a 6-month-old domestic shorthair cat with a left temporomandibular luxation. The condylar process (articular surface) of the mandible *(open arrow)* is distracted rostrally from the mandibular fossa (articular surface) of the temporal bone *(solid arrow).*

Other less common conditions that result in abnormal temporomandibular joint function include osteoarthritis, myositis, retrobulbar abscesses, tetanus, and neoplasia. Causes of osteoarthritis include extension of otitis media, craniomandibular osteopathy, congenital malformation with secondary joint laxity, and trauma. Benign or malignant neoplasms of either bone or soft tissue that occur adjacent to the temporomandibular joints may interfere with normal joint motion and may produce localized bone destruction or proliferation. Radiographic evaluation in cases of myositis, retrobulbar abscess formation, and tetanus would be normal.

References

1. Miller EA, Christensen GC, and Evans HE: Anatomy of the Dog. Philadelphia, WB Saunders, 1964, p.8.
2. Hare WCD: Radiographic anatomy of the feline skull. J Am Vet Med Assoc 134:349, 1959.
3. Ticer JW: Radiographic Technique in Veterinary Practice. Philadelphia, WB Saunders, 1984, pp. 231–259.
4. Morgan JP, and Silverman S: Techniques of Veterinary Radiography. Davis, CA, Veterinary Radiology Associates, 1982, pp. 169–174.
5. Ettinger SJ: Textbook of Veterinary Internal Medicine. Philadelphia, WB Saunders, 1983, pp. 487–490.
6. Burt JK, Bhargava AK, and Prynn RB: Unilateral hydrocephalus with cranial distortion in a cat. Vet Med/Small Anim Clin 65:979, 1970.
7. Krum S, Johnson K, and Wilson J: Hydrocephalus associated with the noneffusive form of feline infectious peritonitis. J Am Vet Med Assoc 167:745, 1975.
8. Becker SA, and Selby LA: Canine hydrocephalus. Comp Contin Ed Pract Vet 2:647, 1980.
9. Hoerlein BF: Canine Neurology. Philadelphia, WB Saunders, 1978, pp. 560–569.
10. Bardens JW: Congenital malformation of the foramen magnum in dogs. SW Vet 18:295, 1965.
11. Wright JA: A study of the radiographic anatomy of the foramen magnum in dogs. J Small Anim Pract 20:501, 1979.
12. Watson AG: The phylogeny and development of the occipitoatlas-axis complex in the dog. MS Thesis, Cornell University, 1981.
13. Ticer JW: Radiographic Technique in Veterinary Practice. Philadelphia, WB Saunders, 1984, p. 256.
14. Haskins ME, Jezyk PF, Desnick RJ, et al: Mucopolysaccharidosis in a domestic short-haired cat—a disease distinct from that seen in the Siamese cat. J Am Vet Med Assoc 175:384, 1979.
15. Cornell Feline Health Center: Veterinary News. Ithaca, NY, Cornell University, Winter, 1983.
16. Kolata RJ: Trauma in dogs and cats: An overview. Vet Clin North Am [Small Anim Pract] 10:515, 1980.
17. Gibbs C: Traumatic lesions of the skull. J Small Anim Pract 17:551, 1976.
18. Phillips IR: A survey of bone fractures in the dog and cat. J Small Anim Pract 20:661, 1979.
19. Gibbs C: Traumatic lesions of the mandible. J Small Anim Pract 18:51, 1977.

20. Roush JC: Orthopedic problems of the cat—a review. Feline Pract 10:10, 1980.
21. Ettinger SJ: Textbook of Veterinary Internal Medicine. Philadelphia, WB Saunders, 1983, pp. 1565–1572.
22. Morgan JP: Radiology in Veterinary Orthopedics. Philadelphia, Lea & Febiger, 1972, pp. 332–335.
23. Watson ADJ, Huxtable CR, and Farrow BR: Craniomandibular osteopathy in Doberman Pinschers. J Small Anim Pract 16:11, 1975.
24. Riser WH, Parkes LJ, and Shiver JF: Canine craniomandibular osteopathy. J Am Vet Radiol Soc 8:23, 1967.
25. Liu SK, Dorfman HD, and Patnaik AK: Primary and secondary bone tumours in the cat. J Small Anim Pract 15:141, 1974.
26. Turrel JM, and Pool RR: Primary bone neoplasms in the cat. Vet Radiol 23:152, 1982.
27. Hardy WD, Brodey RS and Riser WH: Osteosarcoma of the canine skull. J Am Vet Radiol Soc 8:5, 1967.
28. Pletcher JM, Koch SA, and Stedhem MA: Orbital chondroma rodens in a dog. J Am Vet Med Assoc 175:187, 1979.
29. McLain DL, et al: Multilobular osteoma and chondroma (chondroma rodens) with pulmonary metastasis in a dog. J Am Anim Hosp Assoc 19:359, 1983.
30. Selcer BA, and McCracken MD: Chondroma rodens in dogs. J Vet Orthop 2:7, 1981.
31. Richardson RC, Jones MA, and Elliott GS: Oral neoplasms in the dog: A diagnostic and therapeutic dilemma. Comp Contin Ed Pract Vet 5:441, 1983.
32. Rutman MA, Rickardo DA, and Chandler FW: Feline cryptococcosis. Feline Pract 53:36, 1975.
33. Gibbs C: The head. Part III: ear disease. J Small Anim Pract 19:539, 1978.
34. Zontine WJ: Canine dental radiology: Radiographic technic, development, and anatomy of the tooth. Vet Radiol 16:75, 1975.
35. Kealy JK: Diagnostic Radiology of the Dog and Cat. Philadelphia, WB Saunders, 1979, pp. 400–404.
36. Hooft, J, Mattheeuws D, and Van Bree P: Radiology of deciduous teeth resorption and definitive teeth eruption in the dog. J Small Anim Pract 20:175, 1979.
37. Zontine WJ: Dental radiographic technique and interpretation. Vet Clin North Am 4:741, 1974.
38. Gibbs C: The head: Dental disease. J Small Anim Pract 19:701, 1978.
39. Dubielzig RR, Goldschmidt MH, and Brodey RS: The nomenclature of periodontal epulides in dogs. Vet Pathol 16:209, 1979.
40. Gorlin RJ, Barren CN, Chandhry AP, et al: The oral and pharyngeal pathology of domestic animals. A study of 487 cases. Am J Vet Res 79:1032, 1959.
41. Dubielzig RR: Proliferative dental and gingival diseases of dogs and cats. J Am Anim Hosp Assoc 18:577, 1982.
42. Dubielzig RR, Adams WM, and Brodey RS: Inductive fibroameloblastoma, an unusual dental tumor of young cats. J Am Vet Med Assoc 174:720, 1979.
43. Lane JG: Disorders of the canine temporomandibular joint. Vet Annual 21:175, 1982.
44. Ticer, JW: Radiographic Technique in Veterinary Practice. Philadelphia, WB Saunders, 1984, p. 232.
45. Robins G, and Grandage J: Temporomandibular joint dysplasia and open-mouth jaw locking in the dog. J Am Vet Med Assoc 171:1072, 1977.
46. Thomas RE: Temporo-mandibular joint dysplasia and open-mouth jaw locking in a Bassett hound: a case report. J Small Anim Pract 20:697, 1979.
47. Bennett D, and Campbell JR: Mechanical interference with lower jaw movement as a complication of skull fractures. J Small Anim Pract 17:747, 1976.
48. Ticer JW, and Spencer CP: Injury of the feline temporomandibular joint: Radiographic signs. J Am Vet Radiol Soc 19:146, 1978.

CHAPTER 4

THE NASAL CAVITY AND PARANASAL SINUSES

WENDY MYER

RADIOGRAPHIC EVALUATION

Most diseases that affect the nasal cavity have similar clinical signs. Radiography is a noninvasive and effective method to evaluate the location and extent of changes resulting from these diseases. Because radiographic changes are nonspecific, a definitive diagnosis usually depends on diagnostic nasal flushes, nasal biopsies, or both.

A systematic method of evaluation is helpful in accurately assessing radiographic changes that involve the skull. The routine examination should begin with ventrodorsal and lateral views. In addition, open mouth or occlusal views of the nasal cavity (Fig. 4–1) and a rostrocaudal view of the frontal sinuses (Fig. 4–2) are advisable so as to obtain an unobstructed view of these structures. General anesthesia is necessary to achieve good positioning and to allow comparison between the normal and affected sides of the skull. This comparison facilitates evaluation of the complex nasal passages and recognition of minor alterations in contour and radiopacity.

Normal Anatomy

The nasal cavity is the most rostral portion of the respiratory system. It is divided into two symmetric halves called the nasal fossae. These fossae are separated rostrally by a perpendicular cartilaginous nasal septum and caudally by the septal processes of the frontal and nasal bones, the perpendicular plate of the ethmoid, and the sagittal portion of the vomer. The nasal fossae are almost entirely filled by nasal turbinates. The dorsal and ventral conchae are located rostrally and the ethmoidal conchae are located caudally. These structures were formerly called the dorsal nasoturbinates, maxillary turbinates, and ethmoturbinates.[1]

The pattern formed by these delicate bony scrolls and the air surrounding them accounts for the normal radiographic appearance of the nasal passages. On the open mouth view, the nasal conchae appear as fine, semiparallel radiopaque lines that extend caudally from the canine teeth to the level of the third premolars. The ethmoidal conchae form a fine, linear bony pattern fanning out from the cribriform plate to their juction with the nasal conchae.[2] The turbinate pattern can also be seen on the lateral radiograph, but it is not as prominent.

Although the rostral portion of the nasal septum is radiolucent, its location on the open mouth radiograph is marked by the sagittal groove of the vomer (Fig. 4–1).[3] The integrity of the nasal septum is difficult to assess radiographically. In the dog and cat, large areas of

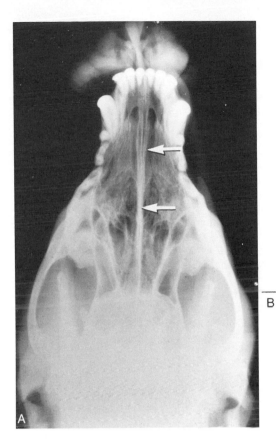

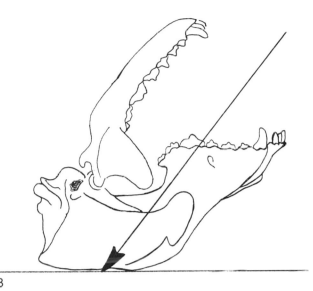

Figure 4–1. *A,* rostroventral-caudodorsal open mouth view of the nasal cavity and ethmoid region of a normal dog. Note the good visualization of the vomer bone *(arrows),* nasal conchae, and ethmoidal conchae. *B,* the head position and direction of the central x-ray beam *(arrow)* used for the open mouth view shown in *A.* With the mouth opened maximally, the cassette is placed parallel to the maxilla, and the x-ray beam is directed roughly parallel to the mandible.

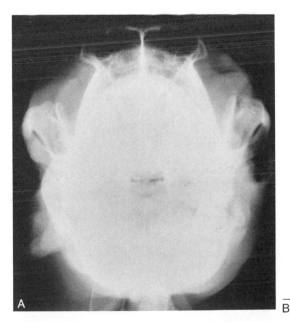

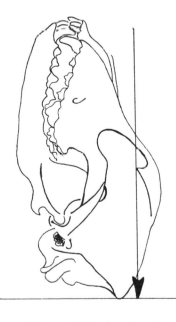

Figure 4–2. *A,* rostrocaudal view of a normal canine skull shows the frontal sinuses. *B,* the head position and direction of the central x-ray beam *(arrow)* used for the view of the frontal sinuses shown in *A.*

the septum can be destroyed and, unless there is concurrent erosion of the vomer or overlying maxilla, this destruction may not be evident radiographically. Positive-contrast rhinography with 30 percent barium was recently recommended as a means of better delineating the nasal septum and evaluating areas of turbinate destruction.[4]

The frontal sinuses are located between the outer and inner tables of the frontal bones. Each sinus has a lateral and a medial portion. The lateral part extends over the orbit as the supraorbital process and may be partially divided by bony septae. The medial portion, which communicates with the ethmoidal conchae, is more variable in size and shape than the lateral compartment. In the cat, the frontal sinuses are small and in Persian cats may be absent.

The maxillary sinuses are lateral diverticuli of the nasal fossae. In the dog, they are more aptly called maxillary recesses, because the openings to the nasal cavity are as large as the sinuses themselves. The maxillary sinuses are absent in the cat.[5]

Alterations in Shape and Contour

Variations in skull shape due to breed and species differences account for most of the congenital alterations in the shape, size, and contour of the nasal passages and sinuses. Changes in the conchal size and shape may occur as the facial portion of the skull is shortened, e.g., in brachycephalic dog breeds and in the cat.

Significant congenital abnormalities that involve the nasal passages are rare. Occasionally, dentigerous cysts may extend into the nasal cavity, causing deformity of the conchae and deviation of the nasal septum. In addition, malformation of these structures may occur with congenital defects in the hard palate. In affected animals, rhinitis may occur owing to the introduction of food into the nasal passages through the defect.

Trauma is the most common cause of acquired facial deformity in the dog and cat. Fractures of the facial portion of the skull frequently involve multiple bones and are more common than fractures of the calvarium. The fractures usually appear as straight or curved radiolucent lines (Fig. 4–3). Occasionally, however, they appear radiopaque due to overlapping bone fragments. Overlying soft-tissue swelling and subcutaneous emphysema are common. Resulting nasal hemorrhage may appear as patchy or widespread areas of increased radiopacity in the nasal fossae.

Facial deformity also may result from neoplastic processes of the skull. The presence of cortical lysis and facial swelling indicates a poorly confined, highly aggressive lesion. Periosteal new bone formation may be seen in conjunction with this cortical lysis.

Alterations in Radiographic Opacity

Virtually all chronic diseases that affect the nasal passages and sinuses result in alterations in their radiographic opacity. Radiographic findings generally conform to one of several patterns. (1) No alteration in the normal radiographic appearance of fine trabecular bone surrounded by air throughout both nasal passages. (2) Areas of *increased* soft-tissue opacity superimposed over the normal turbinate pattern. (3) Areas of *increased* soft-tissue opacity superimposed over areas of turbinate destruction. (4) Areas of *decreased* opacity due to turbinate destruction *without* accompanying soft-tissue opacity. (5) A mixed pattern with areas of turbinate destruction and superimposed soft-tissue opacity interspersed with areas of turbinate destruction alone.

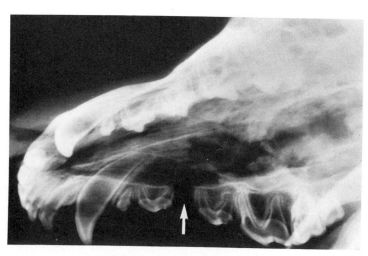

Figure 4–3. Open mouth oblique view of the right maxilla in a 9-month-old male German shepherd with multiple skull fractures after being hit by a car. Note the disruption of the maxillary cortex between the second and third upper premolar *(arrow)*, and the lucent defect extending through the right nasal passage.

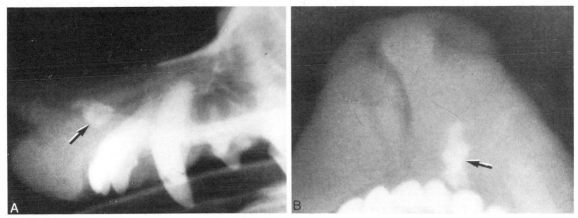

Figure 4–4. Lateral (A) and rostroventral-caudodorsal open mouth (B) radiographs of a 9-year-old female poodle with a history of unilateral nasal discharge and sneezing for 3 weeks. A radiopaque foreign body (arrows) can be seen in the left nostril; note the loss of normal aeration of that nostril.

Although some radiographic changes are more common in certain diseases, the aforementioned radiographic patterns are more a reflection of the aggressiveness and duration of the disease process than an indication of a specific etiology. In some animals, however, the location of an abnormality within the nasal cavity may be helpful in formulating a differential diagnosis. For instance, most nasal neoplasms originate from the region of the ethmoid conchae and cribriform plate.[6] In contrast, destructive rhinitis and hyperplastic rhinitis involve the middle and rostral segments of the nasal passages with equal or greater frequency than the middle and caudal segments. Obliteration of the air passages of one or both nostrils is a common finding in animals with nasal discharge from any cause.

Animals with acute rhinitis frequently have nasal passages that are normal radiographically. Possible causes for rhinitis include foreign bodies, viruses, bacteria, and allergies. Nasal foreign bodies are uncommon in the dog and cat, but should be considered in patients with acute

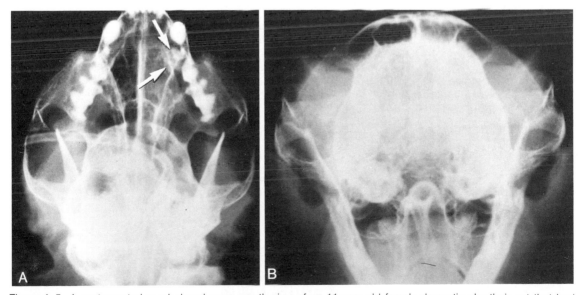

Figure 4–5. A, rostroventral-caudodorsal open mouth view of an 11-year-old female domestic shorthair cat that had respiratory distress for 2 months and unilateral mucopurulent nasal discharge. There is a soft-tissue mass medial to the left upper premolar, which was found to be a nasal polyp (arrow). Note the diffuse opacification of the left nasal passage due to impaired nasal drainage and secondary rhinitis. B, rostrocaudal view of the frontal sinuses shows opacification of the left frontal sinus due to impaired drainage.

onset of violent sneezing, head shaking, and nose rubbing. Unless the foreign body is radiopaque, however, radiographic examination may be unrewarding (Fig. 4–4). Plant awns and other vegetable materials frequently lodge in the rostral portions of the nasal passages. In chronic situations, a focal area of increased soft-tissue opacity may be seen due to the presence of mucopurulent material or to inflammatory response. In some animals, foreign body rhinitis is due to congenital or traumatic defects in the palate coupled with the introduction of food into the nasal passages.

Areas of increased soft-tissue opacity superimposed over the normal turbinate pattern are often seen in animals with chronic rhinitis. This increased opacity may be due to the presence of nasal exudate or to swelling and proliferation of the nasal mucosa (hyperplastic rhinitis) (Fig. 4–5). In the cat, chronic rhinitis is a common sequel to viral upper respiratory tract infections. Frontal sinusitis may be present concurrently in these animals. As previously mentioned, post-traumatic hemorrhage and exudation secondary to chronic radiolucent nasal foreign bodies may also produce this appearance.

Nasal turbinate destruction is an indication of a more aggressive disease process, and occurs primarily with destructive rhinitis or neoplasia. Destructive rhinitis is generally due to fungal infections and most commonly affects mesaticephalic or dolichocephalic dogs of less than 4 years of age.[7] *Aspergillus* sp. (especially *A. fumigatus*) are the most common causative agents.[8] Infections due to *Penicillium* sp. and other fungal agents are noted less frequently.[9] *Cryptococcus neoformans* also may infect the nasal passages, especially in the cat, but this organism usually causes hyperplastic rather than destructive rhinitis.[10] Most cases of destructive rhinitis are characterized by focal radiolucent areas of turbinate destruction. These lesions vary in size from small punctate holes to large, poorly marginated areas of lysis (Fig. 4–6). A mixed pattern of destruction and soft-tissue proliferation may be seen, but is less common. Erosion or deviation of the nasal septum is unusual, except in advanced disease.

Increased soft-tissue opacity superimposed over areas of turbinate destruction, and a mixture of radiopaque areas interspersed with well-defined areas of radiolucency, are patterns typically seen with neoplasia, although they may also occur in destructive rhinitis. In many animals, these areas of increased opacity are due to accumulated nasal secretions. Opacification of the ipsilateral frontal sinus is generally due to impaired sinus drainage, although neoplastic extension into the sinus also occurs.[11]

Neoplasms of the nasal cavity and paranasal

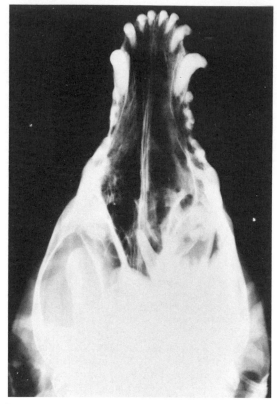

Figure 4–6. Rostroventral-caudodorsal open mouth view of a 6-year-old male Doberman pinscher that had lost weight and had bilateral chronic mucopurulent nasal discharge. There is marked destruction of the normal turbinate pattern in the midportion of both nasal fossae. Destructive rhinitis due to *Aspergillus fumigatus* was diagnosed by culture.

sinuses are rare, and represent approximately 1 percent of all neoplasms in the dog and cat.[12] Studies concerning the biologic behavior of these lesions and their response to various treatment modalities are still in the early stages. A comprehensive discussion of nasal tumors in domestic animals was recently published.[13] Reports to date indicate that 80 percent of nasal neoplasms in dogs are malignant; in cats, 91 percent are malignant.[14] Of these malignant neoplasms, 60 to 75 percent are carcinomas, with adenocarcinomas predominating over other cell types.[15] Older animals are most frequently affected, with a mean age at diagnosis of 8 to 10 years. A marked sex predisposition appears in the cat; males are nearly twice as likely to be affected as females.[16] The few benign neoplasms that do occur are fibromas, adenomas, and papillomas.

The radiographic appearance of nasal neoplasms varies depending upon the type of neoplasm, its duration, and any previous surgical or medical treatment. The more aggressive the neoplasm, the more destructive and less con-

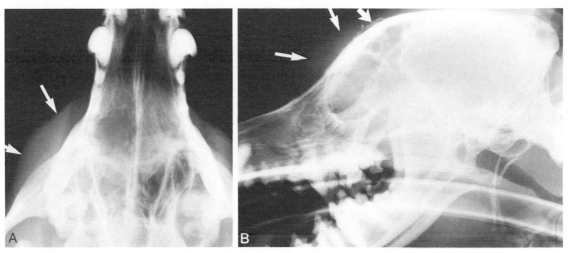

Figure 4–7. Rostroventral-caudodorsal open mouth (A) and lateral (B) views of an 8-year-old male mixed-breed dog with chronic nasal discharge and a history of unilateral epistaxis. Open mouth view shows a large area of turbinate destruction with erosion of the vomer and superimposed soft-tissue opacity in the right nasal passage and frontal sinus. Evidence indicating destruction of the overlying cortical bone includes an external soft-tissue mass (A and B, long arrows) and an irregular periosteal reaction (retouched) over the frontal sinuses (B, short arrow).

fined it appears. Early nasal neoplasms may appear similar radiographically to rhinitis and therefore are difficult to detect. A unilateral increase in nasal opacity with attenuation or obliteration of the normal turbinate pattern is a consistent finding in early nasal tumors of epithelial origin. This homogeneous appearance is due to cellular debris and fluid silhouetting with the turbinates. As the neoplasm grows, the radiographic appearance becomes more heterogeneous due to progressive turbinate destruction (Fig. 4–7). Disruption of the nasal septum is frequently seen with malignant neoplasms. As mentioned previously, the integrity of the nasal septum is difficult to assess radiographically. Recognition of septal penetration is most likely to occur in those animals with destruction of the vomer or marked deviation of the nasal septum (Fig. 4–8).

Peripheral signs of soft-tissue swelling, facial bone destruction, and periosteal new bone formation are usually associated with highly aggressive neoplasms.[17] Areas of bone destruction may be evident on palpation or may cause obvious facial swelling. Superimposition of disrupted overlying bone often contributes to the mixed opacity seen on the open mouth view in many animals with neoplasia (Fig. 4–9). Oblique projections may help to demonstrate defects in the maxillae, the palate, and the nasal and frontal bones.

Radiography is a noninvasive method for evaluating the extent and location of a lesion within the nasal passages. Although radiographic signs tend to be nonspecific, some assessment of the

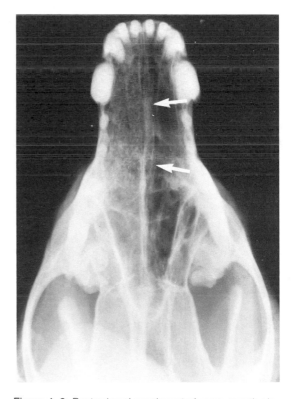

Figure 4–8. Rostrodorsal-caudoventral open mouth view of a 6-year-old male German shepherd with a 4-month history of unilateral epistaxis. There is diffuse opacification of the right nasal passage with many punctate areas of calcification in the middle and rostral portions. There is thinning and apparent deviation of the vomer (arrow). The diagnosis of a chondrosarcoma was made histologically.

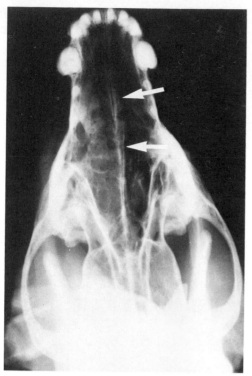

Figure 4–9. Rostrodorsal-caudoventral open mouth view of a 13-year-old female mixed-breed dog with right-sided serosanguinous nasal discharge for 2 months. There was a soft, palpable, fluctuant mass ventral to the right eye. There is a mixed pattern of soft-tissue opacity and turbinate destruction in the right nasal passage with thinning and apparent deviation of the vomer *(arrows)*. The large defect medial to the third upper premolar was due to destruction of the maxilla overlying this nasal adenocarcinoma.

aggressiveness of a disease process can be made. Radiography also allows assessment of treatment response by facilitating periodic re-evaluation of bony changes. A tentative differential diagnosis can be reached based on the location of the radiographic lesion, e.g., unilateral versus bilateral and rostral versus caudal, and on the radiographic pattern of bony destruction or proliferation. Definitive diagnoses should be based on nasal flushes, biopsies, or cultures.

References

1. Evans HE, and Christensen GC: Miller's Anatomy of the Dog, 2nd Ed. Philadelphia, WB Saunders, 1979, p. 158.
2. Sande RD, and Alexander JE: Turbinate bone neoplasms in dogs. Mod Vet Pract 51:23, 1970.
3. Harvey C: The nasal septum of the dog: Is it visible radiographically? Vet Radiol 20:88, 1979.
4. Goring RL, Ticer JW, Gross TL, et al: Contrast rhinography in the radiographic evaluation of diseases affecting the nasal cavity, nasopharynx, and paranasal sinuses in the dog. Vet Radiol 25:106, 1984.
5. Hare WCD: Radiographic anatomy of the feline skull. J Am Vet Med Assoc 134:349, 1959.
6. Bright RM, and Bojrab MJ: Intranasal neoplasia in the dog and cat. J Am Anim Hosp Assoc 12:806, 1976.
7. Bedford PG: The differential diagnosis of nasal discharge in the dog. Vet Annual 18:232, 1978.
8. Lane JG, and Warnock DW: The diagnosis of *Aspergillus fumigatus* infection of the nasal chambers of the dog with particular reference to the value of the double diffusion test. J Small Anim Pract 18:169, 1977.
9. Harvey CE, O'Brien JA, Felsburg PJ, et al: Nasal penicilliosis in six dogs. J Am Vet Med Assoc 178:1084, 1981.
10. Wilkinson GT: Feline cryptococcosis: A review and seven case reports. J Small Anim Pract 20:749, 1979.
11. Gibbs C, Lane JG, Denny HR: Radiological features of intranasal lesions in the dog: A review of 100 cases. J Small Anim Pract 20:515, 1979.
12. Norris AM: Intranasal neoplasms in the dog. J Am Anim Hosp Assoc 15:231, 1979.
13. Reznik G, and Stinson SF: Nasal Tumors in Animals and Man. Boca Raton, FL, CRC Press, 1983.
14. Madewell BR, Priester WA, Gillette EL, et al: Neoplasms of the nasal passages and paranasal sinuses in domesticated animals as reported by 13 veterinary colleges. Am J Vet Res 37:851, 1976.
15. Brodey RS: Canine and feline neoplasia. Adv Vet Sci Comp Med 14:309, 1970.
16. Legendre AM, Krahwinkel DJ, and Spaulding KA: Feline nasal and paranasal neoplasms. J Am Anim Hosp Assoc 17:1038, 1981.
17. Legendre AM, Spaulding KA, and Krahwinkel DJ: Canine nasal and paranasal sinus neoplasms. J Am Anim Hosp Assoc 19:115, 1983.

CHAPTER 5

THE VERTEBRAE

MICHAEL A. WALKER

Prerequisites for accurate radiographic evaluation of the canine and feline spine include knowledge of normal anatomy, proper patient preparation, and good technique. A basic anatomic knowledge includes certain facts.

1. There are 7 cervical, 13 thoracic, 7 lumbar, and 3 sacral vertebrae.

2. The dorsal spinous process of C_2 should be adjacent to or overlap the arch of C_1.

3. On a lateral view, the cervical articular facets are positioned obliquely across the plane of the spinal canal.

4. C_6 has a large lamina ventral to its transverse process.

5. Rib heads are cranial to their corresponding vertebrae.

6. T_{11} is the anticlinal vertebra.

7. The T_{10-11} disc space is normally narrow; adjacent intervertebral disc spaces should be of approximately equal width.

8. The intervertebral foramina serve as "windows" to the spinal canal.

9. Adjacent vertebrae should be approximately equal in size, shape, and radiopacity.

10. The ventral edges of the vertebral bodies of L_3 and L_4, may appear poorly defined due to origins of the diaphragmatic crura.

11. The lumbosacral angle is variable among individuals and varies with flexion or extension of the lumbosacral joint.

12. The spinal canal should be smoothly aligned.

13. Bony hemal arches may be present ventral to several caudal vertebrae.

Because spinal abnormalities are often painful, proper radiographic positioning may require the use of sedation or general anesthesia. General anesthesia also allows the use of positioning blocks and adhesive tape rather than human holders. In cases of suspected spinal fracture, however, loss of the patient's pain perception due to general anesthesia may allow for hazardous manipulation of the unstable spine. Good judgment is necessary in every instance. An improperly positioned, exposed, or processed radiograph of the spine is often nondiagnostic and should be repeated (Fig. 5–1). Short-scale contrast (high mAs, low kVp; black and white radiograph) provides better bone detail whereas long-scale contrast (low mAs, high kVp; gray radiograph) provides for detection of more subtle soft-tissue changes. Choosing a long or short scale of contrast is philosophic and is not as important as achieving a radiograph that is of adequate blackness and is free of artifact.

41

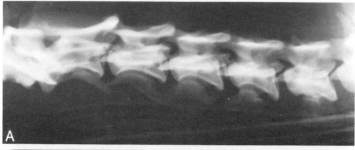

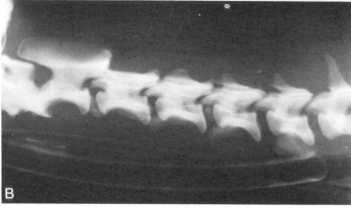

Figure 5–1. *A*, oblique lateral view of the cervical spine demonstrates the difficulty of accurate interpretation. *B*, straight lateral view of same cervical spine. The vertebrae, their articular facets, and the intervertebral disc spaces are now seen clearly.

BASIC ROENTGENOGRAPHIC SIGNS

The signs that apply to the spine are number, alignment, size, shape, and radiopacity. In this chapter, each roentgen sign is presented, followed by definitions of the abnormalities that exhibit that sign. The reader may add to each gamut as experience dictates.

Number. Number abnormalities (Table 5–1) imply an excess or a deficiency of parts. In many instances, these changes are clinically insignificant. Excessive vertebrae is an anomalous condition that is usually manifest as an extra lumbar vertebra. A false impression of excessive lumbar vertebrae may occur if there is agenesis or incomplete formation of the 13th ribs, or if there is a transitional vertebra at the lumbosacral junction. The latter is due to lack of fusion of the first sacral vertebra to the remainder of the sacrum, and is referred to as lumbarization of the sacrum.

TABLE 5–1. **ABNORMALITIES IN THE NUMBER OF VERTEBRAE**

Increased
Anomalous excess
Pseudoincrease due to transitional vertebrae

Decreased
Anomalous lack of normal number
Pseudodecrease due to transitional vertebrae
Manx cat
Tail docking or trauma

Decreased number of vertebrae is an anomaly that occasionally affects either the thoracic or the lumbar spine. It is helpful to count the total number of ribs and to determine the location of the anticlinical vertebra when deciding which part of the spine is anatomically deficient. Again, caution must be used regarding transitional vertebrae, because L_7 may be partially or completely fused with the first sacral vertebra or with the wing of one or both ilia. Sacralization is most frequently encountered in German shepherds, Brittany spaniels, Rhodesian ridgebacks, and Doberman pinschers.[1]

A decreased number of coccygeal vertebrae may be the result of tail docking or trauma. Manx cats may possess few coccygeal vertebrae, "stumpies," or no coccygeal and few sacral vertebrae, "rumpies." Accompanying sacrococcygeal dysgenesis in Manx cats, there may be spina bifida and spinal cord abnormalities, such as meningocele, myelomeningocele, syringomyelia, and spinal dysraphism.[2]

Alignment. Although the bony spine does not lie in one single dorsal plane, the spinal canal should always be smoothly aligned from one vertebra to the next. Numerous causes of abnormal spinal alignment are listed in Table 5–2. Abnormal curvature of the spine may present as scoliosis, a lateral bowing; kyphosis, a dorsal arching; or lordosis, a ventral deviation. Such abnormal contour of the spine may be congenital, idiopathic, or related to another spinal abnormality. Congenital alterations in spinal contour may result from some form of wedge-

TABLE 5–2. **ABNORMAL SPINAL ALIGNMENT**

Scoliosis—postural change
Kyphosis—postural change
Lordosis—postural change
Subluxation/luxation
Atlantoaxial subluxation (odontoid agenesis, fracture,
  fusion failure; ligament rupture)
Fracture
Anomaly (hemivertebra, hemimetameric displacement)
Transitional vertebrae (sacralization, lumbarization)
Muscle spasm—back or abdominal pain
Malunion fracture
Cervical spondylopathy
Lumbosacral instability

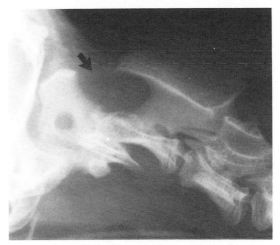

Figure 5–2. Atlantoaxial subluxation. Distance between laminae of C_1 and C_2 is increased.

shaped hemivertebra, including unilateral hemivertebra from hemimetameric displacement, causing scoliosis; ventral hemivertebra from an ossification defect, causing lordosis; and dorsal hemivertebra from an ossification defect, causing kyphosis. The abnormal contour may also be postural as a manifestation of a pain response or as a result of other deforming spinal abnormalities.[3, 4]

Fractures may involve any part of the spine. The most common sites of fracture are the vertebral body, the transverse process, and the dorsal spinous process. Fractures of the vertebral bodies may be accompanied by abnormal spinal alignment, especially when the fracture involves the lumbar spine, and less so with involvement of the thoracic or cervical spine.[5] Fractures may be accompanied by subtle narrowing of the adjacent intervertebral disc space. Two views to determine the degree of fracture displacement should be made. One of the two views may require horizontal-beam radiography to prevent unsafe manipulation of the spine. Malunion fractures may result in permanent abnormal alignment.

Subluxation and luxation, with or without fracture of the spine, may be evident on one radiographic view, but less apparent on a view made 90 degrees to the former. Subluxation may be accompanied radiographically by narrowing of the adjacent intervertebral disc space.

Atlantoaxial (C_{1-2}) subluxation (Fig. 5–2) may be caused by agenesis, fracture, or fusion failure of the odontoid process, or by rupture of the stabilizing ligaments between C_1 and C_2. Normally, the dorsal spinous process of C_2 lies adjacent to or overlaps the caudal aspect of the arch of C_1, and the odontoid process lies on the ventral midline of the spinal canal of C_1. Subluxation of C_2 appears radiographically as caudodorsal displacement of C_2. The position and appearance of the odontoid process varies with the aforementioned pathologic conditions. An oblique lateral radiograph may be necessary to offset the wings of the atlas to the degree that the odontoid process may be seen. A lateral view obtained during flexion demonstrates the subluxation, but care should be taken so as not to overflex the neck; the unstable C_2 could compress the cord by an intact odontoid.[6]

Cervical vertebral malformation-malarticulation, also called canine wobbler syndrome and caudal cervical spondylopathy, can result in abnormal alignment of affected cervical vertebrae to a degree that spinal cord compression results (Fig. 5–3). C_{4-5}, C_{5-6}, and C_{6-7} are the most frequently involved sites, and multiple lesions are often present. Young Great Danes and adult Doberman pinschers are the breeds most frequently affected. Dorsal subluxation of the cranial end of a cervical vertebra may be dynamic or adynamic. Dynamic changes are related to cervical flexion-extension. Adynamic changes occur due to stabilization in malalign-

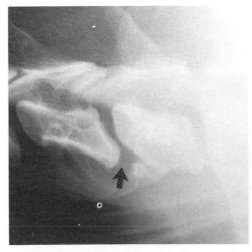

Figure 5–3. Cervical instability with deformity of the cranioventral margin of C_7 vertebral body and spondylosis.

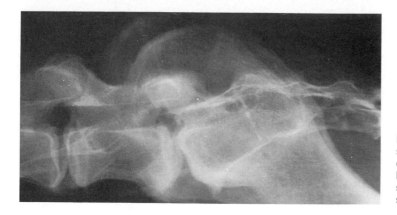

Figure 5–4. Lateral view of the lumbosacral spine in a dog with surgically confirmed cauda equina syndrome. Note the lumbosacral malalignment, spondylosis, and anomalously fused sacrum.

ment by secondary changes, such as spondylosis deformans. Standard lateral views and lateral views during flexion may be helpful when diagnosing the dynamic form of the condition. Other roentgen findings may include misshapened articular facets, an abnormally planed C_7 vertebral body, degenerative joint disease, stenosis of the cranial end of the spinal canal of the affected vertebrae, myelographically determined hyperplasia of the ligamentum flavum, and secondary intervertebral disc herniation.[7–9]

Slight ventral subluxation of the sacrum at the lumbosacral junction, lumbosacral instability, has been associated with cauda equina compression in the dog. This alignment abnormality may be accentuated by extension or flexion of the lumbosacral joint. Additional radiographic changes may include spondylosis (Fig. 5–4) of the lumbosacral spine and lumbosacral disc herniation. The clinical signs of lumbosacral stenosis may be similar to those of lumbosacral instability. Intraosseous venography may reveal evidence of obstructed vertebral sinuses as a result of the narrowed spinal canal. The etiology of these conditions in many dogs is uncertain, but possibilities include developmental, traumatic, and degenerative processes.[10–13]

Size. Vertebrae may be larger or smaller than normal (Table 5–3). One possibility for a vertebra appearing longer than normal is the congenital anomaly of block vertebra (Fig. 5–5). In block vertebra, two or possibly more vertebral bodies, arches, or spines may be fused (Fig. 5–6). The fusion may be partial or complete,

and results from improper segmentation of embryonal somites.[3, 4]

Vertebrae may appear smaller than normal due to traumatic or pathologic fractures, anomaly, or dwarfism. Due to the compacting nature of compression fractures, the vertebrae are often shortened and increased in radiopacity. Hemivertebrae are anomalously short and misshapen as previously described. Primordial dwarfism, manifest by proportionate skull, spine, and limb size decrease, has resulted in distinct miniature breeds. Chondrodystrophic dwarfs have a disproportionate form, with short thick limbs, short cranial base, and short vertebrae.[14]

Shape. There are numerous types and causes of abnormally shaped vertebrae (Table 5–4). Block vertebrae are congenitally fused in part or in whole, and when anatomically junctional are called transitional vertebrae. An anomalously shaped transverse process may result from fusion of a rib with a transverse process at the thoracolumbar junction. The wedge-shaped hemivertebrae (Fig. 5–7) may embryonically result from improper vascularization and there-

TABLE 5–3. **VARIATIONS IN VERTEBRAL SIZE**

Increased
Block vertebrae

Decreased
Fractures (traumatic or pathologic)
Anomaly (hemivertebra)
Dwarfism

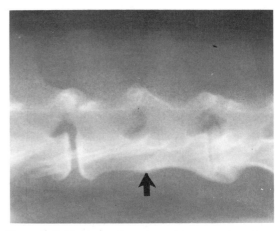

Figure 5–5. Block vertebrae *(arrow)* from two fused lumbar vertebral bodies.

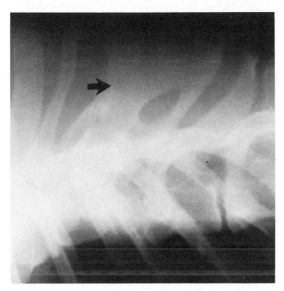

Figure 5–6. Fused dorsal spinous processes *(arrow).*

TABLE 5–4. ABNORMALITIES IN THE SHAPE OF VERTEBRAE

General Shape Alteration
Block vertebrae
Transitional vertebrae
Fused processes
Hemivertebrae
Hemimetameric displacement
"Hooked" dens
Dwarfism
Spina bifida
Fracture
Malunion fracture
Osteomyelitis/discospondylitis
Spondylosis
Neoplasia, primary and secondary
Cervical spondylopathy
Lumbosacral stenosis (acquired, congenital)
Previous surgery
Healed previous disease
Mucopolysaccharidosis

Spondylosis
Spondylosis deformans
Lumbosacral instability
Cervical spondylopathy
Spirocerca lupi infection
Hypervitaminosis A

Periosteal Reaction
Neoplasia, primary and secondary
Osteomyelitis—bacterial, actinomycosis,
  coccidioidomycosis
Spirocerca lupi infection
Healing reaction

Pedicle Changes
Bony proliferation
1. Degenerative joint disease
2. Baastrup's disease
Bone destruction
1 Neoplasia—primary bone, cord, meningeal,
  metastases, marrow
2. Osteomyelitis
3. Hemilaminectomy/dorsal laminectomy

Expansile-Appearing Bone Lesions
Multiple cartilaginous exostoses
Chondroma/chondrosarcoma

Intervertebral Foramen
Enlarged
1. Meningeal or nerve sheath neoplasia—meningioma,
  neurilemoma
Small
1. Intervertebral disc herniation

Spinal Canal
Widened
1. Spinal cord tumor—astrocytoma, ependymoma
Narrowed
1. Cervical spondylopathy
2. Lumbosacral stenosis
3. Healing reaction
4. Subluxated vertebra
5. Space-occupying mass in the canal—herniated disc,
  neoplasm

fore incomplete ossification of the dorsal or ventral portion of the vertebral body, hence the terms dorsal or ventral hemivertebra. Hemimetameric displacement results in unilateral, left and right hemivertebrae. The persistence of sagittal cleavage of the embryonic notochord results in the vertebral end plates having a funnel shape grossly and a butterfly appearance radiographically in the ventrodorsal view. The shapes of the bodies of the butterfly vertebrae and hemivertebrae may be compensated for by adjacent vertebral bodies, but spinal malalignment can also result. Hemivertebrae and butterfly vertebrae occur most frequently in bulldogs, pugs, and Boston terriers.[3, 4]

Other shape anomalies and developmental defects include dorsally angulated odontoid process, dwarfism, and spina bifida. Abnormal dorsal angulation of the odontoid process can result in signs that are similar to those of atlantoaxial subluxation. Chondrodystrophic dwarfism can result in short vertebral bodies that appear to have accordion-like bony protrusions from the ventral surface. Spina bifida is a midline cleavage in the vertebral arch or dorsal spinous process. The arch may be incompletely fused or absent, and the dorsal spinous process may appear in duplicate (Fig. 5–8). Associated spinal cord changes may include meningocele and myelomeningocele. Spina bifida is reported most frequently in the brachycephalic breeds of dogs and in Manx cats.[3, 4, 15] Fractures and malunion fractures of vertebrae can result in innumerable distorted shapes.

Vertebral osteomyelitis, discospondylitis, and spondylosis deformans alter the shape of affected vertebrae. Vertebral osteomyelitis is bony sepsis that is manifest as irregular, poorly

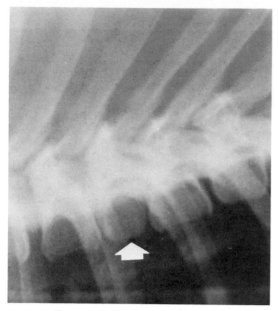

Figure 5–7. Hemivertebra (arrow).

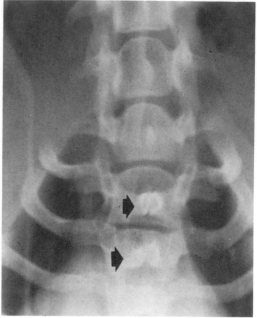

Figure 5–8. Ventrodorsal view of the cervicothoracic spine shows spina bifida with duplication of the T₁ and T₂ dorsal spinous processes (arrows).

marginated bone lysis and production on any or all parts of one or more affected vertebrae. An irregularly shaped periosteal reaction is often present (Fig. 5–9). Both bacterial and mycotic vertebral osteomyelitis can occur. Hematogenous infections are often the cause, but secondary contiguous infection from migrating foreign bodies or other soft-tissue infection is possible. The term vertebral osteomyelitis should not be confused with the term spondylitis. Spondylitis is an all-inclusive term for vertebral inflammation, but it does not necessitate sepsis. Spondylitis may occur as a secondary reaction to neoplasia or other nonseptic insult to the bony spine. Discospondylitis is sepsis of the intervertebral disc space and adjacent ends of the adjoining vertebral bodies (Fig. 5–10). The intervertebral disc space may appear widened and there are areas of bone lysis that often are bounded by bone production in the adjacent vertebral bodies. Discospondylitis most frequently affects the thoracic and lumbar vertebrae of young to middle-aged, large-breed male dogs. Multiple-site lesions occur, but single-site lesions are reported more frequently.[16–19]

Spondylosis deformans is a noninflammatory vertebral body spurring that may vary in extent from small osteophytes to complete bony bridging of adjacent vertebrae (Fig. 5–11). Spondylosis can occur secondary to several spinal abnormalities, including ventral disc protrusions, but often has an idiopathic and clinically insig-

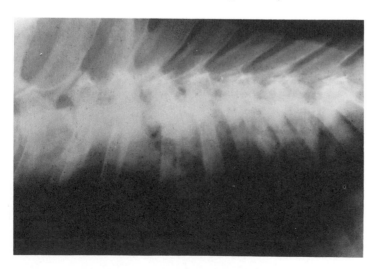

Figure 5–9. Diffuse actinomycosis osteomyelitis of the thoracic spine.

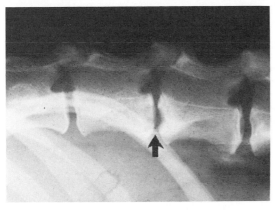

Figure 5–10. *Brucella* discospondylitis *(arrow).*

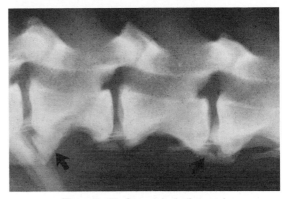

Figure 5–11. Spondylosis *(arrows).*

nificant etiology. The bony spurs may be limited to the vertebral body epiphyses or may extend over the entire length of affected and adjacent vertebrae. Radiographically, the spurs are best seen ventral to the affected vertebrae, but they may occur along the lateral and dorsolateral margins of the vertebral bodies. The dorsolateral spurs may extend to the plane of the intervertebral foramina, but do not usually encroach on the spinal cord. The terms spondylosis deformans and ankylosing hyperostosis have been used in conjunction with the broad category of spondylosis. The term ankylosing hyperostosis has been extrapolated from man; in the dog, it should be reserved for that form of spondylosis in which new bone growth extends the entire length of the vertebral body and results in complete bridging of the intervertebral space.

Spondylosis is most often reported in the thoracic, lumbar, and lumbosacral spine of middle-aged to old male dogs.[20, 21] Spondylosis in the caudal cervical spine of Doberman pinschers and in the lumbosacral spine of all dogs may be associated with, but is not diagnostic of, cervical or lumbosacral instability. Idiopathic spondylosis deformans should not be confused with the ventral vertebral body bony proliferation that may occur with *Spirocerca lupi* infec-

tion in dogs or with hypervitaminosis A in cats. In *Spirocerca lupi* infection, bony proliferation may occur across the ventral surfaces of T_8 to T_{11}, and an esophageal mass is often present. In hypervitaminosis A, ankylosing bony proliferation may occur on the arches and lateral aspects of the bodies of the cervical vertebrae. In addition, bony proliferation may occur on thoracic and lumbar vertebrae, on some of the long bones, and around limb joints.[22] Mucopolysaccharidosis, a lack of degradation of acid mucopolysaccharides before their excretion from the body, may cause multiple bony changes, including partial fusion of cervical vertebrae, irregularly shortened and misshapened vertebrae, partial fusion of lumbar vertebrae, widened intervertebral spaces, and a seemingly widened spine, due to bony proliferation.

Primary or secondary vertebral neoplasia may alter the shape of vertebrae by destroying bone, producing bone, or both (Fig. 5–12). The bony destruction often affects the cortical bone of the vertebra and there may be collapse of the adjacent disc space. A paraspinal, soft-tissue mass may be present. In contrast to discospondylitis, spinal neoplasia does not appear to originate in the intervertebral disc space. Radiographically, the differentiation of neoplasia from osteomyelitis may be difficult if the tumor is

Figure 5–12. Metastatic neoplasia (squamous cell carcinoma) involves L_2 and L_3.

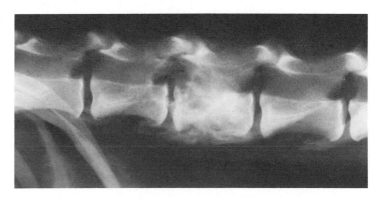

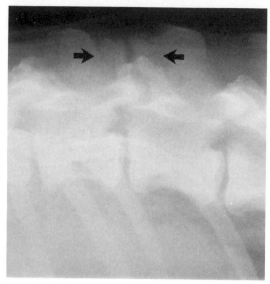

Figure 5–13. Baastrup's disease and possibly osteoarthrosis involves T$_{13}$-L$_1$ *(arrows)*.

producing bone. Osteosarcoma, chondrosarcoma, hemangiosarcoma, fibrosarcoma, carcinoma, and myeloma are some of the more frequently encountered spinal neoplasms.[25–27]

Shape changes in the area of the bony pedicle include degenerative joint disease and Baastrup's disease (Fig. 5–13). Bony proliferation in the area of the articular facets gives the facets an irregularly shaped appearance that is suggestive of spinal osteoarthrosis. Degenerative joint disease of the true vertebral synovial joints is rare and is difficult to demonstrate radiographically. Baastrup's disease is bony proliferation between the bases of adjacent dorsal spinous processes, creating a bony mass and pseudofacets between the vertebral synovial joints. This disease may mimic osteoarthrosis when observed only on a lateral radiograph.[22]

Bone lesions that appear expansile include multiple cartilaginous exostoses and chondroma/chondrosarcoma. Multiple cartilaginous exostoses and chondroma are cartilaginous lesions that create seemingly expansile mineral-stippled masses that are usually benign but can become malignant. The lesions often involve the spinous processes and may eventually compress the spinal cord.[22]

The intervertebral foramen may become enlarged when occupied by a growing neoplasm, such as a meningioma, neurofibroma, or neurilemoma. Although these neoplasms may occur at any level of the spine, they most often involve the cervical spine.[28] A seemingly small intervertebral foramen may be the result of vertebral shifting secondary to intervertebral disc herniation.

The spinal canal may appear widened as a result of soft-tissue expansion from a cord neoplasm, such as astrocytoma or ependymoma.[28] Localized narrowing of the spinal canal may result from cervical spondylopathy, lumbosacral stenosis, a healing reaction, a subluxated vertebra, or a space-occupying mass, such as a mineralized herniated disc or neoplasm in the canal.

Radiopacity. Causes of alterations in radiopacity of the spine are listed in Table 5–5. Increased radiopacity may be artifactual as a result of radiographically underexposed bone, or relative as a result of an excessively short scale of contrast (mAs too high and kVp too low). Because compression fractures compact a given mass of bone into a smaller volume, the radiopacity of the affected vertebra is increased. Bony callus in a healing fracture and the reactive bone in osteomyelitis, discospondylitis, neoplasia, and Schmorl's nodes (disc herniation into a vertebral body) increase radiopacity.[29] Amorphous tumor bone is produced by osteosarcoma of the spine. The rare conditions of osteopetrosis and fluorosis can result in increased vertebral radiopacity. The cause of osteopetrosis in mammals is uncertain, but it may be related to persistence of primitive chondro-osteoid and therefore to interference with the proper development of normal mature bone. The bones are radiopaque and may be hard and chalky. In fluorosis, abnormal bone mineral composition may result in increased radiopacity.[30]

Decreased radiopacity of the spine may be

TABLE 5–5. ALTERATIONS IN RADIOPACITY

Increased
Radiographic technique—underexposure, short scale of contrast (relative)
Compression fracture
Healing fracture/reaction
Osteoblastic metastasis
Osteomyelitis
Discospondylitis
Osteopetrosis
Fluorosis
Schmorl's nodes

Decreased
Radiographic technique—long scale of contrast (relative)
Excessive scatter radiation; obesity
Osteoporosis—senile, disuse
Osteomalacia
Hyperparathyroidism—primary, secondary
Paraneoplastic syndrome
Neoplasia—primary, secondary, myeloma
Osteomyelitis
Discospondylitis
Cushing's disease
Diabetes mellitus
Hypo/hyperthyroidism
Schmorl's nodes

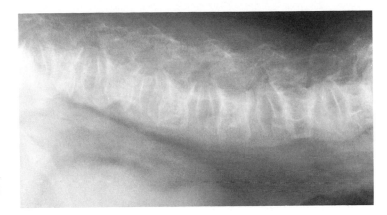

Figure 5–14. Lateral view of the lumbar spine of an African lion with nutritional hyperparathyroidism.

relative as a result of an excessively long scale of contrast (kVp too high, mAs too low). Scatter radiation and obesity diminish radiographic contrast and give the appearance of decreased bony radiopacity. Osteopenia is less than normal bone content for any reason. Osteoporosis is the bone matrix-deficient form of osteopenia that may be a result of aging, malnutrition, estrogen deficiency, Cushing's disease, or the lack of normal stress from disuse. Osteomalacia is the osteoid mineralization-deficient form of osteopenia that may have several etiologies, including calcium deficiency, vitamin D deficiency, phosphorus deficiency, unbalanced calcium-phosphorus ratio, phosphorus excess, and hyperparathyroidism (Fig. 5–14).[31] Primary or secondary hyperparathyroidism may result in a poorly mineralized and weakened spine. On rare occasions, the paraneoplastic syndrome of serum calcium elevation in association with lymphoma or perianal carcinoma may decrease the radiopacity of the spine, resulting in so-called picture frame vertebral bodies.

Areas of decreased radiopacity of the bone may result from tumors, such as myeloma. Neoplasia, osteomyelitis, and discospondylitis often cause both bone production and destruction and therefore create areas of increased and decreased radiopacity within the bone. Osteopenia from Cushing's disease, hyperthyroidism, and diabetes mellitus is not easily recognized in domestic animals. Cushing's disease may cause decreased organic bone matrix due to glyconeogenesis. Hyperthyroidism and diabetes mellitus can cause osteopenia due to overutilization of proteins.[30] Schmorl's nodes are infrequent in domestic animals, but first appear as relatively well-defined areas of decreased radiopacity, which are later bounded by reactive bone. Schmorl's nodes must be differentiated from lesions of discospondylitis.[29]

The radiographic diagnosis of vertebral abnormalities requires proper radiographic technique and a thorough knowledge of normal radiographic anatomy. Differential diagnosis is dependent upon a working knowledge of the diagnostic gamuts based on the roentgen signs of alteration in number, alignment, size, shape, and radiopacity. Preferential diagnosis is aided by compiling and then evaluating the presenting clinical signs, the age, breed, and sex of the animal, and the roentgen signs as perceived by the experienced diagnostician.

References

1. Larsen JS: Lumbosacral transitional vertebrae in the dog. J Am Vet Radiol Soc 18:3, 1977.
2. James CM, Lassman LP, and Tomlinson BE: Congenital anomalies of the lower spine and spinal cord in Manx cats. J Pathol 97:269, 1969.
3. Bailey CS: An embryological approach to the clinical significance of congenital vertebral and spinal cord abnormalities. J Am Anim Hosp Assoc 11:426, 1975.
4. Colter SB: Congenital anomalies of the spine. In Bojrab MJ (Ed). Pathophysiology in Small Animal Surgery. Philadelphia, Lea & Febiger, 1981, p. 729.
5. Feeney DA, and Oliver JE: Blunt spinal trauma in the dog and cat: Insight into radiographic lesions. J Am Anim Hosp Assoc 16:805, 1980.
6. Oliver JE, and Lewis RE: Lesions of the atlas and axis in dogs. J Am Anim Hosp Assoc 9:304, 1973.
7. Chambers JN, and Betts CW: Caudal cervical spondylopathy in the dog: A review of 20 clinical cases and the literature. J Am Anim Hosp Assoc 13:571, 1977.
8. Raffe MR, and Knecht CD: Cervical vertebral malformation—a review of 36 cases. J Am Anim Hosp Assoc 16:881–883, 1980.
9. Trotter EJ, de Lahunta A, Geary JC, et al: Caudal cervical vertebral malformation-malarticulation in Great Danes and Doberman Pinschers. J Am Vet Med Assoc 168:10, 1976.
10. Denny HR, Gibbs C, and Holt PE: The diagnosis and treatment of cauda equina lesions in the dog. J Small Anim Pract 23:425, 1982.
11. Oliver JE, Selcer RR, and Simpson S: Cauda equina compression from lumbosacral malarticulation and malformation in the dog. J Am Vet Med Assoc 173:2 1978.
12. Tarvin G, and Prata RG: Lumbosacral stenosis in dogs. J Am Vet Med Assoc 177:2, 1980.
13. Selcer RR: Lumbosacral instability in the dog. Tenn Vet Med Topics 2:4, 1977.
14. Fetter A: Achondroplasia—lecture notes. Columbus, The Ohio State University, lecture 33.

15. Wilson JW, Kurtz HJ, Leipold HW, et al: Spina bifida in the dog. Vet Pathol 16:165, 1979.
16. Hurov L, Troy G, and Turnwald G: Diskospondylitis in the dog: 27 cases. J Am Vet Med Assoc 173:3, 1978.
17. Johnston DE, and Summers BA: Osteomyelitis of the lumbar vertebrae in dogs caused by grass-seed foreign bodies. Aust Vet J 47:289, 1971.
18. Kornegay JN, and Barber DL: Discospondylitis in dogs. J Am Vet Med Assoc 177:4, 1980.
19. Walker TL, and Gage ED: Vertebral osteomyelitis, discospondylitis, and cauda equina syndrome. In Bojrab MJ (Ed): Pathophysiology in Small Animal Surgery. Philadelphia, Lea & Febiger, 1981, p. 474.
20. Wright JA: A study of vertebral osteophyte formation in the canine spine. I. Spinal survey. J. Small Anim Pract 23:697, 1982.
21. Wright JA: A study of vertebral osteophyte formation in the canine spine. II. Radiographic survey. J Small Anim Pract 23:747, 1982.
22. Morgan JP: Radiology in Veterinary Orthopedics. Philadelphia, Lea & Febiger, 1972, pp. 374, 270–271, 289.
23. Cowell KR, Jezyk PF, Haskins ME, et al: Mucopolysaccharidosis in a cat. J Am Vet Med Assoc 169:3, 1976.
24. Haskins ME, Jezyk PF, Desnick RJ, et al: Mucopolysaccharidosis in a domestic short-haired cat—a disease distinct from that seen in the Siamese cat. J Am Vet Med Assoc 175:4, 1979.
25. Luttgen PJ, Braund KG, Brawaer WR Jr, et al: A retrospective study of twenty-nine spinal tumors in the dog and cat. J Small Anim Pract 21:213, 1980.
26. Morgan JP, Ackerman N, Bailey CS, and Pool RR: Vertebral tumors in the dog: A clinical, radiologic, and pathologic study of 61 primary and secondary lesions. Vet Radiol 21:5, 1980.
27. Wright JA, Bell DA, and Jones DG: The clinical and radiological features associated with spinal tumors in thirty dogs. J Small Anim Pract 20:461, 1979.
28. Gilmore DR: Intraspinal tumors in the dog. Comp Contin Ed Pract Vet 5:1, 1983.
29. Resnick DR, and Niwayama G: Intervertebral disk herniations: Cartilaginous (Schmorl's) nodes. Radiology 126:57, 1978.
30. Aegerter E, and Kirkpatrick JA: Orthopedic Diseases, 4th Ed. Philadelphia, WB Saunders, 1975, pp. 148, 338–339.
31. Smith HA, and Jones TC: Veterinary Pathology, 3rd Ed. Philadelphia, Lea & Febiger, 1966, pp. 821, 826.

CHAPTER 6

INTERVERTEBRAL DISC DISEASE

JAN E. BARTELS

NORMAL ANATOMY OF THE SPINE AND DISC

Anatomic nomenclature of the vertebral column conforms to *Nomina Anatomica Veterinaria*,[3, 8] and is the same for the dog and the cat. The axial skeleton consists of approximately 50 irregularly shaped vertebrae. Ossification centers are mature at approximately 5 to 7 months post partum.[3, 4, 9] The vertebral formula is C_7, T_{13}, L_7, S_3, Cd_{20}–Cd_{25}. The coccygeal component is smaller in the Manx cat and in "screw-tail" breeds of dogs.

Developmental osseous defects of the spine may be incurred during endochondral bone development or during fusion. A knowledge of normal anatomy and variations of respective vertebrae, as well as their radiographic appearance, is a necessity for radiographic interpretation of possible pathologic lesions.[8, 10]

Select anatomic pecularities relating to the axial skeleton are as follows. The normal complement of 13 pairs of ribs is often varied by agenesis or supernumerary ribs. C_6 is unusual in appearance because of the large ventral projection of the transverse processes. There are approximately 30 vertebral bodies (not including the coccygeal segment) with 26 intervertebral spaces. There is no disc between C_{1-2}, S_{1-2}, or S_{2-3}. Disc herniation rarely, if ever, occurs between T_1 through T_{11} due to the strong, binding cross ligaments that attach the rib heads, this group of ligaments is referred to as ligamentum conjugale costarum.[3] At T_{10-11} there is a transition in the direction of the dorsal spinous processes, which serves as an anatomic landmark. The relative diameter of the spinal cord is increased in two locations in which nerves to the limbs arise: the cervical and lumbar enlargements. Caudal to the lumbar enlargement, the cord tapers (conus medullaris). The subarachnoid space is proportionately greater in diameter and is wider in smaller breeds than in larger breeds of dogs.

Canine vertebral bodies can be described generally as nearly square. The following anatomic landmarks can be identified in most vertebrae: lamina, neural arch, dorsal and ventral borders of the vertebral canal, cranial and caudal vertebral end plates, dorsal spinous process, transverse process, and vertebral body. Canine dorsal spinous processes appear round in the ventrodorsal projection. Lumbar vertebrae are generally longer than those in the thoracic spine. Although longer and more massive, the pedicles and laminae of the lumbar vertebra resemble those of typical vertebra in other regions. In the dog, the dorsal spinous process height, when compared to the diameter of the neural canal, has a ratio of approximately 2 to

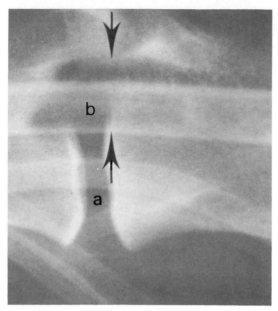

Figure 6–1. Normal metrizamide myelogram, T_{13}-L_1. a: intervertebral disc space; b: vertebral canal. *Arrows,* total extent of the vertebral canal with contrast medium outlining the subarachnoid space. The "space" dorsal to the subarachnoid space is the epidural space, which contains fat.

1. Comparatively, in the cat, this ratio is 1 to 1. In the dog, the transverse processes are directed cranially and have a rounded or club-shaped cranial border. In the cat, vertebral bodies are generally more rectangular and have a coarse, trabecular pattern, which may vary with age; the respective laminae and pedicles associated with the articular processes are less distinct, and the dorsal margin of the intervertebral foramen is more difficult to assess than in the dog.

The vertebral column is supported by numerous ligaments, all of which are of soft-tissue opacity. The intervertebral discs and their ligamentous components hold each pair of vertebrae together. The ridged column formed by this combination (bone, ligament, and discs) provides the superstructure for muscle attachments. The vertebrae articulate with each other at three points: the two diarthroidial components of the lamina and the disc. The normal intervertebral disc is of soft-tissue opacity and is composed of dense fibrous connective tissue, which forms the annulus, and gelatinous material, the nucleus. The latter is closely structured and resembles hyaline cartilage cellularly and biochemically. The cellular, biochemical, and mechanical relationship enhances the elastic properties of the disc (Figs. 6–1 and 6–2).[3]

PATHOPHYSIOLOGY AND INCIDENCE OF SPINE AND DISC DISEASE

Dehydration is the main pathologic change that discs undergo as aging occurs. This condition includes water as well as hyaluronic acid and the mucopolysaccharides. Whether degeneration ultimately results in metaplastic calcification (fibroid-chondroid) is not relevant to this discussion. Disc protrusion is often a catch-all term,[5] whereas herniation implies rupture of the annulus with extrusion or prolapse of the nucleus, calcified or noncalcified, into the epidural space. Herniation is usually chronic and progressive, but occasionally is acute.

The results of clinical surveys and accumulated statistical data are in agreement that the dachshund and other chondrodystrophic breeds are at high risk for disc herniation. Generally, the incidence is dachshund, 65 percent; Pekingese, 5 to 9 percent; poodle, 6 to 10 percent; cocker spaniel, 4 to 8 percent; beagles, 3 to 6 percent; other, 12 percent, and there is no sex predilection. The age at which disc herniation

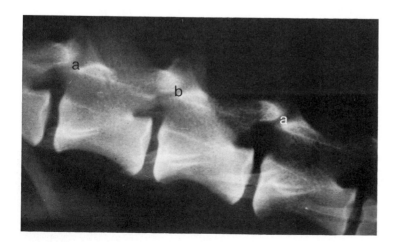

Figure 6–2. Lateral view of lumbar spine. Note intra-articular spaces of adjacent lamina. L_2, L_3, L_4. a: normal width; b: narrowed space with sclerosis. The neural arch and vertebral body bone trabeculation is normal. Assess the respective intervertebral disc spaces, transverse processes, and intervertebral foramen. The L_2-L_3 intervertebral foramen is hazy and is smaller than the adjacent foramen. Diagnosis: disc herniation at L_2-L_3.

occurs is usually between 3 and 7 years (observed in 83 percent of animals). In 55 percent of animals, protrusions are located between the T_{12} and L_1 interspaces; in about 13 percent, herniation occurs between C_2 and C_7; and in 30 percent, protrusions occur from L_{1-2} to L_7-S_1.[5]

RADIOGRAPHIC INTERPRETATION OF SPINAL DISORDERS

Spinal radiography should be technically optimal. The primary x ray beam should be centered on the area at interest. Frequently, multiple projections are required.[7] The intervertebral disc space and foramina in the dog and cat vary in appearance throughout the vertebral column.[5, 6, 10] This variation may necessitate multiple views of the spine (refer to Figs. 6–1 and 6–2 for comparison).

   Disc herniation may be partial, acute, or chronic; it is important to realize that radiography only represents one specific point in time. Previous or subsequent radiographic examinations may yield an entirely different interpretation.

   There are certain radiographic findings that are frequently encountered in patients with possible disc herniation (Figs. 6–3 to 6–7).

   1. Narrowing of the disc space. The space may be narrowed uniformly (compared to adjacent spaces) or it may be wedge shaped. This narrowing is usually accompanied by a decrease in size of the intervertebral foramen.

   2. Narrowing of the intervertebral foramen, with associated narrowing of the space between the articular processes

   3. Calcification of the nucleus with minimal or no calcification of the annular component. Disc mineralization per se is not evidence of herniation but rather of degeneration.

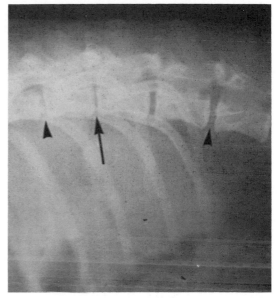

Figure 6–3. Lateral view of the canine spine. There are varying stages of disc calcification (arrowheads). The spine is rotated as evidenced by the asymmetric position of the last pair of ribs. There is a uniformly narrowed (collapsed) intervertebral disc space at T_{12}-T_{13} due to a herniated intervertebral disc (arrow). Note the lack of significant disc calcification at T_{12}-T_{13}. There is chronic chondroid degeneration of nuclear disc components at L_1-L_2 and a calcified annulus at T_{12}-T_{13}.

   4. Calcification of the nucleus, with the annulus being partially or wholly involved. There is no evidence of fusion of disc to end plate. In instances of nuclear protrusion, however, the intervertebral disc space is usually narrowed.

   5. Calcified/radiopaque mass (disc material) in the vertebral canal with correspondent narrowing of the intervertebral foramen. Lateral spondylosis may be similar in appearance to

Figure 6–4. There is calcified intervertebral disc material in the vertebral canal with corresponding narrowing of the intervertebral foramen and lamina. Note the normal size of the space between adjacent articular processes (arrows).

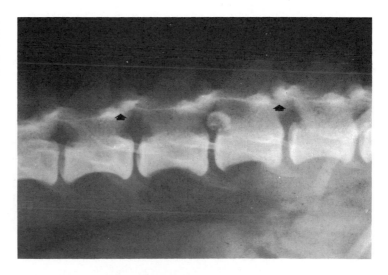

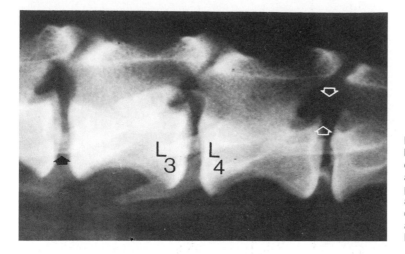

Figure 6–5. There is intervertebral disc herniation at L_3-L_4 with extrusion of the calcified disc material cranially. There are residual calcific portions of the disc present in the intervertebral disc space and foramen. Note the partial calcification of the disc at L_2-L_3 (solid arrow) and the calcified partial protrusion at L_4-L_5 (open arrows).

that of calcified disc material; two views are then necessary for distinction.

6. Collapse of the intervertebral disc space with adjacent end plate sclerosis as well as early osteophyte formation or spondylitic exostosis. This finding is indicative of chronic intervertebral disc herniation.

7. Lateral disc herniation with calcified disc material along a spinal nerve is a rare finding. Ventral disc herniation is also unusual.

The significance of any radiographic finding must be considered with respect to the breed of dog, the age, and the clinical and neurologic signs. A narrow intervertebral disc space without calcification must always be suspect. Calcification of the nucleus is frequently seen in chondrodystrophic dogs 1 year of age or older and is often clinically insignificant. Always compare adjacent intervertebral spaces and articular lamina. Carefully observe the vertebral end plates and foramina. Calcification of disc material is progressive and is usually eccentric due to the location of the nucleus. The ventrodorsal view demonstrates location of disc calcification with reference to the midline, which is important information for surgical intervention.

The more calcific the disc and the more distinct its margins, the longer is the duration of the disc degeneration. When both the annulus and nucleus exhibit calcification, there is limited disc function. This calcification precedes protrusion, although occasionally the reverse is true.

A narrowed intervertebral disc space is a highly significant finding; with rare exception it implies herniation dorsally into the vertebral canal. Dorsal versus ventral herniation is due to weaker dorsal layers of the annulus in contrast to the stronger, thicker layers of the lateral and ventral portions of the annulus. Intervertebral disc space narrowing complemented by a calcific opacity in the vertebral canal implies

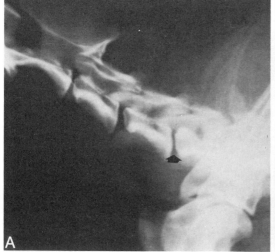
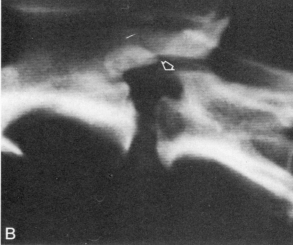

Figure 6–6. A, Cervical intervertebral disc herniation at C_4-C_5 with a narrow intervertebral disc space (arrow) and hazy foramen. B, C_2-C_3 disc herniation with calcified nucleus in the vertebral canal. Do not confuse the cranial articular process of C_3 with disc material (arrow, compare with A).

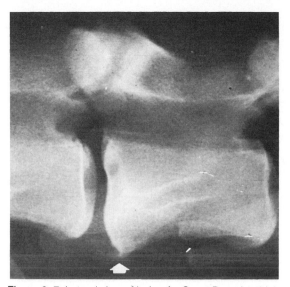

Figure 6–7. Lateral view of L₂-L₃ of a Great Dane in which dural calcification/ossification can be seen; this must not be confused with intervertebral disc disease. Note the early ventral spondylosis on the cranial ventral aspect of L₃ *(arrow)*.

a positive diagnosis, radiographically. The calcific opacity should be identified in two views. Such lesions may, however, be clinically insignificant.

Spondylosis with osteophyte formation is of less significance and indicates chronicity; neurologic sequelae, if present, are usually associated with spinal nerve compression rather than with the cord compression.

It is my opinion that only a small percentage of dogs with intervertebral disc herniation require myelography for diagnosis. Good quality survey radiographs and a complete neurologic examination may obviate this interventional procedure.

CONTRAST-ENHANCED RADIOGRAPHY OF THE SPINAL CORD

After several years of experimentation and practical clinical application, myelography is now an acceptable, realistic approach to contrast medium opacification of the subarachnoid space.[1, 2] Several other techniques, including

Figure 6–8. Extradural, intradural, and intramedullary myelographic patterns.

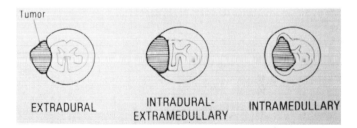

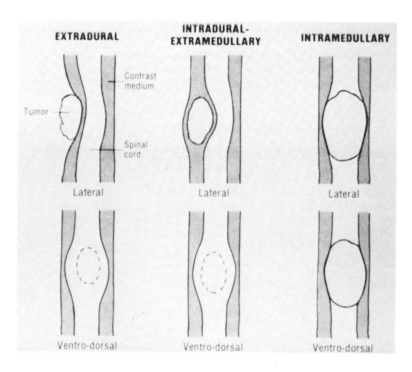

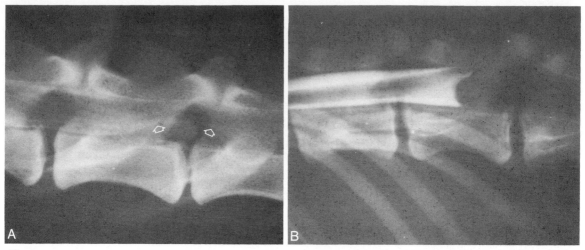

Figure 6–9. *A,* Metrizamide myelogram. There is extradural compression *(arrows)* associated with obvious disc herniation. *B,* Metrizamide myelogram. The intramedullary pattern associated with spinal cord neoplasia can be seen.

epidurography, lumbar venography, venography, and discography, have been suggested as a method for visualization of pathologic processes or abnormalities of the spinal canal.[5] Generally, however, these methods are less specific than myelography. Several types of myelographic contrast media have been utilized and evaluated, from oil-base contrast media to modified aqueous iodine compounds.[2, 6] In clinical practice, Amipaque* (metrizamide) is currently the contrast medium of choice. This product has been available since 1975, and although neurologic sequelae have occurred, it is the most practical contrast medium for myelography in humans and in animals. The technique and neurologic sequelae have been documented.[1, 2, 5] Myelographic changes associated with disc herniation have been reported.[7] The direction of deviation of contrast medium in the subarachnoid space should be characterized because lesions may then be localized in relation to the dura. The anticipated pattern of contrast medium displacement associated with various types of cord compression is illustrated in Figures 6–8 and 6–9.

DISC DISEASE IN CATS

Disc disease in cats has been summarized.[5] Clinically, the process is seen in older cats. A

———————

*Winthrop Laboratories, New York, NY.

low incidence of neurologic dysfunction is noted, although the condition is seen in either the cervical or midlumbar portion of the spine.

References

1. Bartels JE: A retrospective study of five hundred canine myelograms using metrizamide. Unpublished data presented at the 6th International Congress of Veterinary Radiology, University of California. Davis, CA, August 1982.
2. Bartels JE, Braund KG, and Redding RW: An experimental evaluation of a non-ionic agent—Amipaque (metrizamide) as a neurologic medium in the dog. JAV Radiol Soc 28:117, 1977.
3. Evans HE, and Christensen JC: Miller's Anatomy of the Dog. 2nd Ed. Philadelphia, WB Saunders, 1979.
4. Hare WCD: The age at which epiphyseal union takes place in the limb bones of a dog. Wien Tierarztl Mchr Festschrift, Schreiber 47:224, 1960.
5. Hoerlein BF: Canine Neurology: Diagnosis and Treatment, 3rd Ed. Philadelphia, WB Saunders, 1978.
6. Morgan JP: Radiology in Veterinary Orthopedics. Philadelphia, Lea & Febiger, 1979.
7. Morgan JP, and Silverman S: Techniques of Veterinary Radiology. 3rd Ed. Davis, CA, Veterinary Radiology Associates, 1982.
8. Schebitz H, and Wilkins H: Atlas of Radiographic Anatomy of the Dog and Cat, 3rd Ed. Philadelphia, WB Saunders, 1980.
9. Summer-Smith G: Observation of epiphyseal effusion of the canine appendicular skeleton. J Small Anim Pract 7:303, 1966.
10. Wright JA: A study of radiographic anatomy of the cervical spine of the dog. J Small Anim Pract 18:341, 1970.

SECTION 3

AXIAL SKELETON— *EQUIDAE*

CHAPTER 7

THE EQUINE SKULL

R. STICKLE

This chapter is a review of the major radiographic lesions of the equine skull, excluding conditions of the nose and sinuses and dental diseases (see Chapter 8). For a review of the complex anatomy of the skull, which often creates problems in diagnosis, the reader should consult appropriate anatomy texts.[1, 2]

Many areas of the head lend themselves to radiographic examination with the use of relatively low-capacity equipment.[3] The rostral portion of the mandible and the calvarium do not have much soft-tissue covering, and neither do the facial bones, which are relatively thin. The structures that normally contain air (nose, sinuses, pharynx, and guttural pouches) enhance our ability to examine these areas radiographically. In many horses, oblique views are useful for the examination of the head, although basic principles of radiation protection for medical personnel must not be compromised. The use of general anesthesia is often required to obtain a safe and thorough study that could not otherwise be done, including the use of ventrodorsal, oblique, and intraoral views.

FRACTURES

Mandibular fractures, if complete, are usually obvious, especially when they are bilateral. Certain injuries, such as mandibular symphysis separation in foals and trauma to the incisor teeth, are more easily diagnosed by physical examination than with radiography. Fractures that involve the caudal mandible as well as unilateral and fissure fractures of the mandible are more difficult to diagnose. Oblique, ventrodorsal, and intraoral views are more useful than lateral views in these horses (Figs. 7–1 and

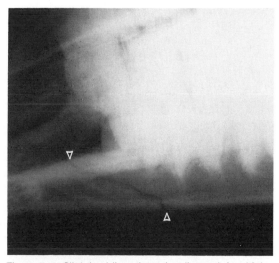

Figure 7–1. Slightly oblique lateral radiograph in which a nondisplaced fracture *(arrowheads)* in the interdental space of one mandibular ramus can be seen.

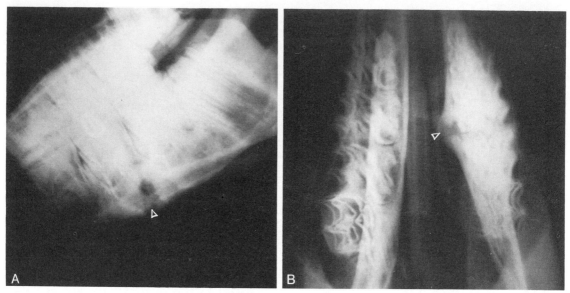

Figure 7–2. *A,* lateral radiograph in which bone remodeling with a central area of radiolucency can be seen *(arrowhead).* Superimposition of both mandibular rami obscures detail. *B,* ventrodorsal view allows better visualization of this chronic fracture *(arrowhead)* and confirms that only one mandibular ramus is involved.

7–2). Tooth alveolar involvement, tooth root fracture, and sequestra formation in chronic cases are important considerations, because complications may result during the course of healing.

Fractures of the face and calvarium may show displacement, soft-tissue swelling, or evidence of hemorrhage into the sinuses. Nondisplaced fractures are often difficult to diagnose, and the normal anatomy must be considered so that normal sutures in young horses are not mistaken for fracture lines (Fig. 7–3). Oblique views are particularly useful in the evaluation of trauma of the face, orbit, and zygomatic arches (Fig. 7–4).

Basilar skull fractures in which the basisphenoid and basioccipital bones are involved have been reported in horses that fall over backwards.[4, 5] These fractures occur in part from tension on the muscle insertions at the base of the skull, and usually produce displacement between the basisphenoid and basioccipital fragments as seen on the lateral view (Fig. 7–5). The displacement is an important diagnostic criterion, because the normal suture line between these bones does not close until up to 3 years of age.[6]

Traumatic fractures of the temporal bone may produce signs associated with the vestibular system and facial nerves.[7] Sclerosis of the involved tympanic bulla may be seen radiographically in instances of long-standing disease. A ventrodorsal view obtained with the horse under general anesthesia is recommended.

Fractures of the petrous temporal bone have also been seen in association with, and possibly secondary to, osseous fusion of the cartilaginous joint between the stylohyoid and temporal bones; fractures of the stylohyoid bone may accompany these lesions. Facial and vestibular nerve signs occur acutely with the temporal fracture, although the stylohyoid lesions may

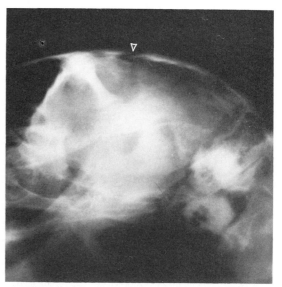

Figure 7–3. Lateral radiograph of a young foal with possible head trauma. The wide lucent line *(arrowhead)* is a normal suture, not a fracture.

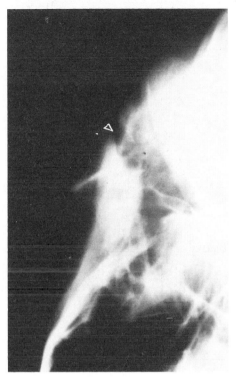

Figure 7–4. Oblique radiograph in which there is evidence of a fracture of the supraorbital process of the frontal bone (arrowhead).

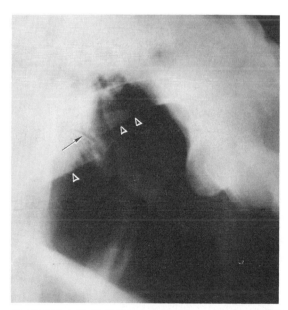

Figure 7–5. Lateral radiograph of an immature horse. The normal suture (arrow) between the basisphenoid and occipital bones is still open. There is a fracture just caudal to this suture. Considerable dorsal displacement of the basilar portion of the occipital bone has occurred (double arrowheads) as compared with the normal position of the basisphenoid bone (single arrowhead).

be chronic. Radiographic signs include periosteal reactivity, which is sometimes accompanied by bone lysis and involves the proximal portion of the stylohyoid bone and the tympanic bulla and surrounding processes (Fig. 7–6).[8] Septic otitis media interna is suspect as being the inciting cause of the hyoid-temporal fusion,[8] although guttural pouch mycosis can also cause fusion of this joint.[4] Stylohyoid fractures have also been reported as primary injuries. These lesions usually involve the distal portion of the bone and are associated with falling or excessive traction on the tongue during examination of the mouth.[4]

Trauma to the temporomandibular joints is difficult to diagnose radiographically. Increased width of the joint space and rostral displacement of the mandibular coronoid processes with subluxations have been reported.[4]

BONE INFECTIONS

Sepsis of the bones of the head often accompanies penetrating wounds, open fractures, tooth root abscesses, and lesions of adjacent soft tissue (e.g., lymph node abscess formation and guttural pouch infection). Radiographically, these lesions usually show bone lysis accompanied by varying degrees of surrounding bone sclerosis and periosteal new bone production. Chronic fistulas associated with the mandibles suggest sequestra and tooth root involvement. Fistulography may be useful in the evaluation of these infections (Fig. 7–7).

NEOPLASIA

Primary bone tumors in the horse are relatively rare, but there appears to be a tendency to the head. Osteomas are usually osteoblastic and well marginated, and often involve the rostral region of the mandible (Fig. 7–8). Bone sarcomas usually originate from the mandible or maxilla. Radiographically, they are poorly marginated, may displace or partially destroy teeth, and show bone lysis as well as areas of new bone production in and around the lesion (Fig. 7–9). Histologically, these are compound neoplasms and their exact classification may be difficult.[9]

Tumors of dental germ origin appear most often in the mandible. These lesions may show irregular areas of osseous opacity within the mass and appear polycystic.[4, 10, 11] Ameloblastic odontomas have been reported in the maxilla of young horses; these tumors contain radiopaque, tooth-like structures.[12]

The various neoplastic and infectious conditions that may affect the bones of the equine

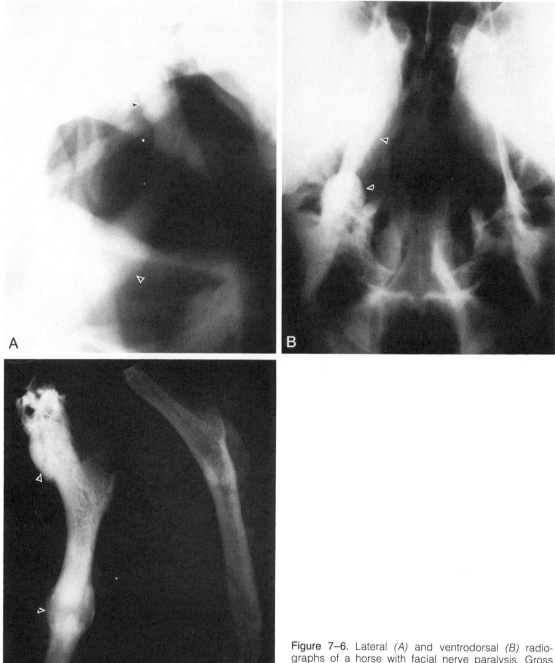

Figure 7–6. Lateral *(A)* and ventrodorsal *(B)* radiographs of a horse with facial nerve paralysis. Gross remodeling of the stylohyoid bone can be seen *(arrowheads)* proximally as well as in the midshaft area. A portion of the rope halter is evident in *A. C,* necropsy specimens. What appear to be old fracture lines can be seen *(arrowheads)*. The affected hyoid bone was fused to the temporal bone, which had fractured, allowing a portion to be pulled away with the hyoid. The opposite normal stylohyoid is included for comparison.

head are difficult or impossible to differentiate in some horses by using either radiography or histopathology alone. A combined diagnostic approach is preferred.

CONGENITAL LESIONS

Malformations of the occipital bone and the first two cervical vertebrae (occipitoatlantoaxial malformations) are common in the Arabian breed

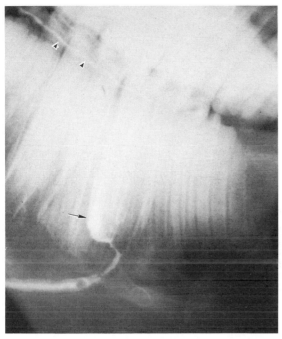

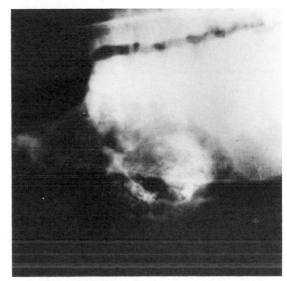

Figure 7–9. Lateral view. Aggressive mandibular lesion due to a large bone sarcoma.

Figure 7–7. Positive-contrast fistulogram obtained with the use of a bulb-tipped catheter. Contrast medium can be seen around the tooth root *(arrow)* and in the mouth *(arrowheads)*. Diagnosis: alveolar periostitis with a secondary draining tract.

(Fig. 7–10). Several variations are reported, but there is usually hypoplasia of the atlas with fusion to the occiput (occipitalization of the atlas) accompanied by hypoplasia of the axis, which may resemble an atlas. These defects exhibit a variety of clinical signs due to compressive myelopathy.[13, 14]

Dentigerous cysts (temporal teratomas) usually develop at the base of the ear from misplaced dental germinal cells. A fistula forms near the ear. Radiography reveals a tooth-like radiopaque structure within the soft-tissue mass (Fig. 7–11).[15]

Polycystic lesions are occasionally seen in the mandible or maxilla in young horses, and are believed to be congenital, non-neoplastic cysts. They may attain considerable size and grossly distort the affected bone. Differentiation of these lesions from dental germ neoplasms is not possible radiographically (Fig. 7–12).[4, 15]

Bilaterally symmetric horn-like bony projec-

Figure 7–8. Lateral view. Osteoma of the rostral mandible.

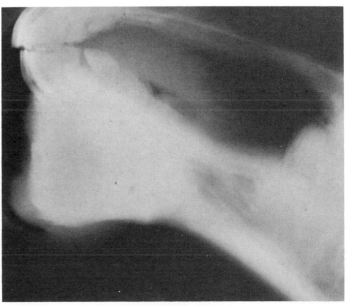

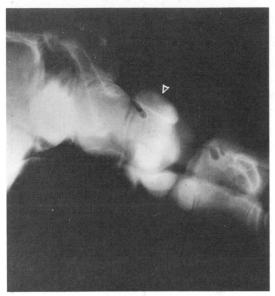

Figure 7–10. Lateral radiograph of a foal born without normal occipital condyles. There is fusion of the atlas *(arrowhead)* to the occipital bone.

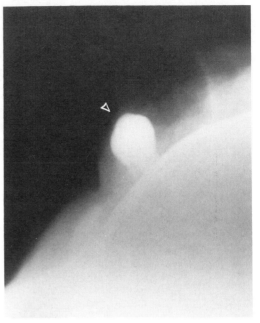

Figure 7–11. Oblique radiograph of the temporal region of a young horse. The radiopaque object *(arrowhead)* just rostral to the base of the ear is a dentigerous cyst.

tions sometimes are found on the nasal and frontal bones. These lesions are thought to be of embryologic origin.[4]

MISCELLANEOUS FINDINGS

Loss of bone radiopacity in the mandible may occur, along with other skeletal manifestations, in cases of severe dietary imbalance. This condition is considered a form of secondary hyperparathyroidism and may result in cyst-like lesions similar to the aforementioned congenital and neoplastic cystic conditions of the mandible.[4, 15] Soft-tissue swelling of the mandible may accompany tooth eruption in young horses. In this instance, smoothly marginated undulations of the edge of the mandible may be evident. The lesions are probably aggravated by abnormal retention of the deciduous premolars ("caps"). Retained deciduous premolars are easily seen radiographically (Fig. 7–13).

Signs of hydrocephalus on survey radiographs

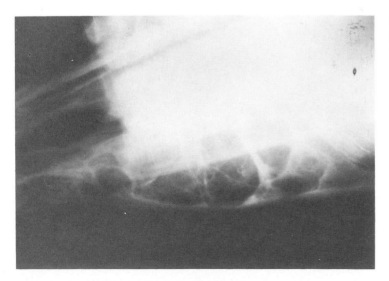

Figure 7–12. Oblique lateral view. Large polycystic lesion in the mandible of a young horse.

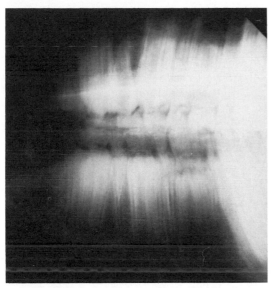

Figure 7–13. Lateral radiograph of a 3-year-old horse. The typical irregular outlines of retained deciduous premolars (caps) can be seen on all premolar teeth.

are reported to be similar to those of other species and include increased size of the cranial vault, thinning of the calvarium, and a homogeneous appearance of the cranial cavity.[4, 14]

SPECIAL PROCEDURES

Fistulography was mentioned in connection with septic bone lesions. This simple technique is useful to identify the extent and depth of draining tracts, the presence of radiolucent foreign bodies, and the involvement of adjacent soft-tissue structures, such as glands or ducts. The use of a catheter with a bulb tip allows injection of contrast medium under moderate pressure. Any water-soluble contrast medium suitable for intravenous injection may be used. Samples for cytologic and microbiologic analysis should be obtained before fistulography. In addition to fistulography, a technique for pa-

rotid duct sialography, and an example of parotid duct obstruction, have been described.[16]

References

1. Getty R (Ed): Sisson and Grossman's The Anatomy of the Domestic Animals, 5th Ed. Philadelphia, WB Saunders, 1975.
2. Schebitz H, and Wilkens H: Atlas of Radiographic Anatomy of the Horse, 3rd Ed. Philadelphia, WB Saunders, 1978.
3. Gibbs C: The equine skull: Its radiological investigation. J Am Vet Radiol Soc 15:70, 1974.
4. Cook WR: Skeletal radiology of the equine head. J Am Vet Radiol Soc 11:35, 1970.
5. Stick JA, Wilson T, and Kunze D: Basilar skull fractures in three horses. J Am Vet Med Assoc 176:228, 1980.
6. Ackerman N, Coffman JR, and Corley EA: The sphenooccipital suture in the horse: Its normal radiographic appearance. J Am Vet Radiol Soc 15:79, 1974.
7. Firth EC: Vestibular disease, and its relationship to facial paralysis in the horse: A clinical study of 7 cases. Aust Vet J 53:560, 1977.
8. Power HT, Watrous BJ, and deLahunta A: Facial and vestibulocochlear nerve disease in six horses. J Am Vet Med Assoc 183:1076, 1983.
9. Gallina AM: Bone and joint pathology. In Mansmann RA, McAllister ES, and Pratt PW (Eds): Equine Medicine and Surgery, 3rd Ed. Vol 2. Santa Barbara, CA, American Veterinary Publications, p. 980, 1982.
10. Hanselka DV, Roberts RE, and Thompson RB: Adamantinoma of the equine mandible. Vet Med/Small Anim Clin 69:157, 1974.
11. Vaughan JT, and Bartels JE: Equine mandibular adamantinoma. J Am Vet Med Assoc 153:454, 1968.
12. Roberts MC, Groenendyk S, and Kelly WR: Ameloblastic odontoma in a foal. Equine Vet J 10:91, 1978.
13. Mayhew IG, Watson AG, and Heissan JA: Congenital occipitoatlantoaxial malformations in the horse. Equine Vet J 10:103, 1978.
14. Mayhew IG, and MacKay RJ: The nervous system. In Mansmann RA, McAllister ES, and Pratt PW (Eds): Equine Medicine and Surgery, 3rd Ed. Vol 2. Santa Barbara, CA, American Veterinary Publications, pp. 1159–1252, 1982.
15. Baker GJ: Diseases of the teeth and paranasal sinuses. In Mansmann RA, McAllister ES, and Pratt PW (Eds): Equine Medicine and Surgery, 3rd Ed. Vol 1. Santa Barbara, CA, American Veterinary Publications, pp. 437–458, 1982.
16. Walters JW, and McGovern MS: Equine parotid duct obstruction. J Equine Med Surg 3:335, 1979.
17. Colles CM, and Cook WR: Carotid and cerebral angiography in the horse. Vet Rec 113:483, 1983.

CHAPTER 8

EQUINE NASAL PASSAGES, SINUSES, AND GUTTURAL POUCHES

JIMMY C. LATTIMER

Radiographic examination of the equine head should be used in combination with endoscopy, physical examination, and clinical pathologic tests to arrive at an accurate diagnosis. The decision to take radiographs should be based on the need to answer specific questions rather than to "see if anything can be found." Used properly in concert with other diagnostic procedures, radiographs can help in establishing an accurate diagnosis, permitting early and definitive treatment of the problem.

Radiographic evaluation of the equine head has received minimal attention in the past, which is probably due, at least in part, to the relative infrequency of radiographically diagnosable diseases of the respiratory tract. Most of the diseases that affect the airways of the equine head are viral or bacterial, and are usually diagnosed on the basis of the results of physical examination and clinical pathologic analysis. It is only the complicated or protracted patient that does not respond to usual treatment procedures that is likely to be radiographed. In addition, the task of radiographing the head of a conscious horse can be formidable. Most horses are somewhat skittish about having cassettes placed near the head. There is also the problem that even the quietest horse is in constant motion while standing, both from the effects of respiration and constant postural shifting of the stay apparatus. In the past, this factor made it virtually impossible for the veterinarian to obtain diagnostic radiographs only with the use of a small portable, hand-held x-ray machine. The need to induce general anesthesia to obtain satisfactory radiographs makes the decision to radiograph the skull difficult, especially in a clinically ill animal.

In recent years, new rare-earth screens and film have been developed, which have greatly decreased the exposure factors when diagnostic radiographs are produced. With these new film-screen combinations, it is possible to obtain diagnostic radiographs in the standing, sedated horse. There are still some views that require general anesthesia (ventrodorsal, for example), but the majority of the standard views are well within the capabilities of the average portable x-ray unit. This fact is especially true if the machine and the cassette are mounted on a stand. Motion of the machine and cassette is then reduced, thus limiting the number of retakes and the amount of radiation exposure acquired by personnel performing the examination.

One of the greatest deterrents to radiography of the equine head is the complexity of the image. The large, multiple, interconnecting air passages and turbinates within the skull, combined with the many sharp and irregular external bone prominences, make any skull radiograph a challenge to interpret. When radiographic anatomy is so complex, it is easy to overlook relatively major lesions. It is therefore imperative that a systematic method of evaluating the radiograph be used. The specific system that is used is not important, only that one is used. It is also necessary that some type of radiographic anatomy reference be consulted, because comparison of the radiograph with a known normal image can usually resolve any questions regarding whether or not a structure in question is abnormal. Remember, however, that there are slight individual variations in anatomy, and minor differences in positioning may radically alter these radiographic-anatomic relationships, making comparisons with reference material difficult. Proper positioning of the subject is mandatory.

NORMAL ANATOMY

Nasal Cavity

The most rostral part of the nasal passage in the horse is composed principally of soft tissue. The rostral one-fourth of the nasal passage is either surrounded completely by soft tissue or is supported by bone only from below (Fig. 8–1). This area is difficult to examine radiographically because of low tissue contrast and markedly reduced opacity when compared to the remainder of the skull. If the rostral nasal passage is to be evaluated, it is necessary to obtain a radiograph for which reduced exposure factors were used. Radiographs of the rostral portion of the nose are occasionally needed, although this area is usually more easily examined by palpation and endoscopy.

The nasal passage caudal to the first maxillary cheek tooth is surrounded by and contains bone structures. The maxillary, nasal, palatine, and vomer bones form the limits of the nasal passage; the dorsal, middle, ventral, and ethmoid turbinates are contained within the passage.[19] Contained within the alveolar recesses of the maxilla are the large cheek teeth. Usually, it is not possible to delineate the individual bones of the face, except possibly in young foals. Likewise, it is difficult to identify the turbinates other than the ethmoid as individual structures. There are, however, a number of external and internal landmarks that serve as reference points (Fig. 8–2).[32]

The most obvious external landmarks on the lateral view of the nasal passage are the large cheek teeth, although they are partially surrounded by the sinuses. These teeth are readily apparent and provide a constant point of reference for lesion placement. It is always advisable to use a field to view of sufficient size so that either the rostral or caudal cheek tooth is identifiable. Another external structure that is usually evident over the caudal portion of the nasal passage is the zygomatic arch, which is also superimposed over the orbit. The shadow of the zygomatic arch continues forward as a line of opacity, which represents the facial crest. Depending on the exact film orientation and exposure factors used, the facial crest may or may not be readily apparent. Identification of the facial crest and the fourth upper cheek tooth are important in that their rostral limits approximately define the rostral limits of the caudal and rostral maxillary sinuses, respectively. Because the two compartments of the maxillary sinus do not usually communicate, except in mules,[19] it is important to determine which of the cavities is affected.

Internal nasal cavity landmarks include the rostral limits of the dorsal and ventral conchal sinuses, the rostral limits of the maxillary sinus, and the ethmoid turbinates (Fig. 8–2). These landmarks basically define the limits of the paranasal sinuses, making it possible to deter-

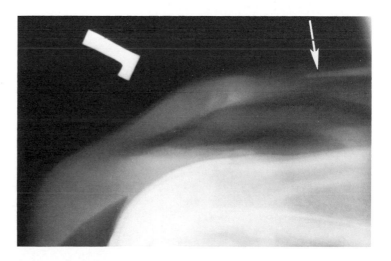

Figure 8–1. Lateral view, rostral portion of the nasal passage. Note that the only bone support for the nares is ventral to these structures. *Arrow,* the long narrow rostral projection of the nasal bone.

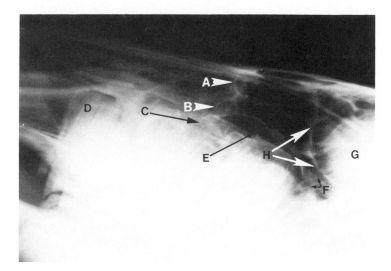

Figure 8–2. Lateral view of the nasal passage of a young horse. A: rostral margin of dorsal conchal sinus; B: rostral margin of ventral conchal sinus; C: rostral margin of maxillary sinus; D: first maxillary cheek tooth; E: intermaxillary septus; F: infraorbital canal; G: ethmoid turbinates; H: rostral margin of the frontal sinus.

mine if the disease process being observed involves the sinuses, the nasal cavity, or both.

The ethmoid turbinates are the most consistently placed of the internal landmarks. They mark the caudal limit of the nasal cavity and are, for radiographic purposes, interposed between the maxillary and frontal sinuses on the lateral projections. The finely scrolled bones of the ethmoids are readily visible as numerous fine, linear opacities that arise from the cribriform plate.

The rostral limit of the maxillary sinus is seen immediately dorsal to the root of the third cheek tooth and may vary somewhat in position from horse to horse and with age; they may be completely obscured in young horses due to tooth overlap. The dorsal and ventral conchal sinuses do not extend as far rostrally as the maxillary sinuses. The thin plates of bone that define their rostral margins are usually seen dorsal to the fourth cheek tooth. The dorsal

sinus is located just below the nasal bone; the ventral sinus is just beneath the dorsal sinus and extends slightly more rostrally.[29, 32] The middle conchal sinus in the horse is small and landmarks attributable to it are not usually observed. The turbinates are not recognized as well-defined structures, and are only represented as multiple scalloped opacities in the dorsal caudal portion of the nasal passage.

In young horses, the long roots of the six large cheek teeth overlap and obscure much of the ventral portion of the nasal passage and paranasal sinuses when seen on the lateral view (Fig. 8–2). Continuous tooth wear as the animal ages results in shortening of these roots. By the time the horse is 15 to 20 years old, the roots of the teeth are quite short and do not obscure as much of the nasal passage and sinuses (Fig. 8–3). Thus, abnormalities of the nasal passage may be more readily apparent in an old animal than in a young one.

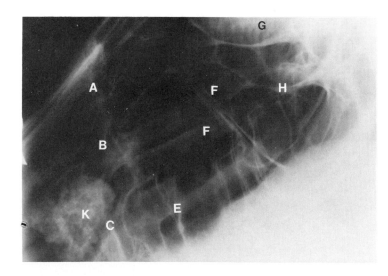

Figure 8–3. Slightly oblique, lateral view of the caudal nasal passage in a 20-year-old horse. A: rostral margin of dorsal conchal sinus; B: rostral margin of ventral conchal sinus; C: rostral margin of maxillary sinus; E: intermaxillary septum; F: infraorbital canal; G: ethmoid turbinates; H: rostral margin of the frontal sinus; K: the abnormal opacity in the nasal cavity was a calcified granuloma, which had no clinical manifestations.

Although the standard lateral projection provides a great deal of information about the condition of the nasal passages, it is advisable that a ventrodorsal projection also be obtained if possible. A disease that uniformly affects one nasal passage may not be discerned on the lateral projection because the uniform increase in opacity is interpreted as underexposure rather than disease. Such an abnormality is readily apparent on the ventrodorsal projection. Likewise, the lateral view is insensitive to lesions of the nasal septum unless they are extremely large. The ventrodorsal projection, however, allows ready detection of even minor lesions of the nasal septum. The major landmarks visible on the ventrodorsal projection are the mandible, the medial wall of the orbit, and the nasal septum (Fig. 8–4). On the ventrodorsal view, a great deal of the nasal passage is obscured by the mandible and cheek teeth. Only 2 or 3 cm of the passage are usually visible on either side of the nasal septum in the rostral portion of the nose; somewhat more is visible in the region ventral to the ethmoid turbinates. Most diseases that affect the nasal passage involve the common nasal meatus, which is immediately adjacent to the nasal septum.

Diseases that affect the common nasal meatus are usually manifested by a marked increase in opacity as the deep nasal cavity fills with fluid

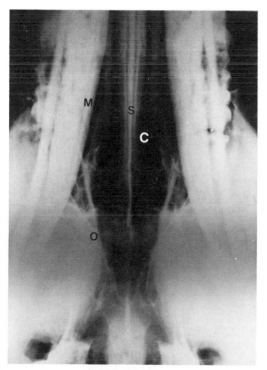

Figure 8–4. Ventrodorsal view of the nasal passage. M: medial border of mandible; S: Nasal septum; O: medial wall of orbit; C: common nasal meatus.

or tissue; the increased opacity may be unilateral or bilateral. Because sequestration of fluid in the nasal passage is unlikely because of the normal nose-down position that is maintained, the opacity usually represents a solid structure. If fluid is truly entrapped in this area, it may be trapped behind an obstruction in the nasal passage, contained within a cyst, or confined to the dorsal conchal sinus, which is superimposed over the nasal passage on the ventrodorsal view. The latter site of confinement should be identifiable on the lateral view.

A second type of lesion seen on the ventrodorsal projection is deviation of the nasal septum. This deviation may result from an intrinsic disease, such as cyst formation, or from pressure by a mass within the nasal passage. The degree and site of the deviation is usually obvious, but the underlying cause may be difficult to determine.

Nasopharynx

The nasopharynx is that portion of the upper airway between the nasal choanae and the glottis. In the horse, the nasopharynx is a single, undivided passage.[29] For radiographic purposes, it extends from about the rostral margin of the vertical ramus of the mandible to the laryngeal cartilages. It is bounded dorsally by the basal bones of the skull and the ventral margins of the guttural pouches. The ventral margin of the nasopharynx is the soft palate, which is indistinguishable from the tongue with which it is in intimate contact. The oropharynx is usually visible in the horse only during deglutition.[17] For the remainder of the time, the tongue is directly in contact with the soft palate, which forces all of the air out of the oropharynx and renders it radiographically undefinable. The dorsal margin of the epiglottis is usually visible just dorsal to the soft palate. Inability to see the epiglottis clearly may be nothing more than a technical or positioning problem, but it may also indicate an abnormality of either the epiglottis or the soft palate. Other than the epiglottis, there are no distinguishing landmarks within the nasopharynx, except the airway itself.

The nasopharynx is almost completely obscured on the ventrodorsal view. Except for the portion just cranial to the larynx, the nasopharynx is superimposed over the heavy bones of the calvarium. Therefore, any lesion within the nasopharynx must be large enough to be visible on the ventrodorsal view.

Paranasal Sinuses

The paranasal sinuses of the horse are large and complex. Together with the nasal cavity, they account for most of the volume of the skull. There are six pairs of sinuses in the horse. The dorsal, middle, and ventral conchal sinuses are within the turbinates of the same name. Lateral to the nasal cavity is the maxillary sinus, which is divided into rostral and caudal compartments. Dorsal and caudal to the nasal cavity is the frontal sinus. Ventral and caudal to the nasal cavity and the ethmoid turbinates is the sphenopalatine sinus. All of the sinus cavities on one side of the skull communicate rather freely, with one exception. In the living animal, the rostral and caudal compartments of the maxillary sinus are separate; this may not be the case in some mules.[19] The frontal sinus communicates with the dorsal conchal and caudal maxillary sinuses; the maxillary sinus communicates with the frontal, middle conchal, and ventral conchal sinuses. The rostral maxillary sinus and the ventral conchal sinus communicate with each other, but there is generally no communication between these two sinuses and the remaining paranasal sinuses.

The septum between the two compartments of the maxillary sinus is usually visible as a thin, angled (vertically to slightly caudally) bone plate dorsal to the fourth cheek tooth (Fig. 8–2).[31] This septum may not be appreciated if there is obliquity to the projection, because the thin

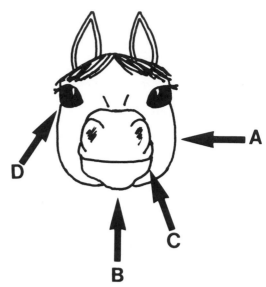

Figure 8–6. Projection angles for examination of the nasal passages and sinuses. A: lateral view; B: ventrodorsal view; C: maxillary sinus view; D: view of orbit.

plate is easily overpenetrated unless it is oriented edge on to the x-ray beam. The septum is also visible on the special projection of the maxillary sinus (Fig. 8–5). This projection is obtained by angling the x-ray beam from 15 to 20 degrees off vertical and shooting from lateral to medial and ventral to dorsal (Fig. 8–6). This view allows most of the lateral portion of the maxillary sinus to be seen in profile without the interference of the overlying teeth. It is always important that both sides be examined to serve as an internal control. It is easy to interpret the opacity of the overlying masseter muscle incorrectly as fluid in the sinus if the projection is slightly off the optimal angle. This special projection usually provides better evaluation of the maxillary sinus than does the lateral view. Identification of the septum allows the determination of which of the two compartments is affected by disease and then to plan treatment accordingly. Fluid is more readily retained within the rostral compartment because the nasomaxillary opening of the sinus is located at the highest point in the sinus.[19] The nasomaxillary opening is common to both the rostral and the caudal maxillary sinuses, but it is divided by the septum. This aperture, which empties into the middle nasal meatus, is usually the sole site of drainage of the sinuses into the nasal cavity; it is not radiographically visible.

The rostral limit of the maxillary sinus is just dorsal to the third cheek tooth and is often obscured on the lateral projection by the cheek teeth in younger animals. This cranial extremity is more readily seen on the special oblique view for the maxillary sinus (Fig. 8–5).

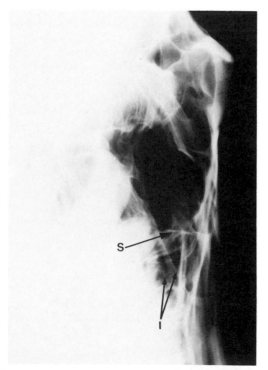

Figure 8–5. Special oblique projection for examination of the maxillary sinus. I: infraorbital canal; S: intermaxillary septum.

The infraorbital canal runs longitudinally through the maxillary sinus, dividing it into lateral and medial portions. The caudal medial compartment communicates with the spheno-palatine and middle conchal sinuses. The in-fraorbital canal is located immediately dorsal to the roots of the teeth; in the young animal, it is virtually in contact with them as they project into the maxillary sinus. The canal is usually seen as a band of increased opacity that runs longitudinally just above the teeth on the lateral view (Figs. 8–2 and 8–3), but is not readily seen on oblique and ventrodorsal projections.[19, 29, 31] The downward growth of the cheek teeth with aging results in better visibility of the maxillary sinus and leaves the infraorbital canal more obviously in the middle of the sinus on the lateral view.

The caudal limits of the maxillary sinus are difficult to recognize radiographically. Its communication with the sphenopalatine sinus, the overlying ethmoid turbinates, and the vertical mandibular ramus make the caudal limits indistinct. Fortunately, identification of the caudal limit is not usually necessary. For the purposes of radiographic interpretation, the maxillary sinus ends at the level of the ethmoid turbinates caudally and at the level of the frontal sinus caudodorsally.

The frontal sinus is dorsocaudal to the nasal cavity; its radiographic limits are not as extensive as its anatomic limits due to the presence of overlying bone. Radiographically, there are essentially two parts to the frontal sinus; the roughly triangular dorsocaudal portion and the portion that is rostral to the orbit. The triangular part is dorsal and caudal to the ethmoid turbinates on the lateral view and tends to be radiolucent in the normal horse. The marked radiolucency is due to the relatively great width of the sinus at this point. This part of the sinus is that which communicates with the maxillary sinus through the frontomaxillary opening.[19] The rostral portion of the sinus is rostrodorsal to the ethmoid turbinates and has a scalloped cranial margin that is dorsal to the fifth cheek tooth.[19] This margin is readily seen on many radiographs. The rostral portion of the frontal sinus communicates openly with and is continued forward by the dorsal conchal sinus. The dorsal conchal sinus usually terminates at the rostral margin of the fourth cheek tooth; it is superimposed over the dorsal one half of the nasal passage and is somewhat tubular. Other than the most caudal portion of the frontal sinus, the dorsal conchal sinus is the most medial of the paranasal sinuses. It virtually touches the midline, owing to the small size of the dorsal nasal meatus. Because it is located so close to midline, it is superimposed over the nasal passage on the ventrodorsal projection. Filling of the dorsal conchal and frontal sinuses with fluid or tissue causes increased opacity in these areas, and incomplete filling may lead to the formation of a fluid level on the standing lateral projection.

The sphenopalatine sinuses are relatively small in the horse and usually are not recognized as separate entities. This fact is due in part to their size and also to the marked opacity of the vertical rami of the mandibles. If recognized, they are small, slight radiolucencies just ventral to the cranial vault and caudal to the ethmoid turbinates. Their caudal termination is usually about the level of the temporomandibular joint.[29]

Guttural Pouches

The guttural pouches are large, ventral diverticuli of the auditory (eustachian) tubes that are unique to *Equidae* among domestic animals. Their function is unknown. It is known, however, that there is a marked increase in the volume of the guttural pouches during deglutition.[17] These large diverticuli are two superimposed air opacities in the area between the vertical ramus of the mandible, the base of the skull, the atlas, and the nasopharynx. The cranial margin of the pouches usually overlaps the caudal half of the mandibular rami, unless the head is abnormally extended.[31]

Each of the pouches has an average volume of approximately 300 ml in the adult animal. Each pouch is divided into a lateral and a medial compartment. This division is formed by the reflection of the mucosa of the pouch over the stylohyoid bone as it courses from the base of the skull to the remainder of the hyoid apparatus, cranioventral to the larynx. Although the medial compartment of the pouch is approximately twice the size of the lateral compartment, the communication between the two compartments is great and it is unlikely that only one compartment is affected by a disease process.

The medial and lateral compartments each give rise to a separate radiographic shadow because of their different size and orientation. Because there is always slightly more air in one pouch than in the other, and the lateral projection is usually slightly oblique under the best of circumstances, it is often possible to see four separate opaque lines attributable to the guttural pouches on this view (Fig. 8–7). If it is possible to see only two of the margins, it may indicate that one of the pouches is filled with fluid.

The guttural pouches are surrounded by many delicate and important structures. A small fold in the dorsal and caudal mucosa of the pouch contains the ninth, tenth, and eleventh cranial nerves. The internal carotid artery

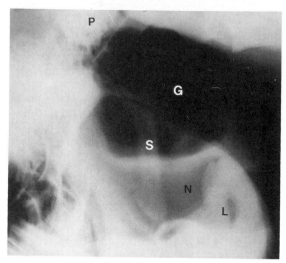

Figure 8–7. Lateral view of guttural pouches. G: guttural pouches; N: nasopharynx; L: larynx; S: stylohyoid bones; P: petrous temporal bone.

crosses the dorsal wall of the guttural pouch; in the normal animal this vessel may be seen through the thin mucosa of the pouch with a fiberoptic endoscope. The external carotid artery, maxillary artery, and maxillary vein cross the lateral surface of the pouch (Fig. 8–8). The facial nerves cross the dorsolateral surface of the guttural pouches after they exit from the skull.[2, 5, 14] Diseases of the guttural pouches may result in injury to any of these structures.

Other less delicate structures that are closely related to the guttural pouches are the dorsal wall of the pharynx, the medial retropharyngeal lymph nodes, and the larynx. The dorsal wall of the pharynx is separated from the guttural pouches by only a layer of connective tissue and two layers of mucosa. Therefore, the division between the two air spaces is only a well-

defined, thin radiopaque line on the lateral view. Marked distention of the guttural pouches may result in partial obstruction of the nasopharynx. The medial retropharyngeal lymph nodes are immediately dorsal to the guttural pouches and are not recognizable as distinct radiographic structures, but they may enlarge and displace the guttural pouches or be a source of infection for them.[6, 24] The larynx is usually not in direct contact with the guttural pouches unless they are distended beyond normal limits. Enlargement or disease of the guttural pouches may cause dysfunction of the larynx by direct interference with its anatomic function or by injury to the motor nerves of the larynx.

The guttural pouches may be seen on the ventrodorsal projection, but it is difficult to evaluate anything other than the symmetry of the air opacities. Gross distention or consolidation of one pouch is readily identifiable, and the ventrodorsal view should be used to determine which pouch is affected if there is doubt after the results of clinical and endoscopic examinations are considered.

RADIOGRAPHIC ABNORMALITIES

Diseases of the Nasal Passage

Infectious, traumatic, inflammatory, developmental, and neoplastic diseases can affect the nasal passage. The clinical signs may consist of nasal discharge, noisy respiration, facial distortion, and epistaxis, in any combination. The list of possible differential diagnoses is long and includes both local and systemic diseases. Diseases such as infectious rhinitis, purpura hemorrhagica, congestive heart failure, emphysema, and pneumonia may cause nasal discharge or epistaxis, but these conditions are unlikely to

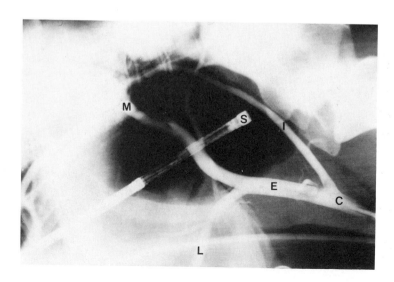

Figure 8–8. Common carotid angiogram shows vessels surrounding the guttural pouch. C: common carotid artery; E: external carotid artery; M: maxillary artery; L: lingual artery; I: internal carotid artery; S: fiberoptic endoscope.

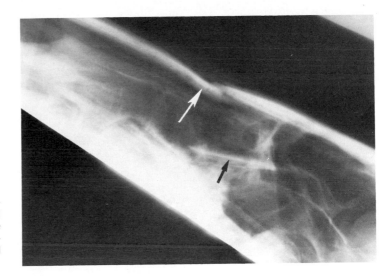

Figure 8–9. Depressed nasal bone fracture. Direct trauma to the nose resulted in slight depression of the nasal bone *(white arrow). Black arrow,* a larger fragment of the maxilla, which was displaced into the nasal cavity.

demonstrate significant radiographic abnormalities unless there is fluid collection in the sinuses.[1, 11, 24]

Fractures of the nasal bones are common and are usually the result of kick or collision injuries. There is often visible facial deformity that is frequently less dramatic than the underlying bony injury. There is usually profuse epistaxis associated with the acute injury. If the fracture is untreated and a piece of depressed bone triggers an infectious or foreign body reaction, a chronic mucopurulent discharge may develop.

Radiographically, a fracture of the nasal bone is recognized as a depressed area in the bone. Occasionally, a large piece of bone is depressed into the nasal passages or into a sinus (Fig. 8–9). The true extent and severity of the fracture is usually difficult to delineate on the radiographs, and the fracture is almost invariably more extensive at surgical exploration. When the nasal passage is examined radiographically, it is a good idea to obtain at least one projection that is tangential to the surface wherein lies the suspected fracture. The bones of the nose are quite thin and if a fracture fragment is not hit virtually edge-on by the x-ray beam, it may be overpenetrated and the lesion may not be recognized. Such a tangential projection has the best chance of outlining fragments that have been displaced into the nasal passage. It may be difficult to recognize a fracture on one view whereas it is quite obvious on another. Therefore, standard lateral and ventrodorsal projections should also be obtained (Fig. 8–10).

Foreign bodies are another source of trauma to the nasal passages, but their occurrence is relatively uncommon. Small foreign bodies do not seem to be much of a problem, but large objects, such as sticks, wire, and bullets, may lodge within the nasal passage and cause a foreign body reaction. Many, but not all, foreign bodies are easily detected and even removed by using endoscopy. In some horses, however, radiography may be needed to localize the problem. The lesion usually appears as a poorly defined area of increased radiopacity somewhere in the nasal passages. The opacity may be caused by exudate, blood, granulomatous proliferation, or a combination. If the foreign body is radiopaque, such as a piece of bone or a bullet, it is generally visible in the middle of the area of increased opacity. Objects such as sticks are usually not recognizable radiographically. Because foreign bodies are usually confined to one side of the nasal passage, their location is readily revealed on the ventrodorsal view.

Uncomplicated rhinitis is unlikely to be seen radiographically. Only if this condition is associated with a sinusitis or some other abnormality, such as a foreign body or a nasal deformity, is it likely to be radiographically obvious. The most one could usually expect to perceive is a slight increase in opacity of the nasal passage and perhaps a slight narrowing of the airways on the ventrodorsal view. These are subtle findings that are highly susceptible to aberrations in technique and positioning and should be supported by other diagnostic procedures before a diagnosis of rhinitis is made.

Neoplasia of the nasal passage may be benign or malignant. The benign lesions are usually osteomas or adamantinomas and occur in young animals.[6, 23] These neoplasms may present as expansile radiolucent lesions (adamantinoma) or as well-defined, bony expansile lesions (osteoma). Benign tumors such as these may be relatively silent clinically, and thus become quite large before a diagnosis is made. If complete resection of the lesion is possible, surgery should be curative.

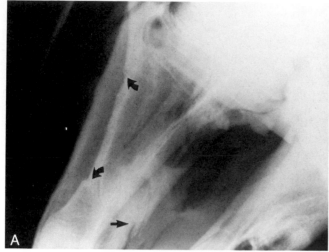

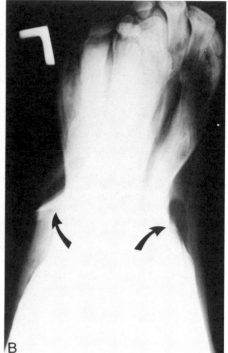

Figure 8–10. Fracture of the maxillary and incisive bones. *A*, lateral view. There appears to be relatively minor displacement of bones, and the fracture lines *(arrows)* are difficult to see. *B*, ventrodorsal view. The marked deformity of the nose and the fracture sites *(arrows)* are obvious.

Malignant lesions, usually adenocarcinomas, occur in older animals and are invasive, grow rapidly, and are ill-defined.[1, 6, 24] The clinical signs are usually unilateral mucopurulent nasal discharge, epistaxis, facial deformities, and upper airway obstruction. The severity of the clinical signs is dependent on the stage of the disease when first evaluated. Radiographically, malignancies are of soft-tissue opacity and are ill-defined (Fig. 8–11). There may be lysis of turbinate and facial bones. Distortion or destruction of the nasal septum may be obvious on the ventrodorsal view, and advanced tumors may have bilateral involvement or may project

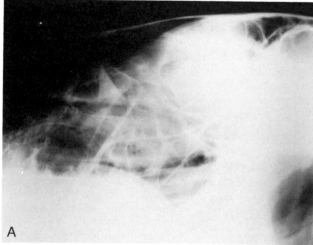

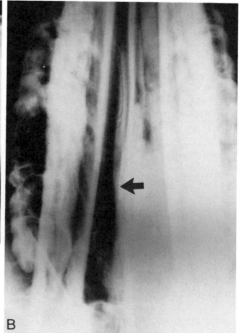

Figure 8–11. *A*, Lateral view. A large, poorly marginated soft-tissue opacity is present in the caudal left nasal cavity of this horse. *B*, ventrodorsal view. Slight displacement of the nasal septum to the right *(arrow)* is evident. Diagnosis: nasal adenocarcinoma.

caudally into the nasopharynx. At present, there is no effective treatment for such advanced lesions.

Intranasal cysts usually occur in young animals and may be congenital.[6] These lesions are large, fluid-filled structures within the nasal passage or sinuses. They may cause facial deformity and nasal discharge, but because of their benign nature intranasal cysts are usually quite large when they are recognized. Radiographically, these cysts appear as large, well-defined areas of increased opacity in the nasal passage; they may be single or multiple, unilateral or bilateral. As they grow, these lesions displace bone structures, especially the turbinates, which is evident radiographically. The ventrodorsal projection may indicate displacement of the nasal septum. There is nothing visible radiographically that distinguishes a cyst from a large, well-defined soft-tissue tumor or ethmoid hematoma, other than possibly the location of the lesion.

Non-neoplastic polyps are often seen in the nasal passage of young horses. These lesions are usually composed of granulation tissue and are probably associated with chronic inflammation.[2, 24] Polyps may be recognized radiographically as relatively well-defined areas of increased opacity in the nasal passage; they vary in size and number. Clinical signs may be delayed until the polyps are of sufficient size or number to interfere with respiration.

A special form of cystic disease occurs in the nasal septum. Varying amounts of the nasal septum in young horses may undergo cystic degeneration due to trauma or infection.[34] The nasal septum widens substantially and interferes with respiration. Both radiographic and endoscopic examination of the nasal passages are needed to evaluate adequately the extent and severity of the problem. Cystic disease is one condition for which the ventrodorsal projection is mandatory. The lateral view is of minimal help in determining the severity of the thickening of the septum, although it may aid in establishing the caudal limit of the problem. Accurate evaluation of the extent of the lesion is imperative, because surgical resection of the affected septal portion is the only effective treatment. Postoperative radiographic evaluation must wait until after the removal of the packing used to control the profuse hemorrhage induced by surgery.

Progressive ethmoid hematoma is newly recognized in the last 15 years, but there is no reason to believe that it is a new disease. It is a slowly enlarging hematoma containing granulomatous reactions, which originates from the submucosa of an ethmoid endoturbinate.[2, 4] It is not known why the mass continues to enlarge,

since it is not neoplastic. Extension into the maxillary, frontal, and sphenopalatine sinuses, as well as into the nasal cavity, is common, as is distortion and destruction of the ethmoid and nasal turbinates and nasal septum. The clinical signs of inspiratory stertor, coughing, choking, excessive salivation, facial deformity, purulent nasal discharge, bad breath, and head shaking are characteristic of this disease. There is usually also a history of a constant trickle of blood from one of the nostrils for weeks to months. Endoscopy reveals a large, smooth-walled greenish mass in the caudal part of the nasal passages.[2, 4] Although the differential diagnoses for these clinical signs are extensive, a thorough physical examination combined with the result of endoscopic and radiographic examinations should make the diagnosis easy to establish.[9]

The radiographic examination of progressive ethmoid hematoma should consist of lateral, ventrodorsal, and special maxillary sinus projections. The lesion is usually confined to one side of the nasal passage, but it may deform the septum and the ethmoid turbinates. It is a round, smooth-walled, soft-tissue mass arising from the region of the ethmoid turbinates (Fig. 8–12).[2, 4] Calcification and air trapping within the lesion have not been described. Because recurrence is common, it is advisable to re-examine the animal at 6-month intervals for at least 2 years after the lesion is removed.

Diseases of the Paranasal Sinuses

Lesions in the paranasal sinuses tend to parallel those seen in the nasal cavity—traumatic fractures, cysts, benign and malignant tumors, and empyema. Ethmoid hematomas also invade the sinuses.[2, 4]

Fractures of the sinuses are manifest in much the same way as nasal bone fractures. Once again, the physical appearance of the face may not indicate the true extent of the lesion. When fracture fragments are depressed into a sinus, there is an even greater likelihood that infection will develop due to reduced drainage and air exchange in the sinus when compared to the nasal passage. The radiographic approach to the diagnosis of paranasal sinus fractures is essentially the same as those into the nasal passage. Whenever it appears that a fracture line enters a sinus, special attention should be given to any increased opacity within the sinuses.

Neoplastic diseases of the paranasal sinuses are either benign or malignant. As with the nasal cavity, the benign tumors are usually osteomas or adamantinomas that arise from or around the roots of the cheek teeth within the maxillary sinus. The malignant neoplasms are either primary (adenocarcinoma) or secondary

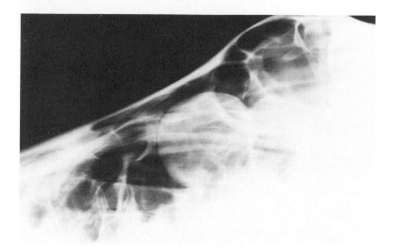

Figure 8–12. This large, well-marginated round opacity protruding rostrally from the nasal passage is an ethmoid hematoma.

(extension of a squamous cell carcinoma from the orbit) lesions.[2, 21] These tumors are ill-defined, soft-tissue lesions. There is usually some lysis of cortical bone and deformity of the facial bones. With primary tumors, much of the opacity within the sinuses may be due to trapped secretions, because the neoplasm obstructs the outflow from the nasomaxillary opening. Thus, the area of increased opacity may be substantially larger than the true area of neoplastic involvement.

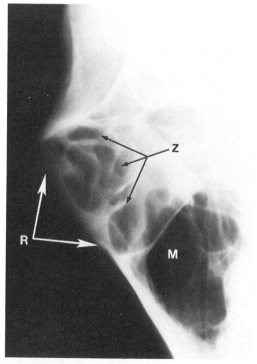

Figure 8–13. Special oblique projection for examination of the orbit. N: maxillary sinus; Z: dorsal margin of zygomatic arch; R: dorsal rim of orbit.

Secondary invasion of the frontal sinus by a squamous cell carcinoma of the orbit is an unusual, but serious, finding. There is usually obvious bone destruction of the orbit. Because of the possibility of orbital tumors extending through the bone into the frontal or maxillary sinus, it is advisable to take a special radiographic projection designed to examine the orbit (Figs. 8–6 and 8–13). The majority of orbital neoplasms do not invade the sinuses, but the prognosis is so much worse for those that do that the examination is warranted.

The most common cause of clinical disease of the sinuses that necessitates radiographic evaluation is empyema. Accumulation of exudate within the sinuses may be the result of many diseases, but the most common is a periapical abscess of one of the last three maxillary cheek teeth. The most commonly affected tooth is the fourth maxillary cheek tooth. Other causes include trauma, fungal granulomas, and neoplasms.[2, 6] The clinical signs of sinusitis are usually poor condition, fetid nasal discharge, bad breath, and sometimes head shaking. There may be evidence of a facial deformity if the infection is secondary to trauma. On physical examination, it may be possible to percuss a dead area in the region of the fluid accumulation.

Endoscopic examination of the sinuses is not possible other than to observe the nasomaxillary opening for drainage of exudate from the sinuses. Therefore, radiography is usually necessary to evaluate lesions indicative of sinus empyema. Sinus fluid is recognized by the presence of a homogeneous fluid opacity in the area of the suspected sinus; it is often possible to identify a fluid line within the sinus (Fig. 8–14). Figure 8–14 demonstrates a substantial variation in the amount of fluid that may accumulate in the sinuses. If the sinus is completely filled with fluid, no fluid line is present. It is

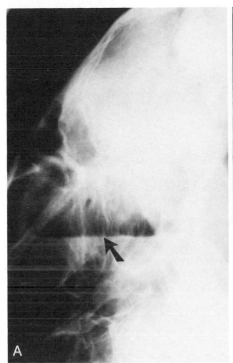

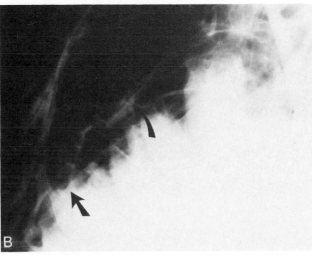

Figure 8–14. Fluid in the maxillary sinus (two different horses). *A,* in one horse there is a large amount of fluid in the caudal maxillary sinus due to empyema. *Arrow,* fluid line. *B,* the other horse has a small amount of fluid in the rostral maxillary sinus due to a periapical abscess of the fourth cheek tooth. *Straight arrow,* fluid line. *Curved arrows,* an area of increased opacity in the sinus just dorsal to the tooth causing the problem.

then necessary to perform the special oblique projections of both sinuses to establish that one sinus is indeed fluid-filled. Both sinuses should be examined to avoid misdiagnosis of the condition because of the mild increase in opacity caused by overlying muscles. Radiography may also reveal the sclerosis around the tooth root, if that is the source of the problem. The periodontal membrane of the tooth is usually widened and decreased in definition. The alveolar bone over the root of the cheek teeth may be so thin in some animals that it is simply absent, due to lysis, with no evidence of proliferation or sclerosis.[5] It is difficult to establish that a tooth is the source of the problem in these horses.

Diseases of the Nasopharynx

Few diseases of the nasopharynx can be diagnosed radiographically; those that can be are often diagnosed more easily by endoscopy. Radiography can, however, play a useful part in the diagnosis of nasopharyngeal disorders, especially if the nasopharyngeal problem is the result of a disease in another area, such as in the guttural pouch or retropharyngeal lymph nodes.

Occasionally, a lateral radiograph of the parotid region indicates the presence of many small radiopacities along the dorsal and lateral borders of the nasopharynx. These small (2 to 4 mm diameter) nodules are caused by severe lymphoid hyperplasia, with lymphoid nodules that project into the nasopharynx where they are surrounded by air. The contrasting opacity of the margins of the nodules with the surrounding air renders them radiographically visible. This appearance, although seen only in the severely affected horse, is a reliable indicator of the disease.

The major nasopharyngeal disorders that can be diagnosed radiographically are epiglottic entrapment and hypoplasia and dorsal displacement of the soft palate. The epiglottis is a curvilinear opacity just cranial to the larynx on the lateral view of the throat in the normal horse. The tip of the epiglottis is usually visible and appears to project above the aryepiglottic folds, which span the distance between the epiglottis and the arytenoid cartilages.[31] When there is epiglottic entrapment, the aryepiglottic folds are dorsally placed over the tip of the epiglottis and the normally curved shape of the tip is lost (Fig. 8–15). This appearance is suggestive of epiglottic entrapment and, when seen, bears further investigation by endoscopy.

Hypoplasia of the epiglottis should be relatively obvious when severe, but the diagnosis is more difficult in the marginal case. If epiglottic hypoplasia is suspected on the basis of the radiographic examination, the study should be repeated after the animal is stimulated to swallow to determine if the position of the epiglottis was causing a false impression of decreased size. These studies should be com-

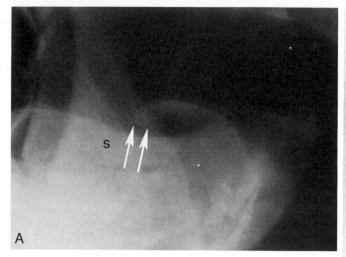
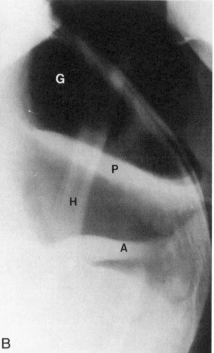

Figure 8–15. *A*, normal epiglottis. *Arrows*, tip of the epiglottis surrounded by air is clearly defined. S: soft palate. *B*, entrapment of the epiglottis. The tip of the epiglottis is no longer visible. The aryepiglottic folds (A) are prominent. H: stylohyoid bone; P: dorsal pharyngeal wall; G: guttural pouches.

pared with a known normal study to evaluate not only the relative size of the epiglottis but also its shape. Some hypoplastic epiglottic cartilages also exhibit substantial deformity.[2]

Dorsal displacement of the soft palate is occasionally the cause of the clinical signs in an animal with dysphagia and intermittent rattling inspiration.[2] It is recognized radiographically by the complete absence of the epiglottic shadow. The floor of the nasopharynx appears to be directly continuous with the floor of the larynx. Some air may also be recognized within the

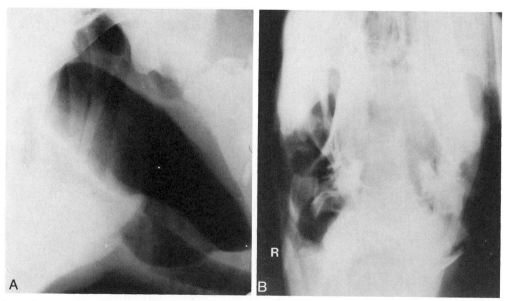

Figure 8–16. Tympanites of the guttural pouch. *A*, lateral view. The margins of the guttural pouch project more caudally over the larynx (compare with Fig. 8–7). Note also that there is compression of the dorsal pharyngeal wall. *B*, ventrodorsal view. Only the right guttural pouch is enlarged. Note the greater radiolucency on the right side.

oropharynx if the displacement of the palate is due to paralysis of the pharyngeal muscles. Pharyngeal paralysis is perhaps the most common cause of dorsal displacement of the soft palate. The paralysis is due to damage to the innervation of the pharynx. Unilateral paralysis is possible and still produces the radiographic and clinical signs.

Guttural Pouch Disease

Tympany is an abnormal accumulation of air within a guttural pouch due to a congenital abnormality of the pharyngeal orifice. The condition, which may be unilateral or bilateral, is apparently caused by a congenital defect in which an abnormal flap of mucosa and sometimes cartilage covers the pharyngeal orifice of the pouch. This flap permits air to enter the pouch but does not allow it to escape. As the amount of trapped air increases, the pressure against the flap increases, reducing the likelihood that any air will escape. The major clinical finding in this disorder is a large, soft, fluctuant, nonpainful mass in the parotid region. The animal usually experiences some degree of dysphagia, particularly if the condition is bilateral. In fact, the major life-threatening problem in

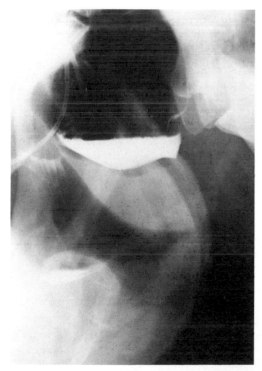

Figure 8–17. Contrast medium (Renografin-76, Squibb and Sons, Princeton, NJ) was used in an attempt to outline a foreign body within the guttural pouches. No such foreign body is seen, but the study clearly demonstrates a fluid line within the air-filled pouch.

foals with this problem is a tendency to develop aspiration pneumonia.[31, 36]

Radiographically, the tympany is manifest as enlargement of the guttural pouch or pouches.[2, 26] If the condition is unilateral, the ventrodorsal view may help to establish which pouch is affected (Fig. 8–16). It is not always easy to determine clinically or on the lateral view which of the pouches is affected or if both are affected. The ventrodorsal view is helpful in these horses. No other abnormalities of the guttural pouches are usually observed and the pouches usually return to normal after surgical resection of the redundant mucosal flaps in bilateral cases or surgical establishment of a communication between the two pouches in a unilateral case.

Trauma to the relatively well-protected guttural pouches is unusual. Occasionally, a foreign body lodges within one pouch.[1] The principal presenting complaint with foreign bodies is profuse unilateral epistaxis, which usually fills the guttural pouch with clotted blood. The blood clots and active hemorrhage from the pouch may preclude endoscopic examination. Radiographic examination is then the most reliable method of evaluating the guttural pouch. If the foreign body is metallic, it is obvious on the radiographic examination. If it is nonmetallic, then it may be necessary to instill water-soluble contrast medium into the guttural pouch to outline the object (Fig. 8–17). Contrast medium is instilled into the pouch through a flexible catheter, which is passed blindly or under endoscopic guidance. Large blood clots within the pouch will appear as filling defects within the contrast medium pool and must be recognized as such. Penetrating foreign bodies are usually sharply angular and rather linear. They are outlined by a contrast halo but are not opacified themselves.

Blunt trauma to the guttural pouch region may result in fracture of the stylohyoid bone. Unilateral epistaxis, pharyngeal swelling, extended head posture, inability to close the mouth or use the tongue, depression, dysphagia, and anorexia are clinical signs of such injuries.[6] Traumatic fractures of the stylohyoid are usually located in the lower one half of the bone. The dramatic clinical signs usually lead to early diagnostic evaluation of the horse. The margins of the fractures should be sharp and clearly defined. It may be necessary to make the film purposely oblique in a rostrocaudal direction so that the two stylohyoid bones are not superimposed and may be examined individually. If the horse is not examined soon after the injury, there may be substantial proliferation on the ends of the fracture fragments. In most horses, this proliferation is a mixture of callus formation and periosteal reaction to infection. Infection may not set in if the injury does not result in a laceration of the guttural pouch mucosa. Horses in which no laceration of the guttural pouch mucosa exists are also less likely to have epistaxis at the time of the original injury and therefore are less likely to be evaluated at the time of injury.

Neoplasms of the guttural pouches have been described but they are rare.[27, 33] Diagnosis is difficult because the signs are indicative of guttural pouch or pharyngeal disease but they are not dramatic. Passage of the endoscope may be difficult or impossible, but the reason for this difficulty may not be discernable from the nasal cavity. Radiographs show only soft-tissue swelling in the region of the guttural pouch and perhaps also decreased volume of the pouches or an irregularity in shape. Blockage of the pharyngeal orifice of the pouch by the tumor may result in retention of sterile or infected mucosal and tumor secretions within the pouch. Radiographs in the latter instance reveal only homogeneous soft-tissue swelling in the area of the guttural pouch. Such swelling is not necessarily indicative of a guttural pouch neoplasm; this radiographic presentation is identical to that of guttural pouch empyema, a more common disease.

The guttural pouches are large, ventral diverticuli of the auditory tubes with pharyngeal orifices located in their dorsal cranial walls (Fig. 8–18). It is difficult for fluid secretion to escape the pouch, except when the animal lowers its head. This anatomic arrangement would appear to favor fluid retention, and subsequently infection, within the pouch. Despite this fact, guttural pouch infections are seen infrequently in clinical practice and are usually observed only in animals that have chronic upper respiratory infections, such as strangles. Horses with bacterial guttural pouch infections also usually have active pharyngitis.[2, 15, 31] Treatment of the pharyngitis may be virtually impossible in these animals until the guttural pouch infection has been brought under control. Instances have also been described in which an animal with empyema had a stenotic pharyngeal orifice of the guttural pouch.[6, 8] This finding is not consistently described and may or may not be a significant predisposing factor in the development of the disease.

Radiographically, guttural pouch empyema is demonstrated as an increase in the opacity of the parotid region on both lateral and ventrodorsal views. Many horses also have a fluid line on the standing lateral view (Fig. 8–18).[2, 5] The presence of a fluid line within the guttural pouch in the absence of profuse epistaxis virtually confirms the diagnosis of guttural pouch empyema, and the animal should be treated accordingly.[10, 15] If the infection has been present for a long time, the exudate may become inspissated and form solid compactions, which are known as gutturoliths or chondroids.[2, 5] These structures are visible radiographically as irregular soft-tissue opacities outlined by air within the guttural pouch. There often is no visible fluid line in horses with extensive gutturolith formation. The gutturoliths may be small or large (Fig. 8–19), and generally must be surgically removed. In chronic guttural pouch infection or after treatment of guttural pouch empyema, there is usually a residual thickening of the floor of the guttural pouch. The result is thickening of the radiographic line that separates the dorsal wall of the pharynx from the guttural pouch; the line may also be roughened and irregular (Fig. 8–20). This roughening and thickening is one of the most consistent findings of chronic guttural pouch disease and should be regarded as diagnostic of past or present infection.

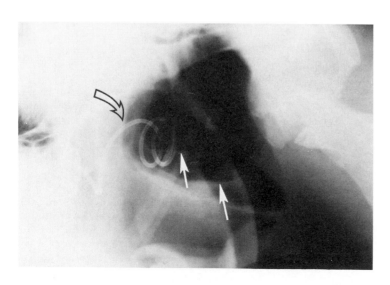

Figure 8–18. Fluid lines are clearly visible within the guttural pouch *(solid arrows)* of a horse with gutturomycosis. The catheter was placed within the pouch for treatment purposes. The point of entry of the catheter *(open arrow)* into the pouch indicates the location of the pharyngeal orifice.

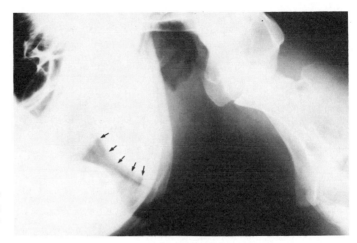

Figure 8–19. An enormous gutturolith virtually obliterates one guttural pouch and causes marked compression of the nasopharynx *(arrows)*.

There are many reports regarding mycotic guttural pouch disease. The high frequency of reports is probably due to the dramatic and catastrophic clinical signs usually associated with the disease and the apparently poor prognosis once the diagnosis is established. There is no breed, age, or sex predilection, and the incidence in the right and left pouches is the same.[7, 28] The only suggested predisposing epidemiologic factors are prolonged stabling of animals during warm months and chronic administration of antibiotics.[7, 25]

The clinical signs described in most horses include slight unilateral nasal discharge for a variable time period followed by an acute episode of tremendous unilateral or bilateral epistaxis.[2, 11, 16, 18, 28] Some horses die of hemorrhage before abnormalities can be observed. Other signs of guttural pouch mycosis are laryngeal hemiplegia, soft palate and pharyngeal paralysis, Horner's syndrome, vocal paralysis, dysphagia, and facial paralysis.[2, 7, 8, 13, 16, 18, 30, 31] Other signs that have been described in asso-

ciation with guttural pouch mycosis are blindness, incoordination, and rupture of the rectus captus ventralis muscles.[16, 22, 35] These instances are associated with extension of the mycotic invasion either directly into the surrounding tissues or along the neurovascular bundles into the orbit and cranial vault.

The clinical signs of mycotic guttural pouch disease are related to invasion of the mycotic infection through the wall of the guttural pouch to destroy the adjacent nerves and vessels. Depending on the area of the pouch wall where the infection is lodged and the size of the mycotic plaque, the signs may vary from minimal or no clinical problem to catastrophic hemorrhage due to rupture of either the internal or the external carotid artery. The most common site for the mycotic plaque to form is in the dorsal medial wall of the medial compartment of the guttural pouch, near the pharyngeal opening of the pouch. This location is also immediately ventral to the tympanic bulla and the point at which the internal carotid artery

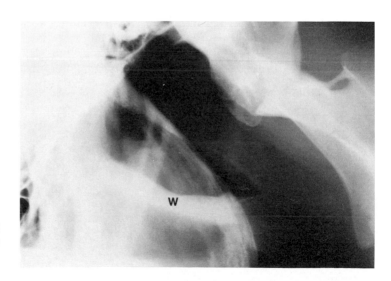

Figure 8–20. Thickening of the dorsal pharyngeal wall *(W)* and floor of the guttural pouches due to chronic guttural pouch infection.

and the ninth, tenth, and eleventh cranial nerves cross the dorsal wall of the pouch. The severe epistaxis that is the most common presenting complaint is usually a direct result of invasion and subsequent rupture of the wall of the internal carotid artery by the mycotic plaque. Although this vessel is the most common site for mycotic plaque formation and the most common structure affected, other areas of involvement have been described. Rupture of both the external carotid artery and maxillary vein have been described.[7, 9, 16, 18, 28] Ulceration of the guttural pouch wall with formation of a fistula to the dorsal wall of the pharynx has also been reported.[20]

The etiologic agent in most cases of guttural pouch mycosis is an aspergillus species; *A. fumigatus* and *A. nidulans* have been isolated.[7, 9, 21] One instance of clinical guttural pouch disease caused by penicillium species fungus has also been reported.[20]

The radiographic findings in cases of guttural pouch mycosis vary from no abnormalities to complete loss of the guttural pouch shadow due to filling of the pouch with blood or exudate. The presence of fluid within the pouch is dependent on whether there has been a recent episode of bleeding or development of a secondary bacterial empyema. In those horses in which only the mycotic plaque is present and there has been no recent bleeding episode, the guttural pouch is usually radiographically normal.[7, 25, 35] One radiographic finding commonly observed in association with guttural pouch mycosis is lysis or sclerosis of either the proximal one third of the stylohyoid bone or the base of the skull and tympanic bulla. Some animals have bony lesions in both places and the stylohyoid bone is fused with the base of the skull (Fig. 8–21).[6, 9] If lysis is present, a pathologic fracture of the stylohyoid may result. These fractures are in the proximal one half of the bone. In contrast, traumatic fractures usually occur in the distal one half of the bone and do not have lysis associated with them. The presence of bone proliferation or apparent pathologic fractures in the proximal one half of the stylohyoid should be considered highly suggestive of guttural pouch mycosis.

Treatment of guttural pouch mycosis usually includes ligation of the vessel in jeopardy. Carotid arteriography should be performed before ligation to locate the site and size of the vascular defect, especially if endoscopic examination of the pouch is not possible or is incomplete. The carotid arteriogram is performed by inserting a 14-gauge polyethylene catheter into the cranial portion of the common carotid artery. It is usually necessary to expose the artery surgically under general anesthesia to allow proper placement of the catheter. Once the catheter is in

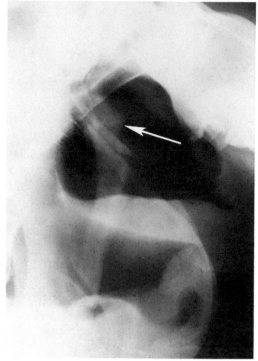

Figure 8–21. Periosteal proliferation causing thickening of the proximal end of the stylohyoid bone *(arrow)*. This animal had a long-standing history of gutturomycosis.

place, a cassette is placed under the parotid region of the throat and the x-ray tube is positioned over the animal. It is advisable that the cassette be placed in some type of tunnel under the head so that it can be placed and removed without moving the animal's head. The proper technical factors for the exposure should be determined before placement of the catheter. Once the film and catheter are in place, approximately 50 ml of contrast medium are infused by hand injection as rapidly as possible. The exposure is made during the last 10 ml of the injection.[6] The vascular anatomy is then studied to determine the site of the vascular blockage or aneurysm (Fig. 8–22). Once the site of the vascular lesion has been determined, the vessel may be ligated or occluded above and below it.

The use of an inflatable-balloon catheter technique to occlude the affected artery above and below the vascular lesion has been described.[12] This technique allows isolation of the diseased vascular segment without the delicate and dangerous surgery required to expose the area of the internal carotid artery where it enters the skull. The technique does, however, require fluoroscopic guidance for catheter placement and experience in handling specialized catheters. These requirements place it beyond the resources of virtually all but teaching hospital practices.

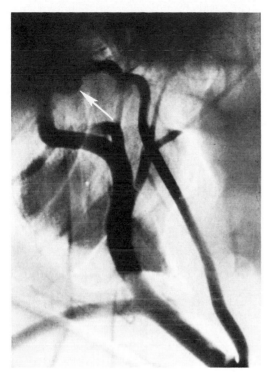

Figure 8–22. Carotid angiogram (similar to that in Fig. 8–8). A large aneurysm *(arrow)* of the internal carotid artery at the dorsal medial wall of the guttural pouch is revealed. The image has been photographically reversed to enhance visibility of the lesion.

References

1. Bayly WM, and Robertson JT: Epistaxis caused by foreign body penetration of a guttural pouch. J Am Vet Med Assoc *180*:1232, 1982.
2. Boles C: Abnormalities of the upper respiratory tract. Vet Clin North Am [Large Anim Pract] *1.89*, 1979.
3. Breuhaus BA, and Brown CM: Dysphagia associated with soft palate thickening. Equine Pract *3*:19, 1981.
4. Cook WR, and Littlewort MCG: Progressive haematoma of the ethmoid region in the horse. Equine Vet J *6*:101, 1974.
5. Cook WR: The auditory tube diverticulum (guttural pouch) in the horse: Its radiographic examination. J Am Vet Med Assoc *14*:51, 1973.
6. Cook WR: Skeletal radiology of the equine head. J Am Vet Radiol Soc *11*:35, 1970.
7. Cook WR: The clinical features of guttural pouch mycosis in the horse. Vet Rec *83*:336, 1968.
8. Daniels L: Endoscopy in the equine. Iowa State Vet *41*:69, 1979.
9. Dixon PM, and Rowlands AC: Atlanto-occipital joint infection associated with guttural pouch mycosis in a horse. Equine Vet J *13*:260, 1981.
10. Dowe JT: Draining the guttural pouch. J Am Vet Med Assoc *170*:384, 1977.
11. Ferraro GL: Epistaxis in race horses. Mod Vet Pract *63*:395, 1982.
12. Freeman DE, and Donawick J: Occlusion of internal carotid artery in the horse by means of a balloon-tipped catheter: Evaluation of a method designed to prevent epistaxis caused by guttural pouch mycosis. J Am Vet Med Assoc *176*:232, 1980.
13. Greet TRC: Observations on the potential role of oesophageal radiography in the horse. Equine Vet J *14*:73, 1982.
14. Habel RE, and King JM: Clinical applications of anatomy: Clinical anatomy of the guttural pouch (diverticulum tubae auditivae). Proceedings of the 20th World Veterinary Congress, Thessaloniki, Greece, *1*:113, 1975.
15. Hackathorn TA: A practical approach to the chronic pharyngitis/guttural pouch problem. Milne FJ (Ed): Proceedings of the 21st Annual Convention, American Association of Equine Practitioners. Boston, 1975.
16. Hatziolos BC, Sass B, and Albert TF, et al: Ocular changes in a horse with gutturomycosis. J Am Vet Med Assoc *167*:51, 1975.
17. Heffron CJ, Baker CJ, and Lee R: Fluoroscopic investigation of pharyngeal function in the horse. Equine Vet J *11*:148, 1979.
18. Hilbert BJ, Huxtable CR, and Brighton AJ: Erosion of the internal carotid artery and cranial nerve damage caused by guttural pouch mycosis in a horse. Aust Vet J *57*:346, 1981.
19. Hillman DJ: In Getty R (Ed.): Sisson and Grossman's The Anatomy of the Domestic Animals. Philadelphia, WB Saunders, 1975, pp. 344–348.
20. Jacobs KA, and Fretz PB: Fistula between the guttural pouches and the dorsal pharyngeal recess as a sequela to guttural pouch mycosis in the horse. Can Vet J *23*:117, 1982.
21. Johnson JH, Merriam JG, and Attleberger M: A case of guttural pouch mycosis caused by *Aspergillus nidulans*. Vet Med/Small Anim Clin *68*:771, 1973.
22. Knight AP: Dysphagia resulting from unilateral rupture of the rectus capitus ventralis muscles in a horse. J Am Vet Med Assoc *170*:735, 1977.
23. Kold SE, Ostblom LC, and Philipsen HP: Headshaking caused by a maxillary osteoma in a horse. Equine Vet J *14*:107, 1982.
24. Larson VL, and Sorenson DK: The respiratory system. In Catcott EJ, and Smithcors JF (Eds.): Equine Medicine and Surgery, 2nd Ed. Wheaton, IL, American Veterinary Publications, 1972, pp. 363–375.
25. Lingard DR, Gossor IIS, and Monfort TN: Acute epistaxis associated with guttural pouch mycosis in two horses. J Am Vet Med Assoc *164*:1038, 1974.
26. Lokai MD, Hardenbrook HJ, and Benson GJ: Guttural pouch tympanites in a foal. Vet Med/Small Anim Clin *71*:1625, 1976.
27. Merriam JG: Guttural pouch fibroma in a mare. J Am Vet Med Assoc *161*:487, 1972.
28. Nation PN: Epistaxis of guttural pouch origin in horses: Pathology of three cases. Can Vet J *19*:194, 1978.
29. Nickel R, Schummer A, Seiferle E, et al: In The Viscera of the Domestic Mammals, Berlin, Paul Parey, 1973, pp. 211–225.
30. Peterson FB, Harmany K, and Dodd DC: Clinicopathologic conference. J Am Vet Med Assoc *157*:220, 1970.
31. Raker CW: Diseases of the guttural pouch. Mod Vet Pract *57*:549, 1976.
32. Schebitz H, and Wilkens H: In Atlas of Radiographic Anatomy of Dog and Horse. Berlin, Paul Parey, 1968, pp. 123–146.
33. Trigo FJ, and Nickels FA: Squamous cell carcinoma of a horse's guttural pouch. Mod Vet Pract *62*:456, 1981.
34. Tulleners EP, and Raker CW: Nasal septum resection in the horse. Vet Surg *12*:41, 1983.
35. Wagner PC, Miller RA, Gallina AM, et al: Mycotic encephalitis associated with a guttural pouch mycosis. J Equine Med Surg *2*:355, 1978.
36. Wheat JD: Tympanites of the guttural pouch of the horse. J Am Vet Med Assoc *140*:453, 1962.

CHAPTER 9

THE EQUINE SPINE

PAT R. GAVIN

Recent advances in film/screen technology have enabled veterinarians to perform a thorough radiographic examination of the equine cervical spine. Universities and major equine referral centers have the ability to radiograph the majority of the remaining spinal column. These studies have increased our understanding of the many conditions that affect the equine spine.

NORMAL ANATOMY

The vertebral formula of the horse is C_7, T_{18}, L_6, S_5, Cd_{15-20}.[1] Common variations from the norm include 17 or 19 thoracic vertebrae and 4 to 6 sacral vertebrae. The first cervical vertebra (atlas) has no spinous process and two large lateral processes, each with two foramina. On a ventrodorsal view, the suture between the lateral arches should not be mistaken for a fracture in a young horse.

The axis (C_2) has a large dorsal spinous process and a protrusion from the body called a dens. Radiography of a young horse demonstrates two growth centers for the dens. By 2 years of age, the osseous projections in the horse fuse and form foramina from the cranial dorsal spine and arch. C_3, C_4, and C_5 are nearly identical in appearance; C_6 has large wing-shaped transverse processes. The caudal or costal aspect of this process has a separate center of ossification in the young horse. C_7 has a more prominent dorsal spine than the preceding vertebra, but it is much smaller than T_1. The author has seen the typical "C_6" transverse process on C_7 in only three of over 300 horses.

Methods of marking the cervical vertebrae with lead markers can be misleading due to misplacement and beam parallax. Proper cassette placement to include the distinctive vertebrae in the field of view (C_1, C_2, or C_6) yields accurate results (Fig. 9–1). The cranial end plate of the vertebral body fuses at about 2 years of age. The caudal end plate first fuses dorsally, but the ventral aspect may still be open at 5 years of age.[2]

The size of the vertebral canal on views obtained in a neutral position and during flexion has been reported.[3] The measurements given are for horses of different sizes. Problems arise when the magnification factor is not considered, and imprecise positioning can lead to erroneous conclusions. The author has generally had unsatisfactory results with radiographic mensuration and does not recommend its indiscriminate use, unless all factors are carefully controlled as initially reported.[3] A false-positive diagnosis of vertebral subluxation can subjectively be made if one fails to realize that the cervical spine is simply made of bony rectangles that must subluxate to some degree when flexed through an arc.

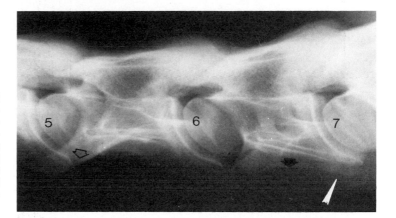

Figure 9–1. Right lateral radiograph of caudal cervical region. *Open arrowhead,* typical transverse spinous process seen on C_3 to C_5. *Solid black arrowhead,* wing-shaped transverse spinous process of C_6. *Solid white arrowhead,* a radiolucent line that represents the physis from the costal growth center of the process. Numbers 5, 6, and 7 correspond to C_5 to C_7.

The majority of midthoracic vertebral bodies are easily visualized because they are overlapped by the dorsal border of the lung. T_2 to T_{10} have large dorsal spinous processes, with the tallest point at T_4 to T_6. Separate centers of ossification develop on the dorsal aspect of the cranial thoracic vertebra at about 1 year of age and persist "unfused" into old age.[4] The anticlinal vertebra is generally T_{15}. Closure of these vertebral end plates takes place at age 3 to 3 1/2 years.[4] The cranial lumbar vertebrae can be visualized on the lateral projection, although the ventrodorsal view is required for visualization of the remaining lumbar spine, sacrum, and cranial coccygeal vertebrae.

The cervical and thoracic spine can be radiographed in the standing animal. Because of the high mAs techniques required for the thicker portions, however, recumbent lateral radiographs should be made. Technical personnel may then be absent during the actual exposures and blurring from patient motion is reduced. The use of anesthesia also allows ventrodorsal projections of the cervical spine, especially cranially, and of the lumbar spine to be obtained. Detailed reviews of the normal anatomy can be found elsewhere.[1–4]

POSITIVE-CONTRAST MYELOGRAPHY

The introduction of a safe water-soluble contrast medium (metrizamide) has permitted the use of positive-contrast myelography in the horse.[5–8] After over 300 myelograms were performed at Washington State University, the mortality rate was approximately 1 percent, although many horses had a transient (24 to 48 hours) worsening of their clinical signs. The size of the equine patient generally limits myelography to the cervical region, except in the foal.

The cervical myelogram is performed by injecting contrast medium in the subarachnoid space at the occipitoatlantal junction. In lateral projections, the dorsal column of contrast medium is slightly wider than the ventral column. The ventral column narrows slightly at the caudal vertebral canal; the dorsal column widens in this region and narrows at the cranial vertebral canal. This stairstep appearance is more pronounced in the caudal cervical region (Fig. 9–2).

Positional films may be of help in survey radiography of the spine, whereas they are extremely beneficial with myelography. Upon flexion, the normal dorsal canal has a uniformly wide appearance, whereas the ventral column narrows to a thin line at the intervertebral region in the midcervical area (Fig. 9–2). In hyperextension, there should be no significant changes in the above sites radiographically. Positional films do not show significant changes in the normal horse at C_{1-2}, C_{5-6}, and C_{6-7}. Appropriate muscular relaxation under general anesthesia is needed so as to flex or extend the neck properly. Attention to accurate positioning is mandatory to prevent equivocal diagnoses.

CONGENITAL ANOMALIES

Recent reports have detailed an apparently inherited congenital disorder of the Arabian foal, termed occipitoatlantoaxial malformation.[9, 10] The neurologic disease is recognized at birth in some animals and as progressive ataxia in others. The radiographic appearance is one of symmetric occipitalization of the atlas and atlantalization of the axis, with varying degrees of fusion of these structures. The dens may be luxated or fractured. Similar but nonsymmetric malformations have been reported in other breeds. The lack of symmetry suggests this may be a sporadic, nonheritable congenital defect in the non-Arabian breeds (see Fig. 7–10).

Conformational defects of scoliosis, lordosis, and kyphosis are occasionally seen in the foal, associated with fused or block vertebrae and hemivertebrae.[11] Similar conformational prob-

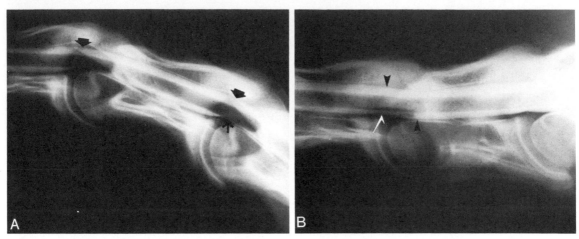

Figure 9–2. *A,* right lateral myelogram of the cranial cervical region during flexion. *Arrowheads,* the dorsal contrast medium column is of uniform width. *Small arrow,* thinning of the ventral column that occurs normally during flexion. (The vertebrae are C_3 to C_5.) *B,* normal right lateral myelogram of caudal cervical region in extension. The contour of contrast medium column changes as the cord passes in a slightly stairstepped manner through the caudal cervical canal. Note that the thinned ventral column *(arrow)* is directly across from the wide dorsal column; hence there is no compression. (The wing-shaped transverse spinous process of C_6 is used for orientation.)

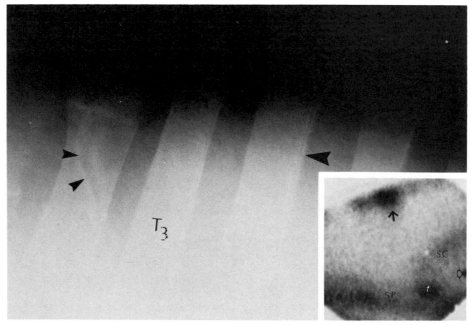

Figure 9–3. Right lateral radiograph of the thoracic spinous processes of a horse with fistulous withers. There is an area of decreased opacity with sclerotic margin over the T_2 dorsal spinous process *(small arrowheads)*. Without an orthogonal view, it is difficult to confirm this finding. *Large arrowhead,* normal periosteal proliferation at the attachment of the tendons from the epaxial musculature. Culture of a surgical specimen of the area revealed *Brucella abortus.* *Inset*: Left lateral oblique bone scan of the same area. The increased uptake *(black arrow)* indicates osseous involvement of the T_2 dorsal spinous process. Increased activity in the regions of T_3 and T_5 may indicate normal activity in the growth centers. *Open arrow,* a radioactive marker placed on the right scapular region. SP: spine; SC: right scapula.

lems may be encountered in the adult horse, but these defects are usually related to muscle spasms or acquired fusions. Other deviations from normal anatomy include prominent dorsal spinous processes in the cervical vertebrae, cervical ribs, and congenital fusion of the dorsal spinous processes in the thoracolumbar spine. These conditions may be associated with a clinical problem, but are most often clinically benign.

INFECTIOUS LESIONS

The various diarthrodial joints of the spine can become involved in cases of "joint ill" or septicemia in the foal. Other vertebral osteomyelitis may result from direct extension or hematogenous spread of a bacterial and, rarely, a fungal infection. The radiographic appearance is generally one of lysis of bone. The more chronic lesions have a mixed pattern of lysis and periosteal new bone formation.

The most common infectious osteomyelitis of the equine spine involves the dorsal spinous processes of the cranial thoracic vertebrae; it is commonly called fistulous withers. In many horses, involvement is limited to the supraspinous bursa and surrounding soft tissues, and it becomes a diagnostic challenge to ascertain the extent of involvement of the spinous processes. The difficulty arises because the separate center of ossification of these processes is normally irregular and mottled in appearance, and there is often a smooth periosteal proliferation on the spinous processes at the insertions of tendons and ligaments. Lysis of the main shaft of the process or an irregular periosteal proliferation are indications of osteomyelitis. If available, the use of nuclear medicine bone scans of the skeletal region increase the accuracy of this diagnosis. *Brucella* sp. should be ruled out due to the possible zoonotic problem (Fig. 9–3).

TRAUMATIC LESIONS

Fractures of the spine after trauma can occur virtually anywhere along the spinal column. Equine patients with fractures of the cervical vertebrae and dorsal arch displacement may recover to varying degrees; myelography is indicated in horses with residual neurologic disease to ascertain if compressive forces on the spinal cord remain.

The dorsal spinous processes of the thoracic vertebra in the withers area may fracture after a backwards fall (Fig. 9–4). Fractures of the vertebral bodies of the remainder of the spinal column are infrequently encountered; when they occur, the area most often affected is T_{11-13}.[12] The lack of proper radiographic detail in the caudal lumbar region causes difficulty in visualizing fractures in the area. An abrupt change in the longitudinal axis at a single vertebra or intervertebral space may be the only radiographic sign of a fracture.

ACQUIRED LESIONS AND LESIONS OF UNKNOWN ETIOLOGY

Subluxation of the spine, especially the sacroiliac region, may cause back pain in the horse. This condition is generally not detectable radiographically, although a proliferative response may be detected on a ventrodorsal view. The horse may develop degenerative spondylosis of the vertebral bodies in the thoracolumbar spine. This lesion is generally seen in the aged horse, and it may be an incidental finding. The condition has been associated with back pain in the horse,[12] and it is rarely associated with an

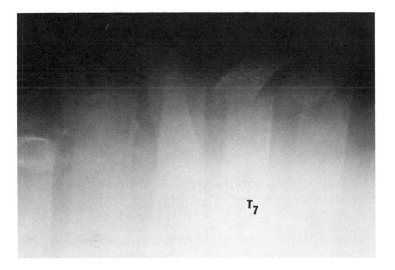

Figure 9–4. Left-to-right standing lateral radiograph. The dorsal spinous processes of T_4 to T_8 are fractured, the result of a fall on the withers.

infectious agent. Due to the difficulty in obtaining satisfactory lateral radiographs of the lumbosacral region, the radiographic diagnosis of cauda equina syndrome is even more difficult than in the dog.

Overlapping of the dorsal spinous processes in the thoracolumbar region is rather common. The overlapping may be an incidental finding in a clinically normal horse or it may be responsible for back pain. The condition has been graded by some veterinarians in an attempt to correlate the radiographic appearance with the clinical signs.[4] The degree of involvement varies from simple impingement to fusion of adjacent spinous processes. The condition generally occurs in the spine beneath the saddle area and is most commonly detected in hunters and jumpers.[12] Any of the numerous spinal articulations may become arthritic in the horse. Clinical improvement after the administration of local anesthetic in the area aids in diagnosing this condition and prevents the placement of undue significance to a radiographic lesion that may be associated with the normal aging process.

The etiologies of spinal ataxia in the horse are many and varied; some form of cervical vertebral malformation, however, is commonly encountered. It has been suggested that the "wobbler" condition is a congenital or inherited process. Current breeding studies at Washington State and Oregon State Universities are not complete, but to date they have failed to define an inherited mode. Certainly the condition is rather common in the species and has been detected in many breeds.

In spinal ataxia, there is usually a history of an acute traumatic event followed by the development of ataxia. The physical examination should include a thorough neurologic assessment. If a vertebral fracture is suspected, standing survey radiographs of the cervical spine should be obtained. Most often, the horse is ataxic, and the condition leads to the fall. The ataxic horse may be of any age, although most are affected and subsequently evaluated at the time that they enter training.

The radiographic and myelographic examination of the ataxic horse has been reviewed extensively in recent articles.[2, 5, 8, 13] General anesthesia and lateral recumbent films are needed for accurate positioning, to obtain cerebrospinal fluid, and to perform the myelogram. Care should be exercised in the selection of preanesthetic or anesthetic induction agents; any substances that lower the seizure threshold should be avoided. A low kVp technique improves radiographic contrast as well as visualization of the spine and contrast medium.

The lesions fall into two main categories: those of vertebral instability in the cranial cervical spine, which are best visualized on flexion studies, and those of the caudal cervical spine, which are best evaluated on normal and hyperextended views. The cranial lesions are most often seen at C_{3-4} and C_{4-5}. Survey radiographs reveal a remodeling of the vertebra that is best appreciated on the caudal aspect of the ventral spinal canal border on the cranial vertebra. Ronald Sande has termed this change the "ski jump" sign (Fig. 9–5). This proliferation results in a relatively stenotic vertebral canal that is best seen during flexion of the neck. Our attempts to quantify the change have failed, and the survey radiographic findings should be interpreted as tentative. If the change is severe and the canal appears stenotic without flexion, care should be exercised in the manipulation of the horse under anesthesia. In all horses, contrast myelography should be used to confirm tentative findings. Several horses with the "ski jump" sign were myelographically normal.

Myelographic examinations have shown cervical cord compression when no such compression was suspected on the basis of the results of survey radiographs. An objective evaluation of the change in the contrast medium column to quantify cervical cord compression has eluded us after hundreds of cases. Flexion of the spine normally reduces the ventral contrast medium column to a thin line at C_{3-4} and to a slightly lesser extent at C_{4-5}. Think of the spinal cord as delicate tissue floating in a cylinder of fluid. To damage the tissue, the cord could not just be touched ventrally as it floats upwards. Therefore, there must be "significant" compression of opposing contrast medium columns. Both contrast medium columns must be reduced to ≤ 50 percent of the normal width. The reference normal width can be from the column cranial or caudal to the narrowed area, or comparisons to the cranial and caudal intervertebral sites can be made (Fig. 8–5). It must be stressed that the changes in the opposing contrast medium column must be made at the same level and not in a stairstep arrangement. Because the ventral contrast medium column is more visibly compressed, these lesions are often termed cranial cervical ventral compressive lesions. These subjective guidelines have led to excellent diagnostic accuracy when compared to postmortem findings. To date, a false-positive diagnosis in the cranial cervical region has not been detected at our institution. The area involved is equally divided into C_{3-4} and C_{4-5}, with infrequent instances at C_{2-3} and C_{5-6}; occasionally, double and even triple level compressions occur.

The diagnosis of caudal cervical lesions is more difficult. Excellent radiographs of the caudal region are more difficult to obtain due to the increased thickness of the patient and the

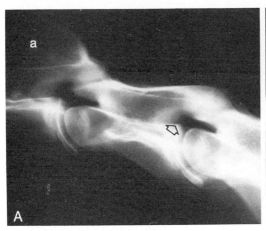
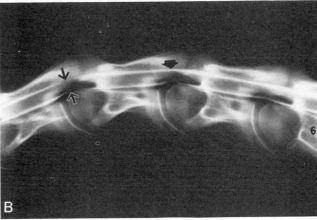

Figure 9–5. *A*, right lateral radiograph of the cranial cervical region of an ataxic yearling Arabian filly. a: dorsal spinous process of the axis. *Open arrow,* remodeled ventral caudal spinal canal of C_3. This change has been termed the "ski jump" sign, and results in a stenotic vertebral canal. *B,* lateral myelogram of the area in flexion. The results of the standard myelogram, in extension, were within normal limits. With the region in flexion, a narrowed dorsal and ventral contrast medium column can be seen at C_3-C_4 *(arrows).* Compare this finding with the narrowed ventral but normal dorsal contrast medium column *(arrowhead)* at C_4-C_5.

normally overlying shoulders. Attention to proper technique, however, should result in radiographs of good to excellent quality to the level of C_7-T_1 in all horses. The survey study of affected horses often reveals a lack of detail in the articular process region of C_{5-6} or C_{6-7}, which is often due to a proliferative reaction of one or more articular processes (Fig. 9–6). Interpretation of the survey radiographs alone would again lead to several false-positive and negative diagnoses. Soft-tissue lesions may cause cord compression with no visible evidence on the survey radiographs. Synovial cysts causing such compression in this region are uncommon.[11]

To obtain a high quality myelogram in this region, adequate contrast medium must be given and the head must be elevated for a few minutes to allow the contrast medium to gravitate to the caudal cervical region. The normal contrast medium columns have a stairstep appearance in this region, making the judgment of "significant" compression difficult. Again, it must be stressed that the narrowed contrast medium columns must be directly opposite each other for cord compression to occur. Often the dorsal contrast medium column is displaced by an apparent soft-tissue extradural mass. In most instances, this mass may be evident in the normally positioned radiograph, but it is more apparent during hyperextension of the neck (Fig. 9–6). Some of these lesions improve upon flexion, although it is difficult to obtain much flexion in the caudal cervical spine. Because the dorsal column is more visibly compressed, these findings are often called caudal cervical dorsal compressive lesions. Postmortem examination of the lesions in the caudal cervical region often reveals the affected articular processes have changes compatible with osteochondrosis. In

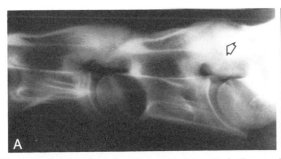
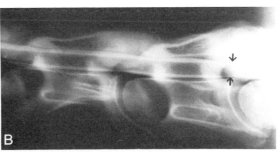

Figure 9–6. Right lateral radiograph of an ataxic 2-year-old Hanoverian stallion. C_5 to C_7 are visualized. The articular process articulation at C_6-C_9 is not visualized and there is increased opacity in this region *(open arrow)*. *B,* right lateral myelogram. The dorsal and ventral contrast medium columns are narrowed at C_6-C_7 *(arrows)*. The contrast medium column is compressed more from its dorsal aspect than from its ventral aspect.

addition, articular process fractures (primary or pathologic) are seen. These fractures cannot usually be visualized, even on retrospective examination of the radiographic study. Ventro-dorsal projections of this area are possible, but substandard quality prevents accurate assessment. Oblique ventrodorsal views may be rewarding, but the two obliques are difficult to match technically and the ability to compare the radiographs for loss of symmetry is correspondingly hampered. Occasionally, these caudal cervical dorsal compressive lesions are multiple and may be found in conjunction with the cranial cervical ventral compressive lesions.

Many ataxic horses have normal survey radiographic and myelographic findings. It should be remembered that there are numerous other causes of cervical cord disease and ataxia in the horse.

References

1. Getty R (Ed): Sisson's and Grossman's The Anatomy of the Domestic Animals, 5th Ed. Philadelphia, WB Saunders, 1975.
2. Rendano VT, and Quick CB: Radiographic interpretation: Equine radiology—the cervical spine. Mod Vet Pract 59:921, 1978.
3. Mayhew IG, Whitlock RH, deLahunta A: Spinal cord disease in the horse. Cornell Vet 68:44, 1978.
4. Jeffcott LB: Radiographic features of the normal equine thoracolumbar spine. Vet Radiol 20:140, 1979.
5. Rantanen NW, Gavin PR, Barbee DD, et al: Ataxia and paresis in horses. Part II. Radiographic and myelographic examination of the cervical vertebral column. Comp Contin Ed Pract Vet 3:S161, 1981.
6. Nyland TG, Blythe L, Pool R, et al: Metrizamide myelography in the normal horse: Clinical, radiographic, and pathologic findings. J Am Vet Radiol Soc 20:66, 1979.
7. Beech J: Metrizamide myelography in the horse. J Am Vet Radiol Soc 20:22, 1979.
8. Stowater JL, Kneller SK, Froehlich PS: Metrizamide myelography in two horses. Vet Med/Small Anim Clin 73:177, 183, 1978.
9. Mayhew IG, Watson AG, Heissan JA: Congenital occipitoatlantoaxial malformations in the horse. Equine Vet J 10:103, 1978.
10. Whitwell KE: Cranovertebral malformations in an Arab foal. Equine Vet J 10:125, 1978.
11. Jeffcott LB: Disorders of the thoracolumbar spine of the horse—a survey of 443 cases. Equine Vet J 12:197, 1980.
12. Jeffcott LB: Disorders of the equine thoracolumbar spine. A review. J Equine Med Surg 2:9, 1978.
13. Wagner PC: Disorders of the spine. *In* Mansmann RA, McAllister ES, and Pratt PW (Eds): Equine Medicine and Surgery, 3rd Ed. Santa Barbara, American Veterinary Publications, 1982.
14. Fisher LF, Bowman KF, MacHarg MA: Spinal ataxia in a horse caused by a synovial cyst. Vet Pathol 18:407, 1981.

SECTION 4

APPENDICULAR SKELETON— COMPANION ANIMALS

CHAPTER 10

DISEASES OF THE IMMATURE SKELETON

MICHAEL R. METCALF

Because the immature skeleton develops rapidly in the first year of life, it is subject to stresses not present in adult life. Heredity has determined the basic formation of the skeleton, but hormonal and nutritional stresses can alter skeletal development. The purpose of this chapter is to discuss the radiographic abnormalities seen with diseases of the immature skeleton due to genetic, hormonal, or nutritional stresses. Abnormalities due to trauma, infection, or neoplasia are discussed elsewhere. With the exception of accidental trauma or infection, these diseases are the most common cause of lameness in the young animal. The etiology of these diseases, however, is often poorly understood or is not known at all. The roentgen sign approach is the surest way to correct radiographic interpretation. Because many of these diseases have "classic" roentgen signs, however, this discussion is organized with attention to the disease entity.

OSTEOCHONDROSIS

Osteochondrosis is a disturbance of enchondral ossification, which is the formation of bone by way of cartilage. This disturbance leads to increased thickness of the cartilage. Because nutrients are primarily supplied to chondrocytes via synovial fluid, cells in the thicker areas of cartilage can become necrotic. Several problems may then result. If a cleft forms in the region of necrosis and reaches the surface of the cartilage, creating a flap or defect, osteochondritis dissecans results.

Fragmented coronoid process results from separation of the coronoid process from the remainder of the ulna, possibly due to osteochondrosis.[1-3] The actual cause of the separation is not known, but it may be due to mechanical or traumatic factors.[4] Some individuals believe that ununited anconeal process is also due to osteochondrosis.[1] The radiographic appearance of these conditions is addressed separately.

Osteochondritis Dissecans. The radiographic signs of this condition are based on the visualization of either a subchondral bone defect or cartilage flap. This abnormality is most often seen in the caudal aspect of the humeral head (shoulder),[5, 6] but it is also found in the medial humeral condyle (elbow),[1-3, 6] the medial or lateral femoral condyle (stifle),[5, 6] and the proximal aspect of the medial trochlea of the talus (tarsus).[6] The disease occurs in large and giant breeds, usually between 4 and 10 months of age. Osteochondritis dissecans is frequently present in more than one joint and is commonly bilateral.

The defect in the shoulder is best visualized on a lateral radiograph; other projections are rarely beneficial. A craniocaudal projection or a

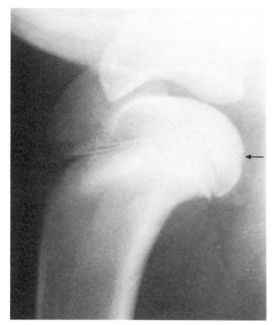

Figure 10–1. Lateral view of the shoulder of a dog with osteochonditis dissecans of the humeral head. Note the broad, shallow defect in the caudal aspect of the articular surface. (Courtesy of Dr. Michael Walker, University of Tennessee. Knoxville, TN.)

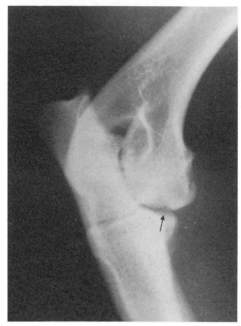

Figure 10–2. Craniolateral-caudomedial oblique radiograph of the elbow of a dog with osteochondritis dissecans of the medial humeral condyle. There is an articular defect in the medial (nonsuperimposed) condyle of the humerus. (Courtesy of Dr. Michael Walker, University of Tennessee, Knoxville, TN.)

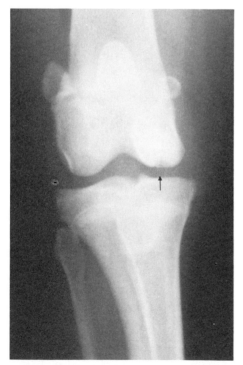

Figure 10–3. Craniocaudal radiograph of the stifle of a dog with osteochondritis dissecans of the medial femoral condyle. There is a defect in the articular surface of the medial femoral condyle. A mineralized cartilage flap covers the defect. (Courtesy of Dr. Michael Walker, University of Tennessee, Knoxville, TN.)

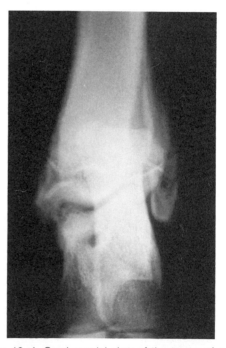

Figure 10–4. Craniocaudal view of the tarsus of a dog with osteochondritis dissecans of the medial trochlea of the talus. There is an articular defect in the proximal, medial aspect of the medial trochlea. A piece of mineralized cartilage is superimposed over the defect. (Courtesy of Dr. Michael Walker, University of Tennessee, Knoxville, TN.)

slightly oblique craniocaudal projection is necessary to visualize a lesion in the elbow, stifle, or tarsus. The tarsal radiograph must be obliqued to move the image of the calcaneus to a nonsuperimposed position relative to the medial trochlea of the talus. A comparison radiograph of the opposite extremity may be helpful.

The primary radiographic sign of osteochondritis dissecans is common to all locations. There is a defect in the subchondral bone that causes a flattening or concavity of the articular surface. This defect may have a sclerotic margin. The subchondral defect in the humeral head is usually broad-based and shallow (Fig. 10–1). The cartilage flap may become calcified and in such instances is radiographically apparent as a thin, linear mineral opacity covering the defect. If the cartilage flap separates, it often calcifies and it is then recognizable radiographically. This calcified cartilage can be visualized in any part of the joint. Arthrography can be helpful in identifying the cartilage flap or free joint body when there has been no calcification. Examples of the radiographic changes in the elbow, stifle, and tarsus are shown in Figures 10–2, 10–3, and 10–4, respectively.

Fragmented Coronoid Process. Because the medial coronoid process of the ulna does not develop as a separate ossification center, the previous designation for this disease—ununited

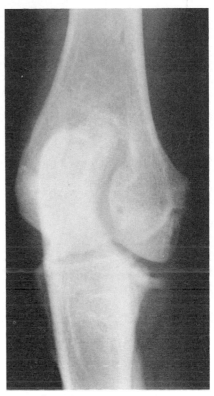

Figure 10–6. Craniolateral-caudomedial oblique radiograph of the elbow of a dog with a fragmented medial coronoid process. There is a large osteophyte on the medial aspect of the ulna at the humoroulnar joint. Partially superimposed on the osteophyte is a mineral opacity, representing the fragmented coronoid process, separated from the remainder of the bone. It is uncommon to actually visualize a fragmented coronoid process as a separate opacity on a radiograph.

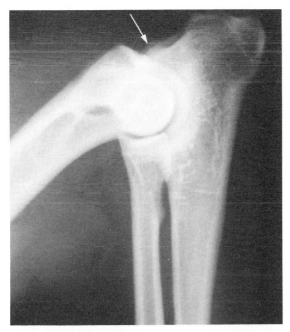

Figure 10–5. Lateral radiograph of the flexed elbow of a dog with a fragmented medial coronoid process. There is degenerative change as shown by a broad rim of osteophytes on the proximal aspect of the anconeal process.

coronoid process—is a misnomer. Fragmented coronoid process may be another manifestation of osteochondrosis.[1–3] Another theory is that mechanical stress is placed on the coronoid process from a subluxated humeroradial joint caused by growth retardation of the distal radial physis.[4] This condition occurs primarily in medium to large-breed dogs of 4 to 10 months of age, and particularly in fast-growing animals. The disease is often bilateral.

Radiographically, fragmented coronoid process is most often diagnosed by the secondary changes it causes. The earliest point at which these changes can be detected is 7 to 8 months of age. The actual fragmented coronoid process is usually not apparent radiographically. The earliest sign of secondary degenerative joint disease is the presence of osteophytes on the proximal and lateral aspects of the anconeal process (Fig. 10–5). Degenerative changes on the medial humeral epicondyle and medial aspects of the joint follow (Fig. 10–6).[1–3, 6] Sclerosis between the proximal radius and ulna and pos-

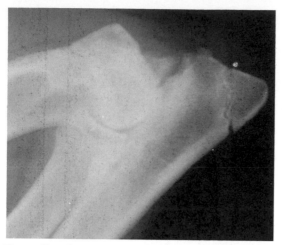

Figure 10–7. Lateral radiograph of the flexed elbow of a dog with an ununited anconeal process. A radiolucent line of separation is apparent between the olecranon and the anconeal process. Note that the medial epicondyle of the humerus is not superimposed over the anconeal process. (Courtesy of Dr. Michael Walker, University of Tennessee, Knoxville, TN.)

sibly an increased humeroradial joint space may be seen on the lateral projection.[4]

Ununited Anconeal Process. The etiology and pathogenesis of this condition have not yet been determined, although osteochondrosis is believed to be a factor in its occurrence.[1] The incidence is highest in large dogs and its occurrence is often bilateral.

The normal anconeal process develops as a separate center of ossification that fuses with the olecranon at 4 or 5 months of age. If the anconeal process is separated from the olecranon along the fusion line at an age greater than 5 months, the separation is abnormal. Before this time, an assessment cannot be made.[2, 5, 6]

The radiographic signs are based on the appearance of a radiolucent line of separation between the olecranon and the anconeal process (Fig. 10–7). It is important to obtain a lateral radiograph of the elbow in extreme flexion. If not flexed, the distal, caudal aspect of the medial epicondyle of the humerus is superimposed on the anconeal process, which can be confused with a separation line. With time, sclerosis can be visualized along the margins of the separation. Degenerative changes subsequently appear, although this occurrence is not likely before 7 to 8 months of age.

HYPERTROPHIC OSTEODYSTROPHY

This is a condition of rapidly growing, large to giant dogs, 3 to 7 months of age. The changes are usually found in the distal aspects of the radius, ulna, and tibia, although any bone of the appendicular skeleton may be affected. The condition is frequently bilaterally symmetric. The etiology of the disease is unknown, but it has been hypothesized that dietary factors are involved, including nutritional oversupplementation, dietary calcium and phosphorus imbalance, or vitamin C deficiency.[6] It is also hypothesized that the radiographic changes are due to metaphyseal inflammation, which causes a transverse band of necrosis across the metaphysis.[7] Extraperiosteal changes may be due to mineralization of cellular debris or hematomas. That inflammation is involved is supported by the clinical appearance of painful and swollen affected metaphyses. In addition, the dog is usually febrile.

The early radiographic changes consist of mixed sclerotic and radiolucent regions in the affected metaphysis, which progress to a radiolucent line or band parallel to and just proximal to the physis.[5, 6] Adjacent to the radiolucent zone is a zone of sclerosis (Fig. 10–8), which is accompanied by soft-tissue swelling. Secondarily, extraperiosteal tissues surrounding the metaphysis become mineralized, which is radio-

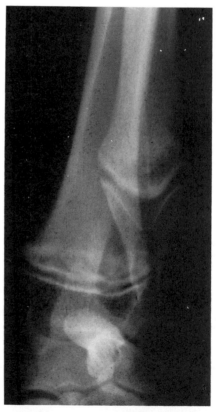

Figure 10–8. Craniocaudal radiograph of the distal radius and ulna in a dog with hypertrophic osteodystrophy. There is a heterogeneous appearance just proximal to the distal radial and ulnar physes consisting of mixed sclerotic and radiolucent regions. (Courtesy of Dr. Michael Walker, University of Tennessee, Knoxville, TN.)

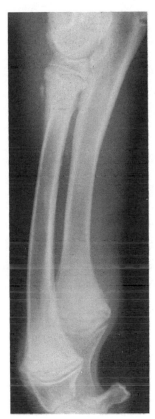

Figure 10–9. Lateral radiograph of the antebrachium of a dog with hypertrophic osteodystrophy. There is sclerosis of the metaphyseal regions, which includes a radiolucent zone just proximal to the distal physes. There is early extraperiosteal soft-tissue mineralization cranial to the proximal radial metaphysis, a process that often progresses to form a "cuff" around the metaphyses. (Courtesy of Dr. Michael Walker, University of Tennessee, Knoxville, TN.)

ease characterized clinically by a shifting leg lameness and a chronic course. The primary sites are the humerus, ulna, and femur. The diaphysis is more often affected than the metaphysis. The cause and pathogenesis of the disease are unknown.

Radiographically, there is an increase in medullary opacity.[5, 6] The trabeculae become blurred, with eventual loss of visualization. The increased medullary opacity can be either diffuse and patchy or well-defined sclerotic areas that may become as radiopaque as the cortex. The changes are first seen near the nutrient foramen, but they may progress to other areas of the bone. Secondarily, the endosteal cortex thickens and becomes roughened. Periosteal new bone is stimulated, which appears as laminar thickening of the cortex (Fig. 10–10).

These changes continue for 4 to 6 weeks in a single bone and then gradually disappear. The residual changes include decreased radiopacity

graphically visualized as a cuff of smooth or irregular ossification around the metaphysis, separated from the cortex by a radiolucent line (Fig. 10–9). This extraperiosteal ossification may progress to involve the diaphysis, probably occurring as the bone lengthens. In the advanced stages, the radiolucent line between newly ossified extraperiosteal tissue and bone disappears. The metaphysis may then appear enlarged.

Although usually self-limiting, the disease may cause permanent bone deformities. These defects include enlarged metaphyses and inhibition of the distal ulnar physis, resulting in carpal valgus deformity.

PANOSTEITIS

Panosteitis is a disease of large dogs, 5 to 24 months of age; mature dogs may also be affected. It is most common in the German shepherd dog. Panosteitis is a self-limiting dis-

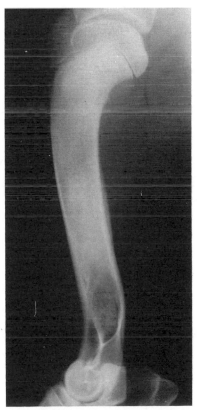

Figure 10–10. Lateral radiograph of the humerus in a dog with panosteitis. Medullary sclerosis is visualized in the mid-diaphyseal region of the humerus, in contrast to the more radiolucent, normal areas proximal and distal to the sclerotic area. A smooth periosteal reaction is present on the caudal, mid-diaphyseal cortex adjacent to the sclerotic region. Note the lesion in the caudal articular surface of the humeral head due to osteochondritis dissecans. (Courtesy of Dr. Michael Walker, University of Tennessee, Knoxville, TN.)

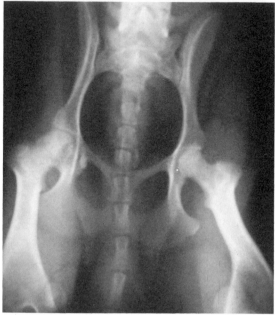

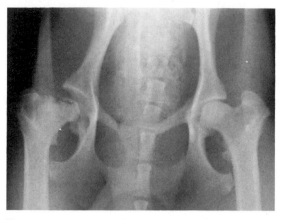

Figure 10–12. Ventrodorsal view of the pelvis of a dog with the later stages of aseptic idiopathic necrosis of the right femoral head. Extensive remodeling and fragmentation have substantially changed the normal size and shape of the femoral head. There is no longer continuity of the coxofemoral articular surfaces. Degenerative change is evidenced by osteophytes on the femoral neck. (Courtesy of Dr. Michael Walker, University of Tennessee, Knoxville, TN.)

Figure 10–11. Ventrodorsal radiograph of the pelvis of a dog with aseptic idiopathic necrosis of the right femoral head. The early stages of the diseases are indicated by the irregular areas of lysis in the femoral head. The femoral head has lost its normal shape.

of the medullary canal with coarse trabeculations, roughened endosteum, and a thickened cortex.

ASEPTIC IDIOPATHIC NECROSIS OF THE FEMORAL HEAD

This condition, which is also known as Legg-Calvé-Perthes disease, occurs in small dogs, 3 to 11 months of age. It is usually unilateral, but may be bilateral. The cause is unknown. The early radiographic changes consist of irregular areas of lysis in the femoral head and a widening of the articular space (Fig. 10–11)[5, 6] followed by flattening and collapse of the femoral head. Partial fragmentation of the femoral head may occur (Fig. 10–12). Because of disruption of the normal outline of the femoral head and discontinuity of the joint space, remodeling of the femoral neck and the acetabulum occur as secondary degenerative changes.

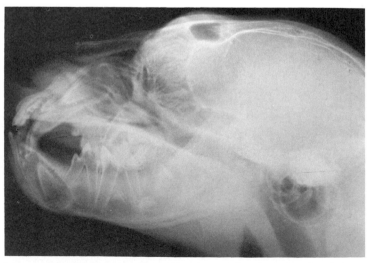

Figure 10–13. Lateral view of the skull of a cat with nutritional secondary hyperparathyroidism. There is a generalized decrease in bone opacity and decreased visualization of the lamina dura around the apical aspects of the mandibular tooth roots. (Courtesy of Dr. Michael Walker, University of Tennessee, Knoxville, TN.)

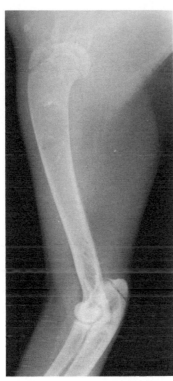

Figure 10–14. Lateral radiograph of the humerus of a cat with nutritional secondary hyperparathyroidism. Bone cortices are abnormally thin. The trabecular appearance in the distal humerus is coarse. These signs occur because of generalized increased bone resorption. (Courtesy of Dr. Michael Walker, University of Tennessee, Knoxville, TN.)

NUTRITIONAL SECONDARY HYPERPARATHYROIDISM

An imbalance of dietary and resulting blood levels of calcium and phosphorus causes the parathyroid gland to release excess amounts of parathormone, which in turn causes increased resorption of bone. Hyperparathyroidism due to nutritional imbalance is termed nutritional secondary hyperparathyroidism. This condition can occur at any age if an animal is improperly fed. Because the young animal is growing rapidly and has additional nutritional needs, however, it is most likely to occur in the immature animal.

Radiographically, there is a generalized decrease in bone opacity. This decrease is often best visualized in the mandible, where there is loss of visualization of the lamina dura.[5] In addition, there is increased contrast between the teeth and the remainder of the mandible (Fig. 10–13). The cortices of the long bones become thinner and the trabeculae become coarse and prominent (Fig. 10–14).[5, 6] If not remedied, secondary signs of osteoporosis occur, including folding fractures of long bones, compression fractures of vertebrae, and pelvic malformation.

References

1. Boudrieau RJ, Hohn RB, and Bardet JF: Osteochondritis dissecans of the elbow in the dog. J Am Anim Hosp Assoc 19:627, 1983.
2. Fox SM, Bloomberg MS, and Bright RM: Developmental anomalies of the canine elbow. J Am Anim Hosp Assoc 19:605, 1983.
3. Olsson S-E: The early diagnosis of fragmented coronoid process and osteochondritis dissecans of the canine elbow joint. J Am Anim Hosp Assoc 19:616, 1983.
4. Wind AP: Incidence and radiographic appearance of fragmented coronoid process. Calif Vet 36:19, 1982.
5. Morgan JP: Radiology in Veterinary Orthopedics. Philadelphia, Lea & Febiger, 1972.
6. Owens JM: Radiographic Interpretation for the Small Animal Clinician. St. Louis, Ralston Purina Co., 1982.
7. Woodard JC: Canine hypertrophic osteodystrophy, a study of the spontaneous disease in littermates. Vet Pathol 19:337, 1982.

CHAPTER 11

FRACTURE HEALING AND COMPLICATIONS

ROBERT L. TOAL

INITIAL RADIOGRAPHS

If a limb fracture is suspected, at least two radiographs taken at a 90 degree angle to each other should be made. The joints above and below the affected bone should be included in the field of view; this allows for the assessment of joint involvement and degree of fragment rotation. The use of sedation or anesthesia is helpful so the animal may be positioned properly, if its use is not contraindicated medically. A horizontal beam craniocaudal radiograph may be obtained when patient condition, limb swelling, or decreased range of motion prevents the use of standard views of the limb in extension.[1] If patient status precludes sedation and sufficient help is not available, a single lateral radiograph can be obtained initially to provide an idea of the extent of the lesions. Supplemental radiographs can be made at a more opportune time. Techniques such as stressed views, oblique projections, and opposite limb comparison radiographs are helpful in some patients.

FRACTURE RECOGNITION

Radiographically, a fracture is identified as a disruption in bone continuity. Alterations in bone size, shape, position, and function are usually present to some degree. One or more radiolucent fracture lines may be seen.

Occasionally, a fracture may be present but bone distraction is minimal, making radiographic detection difficult (Fig. 11–1). Reasons for fracture nonvisualization include poor quality radiographs; a fracture line not tangential to the x-ray beam; early cortical stress fractures; minimal displacement, as in physeal fractures; and obscured visualization by overlying structures. Repeat radiographs obtained with the use of proper technique or oblique projections may help. In some instances, radiographs taken 1 to 2 weeks later show a more apparent fracture line or early callus formation. In certain instances, such as in early cortical stress fractures, nuclear scintigraphy is indicated because of its inherent sensitivity in detecting bone lesions when compared with conventional radiography (see Chapter 47).

Occasionally, normal or variant anatomy may simulate fracture. This situation occurs with normal or ectopic nutrient foraminae,[2] normal and accessory ossification centers, inconstant and multipartite sesamoids, open physes, and syndesmoses (Fig. 11–2).

FRACTURE DESCRIPTION

The radiographic evaluation of a fracture should be systematic to ensure that important information is not overlooked. A radiographic de-

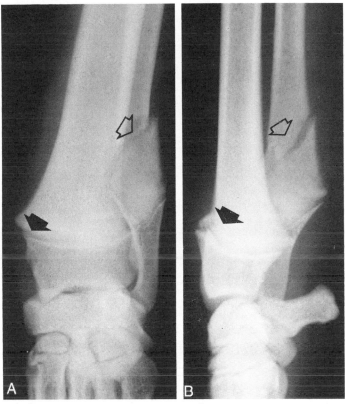

Figure 11–1. Craniocaudal *(A)* and lateral *(B)* radiographs of an oblique fracture of the distal ulnar metaphysis with slight lateral and caudal displacement *(open arrows)*. In addition, there is a fracture of the distal radial physis with slight lateral and cranial displacement *(solid arrows)*. Minimal displacement makes radiographic detection of the distal radial physeal fracture difficult.

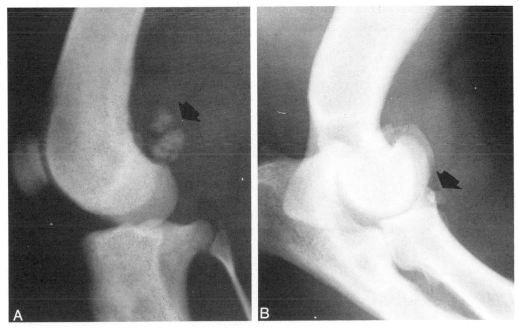

Figure 11–2. Examples of pseudofractures. *A*, multipartite lateral gastrocnemius fabellae *(arrow)*; *B*, inconstant sesamoid bone associated with the ulnar collateral ligament *(arrow)*.

scription begins with the fracture type, the bone involved, and the location within the bone.[3] The direction of fissure fractures and the presence of any joint involvement are noted, and the presence of intra-articular fragments is carefully assessed. These fragments may be associated with luxations, subluxations, or any joint trauma. Next, the positional changes of the major distal fragment relative to the proximal fragment should be characterized. The direction of displacement and angulation of the fracture fragments should be evaluated. Alterations in bone length are described as overriding (bone shortening) or distraction (bone lengthening). Rotational deformities should be noted, although unstable distal fragments that are fully moveable vary markedly in rotational direction. Lastly, the amount of soft-tissue change should be characterized in terms of size (swelling or atrophy) and opacity (emphysema, opaque foreign objects).

FRACTURE CLASSIFICATION

The fracture type can influence the therapeutic plan, the rate of fracture healing, the appearance of fracture callus and the possibility of postoperative complications. Most fractures can be classified according to one or more of the types.

Open Versus Closed. Open fractures have a skin defect in the region of the fracture site.

The loss of the protective skin barrier may result in wound contamination and possible infection. Radiographically, the bone may or may not protrude from the skin. Occasionally, foreign debris, metallic opacities, or tissue emphysema are identified. Frequently no radiographic clues are seen, making clinical assessment important. A closed fracture does not have a skin defect in the region of the fracture site. The categorization of a fracture as open or closed is a basic first step in fracture classification. The method of fracture repair, patient management, and prognosis are directly influenced by this information.[4]

Number and Extent of Fracture Lines. *Simple complete* fractures have one fracture line, which extends through the bone. The direction may be characterized as transverse, spiral, or oblique. In an *incomplete* fracture, only a portion of the bone or a single bone cortex has a fracture line. Incomplete fractures are frequently seen as fissure fractures, which may be seen originating with the main fracture site and radiating into the major fragments or even a joint (Fig. 11–3). Other examples of incomplete fractures include greenstick fractures in immature animals, folding (pathologic) fractures in osteoporotic bone, and stress fractures.

Stress (fatigue) fractures are microfractures in the bone cortex from cyclic loading, resulting in local strain of bone tissues.[5] Initially, no radiographic signs are found although increased

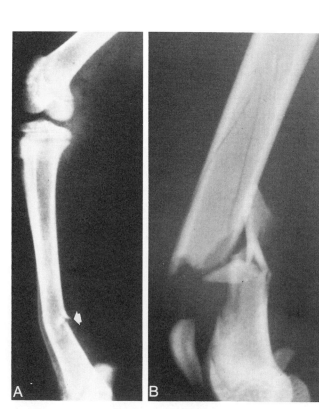

Figure 11–3. *A,* incomplete fracture in a cat. An obvious fracture line is not seen, although discontinuity of the bone cortex is present *(arrow). B,* lateral femoral radiograph of a comminuted distal femoral fracture in a cat. Several fissure fractures radiate into the proximal fragment.

radiotracer uptake may be seen scintigraphically (see Chapter 47). When present, roentgen signs include focal bone porosity, faint periosteal reaction, and oblique to dish-shaped fracture lines that involve a single cortex. *Comminuted* fractures have multiple fracture lines that communicate to a single plane or point. *Multiple* fractures have more than one fracture line within a bone and the fracture lines do not communicate. *Impacted* fractures result from compression forces that shorten bone length by crushing bone tissue. These injuries may occur in vertebral bodies or open physes.

Avulsion Versus Chip Fractures. Avulsion and chip fractures result in fragments of variable size with a defect or fracture "bed" in the parent bone. Avulsion fractures are associated with excessive traction by a muscle, ligament, or tendon; they are usually periarticular, intra-articular or involve traction epiphyses. Chip fractures are small fragments that usually result from direct bone trauma or hyperextension. In a general sense, chip fractures may describe any small fracture fragment. Periarticular chip fractures should be distinguished from accessory ossification centers and soft-tissue dystrophic mineralization. Differentiation is not always possible radiographically; findings should thus be correlated with the clinical signs.

Salter Fractures. The various combinations of metaphyseal-physeal-epiphyseal fractures in growing bone are called Salter fractures. Six classes have been described that relate fracture type to prognosis (Fig. 11–4).[6–7, 8] Important clinical factors include the age of the patient at the time of injury (remaining growth potential)

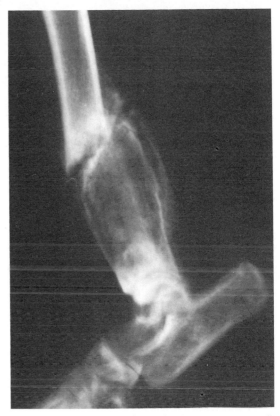

Figure 11–5. Lateral radiograph shows an expansile lesion of the distal tibia with cortical thinning and generalized osteolysis. There is a pathologic fracture at the junction of the expansile lesion and the normal tibial shaft. A cuff of periosteal bone is present subjacent to the fracture. Histologic diagnosis: fibrosarcoma.

and the specific physis involved (percentage contribution to overall bone length). Serious complications of Salter fractures include clinically evident growth disturbances and joint abnormalities. Type II injuries are the most common type of Salter fracture. Salter V injuries most often result in growth deformities, especially when the distal ulnar physis is involved.

Some physeal fractures are minimally displaced, making initial detection difficult (Fig. 11–1). Quality radiographs of both limbs should be obtained and then compared. Malalignment of the epiphysis relative to the diaphysis or a disruption of the radiolucent physis when compared to the normal opposite limb may be the only detectable signs of fracture. If a physeal fracture is identified and the potential for growth disturbance is high, repeat evaluation every 10 to 14 days is indicated.

Pathologic Fractures. This type is a spontaneous fracture that occurs without history of overt trauma in bone weakened by a pre-existing lesion. It may occur, for example, in hyperparathyroidism and is suspected when a fracture

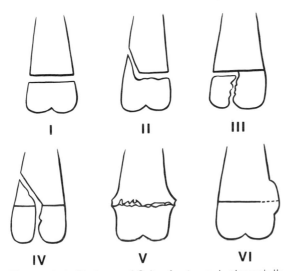

Figure 11–4. Six types of Salter fractures. I; physeal; II: physeal-metaphyseal; III: physeal-epiphyseal; IV: physeal-epiphyseal-metaphyseal; V: impacted physis; VI: eccentric physeal impaction resulting in transphyseal bridging.

occurs in bone that radiographically is less opaque and has narrow cortices and thin and scant trabeculae. Impacted fractures in vertebral bodies and folding fractures in long bones are examples of pathologic fractures. A folding fracture in a long bone is analogous to a soda straw that has been bent. Bone discontinuity is not identified, although malalignment is present and there is a thin sclerotic crease of bone where the cortex has collapsed. Pathologic fractures may also occur in bones weakened by tumor, congenital cysts, or infection; a fracture in the presence of an aggressive or expansile bone lesion is indicative (Fig. 11–5).

FRACTURE HEALING

Three distinct histologic patterns of bone healing have been identified: (1) direct healing of bone by osseous tissue; (2) union of fragments by fibrous connective tissue, which is later converted to bone (intramembranous ossification); and (3) callus formation that matures through a sequence of granulation tissue, cartilage, mineralized cartilage, and finally replacement by bone (endochondral ossification).[9]

Primary Bone Healing. Direct healing of a fracture by the initial formation of bone tissue has been termed primary bone healing.[10, 11] Primary bone healing can occur under conditions of rigid fixation in which micromotion of a contact or gap area results in less than 2 percent strain. This degree of stability is usually achieved only by anatomic reduction and compression fixation. In areas of stable bone contact, direct extension of haversian osteons unites the fragments. In minute fracture gaps that are rigidly stabilized, lamellar bone forms after granulation tissue or woven bone deposition. The process in each instance is bony union through direct bone formation; callus formation is not involved in the process. Although this repair is exclusively of bone tissue, it is mechanically inferior to normal cortical bone. Normal strength is attained through extensive remodeling, which may take months to complete.

Primary bone healing is characterized radiographically by a lack of periosteal callus, a gradual loss in opacity of the fragment ends, and a progressive disappearance of the fracture line. The re-establishment of cortex and medullary cavity continuity occurs quickly (Fig. 11–6). If anatomic reduction is not achieved and micromotion is uncontrolled, secondary bone healing will predominate.

Secondary Bone Healing. This process involves fibrous connective tissue or fibrocartilaginous callus, which is replaced by bone. The cells participating in the healing process are pluripotential mesenchymal elements, which differentiate into osteoblasts, fibroblasts, or chondroblasts depending on the specific microenvironment at the time. Bone cannot form in an unfavorable environment (motion). Therefore, under conditions of instability, the mesenchymal cells of the periosteum respond by the production of a fibrous to fibrocartilaginous callus. With time, this callus bridges the fragments and increases stability. The stable environment permits vascularization of the callus, resulting in callus ossification and thus bony union. Callus size is determined by a host of factors: fracture type, the degree of stability, width of the fracture gap, and the condition of the regional soft tissues (vascularity).

The following radiographic description of uncomplicated secondary bone healing is of a simple, long-bone diaphyseal fracture that has been stabilized with an intramedullary pin.[12] By the first week, fragment ends begin to lose their sharp margins and the fracture gap increases slightly in width. These changes are due to a combination of interfragmentary motion and vascular ingrowth. Within the next 2 weeks, variable amounts of periosteal, endosteal, and intercortical callus appear. Initial periosteal cal-

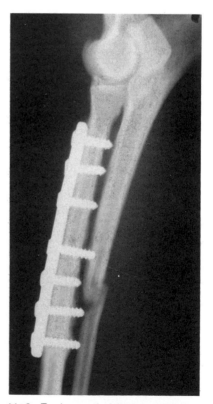

Figure 11–6. Twelve-week follow-up radiograph of a healed proximal radial fracture. The fracture line is no longer evident and there is continuity of the cortex and medullary cavity. Anatomic reduction and stable fixation resulted in bone healing without the formation of a periosteal callus. The ulnar fracture is still evident.

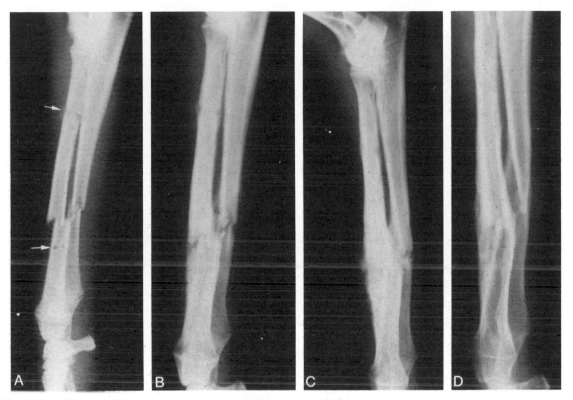

Figure 11–7. Sequential lateral radiographs of a midshaft antebrachial fracture demonstrating secondary bone healing. A, initial post-reduction radiograph shows approximately 50 percent purchase of the fracture fragments. The limb is casted. Pins were used with a reduction apparatus causing the pin tracts in the radius *(arrows)*. B, poorly mineralized immature callus (2-week follow-up). C, mature callus begins to bridge the fracture (4-week follow-up). D, healed fracture (10-week follow-up).

lus is faintly mineralized and has irregular margins; it is located subjacent to the cortex on each fragment a slight distance from the fracture gap. By 4 weeks, the callus is smoother and more opaque and is visualized as a cuff of bone beginning to bridge the fracture gap; the fracture line should be smaller in size. After 4 weeks, the fracture line is slowly obliterated and the bony callus bridges the fracture area. At this point, the callus should be as opaque as normal bone. After 12 weeks, the external callus remodels until the continuity of the cortex and medullary cavity is re-established. This final process may take several months to years. Healing in individual patients varies from this description, depending on several factors (Fig. 11–7).

FACTORS THAT MODIFY FRACTURE HEALING

In the evaluation of fracture healing the many factors that influence healing or contribute to complications must be considered. Understanding their role in part explains the radiographic appearance in follow-up evaluations.

Vascular Integrity. Normal vascular ingrowth at the fracture site occurs within the first 10 days after injury. Radiographically, this ingrowth is seen as slight demineralization of fragment ends that results in slight widening of the fracture gap and fuzzy fragment margins. Isolated bone fragments that are revascularizing respond similarly. Regional vascular status also influences callus characteristics because of the effects of relative tissue hypoxia on stem cell differentiation.[13] A rich vascular network results in pluripotential daughter cells that become osteoblasts. Decreased vascularity below a critical point results in chondroblasts or fibroblasts. The produced bone or fibrocartilage differs in radiographic opacity. Because of compromised circulation, the initial callus formation at the fracture site is fibrocartilaginous (soft-tissue opacity). Initial mineralized callus forms at a slight distance from the fracture gap where the circulation is less compromised. With subsequent vascular ingrowth, the entire callus mineralizes.

The temporal sequence of revascularization after a fracture and the associated roentgen findings vary for each fracture. This variation is the result of differences in the extent of the initial circulatory compromise, post-reduction fragment stability, and the available soft tissue in the region, which is a principal source of neovascularization for healing bone (extraosseous blood supply of healing bone).[14]

Fracture Location. The anatomic location of a fracture can influence the healing response. This fact is best demonstrated by metaphyseal fractures, which have an early onset of mineralized callus when compared with diaphyseal fractures; this is due to the rich blood supply in the metaphyseal region and to the abundant trabecular bone with its increased surface area. In general, metaphyseal fractures heal more rapidly than diaphyseal fractures. Antebrachial diaphyseal fractures in miniature breeds and tibial shaft fractures in mature dogs heal more slowly and have a greater incidence of complication than other diaphyseal fractures, because there is decreased soft-tissue support and poor vascular recruitment in the region.[15, 16] Healing capital femoral physeal fractures and femoral neck fractures will undergo rapid revascularization if they are adequately reduced and stabilized. In some cases, an exuberant fibrovascular response can occur, which causes local osteolysis of the femoral neck.[17] Radiographically, this response results in femoral neck thinning, which can proceed to an apple-core appearance (Fig. 11–8).

Degree of Motion. Stability and adequate blood supply are related factors that are essen-

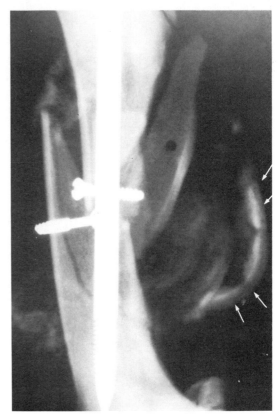

Figure 11–9. Lateral radiograph of a comminuted femoral fracture 3 weeks after surgery. The surgical devices have not maintained stability and the main fracture fragments are telescoping. There is a mineralized periosteal reaction in the soft tissue typical of stripped periosteum (arrows). Radiographically, the fracture fragments are sharply marginated, suggesting deficient regional microvasculature.

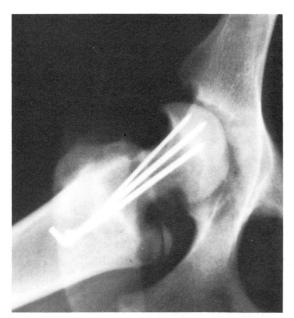

Figure 11–8. Follow-up radiograph of a capital femoral physeal fracture 1 month after repair. Bone resorption in the femoral neck. An exuberant fibrovascular healing response resulted in local osteolysis, producing an "apple core" appearance.

tial for normal fracture healing. An unstable fracture results in damage to the microvasculature in the region. Radiographically, fracture fragments may retain their sharp margins longer than usual. Initial callus at the fracture site is usually poorly mineralized and nonbridging (Fig. 11–9). Periosteal stimulation due to fragment motion may result in callus formation at a point distant from the fracture site. The callus initially presents as ill-defined, poorly marginated periosteal new bone that extends over a large portion of the diaphysis. This later finding, however, is not specific for fragment motion; it can occur secondary to periosteal stripping at the time of injury or surgery, or to early osteomyelitis. Clinical signs may help in this distinction.

Persistent motion results in exuberant fibrocartilaginous callus formation, which is an attempt by the body to provide stability. If the callus later mineralizes, it usually does not bridge the fracture gap. Intramedullary pin migration may also be present (Fig. 11–10). If

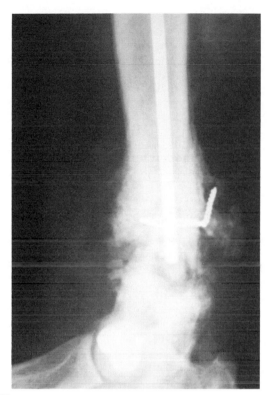

Figure 11–10. Follow-up lateral radiograph of a "Y"-type distal humeral fracture 2 months after repair. There is migration of the large intramedullary pin in a proximal direction. An exuberant non-bridging periosteal and endosteal callus is visualized. These changes suggest instability at the fracture site and infection.

Periosteal stripping alone can stimulate the production of new bone. In these instances, the extent of the periosteal reaction often exceeds the anatomic limit of the fracture itself. Damaged regional vasculature regenerates with time as stability improves.

Poor post-reduction apposition may adversely affect stability and thus callus characteristics and healing time. Large fracture gaps require more callus and time to bridge the fragments. Good reduction and alignment minimize the callus requirement and promote anatomic restoration. Good alignment is also important for proper joint function and helps to prevent fracture disease and osteoarthrosis.

Age. An immature skeleton is rapidly growing and has a more extensive blood supply than the adult. Because of these factors, juvenile bone heals more rapidly (2 to 4 weeks) and with more exuberant callus formation than mature bone. In addition, the young animal exhibits a periosteal reaction after injury that is especially evident at sites where heavy fascial attachments

motion is severe, complications such as delayed union or non-union may result.

Adequate stabilization and vascular integrity lead to the early formation of a well-mineralized callus. The callus is small to moderate in size, sharply marginated, and limited to the fracture site. Rigid fixation results in minimal to no callus formation (Fig. 11–6).

Fracture Type and Degree of Post-Reduction Apposition. The type of fracture, degree of initial displacement, and accuracy of reduction influences fracture healing characteristics. Spiral and long, oblique diaphyseal fractures heal with more callus than do transverse fractures. Comminuted fractures with multiple fragments may heal more slowly and with more variable callus than do simple fractures. Gunshot fractures with severe soft-tissue injury are frequently associated with delayed union (Fig. 11–11).[18] Open fractures have a greater tendency for osteomyelitis and complications than do closed fractures.

Severe displacement of fragments with marked overriding indicates severe disruption of the periosteum and regional vasculature.

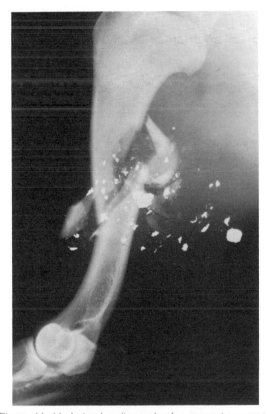

Figure 11–11. Lateral radiograph of a severely comminuted gunshot fracture of the humerus. Multiple metallic fragments are identified within the soft tissues. Gunshot fractures are open fractures that usually have extensive regional soft-tissue trauma due to the projectile. Both of these factors contribute to complications in the healing process. This fracture was stabilized by using a Kirschner device, and eventually healed 1 year later.

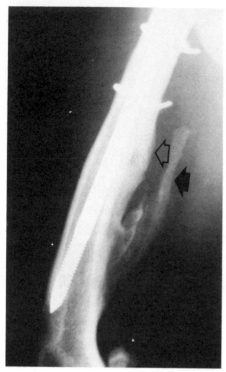

Figure 11–12. Lateral radiograph of a pinned femoral fracture. There is mineralization in the area of attachment of the adductor muscle *(solid arrow)*. Mature callus is present at the fracture site *(open arrow)*.

deformities can then result, especially if the distal radius and ulna are involved (Figs. 11–13 to 11–15). Physeal growth disturbances may occur after soft-tissue trauma alone, without the presence of a fracture.[19] The clinician should be aware of this fact. Radiographs obtained after 2 weeks should be considered if growth deformity is suspected.

POST-REDUCTION AND FOLLOW-UP RADIOGRAPHIC EVALUATION

Initial Postoperative Evaluation

The initial postoperative radiographs should be evaluated for the quality of fracture reduction, fragment alignment, and proper placement of orthopedic fixation devices. The degree of fracture reduction refers to the amount of fragment ends that are in contact with each other. For simple fractures, 50 percent contact is the acceptable minimum for adequate healing, but more is desirable. Joint fractures require more accurate reduction for adequate function. Joint incongruities are identified as "step" deformities or fracture gaps that disrupt articular contour.

Fragment alignment and rotation should also be assessed. Exact anatomic alignment is desirable but is impossible to accomplish in all fractures for all fragments. Rotation of the distal fragment relative to the proximal fragment is an important finding that may have serious consequences if not identified and corrected. The accurate assessment of alignment and rotational deformities, however, requires the use of good radiographic positioning techniques. Excess abduction or torsion of the distal limb by the holder during radiography may simulate rotational or angular malalignment of the distal fragment in the postoperative radiograph. In addition, changes in the angle of the x-ray beam relative to the fracture may project fragments differently. These artifacts can be avoided if the animal is carefully positioned.

are stripped from bone, such as the adductor muscle attachment to the caudal femur (lateral lip of the facies aspera). In this instance, a prominent spike of new bone formation coursing proximally in the caudal musculature can occur. This finding is seen to a variable degree in all dogs but seems to be more prominent in the younger animal (Fig. 11–12).

Fractures to the growing physis usually involve the zone of hypertrophied chondrocytes. Regional trauma may be sufficiently severe to compromise the epiphyseal vasculature or to disrupt the germinal layer directly. Growth

Figure 11–13. *A,* craniocaudal radiograph of the antebrachium of an immature dog. Distal radial and ulnar fractures are apparent. *B* and *C,* 6 weeks after application of external fixation. There was clinical evidence of valgus deformity of the manus when the fixation device was removed. The fractures appear to be healing but the manus valgus is apparent and there is caudal angulation of the distal radial epiphysis. These deformities were not treated. *D* and *E,* 5 months later. There is extensive valgus deformity and cranial bowing of the radius. These changes resulted from insufficient longitudinal ulnar growth due to physeal trauma, which occurred at the time of the original fracture. Had proper therapy been instituted when these deformities were detected (*B* and *C*), the development of these severe changes would have been prevented.

Figure 11–14. *A,* elbow of a dog with insufficient longitudinal ulnar growth, which resulted in subluxation of the humeroulnar articulation. This is the third radiographic sign associated with insufficient longitudinal ulnar growth (see Fig. 11–13 for illustration of manus valgus and radial bowing). *B,* after distal ulnar diaphyseal ostectomy. Release of ulnar tension allowed the proximal ulna to assume its normal articular relationship with the humerus.

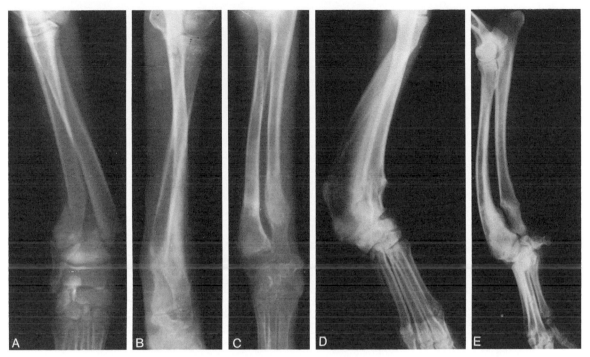

Figure 11–13. *See legend on opposite page*

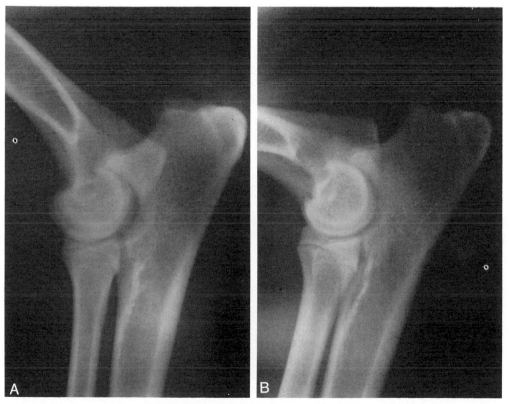

Figure 11–14. *See legend on opposite page*

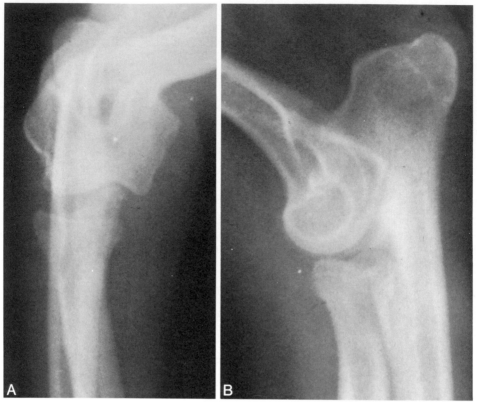

Figure 11–15. *A* and *B,* elbow of a dog with insufficient longitudinal radial growth, which resulted in distal subluxation of the radius and proximal subluxation of the ulna from the humerus, a change frequently observed in dogs with this condition.

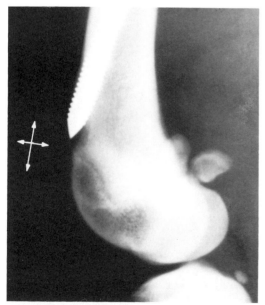

Figure 11–16. Immediate post-reduction radiograph of a midshaft femoral fracture. Notice that the pin encroaches upon the joint. The pin should be retracted slightly. *Crossed arrows,* position of the patella.

Next, the orthopedic fixation device is evaluated for placement and the ability to maintain reduction and to prevent motion throughout the healing phase. Weakness in fixation placement, if caught early, can be corrected and disastrous complications may be avoided. Intramedullary pins should be seated deeply and should span the fracture gap adequately. The pins should be of sufficient size for the bone involved and should not penetrate the joint (Fig. 11–16). The far and near pins of a two-pin Kirschner apparatus should be properly angled toward the bone, just penetrating both cortices. Wires should be of adequate size, should not be kinked or broken, and each arm should be twisted equally. The wire should be seated snugly against the cortex with a minimum of space between it and the bone. Bone plate size is important to evaluate. Excessively large plates may result in stress protection of the bone and osteoporosis. Implants that are too small may result in instability at the fracture site, with delayed union or non-union as a possible sequela. Bone plates should be anchored securely to the bone, with a minimum of six cortices engaged by the bone screws above and below the fractures. Bone screws should be solidly seated and fully engaged in each cortex. The orthopedic devices should not cause fragment distraction or be interposed between major fragments.

Follow-up Evaluations

Soft-tissue thickness influences beam attenuation and thus radiographic opacity. The limb should be remeasured during each radiographic evaluation and appropriate kVp and ma factors should be selected on the basis of an established technique chart. Limb atrophy changes the thickness measurement significantly during fracture healing. Follow-up studies in which the same exposure factors were used as were for the initial fracture radiograph may vary markedly in tissue opacity.

Bandages, casts, and external fixation rods should be removed if possible before radiography. A clear, unobstructed view of the fracture area is then assured. If cast removal is impractical, the following technical alterations are suggested. For plaster casts, measure the cast limb and increase the normal kVp by 10 percent. For fiberglass casts and heavy bandages, measure the cast limb and use that kVp.

The protocol for repeat radiographs in fracture healing varies with the clinician and with the clinical circumstances of each case. Obviously, every follow-up office visit of a fracture patient need not include a radiographic examination. Good clinical judgment should be exercised in this regard. In general, a basic radiographic plan should be followed and modified when appropriate.[20] Radiographs should be made immediately after initial fracture reduction or after any major alterations (removal, adjustments, or additions) of stabilization devices. Routine follow-up radiographs are made every 3 to 4 weeks (or longer) to assess healing. If the clinical signs and history suggest complications, immediate re-examination is indicated. Revision of the routine follow-up schedule may be necessary if complications are seen that necessitate more frequent monitoring.

Follow-up radiographs should be evaluated for progression in the fracture healing process or the possible development of complications. This evaluation is facilitated by comparing current radiographs with previous studies, especially the immediate postoperative and the most recent follow-up examination. To assure that vital information is not overlooked, the ABCDS mnemonic system can be used when evaluating post-reduction films (G. Boring, personal communication). The five letters in the mnemonic stand for Alignment, Bone, Cartilage (joints),

Device (orthopedic appliance or device), and Soft tissues. By utilizing this system, a complete radiographic evaluation is assured.

Alignment. The major and minor fracture fragments should be evaluated for any changes in alignment, reduction, or rotation since the previous study. This evaluation is especially important for poorly reduced fractures or for those stabilized with intramedullary pins in which rotational forces are not adequately controlled.

Bone. The bone should be evaluated for the progression of fracture healing and callus formation. All fragments should be involved in the healing response and should be in the same location as in previous radiographs. Fragments that are poorly vascularized retain their sharp margins radiographically. With time, they can revascularize and become incorporated into the healing process or they can become ischemic and develop into a sequestrum. Persistence of sharp margins and an increased opacity of the fragment on subsequent radiographs indicate sequestral formation.

Fragments removed surgically create defects in the region of the fracture. Large defects seldom fill in completely and may serve as a point of stress concentration, rendering the implant vulnerable to mechanical failure (bending or breaking). The bone may also be weaker at this site when the implant is removed.

The overall bone opacity and architecture should also be evaluated. Complications such as osteomyelitis and osteoporosis, if gone unsuspected, may be well advanced by the next follow-up examination. The routine evaluation of bone opacity and architecture can help to identify suspect areas and thus to plan treatment accordingly.

Excessive periosteal reactions are frequently seen either at or distant from the fracture site. These reactions can result from a number of possibilities: normal callus for that fracture, rotational instability, infection, and periosteal stripping at the time of injury or surgery (Figs. 11–12 and 11–17). On follow-up studies many plated bones have a variably sized callus. This finding may suggest some instability, but other possibilities include interfragmentary callus formation due to the size of the fracture gap, cancellous grafting with new bone production, and periosteal trauma during surgery.

Situations in which no to minimal callus formation is evident are occasionally encountered. Possibilities for such scant formation include too short an interval since fixation, primary bone healing (must have anatomic reduction and compression fixation), stable fixation resulting in minimal callus formation, compromised vascularity with poorly mineralized callus, and

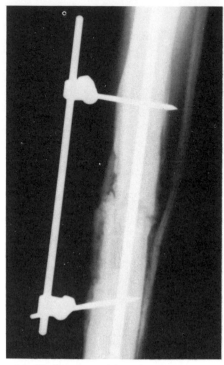

Figure 11–17. Craniocaudal radiograph 4 weeks after treatment of a midshaft tibial fracture. There is a smoothly marginated, continuous periosteal reaction surrounding the fragments distal to the fracture site. Periosteal stripping at the time of injury and slight rotational instability could account for the finding. The smooth margins suggest chronicity. When examined 2 weeks later, there was complete fragment union and the orthopedic devices were removed.

atrophic non-union. Clinical signs, history, and serial radiographs are helpful in distinguishing among these possibilities.

Cartilage. It is important to evaluate the joint spaces near the fracture. For articular fractures,

the apposition of fragments should be carefully evaluated on standard and oblique views. Joints should be scrutinized for evidence of migration of the orthopedic device into the joint space. The development of joint effusion, an irregular periosteal reaction, and subchondral bone lysis may signal septic arthritis. Joint effusion in the presence of osteophytes is suggestive of degenerative joint disease. The range of motion of the joint may be better evaluated clinically than radiographically.

Orthopedic Device Evaluation. The placement and position of the orthopedic implants should be compared with those on previous radiographs. Always check for movements, bending, or breakage of pins, wires, plates, and screws. Minimal implant bending can be detected by placing a straight edge on the radiograph. A loose implant is painful and does not provide the structural support for which it was intended. A radiolucency is often noted in bone at the point where a metallic device is located (Fig. 11–18). The radiograph "rule out" list for this finding includes motion of the implant or fracture fragments, osteomyelitis, and bone necrosis secondary to heat generated by high speed drills. It should be realized that bone loss around an implant may be sufficient to result in loosening, but should not result in detectable radiopacity changes; 50 percent of bone matrix must be lost before a lytic area is detectable radiographically.

The time to remove a surgical implant varies with each patient and should depend on a blend of clinical and radiographic information, but mostly good clinical judgment. Clinically, the limb should be palpably firm, nonpainful, and weight-bearing to some degree. Radiographically, pin implants are removed if the fracture line is not visible and normal callus bridges all or most of the fracture. Removal of plate im-

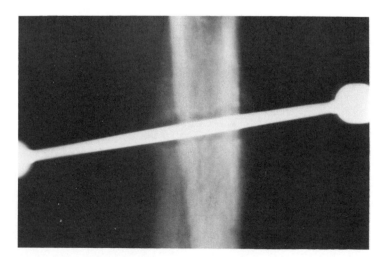

Figure 11–18. There is an obvious radiolucent tract surrounding this transverse Kirschner pin. This amount of bone loss is sufficient to result in implant loosening. Many of these pin tracts are infected, albeit subclinically.

plants follows similar principles, although callus is more variable, depending on the type and severity of the fracture and the rigidity of fixation. Suggested timetables for plate removal have been published.[21, 22] In one study 3 to 5 months for young animals and 5 to 14 months for adults were the recommended intervals.[23] Removal of screws and pins penetrating the cortex leaves defects in the bone. Although these areas fill with bone, the new bone is less opaque, and thus the defect remains radiographically apparent for months to years.[23] If an implant is removed prematurely or physical activity is too vigorous shortly after removal, refracture through the original fracture site may occur. Caution in implant removal is advised until experience is gained.

Soft Tissues. Post-surgical emphysema and soft-tissue swelling are usually gone or are significantly decreased within 7 to 10 days. Subcutaneous and fascial emphysema is recognized as rounded or linear air opacities within the soft tissues. Soft-tissue swelling is characterized by the loss of fascial plane visualization and increased limb size. Air pockets with soft-tissue swelling that recurs after initial subsidence indicate infection. Chronically, soft-tissue atrophy results in loss of fascial plane visualization with a decrease in muscle mass. Calcification of soft tissues in animals with a fracture is occasionally seen, possibly resulting from an isolated bone fragment or cancellous grafts within the soft tissue, dystrophic mineralization, mineralization of hematoma, and myositis ossificans. Soft-tissue mineralization can also occur in conjunction with an aggressive bone lesion secondary to osteomyelitis or fracture-associated sarcoma.

Fracture Complications

Malunion is defined as bone healing in an abnormal position. In long bones, malunion may be characterized as end to end, side to side, end to side, and cross-union with adjacent bones. These configurations are associated with variable degrees of angular and rotational deformity (Fig. 11–19). If deformity is severe, functional impairment may ensue or abnormal weight-bearing may result in joint arthrosis. When malunion occurs within a joint, the incongruity quickly leads to degenerative changes.

Delayed union is present when a fracture has not healed in the time that would be expected for the bone involved and the type of fracture (Table 11–1). Radiographically, fracture lines remain evident with minimal callus bridging the fracture gap. In addition, there may be minimal change in sharpness of fragment margins. Fragment motion due to instability is the most frequent cause of delayed union. If the

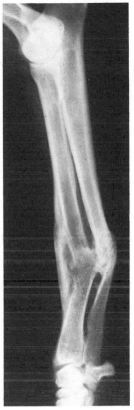

Figure 11–19. Lateral radiograph reveals a malunited fracture of the distal radius and ulna.

underlying cause is adequately corrected, healing will ensue. If the situation is not remedied, non-union may result (Fig. 11–20).

Non-union is the situation in which all evidence of fracture healing has ceased and the fragment ends have not united. Sequential radiographs are helpful in making this assessment.

Radiographically, non-union has been classified as hypertrophic and atrophic (Fig. 11–21). Clinically, it may be important to distinguish between the two types.[24] Hypertrophic non-

TABLE 11–1. APPROXIMATE TIME TO REACH CLINICAL UNION IN A NONCOMPLICATED DIAPHYSEAL FRACTURE*

Age of Animal	External Skeletal and Intramedullary Pin Fixation	Fixation with Plates
Under 3 mo	2–3 wks	4 wks
3–6 mo	4–6 wks	2–3 mo
6–12 mo	5–8 wks	3–4 mo
Over 1 yr	7–12 wks	5–8 mo

*From Brinker, WO, Hohn RB, and Prieur WD (Eds): Manual of Internal Fixation in Small Animals. New York, Springer Verlag, 1983, with permission.

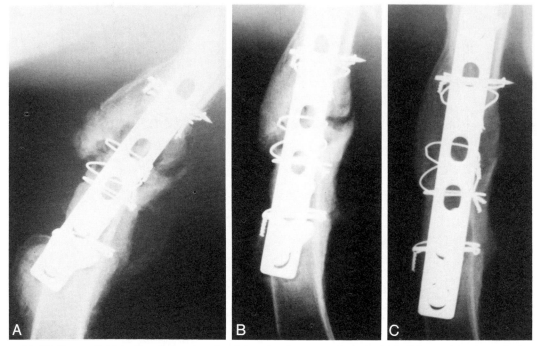

Figure 11–20. Sequential lateral radiographs of a delayed union, comminuted midshaft femoral fracture. *A,* 4-month follow-up radiograph shows malalignment of fragments, reactive nonbridging callus formation, and a visible fracture gap. *B,* 5 months later. There is an organized callus. Clinically, the limb was stable and not painful; the animal was bearing weight. *C,* 9 months later. Bridging callus obliterates the fracture gap. The fracture has healed.

union has a well-defined fracture gap, a small to large (elephant foot) nonbridging callus, sclerotic fracture ends with a closed marrow cavity, and fragment ends that are smooth, rounded, and well defined. Atrophic non-union has minimal if any callus formation, a well-defined fracture gap, and sharply marginated to tapered fragment ends with a sclerotic marrow cavity. Osteoporosis and soft-tissue atrophy may be present in each instance to varying degrees.

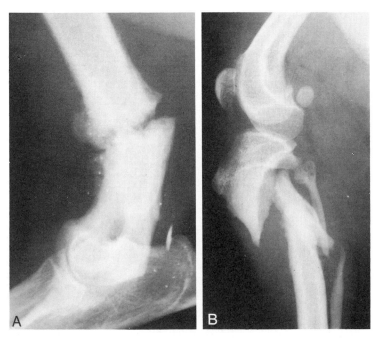

Figure 11–21. *A,* hypertrophic non-union. Lateral view of a chronic distal humeral fracture shows a well-defined fracture gap, nonbridging callus formation, and a sclerotic marrow cavity of the fragment ends. *B,* atrophic non-union. A 3-month follow-up radiograph of a proximal tibial fracture. There is fragment distraction with a well-defined fracture gap, no visible callus formation, sharply marginated fragment ends, and a sclerotic marrow cavity.

In some cases of non-union, a pseudoarthrosis (false joint) may form. Bone ends are connected by a fibrous tissue structure resembling a joint capsule that contains mucinous synovium-like fluid. Radiographically, presumptive evidence of a joint may be seen as a soft-tissue mass at the fracture site with focal bone fragments appearing in a flexed position.

When non-union is suspected, osteomedullography may be helpful to substantiate a diagnosis.[25] This technique is painful, and thus the animal should receive general anesthesia and not sedation. An 18 to 20 gauge sternal biopsy needle is placed into the medullary cavity of the distal fragment proximal to the physis. Three to five milliliters of water-soluble contrast medium are forcefully injected and a radiograph is made at the end of the injection. It is of utmost importance to compress the soft tissues at the level of the fracture site with a blood pressure cuff or elastic bandage. This pressure prevents the escape of contrast medium into the soft tissues, which leads to erroneous results. Demonstration of medullary vessels crossing the fracture gap into the proximal fragment suggests that healing is occurring. In man, these connections should be present by the 10th week at the latest. Lack of intramedullary vascular connections between the fracture fragments is compatible with non-union, and surgical intervention may then be necessary.

Osteomyelitis as a complication in bone healing is usually due to local infection rather than to hematogenous spread and localization. Potential causes include contamination from open fractures, long surgical procedures with wide exposure, excessive tissue damage in surgery (desiccation or trauma) and foreign objects (sequestra, sutures and sponges, and occasionally the implant itself). Clinical signs of acute osteomyelitis are fever, local heat, swelling, and pain. Initial radiographs may reveal soft-tissue swelling with or without subcutaneous emphysema. Repeat radiographs 7 to 10 days after the onset of clinical signs show a generalized irregular periosteal reaction. As the bone infection progresses, radiographic signs of an aggressive bone lesion may develop (Fig. 11–22) (see Chapters 2 and 12). A combination of cortico-medullary osteosclerosis with areas of osteolysis surrounding pin metallic implants is highly suggestive of pin tract osteomyelitis. A pin tract osteomyelitis is frequently associated with Kirschner pins (Fig. 11–18). Irregular periosteal reactions are often at the pin cortex junction.

Chronic osteomyelitis may first be noted as a purulent draining tract from an open wound. The persistent inflammation is usually due to a foreign object, most notably a sequestrum. A dead bone fragment is called a sequestrum. It may be paraosteal, cortical, or intramedullary in location. Classically, an infected sequestrum

Figure 11–22. *A,* lateral view 4 weeks after repair of a proximal femoral fracture. There is abundant periosteal reaction, cortical thinning, and permeative osteolysis of the distal femoral fragment. There is minimal callus formation associated with the fracture site. Radiographic diagnosis: osteomyelitis. *B,* lateral view 6 weeks after repair of a distal tibial fracture. There is abundant smooth to irregular periosteal reaction involving the entire diaphysis of the tibia. The proximal intramedullary pin encroaches on the stifle joint. Radiographic diagnosis: chronic osteomyelitis with encroachment of the implant on the stifle joint.

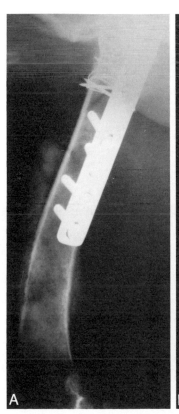
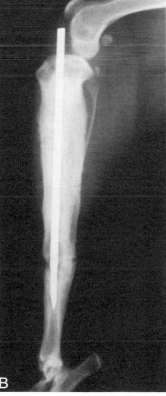

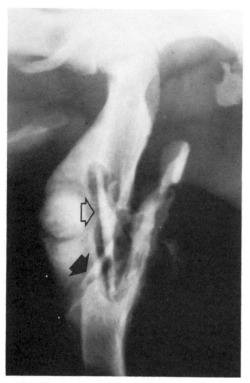

Figure 11–23. A, chronic midshaft femoral fracture had an associated draining tract for several months (cloaca). Two well-marginated radiopaque cortical fragments (sequestra) were identified *(arrows).* The largest fragment *(open arrow)* is surrounded by a zone of radiolucency and an outer rim of sclerotic bone (involucrum).

is recognized as a sharply marginated sclerotic fragment separated from the parent bone by a zone of radiolucency and an outer rim of sclerotic bone (involucrum) (Fig. 11–23). In some instances, the draining tract is evident (cloaca). Bone sequestra may be associated with infections or draining tracts. Failure of any isolated bone segment to be resorbed or revascularized may result in a sterile sequestra. In these instances, reaction of surrounding bone tissue is less exuberant and clinical signs of osteomyelitis are not present.

Nerve injury may be associated with the initial fracture (radial nerve in spiral humeral fractures) or with fracture repair and healing (sciatic nerve in femoral fracture pinning). Fracture-related sciatic palsy is related to surgically induced trauma, scar formation in the region of the nerve, and the proximal placement of the pin in the femur.[26] The more medial is the exit of the pin relative to the greater trochanter and the longer is the exposed proximal portion of the pin, the more likely is the occurrence of sciatic entrapment (Fig. 11–24). Thus, postoperative femoral radiographs should be evaluated for proximal pin location.

Osteoporosis may result from chronic disuse

of the limb or from stress protection by the orthopedic device. A generalized decrease in bone opacity with coarse trabeculation involving the entire limb signifies disuse osteoporosis. The bone may become hypoplastic. Osteoporosis may occur within 2 to 3 weeks in very young animals, but takes longer in the adult. A focal decrease in bone opacity and cortical thickness subjacent to an orthopedic implant suggests osteoporosis due to stress protection by the implant. Stress protection is related to increased implant size and stiffness and not to implant type (plate or pin) (Fig. 11–25A).

Joint complications after fractures include degenerative joint disease, ankylosis, and soft-tissue muscular and capsular contracture. Physeal growth deformities can follow direct trauma to the physis or may result from radioulnar synostosis (Fig. 11–13 to 11–15).

Fracture-associated sarcomas in the dog have been reviewed.[27] The etiology is unknown, but theories include coincidental spontaneous os-

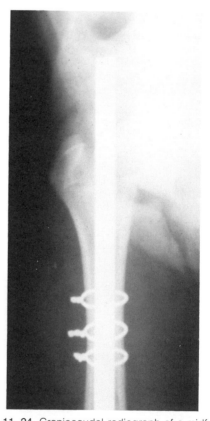

Figure 11–24. Craniocaudal radiograph of a midfemoral fracture immediately after repair with three full cerclage wires and a large intramedullary pin. There is a more medial exit of the proximal pin relative to the greater trochanter and a long, exposed proximal portion of the pin. Both of these factors contribute to a reactive tissue scar that could entrap the sciatic nerve. The therapeutic plan would include cutting the pin to decrease its length.

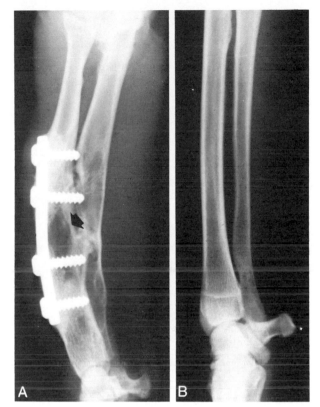

Figure 11-25. *A*, lateral view of the antebrachium of a 2-year-old dog 1 year after corrective osteotomy for radius curvus. The dog was moderately lame and exhibited elbow pain. A large bone plate with four bone screws is affixed to the radius. There is medullary sclerosis surrounding the bone screws and a focal area of osteopenia involving the radius subjacent to the bone plate and two innermost screws *(arrow)*. These findings are compatible with osteoporosis secondary to stress protection. In addition, the entire distal limb exhibits a generalized decrease in bone opacity, cortical thinning, and a coarse texture of the trabecular bone, indicating osteoporosis. *B*, the distal antebrachium of a normal dog. Compare the cortical thickness and trabecular bone with that in *A*.

teosarcomas, carcinogenesis due to metallic implants, and the cocarcinogenic effects of chronic inflammation in an environment in which stem cells are proliferating (fracture healing). Current evidence suggests that the latter is the most likely cause. The overall incidence is low and a variable post-fracture latency period is usually present (mean, 5.8 years). The femoral diaphysis is the most frequently involved site of fracture-associated sarcoma. The roentgen signs are those of an aggressive bone lesion with soft-tissue mineralization, which occurs in the location of a previous fracture that had experienced complications when healing (osteomyelitis). A draining fistula may be present in some instances, and thus osteomyelitis may be present simultaneously. The lungs should always be examined radiographically for potential metastatic disease when limb neoplasia is suspected.

References

1. Walker M: Horizontal beam radiography as a diagnostic aid for trauma of the abdomen and extremities. *In* Scientific Proceeding, Vol. II. 42nd Annual Meeting of American Animal Hospital Association, Cincinnati, OH, 1975, pp. 254–256.
2. Orsini PG, Rendano VT, and Sack WO: Ectopic nutrient foramina in the third metatarsal bone of the horse. Equine Vet J *13*:132, 1981.
3. Pitt M, and Speer D: Radiologic reporting of orthopedic trauma. Med Radiogr Photogr *15*:14, 1982.
4. Nunamaker D: Management of infected fractures—osteomyelitis. Vet Clin North Am [Small Anim Pract]: 5:259, 1975.
5. Carter D, and Spengler D. Biomechanics of fracture. *In* Sumner-Smith G (Ed): Bone in Clinical Orthopedics. Philadelphia, WB Saunders, 1982, pp. 315–316.
6. Salter RB, and Harris WR. Injuries involving the epiphyseal plate. J Bone Joint Surg 45:587, 1963.
7. Llewellyn HR. Growth plate injuries—diagnosis, prognosis and treatment. J Am Anim Hosp Assoc *12*:77, 1976.
8. Marretta SM, and Schrader SC. Physeal injuries in the dog: A review of 135 cases. J Am Vet Med Assoc *182*:708, 1983.
9. Peacock E, and Van Winkle W: Wound Repair. Philadelphia, WB Saunders, 1976, pp. 547–606.
10. Perren SM: Primary bone healing. *In* Bojrab MJ (Ed): Pathophysiology in Small Animal Surgery. Philadelphia, Lea & Febiger, 1981, pp. 519–528.
11. Rahn B: Bone healing: Histologic and physiologic concepts. *In* Sumner-Smith G (Ed): Bone in Clinical Orthopedics. Philadelphia, WB Saunders, 1982, p. 366.
12. Braden TD, and Brinker WO. Radiologic and gross anatomic evaluation of bone healing in the dog. J Am Vet Med Assoc *12*:1318, 1976.
13. Dingwall JS: Fractures. *In* Archibald J (Ed): Canine Surgery. 2nd Ed. Santa Barbara, CA, American Veterinary Publications, 1974, pp. 949–956.
14. Rhinelander FW, and Wilson JW. Blood to developing, mature, and healing bone. *In* Sumner-Smith G (Ed): Bone in Clinical Orthopedics. Philadelphia, WB Saunders, 1982, pp. 81–158.
15. Lappin MR, Aron DN, Herron HL, et al. Fracture of the radius and ulna in the dog. J Am Anim Hosp Assoc *19*:643, 1983.

16. Heppenstall RB: Fractures of the tibia and fibula. *In* Heppenstall RB (Ed): Fracture Treatment and Healing. Philadelphia, WB Saunders, 1980, pp. 777–802.

17. Hulse DH, Abdelbaki YZ, and Wilson J. Revascularization of femoral capital physeal fractures following surgical fixation. J Vet Orthop 2:50, 1981.

18. Swan KG, and Swan RC: Gunshot Wounds—Pathophysiology and Management. Littleton, MA, PSG Publishing, 1980, p. 211.

19. O'Brien TR, Morgan J, and Suter P. Epiphyseal plate injury in the dog: A radiographic study of growth disturbance in the forelimb. J Small Anim Pract 12:19, 1971.

20. Morgan JP: Radiographic diagnosis of fractures and fracture repair in the dog. Bi-weekly Small Anim Vet Med Update Series 19:1, 1978.

21. DeAngelis M: Causes of delayed union and nonunion of fractures. Vet Clin North Am [Small Anim Pract] 5:251, 1975.

22. Brinker W, Flo G, Braden T, et al. Removal of bone plates in small animals. J Am Anim Hosp Assoc 11:577, 1975.

23. Rahn B: Bone healing: Histologic and physiologic concepts. *In* Sumner-Smith G (Ed): Clinical Orthopedics. Philadelphia, WB Saunders, 1982, p. 377.

24. Brinker WO, Hohn RB, and Prieur WD: Manual of Internal Fixation in Small Animals. New York, Springer-Verlag, 1984, p. 243.

25. Punto L, Puranen J, and Mokka R: Osteomedullography in tibial shaft fractures of the dog and pig. J Am Vet Radiol Soc 18:102, 1977.

26. Fanton JW, Blass CE, and Withrow SJ: Sciatic nerve injury as a complication of intramedullary pin fixation of femoral fractures. J Am Anim Hosp Assoc 19:687, 1983.

27. Stevenson S, Hohn R, Pohler O, et al. Fracture-associated sarcoma in the dog. J Am Vet Med Assoc 180:1189, 1982.

CHAPTER 12

NEOPLASIA

DONALD E. THRALL

Most neoplastic bone lesions can be characterized radiographically as having an aggressive appearance. The radiographic signs of aggressive versus nonaggressive bone lesions were discussed in Chapter 2. It is impossible to make a definitive diagnosis of an aggressive bone lesion by radiographic means alone. The radiographic features of the lesion must be considered with the signalment, anamnesis, and physical and laboratory findings before a list of differential diagnoses is formulated. Histologic evaluation of the lesion is usually necessary before a definitive diagnosis can be made.

PRIMARY BONE TUMORS

The most common primary tumor of the appendicular skeleton is osteosarcoma. Osteosarcomas most commonly affect giant and large breeds of dogs. Average age of affected dogs is approximately 7 years; however, osteosarcomas are occasionally detected in young dogs (1 to 2 years).[1] Primary appendicular osteosarcomas are generally solitary, aggressive lesions that originate in the metaphysis of long tubular bones. Common sites of osteosarcomas in the pectoral limb are the proximal humerus and distal radius. In the pelvic limb, the distal femur, proximal tibia, and distal tibia are commonly affected. The radiographic appearance of osteosarcomas can be quite variable; they may be predominantly osteolytic (Fig. 12–1), mixed osteolytic/osteoblastic (Fig. 12–2), or predominantly osteoblastic (Fig. 12–3), and the associated periosteal reaction may be active (Fig. 12–4) or inactive (Fig. 12–3). It has been suggested that active periosteal spicules associated with malignant processes are long and thin (Fig. 12–4), whereas those associated with benign processes are short and squat (Fig. 12–5). There are instances, however, in which the periosteal spicules found with osteosarcomas are short and squat (Fig. 12–6). Thus, in dogs, the type of periosteal reaction cannot be used as a means to differentiate between neoplasia and infection.

The diaphyseal margin of the periosteal reaction in osteosarcoma is sometimes triangular. Such a shape has been referred to as Codman's triangle (Fig. 12–6) and has been interpreted by some individuals as being seen only in osteosarcoma. Codman's triangle, however, can be seen with any lesion that results in periosteal elevation and is not specific for osteosarcoma.

Although most osteosarcomas begin as monostotic lesions, they may not remain monostotic for the duration of their existence. As they progress, the tumor may metastasize to other bones, or periosteal proliferation may be induced on adjacent bones by direct infiltration or mechanical irritation of adjacent periosteum.

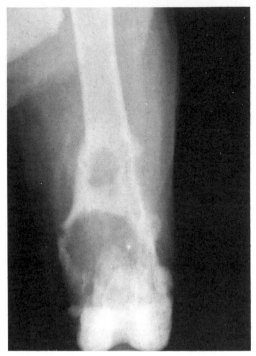

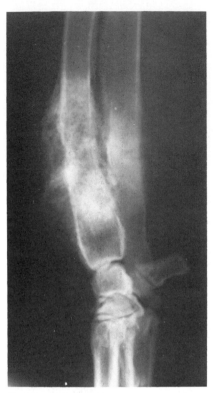

Figure 12–1. Craniocaudal femoral radiograph. An aggressive, primarily osteolytic lesion is present in the distal part of the bone. Foci of periosteal proliferation are present and the medial cortex is expanded. Diagnosis: osteosarcoma. (All figures From Newton CD and Nunamaker DM: Textbook of Small Animal Orthopedics. Philadelphia, Lippincott/Harper & Row, 1985, with permission.)

Figure 12–2. Lateral view. A mixed osteolytic/osteoblastic aggressive lesion is in the distal radius. Diagnosis: osteosarcoma.

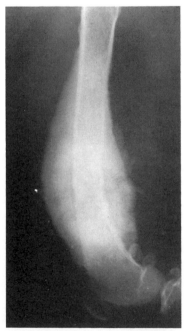

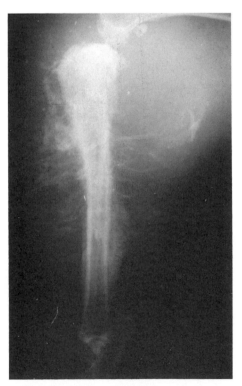

Figure 12–3. Lateral view. A predominantly osteosclerotic lesion can be seen in the femur. The periosteal reaction is relatively inactive (smooth). Diagnosis: osteosarcoma.

Figure 12–4. Lateral view. There is an extensive, aggressive lesion with active periosteal reaction in the tibia. Diagnosis: osteosarcoma.

are smaller (Miniature Schnauzers being a representative breed) with a lower ratio of pectoral to pelvic limb site of tumor involvement.

The second specific situation in which osteosarcoma is associated with another osseous abnormality is the association of tumorogenesis and an internal fixation device. Multiple case reports have been published in which the development of malignant tumors adjacent to long-standing internal fixation devices has been described. This association was discussed in Chapter 11.

Primary bone tumors of the appendicular skeleton other than osteosarcoma are not common. Those lesions occasionally encountered include fibrosarcoma, chondrosarcoma, and hemangiosarcoma. These neoplasms are generally similar in appearance to osteosarcoma (Fig. 12–8) and a biopsy is necessary for diagnosis.

In addition to neoplasia, the major diagnostic consideration for monostotic aggressive lesions

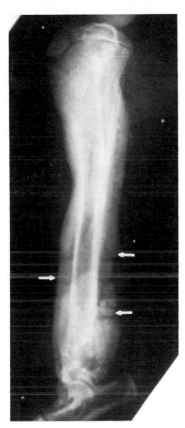

Figure 12–5. Lateral radiograph of the tibia of a dog. An extensive periosteal reaction can be seen. In some areas, the reaction is smooth, whereas in others it has an irregular, "short and squat" appearance *(arrows)*. Diagnosis: bacterial osteomyelitis.

In young animals with osteosarcoma, physeal cartilage acts as a barrier preventing metaphyseal tumor from spreading to the epiphysis. In adult animals, or in young animals after the physis closes, metaphyseal tumors readily progress to involve the epiphysis. Articular cartilage may act as a barrier to prevent tumors from invading opposing articular surfaces. With advanced tumors, however, opposing articular surfaces may become affected.

Two specific situations in which the development of osteosarcoma is associated with another osseous abnormality deserve consideration. The first is the association of osteosarcoma with idiopathic polyostotic bone infarction, which is a rare condition in dogs characterized by multifocal medullary necrosis and endosteal osteogenesis (Fig. 12–7). Many of these dogs also develop bone sarcoma.[2] The relationship between the bone infarction and bone sarcoma is unknown. Dogs that develop bone sarcoma associated with medullary bone infarction differ in their breed, weight, and primary tumor site from other dogs with bone tumors. Such dogs

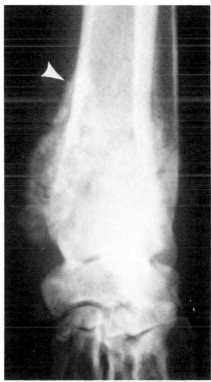

Figure 12–6. Craniocaudal radiograph of the distal antebrachium. There is an aggressive, predominantly osteoblastic lesion of the distal radius. Medially, portions of the periosteal reaction have a "short and squat" appearance. The proximal aspect of the periosteal reaction on the medial side of the radius forms a triangular junction with the radius *(arrow)*; this has been referred to as Codman's triangle. Codman's triangle can be found in periosteal reactions resulting from many different primary lesions, e.g., neoplasia, inflammation, and trauma. Diagnosis: osteosarcoma.

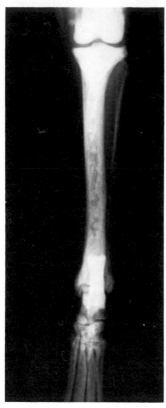

Figure 12–7. Craniocaudal radiograph of the tibia reveals numerous medullary radiopacities. These opacities represent endosteal osteogenesis associated with bone infarcts.

is osteomyelitis. Bacterial osteomyelitis is most often the result of direct contamination of the bone, e.g., surgery or external trauma, rather than being hematogenous. Thus, the location of bacterial osteomyelitis in the bone is more variable than the location of primary tumors, which are primarily metaphyseal. Nevertheless, appearances may be similar. In dogs in which the radiographic appearance of osteomyelitis is consistent with neoplasia, there is usually an event in the clinical history, such as surgical intervention, or physical evidence, such as draining fistulas, that suggests infection rather than tumor (Fig. 12–9). Because the radiographic appearance can be similar, diagnosis must not be based solely on these findings.

Mycotic osteomyelitis is generally of hematogenous origin and therefore is usually characterized by polyostotic lesions, which are frequently metaphyseal. Mycotic bone lesions, however, may be monostotic or only one lesion may be detected. In such instances, the tentative diagnosis may be neoplasia. Because the appearance of mycotic bone lesions may be

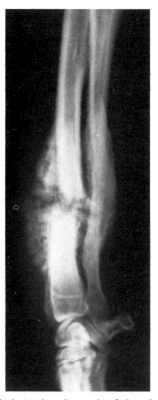

Figure 12–9. Lateral radiograph of the distal antebrachium of a 2-year-old dog 2 months after it was attacked by another dog. There are aggressive lesions of the distal radius and ulna and a radial fracture. The radiographic findings are consistent with neoplasia, but the history is more suggestive of infection. Diagnosis: bacterial osteomyelitis.

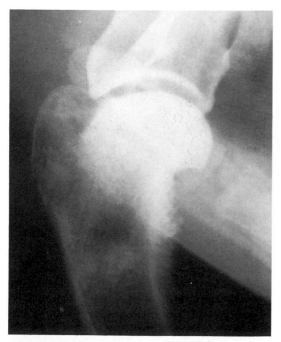

Figure 12–8. Lateral view of the shoulder. An aggressive humeral lesion can be seen. Diagnosis: hemangiosarcoma.

eton arise hematogenously, they tend to have a polyostotic distribution (Fig. 12–12); diaphyseal and metaphyseal locations are common. Metastatic bone tumors have an aggressive appearance and may be predominantly osteolytic, predominantly osteoblastic, or mixed osteolytic/osteoblastic. Diagnosis of suspected bone metastasis by clinical signs and radiographic analysis is impossible; histologic evaluation is necessary.

DIRECT TUMOR EXTENSION TO BONE

Soft-tissue neoplasms of the extremities may invade underlying bone, resulting in detectable radiographic change. Such change may be primarily osteoblastic, osteolytic, or mixed, but it nevertheless is usually aggressive and is rarely specific. Bone changes from adjacent soft-tissue tumors can result from mechanical stimulation

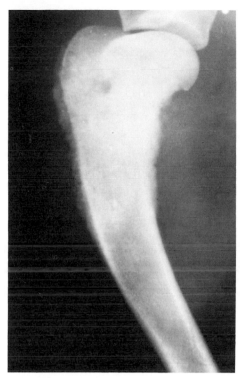

Figure 12–10. Lateral radiograph of the proximal humerus reveals an aggressive lesion. Other bone lesions were not detected. The appearance of the humeral lesion is consistent with neoplasia; *Actinomyces sp.* was identified after biopsy and culture. The bone lesion resolved after appropriate chemotherapy. Inflammatory bone disease and neoplastic bone disease can be similar in appearance.

identical to that of osteosarcoma or other tumors (Fig. 12–10), diagnosis must not be based on the radiographic findings.

Traumatic bone lesions can have an aggressive radiographic appearance, and in some instances neoplasia will be considered in the differential diagnosis (Fig. 12–11). In other instances, known previous trauma will influence radiographic evaluation, and neoplasia may not be considered strongly. In either situation, the definitive diagnosis cannot be substantiated radiographically, and if the diagnosis is in doubt, the use of more interventional techniques should be considered.

METASTATIC BONE TUMORS

In dogs, primary bone tumors are more common than metastatic lesions. Nevertheless, as cancer patients are kept alive longer, more patients with metastatic bone tumors are encountered. Any malignant tumor has the potential to metastasize to the skeleton, but epithelial metastases are more common than mesenchymal ones.[3] Because metastatic sites in the skel-

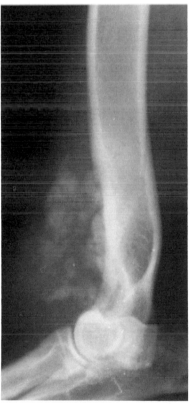

Figure 12–11. Lateral radiograph of the distal humerus of a 9-month-old Irish setter with a 30-day history of lameness and progressive localized swelling. There is an area of soft-tissue swelling that contains foci of mineralization. There is also an area of smooth periosteal reaction on the cranial humeral diaphysis. Some cortical irregularity is also present. The lesion is aggressive and neoplasia should be considered. Diagnosis: calcifying hematoma associated with avulsion of the extensor carpi radialis.

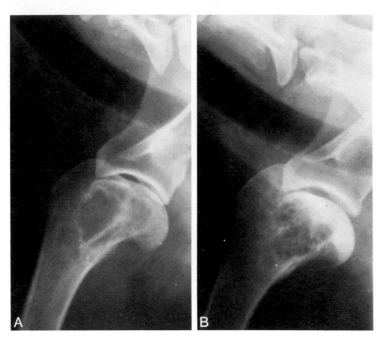

Figure 12–12. *A* and *B*, lateral views of both shoulders of a dog. Aggressive bone lesions are evident. The appearance of each lesion, considered individually, is consistent with primary bone tumor. Because of the polyostotic distribution, however, metastatic neoplasia or hematogenous infection is a more likely diagnosis. Diagnosis: metastatic mammary adenocarcinoma.

of the periosteum or actual tumor infiltration into the bone.

References

1. Alexander JW, and Patton CS: Primary tumors of the skeletal system. Vet Clin North Am *13*:181, 1983.
2. Dubielzig RR, Biery DN, and Brodey RS: Bone sarcomas associated with multifocal medullary bone infarction in dogs. J Am Vet Med Assoc *179*:64, 1981.
3. Russell RG, and Walker M: Metastatic and invasive tumors of bone in dogs and cats. Vet Clin North Am *13*:163, 1983.

CHAPTER 13

RADIOGRAPHIC SIGNS OF JOINT DISEASE

GRAEME ALLAN

Signs of joint disease that can be distinguished radiographically are listed in Table 13–1. Many signs are seen in more than one type of joint disease. Animals with joint diseases that are progressive may have different signs when examined during different phases of the disease.

The examining clinician must determine whether lameness is due to a mono- or multiarticular problem. A hallmark of immune-mediated joint diseases is their polyarticular distribution. The same finding applies to hematogeneously disseminated septic arthritis. Most other joint diseases are mono- or pauci-articular.

Are there systemic signs of illness? Cats with feline chronic progressive polyarthropathy, or mycoplasma arthritis, suffer systemic signs of illness, which include transient fever, malaise, and stiffness as well as lameness. Animals with signs of bleeding disorders and concurrent joint pain should be examined for signs of hemarthrosis. Systemic lupus erythematosus is a multiorgan disease, of which polyarthropathy may be a mild clinical sign. These points are mentioned only to underscore that sound knowledge of joint pathophysiology is as important in the diagnosis of joint diseases as is the ability to take and interpret radiographs of joints.[85]

Increased Synovial Mass. Any moderate increase in joint capsular or intracapsular soft-tissue mass may be detected on good quality radiographs. The joint cartilage, synovial fluid, synovium, and joint capsule cannot be differentiated by using survey radiographs, because they are of equal radiopacity. In most joints, any increase in synovial mass appears as periarticular swelling; this is identified radiographically by the increased radiopacity of affected soft tissues. When the stifle is involved, the infrapatellar fat pad sign can be used. The infrapatellar fat pad is readily identified on lateral radiographs of a normal stifle. When the stifle synovial mass increases, a combination of inflammatory response, edema, and compression causes the fat pad to become less visible.

TABLE 13–1. **RADIOGRAPHIC SIGNS OF JOINT DISEASE**

Increased synovial mass
Altered thickness of the joint space
Subchondral osteolysis
Subchondral osteosclerosis
Subchondral bone "cyst" formation
Perichondral osteolysis
Perichondral bone proliferation
Mineralization of joint soft tissues
Joint "mice"
Joint displacement
Joint malformation

If necessary, the joint cartilage and the synovium can be silhouetted by using contrast arthrography. This technique has been used to aid in the identification of chondral flaps and tears in osteochondritis dissecans in dogs,[105] and in synovial hypertrophy in villonodular synovitis in horses.[76]

Altered Thickness of the Joint Space. The joint space is the radiolucent space between the subchondral bone of opposing weight-bearing surfaces of a joint. This radiolucent space consists of two layers of articular cartilage separated by a microfilm of synovial fluid. In the early stages of joint disease, synovial effusion may cause widening of the joint space. As joint disease progresses, attrition of articular cartilage results in the radiolucent joint space appearing thinner. Radiographs taken while the patient is weight-bearing on an affected joint are required if changes in the thickness of the joint space are to be properly assessed. Radiographs taken of the recumbent animal are not regarded as adequate for this purpose. The one exception to this rule may be when there is muscle contracture, as in contracture of the infraspinous muscle. Such contracture causes noticeable diminution of the articular joint space of the shoulder joint.[111]

Subchondral Osteolysis. The subchondral bone is separated from the synovial fluid by an intact layer of joint cartilage. Any disease process that changes the character of the synovial fluid, causing the joint cartilage to erode, potentially threatens the integrity of the subchondral bone. In inflammatory joint diseases, inflammatory exudates can cause pronounced subchondral osteolysis. Infectious arthritis can extend into subchondral bone. Subchondral osteolysis initially appears as a ragged margin of subchondral bone, but can extend to cause marked destruction of bone. When osteolysis affects smaller carpal and tarsal bones, these small cuboidal bones can be dramatically reduced in mass.

Subchondral Osteosclerosis. In benign joint diseases, such as degenerative joint disease, the subchondral bone may appear sclerotic. Subchondral osteosclerosis appears as a subchondral zone of increased opacity or whiteness that is 1 to 2 mm wide.

Subchondral Bone "Cyst" Formation. Subchondral bone cysts, a feature of degenerative joint disease in humans, are occasionally encountered in animals with joint disease.

Perichondral Osteolysis. At the chondrosynovial junction, articular cartilage merges with the synovium. The highly vascular synovium is sensitive to inflammation. Synovial inflammation, or hypertrophy, can result in erosion of the bone adjacent to the synovium. Early inflammation causes the adjacent bone to appear ragged and spiculated. Long-standing or severe synovial inflammation or hypertrophy can cause pronounced bone erosion. Perichondral bone erosion is a characteristic of some immune-mediated joint diseases and of villonodular synovitis.

Perichondral Bone Proliferation. In degenerative joint disease, fibrocartilage elements form at the chrondrosynovial junction. Gradual ossification of this fibrocartilaginous periarticular "collar" produces osteophytes. Progressive enlargement of osteophytes can result in their incorporation in the adjacent joint capsule. Osteophyte formation is a characteristic of many chronic joint diseases, but it is most prevalent in degenerative joint disease.

Articular Soft-Tissue Mineralization. As a consequence of many chronic joint diseases, mineralization may involve the joint capsule or synovium or it may be free within the synovial fluid. Additionally, large accumulations of articular or periarticular calcific material may occasionally be observed. Ellison and Norrdin reported a case of multicentric calcinosis,[30] and Gibson and Roenigk described a case of pseudogout.[34] In both instances, the subject was a dog. Large osteochondromas have been reported within the joints of dogs[98] and cats.[52]

Joint "Mice." Small, well-defined articular and periarticular accumulations of calcific material are occasionally observed in dogs and cats. Such mineralized fragments are called joint mice. Not all such fragments are free within the joint, although they may appear so radiographically. As in humans,[68] joint mice usually fall into three fairly distinct categories. They are either avulsed fragments of articular or periarticular bone, osteochondral components of a disintegrating joint surface, or small synovial osteochondromas (see Table 13–2). Joint mice must be differentiated from sesamoid bones adjacent to the elbow, stifle, tarsus, and metacarpophalangeal and metatarsophalangeal joints.

Joint Displacement. When the normal spacial relationship between the adjacent osseous components of a joint is disturbed, some type of displacement has occurred. A good example is the cranial drawer sign in a stifle with a ruptured cranial cruciate ligament. Clinically detectable displacement is not always easy to illustrate radiographically. Stress radiography may be employed to reproduce displacement so that it can be recorded radiographically. Joint displacement is usually a consequence of trauma to fibrous or ligamentous supporting structures.

Joint Malformation. Joint malformation represents the end product of osseous remodeling, and is usually the result of malunion of bones of traumatized joints, chronic degenerative joint disease, or congenital joint disease.

TABLE 13–2. SOME COMMON JOINT MICE*

Joint	Etiology
Shoulder	Osteochondritis dissecans of the head of the humerus
	Mineralization of the bicipital tendon
	Synovial osteochondroma
Elbow	Ununited anconeal process
	Fragmented coronoid process
	Osteochondritis dissecans of the humeral medial condyle
	Avulsion fractures of the humeral medial epicondyle
Hip	Avulsion epiphyseal fractures after femoral luxation
	Avascular necrosis of the femoral head
Stifle	Osteochondritis dissecans of the femoral condyles
	Avulsion fractures of the:
	• origin of the long digital extensor tendon
	• origin or insertion of the cruciate ligaments
	Synovial osteochondroma
Hock	Osteochondritis dissecans of the talus

*In all joints, soft-tissue periarticular mineralization may occur secondary to degenerative joint disease.

DEGENERATIVE JOINT DISEASE

Degenerative joint disease is the most common joint abnormality seen in small animal practice. The disease occurs most frequently in the large, weight-bearing joints of medium to large-sized dogs, but it can afflict any synovial joint. The best example of canine degenerative joint disease is that which occurs secondary to canine hip dysplasia. The incidence of hip dysplasia varies from breed to breed. In many large breeds, the incidence exceeds 50 per cent. The next most frequent locations are the canine shoulder and stifle joints. Ljunggren and Olsson identified signs of shoulder degenerative joint disease in 33 percent of a group of dogs examined at necropsy.[59] Tirgari and Vaughan reported that in a necropsy survey of 150 dogs, 20 percent of the dogs had stifle degenerative joint disease.[106] In both groups, the dogs were randomly selected.

Degenerative joint disease may be primary (idiopathic) or secondary to a developmental or acquired disorder. Examples of developmental disorders include osteochondrosis, fragmented coronoid process, ununited anconeal process, hip dysplasia, patellar luxation, achondroplasia, and conformational disorders, such as valgus and varus deformities of the carpus. Acquired disorders capable of causing degenerative joint disease include trauma, joint instability, epiphyseal aseptic necrosis, and acquired postural or conformational defects, such as joint malalignment after fracture repair.[66, 79, 85]

The initial stages of the disease are asymptomatic and escape radiographic detection. The first pathologic change is a mild nonsuppurative synovitis, accompanied by a significant increase in the volume of synovial mass. Focal articular degeneration follows. The radiolucent joint space may appear widened during this stage[2, 63, 77] In the coxofemoral joint, the increased synovial mass in severe cases may appear as joint laxity or subluxation.[77]

Radiographic changes vary according to the stage of the disease. As the joint cartilage becomes thinner, several pathologic changes take place. The most readily recognizable change is osteophyte formation, which follows neovascularization of the chondrosynovial junction with resultant fibrocartilage formation. This fibrocartilage collar gradually ossifies with the formation of characteristic perichondral osteophytes (Fig. 13–1A). Osteophyte formation is always on a non–weight-bearing surface. Osteophytes may eventually grow into adjacent ligamentous or capsular attachments, or may protrude directly into the joint spaces.[2, 17, 104] Osteophyte formation was identified radiographically within a few months of severence of the cranial cruciate ligament in one group of dogs.[67]

Continued attrition of the articular cartilage may be detected on radiographs obtained during weight-bearing as thinning of the radiolucent joint space. Pathologic alteration of the subchondral bone shelf, including eburnation, compression, and necrosis, may be detected radiographically as subchondral sclerosis of the weight-bearing surface.[72, 80, 87, 109] Subchondral cyst formation, a feature of degenerative joint disease of the human femoral head, has rarely been reported in small animals.[104]

Affected joints exhibit decreased range of movement, which results in increased loading of the diminished weight-bearing surface. The combination of increased load, diminished subchondral strength, and loss of shock-absorbing cartilage results in alteration in the shape of the subchondral bone table (Fig. 13–1B). This remodeling of the subchondral bone is complemented by the addition of peripheral new bone in the form of perichondral osteophytes. The altered shape of the osseous components of affected joints is readily identified radiographically.[104, 109] The gamut of the radiographic changes seen in degenerative joint disease is outlined in Table 13–3.

HIP DYSPLASIA

The term hip dysplasia means abnormally formed hip joints. The condition occurs principally in large dogs, but it also affects small dogs and cats. Male and female animals are equally affected. Unilateral hip dysplasia occurs and is reported in approximately 11 percent of dogs.[55]

Hip dysplasia is an inherited disorder. Heritability estimates range from 0.2 to 0.6.[45, 48, 50,

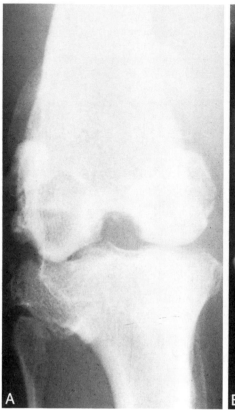
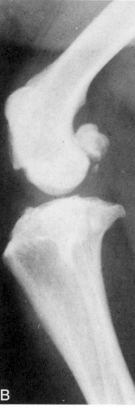

Figure 13–1. An 11-year-old mixed-breed canine that had chronic weight-bearing lameness of the right hind leg. With exercise the dog became less lame. *A*, perichondral osteophytes are present on the distal femur and proximal tibia. Medial patella luxation was palpable. *B*, note the altered shape of the caudal aspect of the proximal tibia, which represents remodeling. Diagnosis: degenerative joint disease, secondary to patellar luxation.

[56, 60] More recent estimates for the German shepherd breed indicate a heritability value of 0.46.[44] Environmental factors influence the phenotypic expression of hip dysplasia. The role of nutrition has been studied extensively. Overnutrition is regarded as one of the principal nongenetic factors that influence the expression of canine hip dysplasia.[43, 51]

Radiography is used to diagnose hip dysplasia. Animals may be examined because they have a clinical problem related to their coxofemoral joints, or because their owners want the hip joints evaluated for breeding purposes. With respect to the latter, it is important to remember that radiography provides only a record of the animal's hip dysplasia phenotype. Selective breeding, based on pelvic radiogra-

TABLE 13–3. RADIOGRAPHIC SIGNS OF DEGENERATIVE JOINT DISEASE

Synovial effusion
Initial widening, then thinning, of the radiolucent joint space
Osteophyte formation on non–weight-bearing surfaces
Subchondral sclerosis
Remodeling of subchondral bone
Mineralization of intra- and periarticular soft tissues
Subchondral cyst formation (rare)
Subluxation (of the coxofemoral joint)

phy, has reduced the incidence of hip dysplasia in one closed colony of German shepherd dogs from 46 to 28 percent in 5 years.[44]

Hip dysplasia is a developmental, age-related disorder; it is not present at birth. A variable amount of time must elapse before radiographic changes are manifest. Once present, these changes usually progress as the animal ages. If radiographs are made before recognizable dysplastic changes are apparent, the animal may erroneously be classified as normal. Signs of hip dysplasia in a young animal may be described as mild, but subsequent examinations may reveal a more severe grade of hip dysplasia. So that a uniform classification of hip dysplasia may be applied and that diagnostic errors are minimized, it is recommended that the radiographic classifications of canine coxofemoral joints be made at a set age. The chance of diagnostic error diminishes with increasing age (Table 13–4).[50, 55, 107] Accordingly, it is recommended that dogs should not be certified as free of radiographic signs of hip dysplasia before they are 24 months of age.

Radiography has limited sensitivity to detect early joint changes, which consist of mild, non-suppurative synovitis and focal degenerative articular lesions.[63] As the volume of synovial fluid and the ligamentum teres increases, it may be detected radiographically as coxofem-

TABLE 13–4. **ACCURACY OF RADIOGRAPHIC DIAGNOSIS OF HIP DYSPLASIA, RELATED TO AGE**

Age (months)	Percent of Dysplastic Dogs Diagnosed Radiographically
6	25
12	70
18	78
24	95
36	96

*Data for German shepherd and Visla breeds, compiled by Jessen and Spurrell.[50]

oral subluxation.* This finding is regarded as the earliest radiographic sign of hip dysplasia (Figs. 13–2 and 13–3).[61, 62]

Subsequent radiographic changes are those of degenerative joint disease (Fig. 13–4). The

*Subluxation can be detected clinically as joint laxity. For years investigators have attempted to use palpable laxity as a method of early selection of dogs who are free of hip dysplasia. Despite a fairly strong correlation between palpable laxity and the ultimate radiographic diagnosis of hip dysplasia,[35, 113] hip joint palpation of young dogs has not proven a reliable technique in practice.

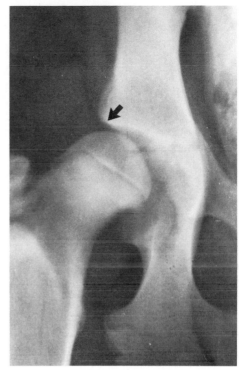

Figure 13–3. Moderate hip dysplasia. Subluxation of the femoral head is accompanied by remodeling of the acetabulum. The cranial effective acetabular margin is rounded *(arrow)* and the acetabulum is shallow. Note the wedge-shaped joint space.

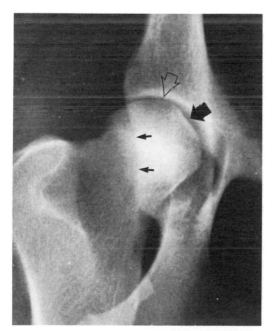

Figure 13–2. Normal mature coxofemoral joint. Note that two thirds of the femoral head lies medial to the shadow of the dorsal effective acetabular margin *(small arrows)*. The cranial margin of the femoral head is separated from the adjacent acetabulum by a fine radiolucent line, which represents the radiolucent joint cartilage and a microfilm of synovial fluid *(open arrow)*. The flattened portion of the femoral head is normal and represents the fovea capitis femoris *(solid arrow)*.

order of changes is: (1) perichondral osteophyte formation; (2) remodeling of the femoral head and neck; (3) remodeling of the acetabulum; and (4) sclerosis of subchondral bone of the femoral head and acetabulum. During the degenerative phase, the femoral head loses its spheroidal shape and becomes flattened along its articular surface. The femoral neck becomes thickened and the surface of the neck becomes irregular, due to the growth of a collar of perichondral osteophytes. The acetabulum loses its cup-like shape, and becomes shallow. Sclerosis of subchondral bone is a response to thinning or loss of articular cartilage. A variable degree of coxofemoral subluxation is always present and coxa valga is common. Subchondral cyst formation is an infrequent manifestation of degenerative joint disease in small animals, but it may occasionally be observed.[93, 102] Hip dysplasia is usually bilateral, but the unilateral variety has been reported.[55]

Because hip dysplasia control programs require a high standard of radiographic diagnosis, different investigators have examined objective criteria taken from radiographs in an attempt to reduce the subjective nature of interpretation. A ratio of pelvic width to acetabular depth was an early attempt to measure changes that might

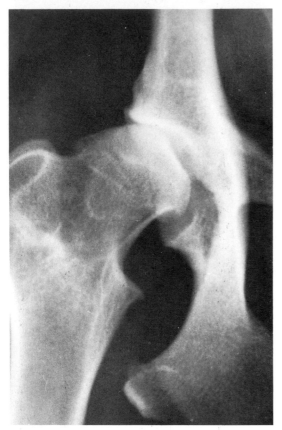

Figure 13–4. Advanced hip dysplasia. The acetabulum and femoral head show advanced signs of remodeling. Osteophytes are forming on the femoral neck and head, as well as on the cranial effective acetabular margin. The subchondral bone of the acetabular articular surface is sclerotic. These are easily recognized signs of degenerative joint disease.

be diagnostic.[92] Another was "Norberg's angle," which quantified the acetabular depth by measuring the location of the center of the femoral head in relation to the acetabular rim.[78] The search for objective diagnostic tests continues,[10, 110] but to date no fool-proof test has emerged. Veterinarians are therefore encouraged to develop expertise in radiographic interpretation or to rely on those individuals of greater expertise. Hip dysplasia is a disease of economic importance, and dog fanciers and breeders deserve the best diagnostic services available. For this reason the Orthopedic Foundation for Animals (OFA) has established a film reading service for veterinarians. Radiographs that are submitted to the service are read by three qualified veterinary radiologists, and a consensus report is returned to the referring veterinarian.*

*For further information, write to The Orthopedic Foundation for Animals, Inc., University of Missouri-Columbia, Columbia, MO 65211.

TRAUMA THAT INVOLVES THE OSSEOUS COMPONENTS OF JOINTS

Any fracture in which there is communication between the joint space and fractured intracapsular osseous components is an articular fracture (Fig. 13–5). Articular fractures must be accurately diagnosed to ensure appropriate surgical reduction and stabilization. Radiographic examinations should include two projections taken at right angles to one another. The standard projections are the craniocaudal (or caudocranial, dorsopalmar, dorsoplantar) and lateral views. To these should be added the oblique view and projections during flexion and stress when needed. These additional projections are of most value when chip or avulsion fractures are suspected, or when the osseous structures of interest are superimposed on other osseous structures.[90, 94]

Articular fractures occur frequently in immature animals because of the high incidence of physeal and epiphyseal trauma in these patients. Physeal fractures that are articular are

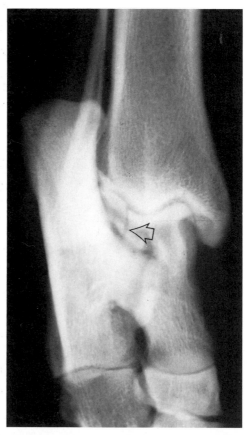

Figure 13–5. A 3-year-old German short-haired pointer with acute onset of non–weight-bearing lameness of the left hind leg. Radiography revealed a fracture through the lateral trochlear ridge of the talus (arrow). Diagnosis: articular fracture of the tibial tarsal bone. (Courtesy of A. K. W. Wood.)

usually classified as Salter type III or IV fractures.[97] Because the proximal femoral physis is intracapsular, all proximal femoral physeal fractures are articular fractures. In a retrospective study of femoral head and neck fractures, Daly reported that 77 percent of lesions were intracapsular, 59 percent of which were physeal.[23]

Premature physeal closure sometimes follows repair of Salter fractures, and may be observed within 2 to 3 weeks of surgery.[20, 23, 65] It should be regarded as an expected finding, regardless of the type of physeal trauma, and should be included in the prognosis. Although many dogs in the aforementioned study had significant growth potential remaining at the time of injury, clinical signs related to premature physeal closure were rare.

The proportion of physeal trauma that is articular is lower for joints other than the coxofemoral joint. Grauer et al. reported that 9 of 57 distal femoral physeal fractures were classified as Salter type III or IV.[37] Distal humeral fractures are classified as condylar or intercondylar. Lateral condylar fractures predominate, and are most frequently reported in immature dogs.[26] Fractures that involve the carpal and tarsal bones occur frequently, particularly in racing greyhounds.[25]

SPRAINS: CAPSULAR, LIGAMENTOUS, AND TENDINOUS INJURY TO JOINTS

Supporting soft-tissue structures of joints are relatively radiolucent and therefore are not visualized clearly on a radiograph. Mild sprains are difficult to diagnose, because the only radiographic sign is minimal soft-tissue swelling. The radiographic features of severe sprains include periarticular soft-tissue swelling, avulsion fractures at points of attachment of ligaments, tendons, and capsules to bone, joint instability or subluxation, and spacial derangement of the osseous components of a joint.[31, 111] It is important to diagnose sprains promptly. In many instances, appropriate medical or surgical therapy ensures normal joint function in moderate to severe sprain injuries.[19, 25, 27, 31, 54, 88] Many patients with profound sprains, such as carpal hyperextension injuries, can be effectively salvaged, thus allowing the affected animal to ambulate satisfactorily instead of surviving as a cripple.[33]

The clinical assessment (palpation, manipulation) of a sprained joint is usually the best diagnostic tool. Radiography adds information that is useful for treatment planning, documents the presence and magnitude of the sprain, and identifies avulsed osseous fragments.[31] A useful technique for radiographic assessment of a sprained joint is stress radiography (Fig. 13–6). In practice, this technique involves application of force to the joint in question, to demonstrate displacement of its osseous components. The forces applied are the same stresses to which the joint would be subject in normal daily activity, and are defined as compressive, rotational, traction, shear, and wedge forces.[32]

An excellent example of a compressive stress is a radiograph of a joint during weight-bearing. Ligamentous trauma, as in carpal hyperextension injuries, is readily demonstrated by this technique. The cranial drawer sign seen in cranial cruciate ligament trauma is a practical example of a shearing stress. It is stress that is used routinely in clinical examination of the stifle. The same manipulative procedure can be applied to the stifle during radiography. Traction stress involves pulling the osseous components of the joint away from one another. One useful application of traction stress involves capital physeal fractures of the femoral head. By applying traction to the femur in the extended ventrodorsal position, capital fractures are easy to identify. Traction and wedge stresses are useful to examine joints for small avulsion fractures and intra-articular joint mice. Unilateral trauma to collateral ligaments of the elbow and stifle are lesions that can be uncovered by using wedge stresses. Because stress radiography involves personnel holding the patient during x-ray exposure, utmost care must be taken to ensure that such individuals wear appropriate protective clothing.

HEMARTHROSIS

Intra-articular hemorrhage may occur in dogs with coagulopathies or after joint trauma. Hemarthrosis was recently reported in a dog with suspected warfarin toxicosis.[6] Other coagulopathies in the dog that could cause hemarthrosis include hemophilia A and B, von Willebrand's disease, deficiencies in factors VII, X, and XI, and liver disease.[29] Isolated, infrequent episodes of intra-articular bleeding do not significantly alter the articular cartilage. Repeated hemorrhage can lead to severe damage to this cartilage as well as to the subchondral bone.[47, 109]

Animals suffer severe non–weight-bearing lameness of affected limbs. Affected joints are swollen and painful. Radiography in acute cases reveals joint soft-tissue swelling, which may be extensive.[6] With chronic intra-articular hemorrhage, the joint cartilage may be eroded and thin, causing the appearance of decreased articular joint space on weight-bearing radiographs. The subchondral bone appears irregular if it is involved in the destructive process. Remodeling of bones adjacent to affected stifles was

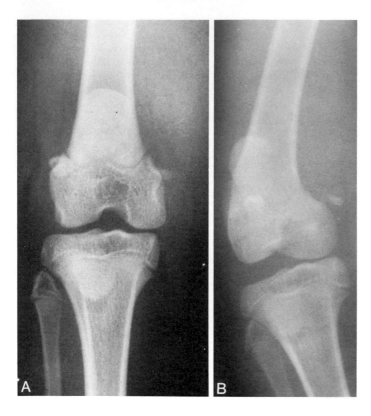

Figure 13–6. An 8-month-old Burmese kitten was lame in the left hind leg. Results of a standard craniocaudal projection *(A)* appeared normal. A stressed craniocaudal projection *(B)* revealed widening of the lateral radiolucent joint space. Diagnosis: ruptured lateral collateral ligament of the stifle joint. (Courtesy of A. K. W. Wood.)

reported in dogs after repeated intra-articular injections of whole blood.[47] In advanced cases, signs similar to degenerative joint disease may be present.[109]

INFECTIOUS ARTHRITIS

Infectious arthritis is a relatively infrequently diagnosed joint disease in small animals. According to Pedersen, the incidence of infectious arthritis is lower than that of immunologic joint disease.[81] Infectious arthritis is difficult to diagnose radiographically. Initial radiographic changes are similar to those seen in any effusive, nonerosive joint disease. Irreversible joint damage has occurred by the time a definitive radiographic diagnosis can be made. Ideally, the patient should be diagnosed and successfully treated without definitive radiographic changes becoming apparent.[12]

Polyarticular infectious arthritis can occur secondary to bacteremia caused by an isolated focus of infection (endocarditis, discospondylitis, or omphalophlebitis) or in conjunction with some systemic diseases (mycoplasma arthritis, canine leishmaniasis, or feline caliciviral lameness).[7, 14, 18, 71, 81] Monoarticular infectious arthritis most likely results from an extension of focal osteomyelitis into an adjacent joint, direct joint trauma, foreign body penetration (grass seed awns), or it may occur after joint surgery or intra-articular therapy.[11, 73, 80, 95] Polyarticular

infectious arthritis must be differentiated from immunologic joint disease.

The earliest radiographic changes are synovial effusion and increased synovial mass, which

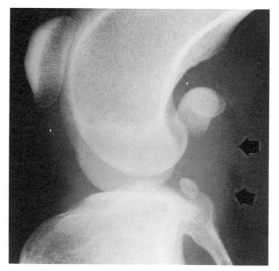

Figure 13–7. An 8-year-old male Australian cattle dog had neurologic signs related to the hindquarters as well as pain in the right stifle. Lateral view demonstrates that the infrapatellar fat pad is compressed by synovial effusion into the right stifle joint. Note the bulging caudal compartment of the stifle joint *(arrows)*. Radiography of the thoracic spine revealed discospondylitis. Laboratory diagnosis: septic arthritis, based on isolation of *Staphylococcus aureus* from the synovial fluid.

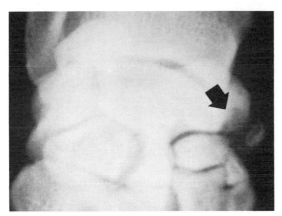

Figure 13–8. A 2-year-old male mixed-breed dog had acute onset lameness of the right carpus. Radiographically, subchondral osteolysis of the radial carpal bone *(arrow)* can be identified adjacent to the carpal sesamoid bone. Laboratory diagnosis: septic arthritis.

TABLE 13–5. PROGRESSION OF RADIOGRAPHIC SIGNS OF INFECTIOUS ARTHRITIS

Increased synovial mass, indicating synovial effusion and widened radiolucent joint space

Diminished radiolucent joint space, indicating destruction of articular cartilage

Loss of the smooth surface of the subchondral bone plate, an early sign of infectious penetration of subchondral bone

Osteolytic destruction of subchondral and perichondral bone, which is usually highlighted by a peripheral border of osteosclerosis

In advanced cases, weight-bearing surfaces may collapse, causing distortion of joint architecture

represent an inflammatory response of the synovium (Fig. 13–7). There is soft-tissue swelling, which is usually demarcated by the distended joint capsule. Joint capsular distention is best identified in carpal, tarsal, and stifle joints. A useful landmark in the stifle is the infrapatellar fat pad. When the fat pad silhouette becomes unclear or lost, synovial effusion is present (Fig. 13–7).[12]

In untreated infectious arthritis, joint cartilage destruction follows synovial effusion, which is itself followed by subchondral and perichondral bone destruction (Figs. 13–8 and 13–9).[21, 22]

Specific radiographic features of infectious arthritis become prominent after the articular cartilage is destroyed and subchondral osteomyelitis is established.[1, 73] Schrader reported that destruction of the femoral head was noted radiographically 4 weeks after the onset of clinical signs of coxofemoral infectious arthritis.[99] The width of the radiolucent joint space is progressively reduced as the articular cartilage is destroyed. Radiographs obtained during weight-bearing are needed to demonstrate this change. Destruction of the subchondral bone plate and subsequent subchondral osteomyelitis cause the margins of the joint space to appear uneven or ragged. Continued subchondral bone destruction produces large cystic subchondral radiolucent spaces. Bone sclerosis adjacent to the osteolytic bone is a sign of osseous inflammatory response to the infection (Table 13–5).

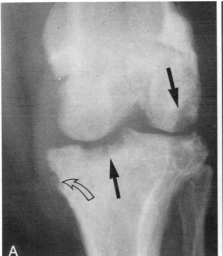
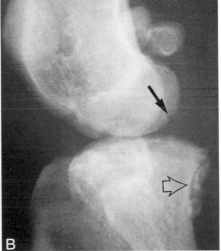

Figure 13–9. An 8-year-old male Australian cattle dog had stifle swelling and pain that persisted after repair of a ruptured cranial cruciate ligament. *A* and *B*, subchondral bone erosion involves the medial condyle of the tibia and the femoral condyles *(solid arrow)*. Note the concurrent medial patellar luxation. Laboratory diagnosis: septic arthritis, based on isolation of *Staphylococcus aureus* from the synovial fluid.

TABLE 13–6. DIAGNOSTIC GUIDELINES IN CANINE RHEUMATOID ARTHRITIS

Morning stiffness
Pain or tenderness in one or more joints
Soft-tissue swelling or effusion in one or more joints
Swelling of any other joint
Symmetric onset of joint symptoms and swelling
Radiographic signs consistent with rheumatoid arthritis
Positive rheumatoid factor test
Poor mucin precipitate of synovial fluid
Characteristic histologic changes in the synovium

(From Barrett RE: Canine polyarthritis. *In* Kirk RW (Ed.): Current Veterinary Therapy VII. Philadelphia, WB Saunders, 1980, p. 800, with permission.)

RHEUMATOID ARTHRITIS

Rheumatoid arthritis is a severe, progressive, erosive polyarthritis, which has been reported in dogs.[3, 8, 39, 46, 58, 75, 83, 100] To date, there are no reports of this disorder affecting cats, although it has been suggested that feline chronic progressive polyarthritis may be a feline form of rheumatoid arthritis.[41] Diagnostic criteria for human rheumatoid arthritis have been established.[96] These criteria have been modified for the canine.[5] Nine criteria must be evaluated; six of the nine should be satisfied for a diagnosis of classic rheumatoid arthritis to be made in the dog (Table 13–6).

Radiographic changes usually occur in distal joints of the extremities. The more proximal large joints (stifle and elbow) are occasionally affected. Synovial effusion occurs initially. Radiographs taken early in the course of the disease detect nonspecific soft-tissue swelling around affected joints. The joint capsule may be distended.[75] The first radiographic signs of an osseous pathologic process may be detected several weeks after the onset of clinical signs. Initial changes are mild, but as expected in a progressive disease, the magnitude of radiographic abnormalities becomes marked as the disease progresses.[3, 8, 75, 80, 83]

The progression of radiographic changes includes perichondral osteopenia; subchondral bone destruction/cyst formation (Fig. 13–10A); perichondral osteolysis and erosion (Fig. 13–10B); narrowing of the joint space; progressive osteopenia of epiphyses adjacent to affected joints; destruction of subchondral and perichondral bone; "mushrooming" of the ends of metacarpi and metatarsi, which occurs in advanced cases and represents collapse of subchondral bone; and varying degrees of joint subluxation and luxation in advanced cases. Other changes, more characteristic of degenerative joint disease (perichondral osteophytes, subchondral sclerosis, and calcified periarticular tissues) may also be present at this stage.

SYSTEMIC LUPUS ERYTHEMATOSUS

Systemic lupus erythematosus is a multisystemic disease of unknown origin. It affects dogs of all breeds as well as cats.[84] The disorder has a variety of clinical manifestations, including polyarthritis, anemia, nephropathy, skin disease, pericarditis/myocarditis, and lymphadenopathy.[38] The diagnosis of systemic lupus ery-

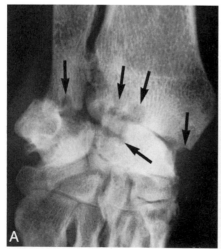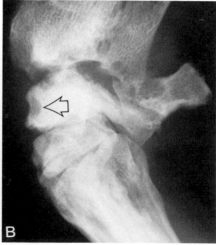

Figure 13–10. An 8-year-old male (neutered) corgi cross-breed had non—weight-bearing lameness of the right foreleg, valgus deviation of the left paw, and left carpal joint swelling and crepitus. *A,* dorsolateral-palmaromedial projection (right carpus). There is extensive subchondral erosion of the styloid process of the ulna and of the articular surfaces of the distal radius and radial carpal bone *(arrows). B,* lateral projection during flexion. In addition to the changes seen in *A,* note lysis of the non—weight-bearing dorsal surface of the radial carpal bone *(arrow).* Laboratory diagnosis: canine rheumatoid arthritis. (Courtesy of A. K. W. Wood.)

TABLE 13–7. **DIAGNOSTIC CRITERIA FOR CANINE SYSTEMIC LUPUS ERYTHEMATOSUS**

Diagnosis of canine systemic lupus erythematosus is justified if the patient exhibits two of the following clinical syndromes, and if there is serologic evidence of the disease (antinuclear antibody positive, strongly positive L.E. preparation, or both).

- Skin disease, with clinical and histologic resemblance to lupus
- Polyarthritis, with shifting lameness and slow progression
- Coombs'-positive hemolytic anemia
- Thombocytopenia
- Protein-losing nephropathy

(From Halliwell REW: Autoimmune disease in the dog. Adv Vet Sci Comp Med 22:221, 1978, with permission.)

thematosus is complicated, based on the concurrence of clinical manifestations and serologic evidence of the disease. The most valuable serologic screening test for lupus is the antinuclear antibody test (Table 13–7).

The relative frequency of the different clinical manifestations varies according to different authors. Grindem and Johnston reviewed 121 cases of systemic lupus erythematosus, and reported that joint disease was the most frequent clinical sign (69 per cent), followed by hematologic (53 per cent), renal (50 per cent), cutaneous (33 per cent), and intrathoracic (17 per cent) manifestations.[38] Scott et al. found that skin disease was the most frequent manifestation (54 per cent), with polyarthritis present in 39 per cent of cases.[101]

Arthritis that occurs in this disease is described as nonerosive and effusive. Polyarthritis (five or more joints affected) is usual, but mono- and pauciarticular arthritis has been reported. Clinically, affected animals demonstrate reluctance to move as well as shifting lameness. Affected joints may be swollen, painful, and warm. The joints most commonly affected are the carpus, tarsus, metatarsus, stifle, and elbow.

Radiographic signs are usually absent or are minimal. In chronic cases, the radiolucent joint space of affected joints may be narrowed, and the joint capsule is distended. A mild periosteal response has been reported at the junction of the joint capsule and the bone. Contrast arthrography has been used to demonstrate distention of the joint capsule. The synovial margin outlined by arthrography was reported as being irregular and indistinct.[84]

FELINE CHRONIC PROGRESSIVE POLYARTHRITIS

Feline chronic progressive polyarthritis[70, 82, 86, 112] is a recently described disease of young to middle-aged cats. In all cases reported to date, all animals affected are male cats. The disease is manifested as one of two syndromes.

The Periosteal Proliferative Form. This is the most prevalent form of the disorder. Affected cats display clinical signs characterized by fever, malaise, and stiffness, which is followed by periarticular soft-tissue swelling and regional lymphadenopathy. Radiographic changes can be identified in affected joints after a few weeks of clinical illness. The joints most commonly affected are the small joints of the fore and hind feet, particularly the carpi and tarsi. The stifle, elbow, shoulder, and hip joints are affected to a lesser extent.

During the first month, periarticular soft-tissue swelling is the predominant sign. Swelling may be either intra- or extracapsular. One to three months after the onset of clinical signs, periosteal new bone production at points of joint capsular attachment can be identified. During this phase, the bone adjacent to affected joints may show signs of osteopenia, such as decreased bone opacity and a coarse trabecular

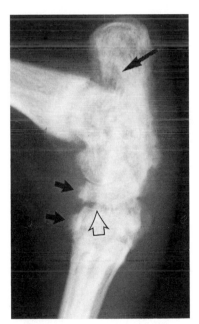

Figure 13–11. A 2-year-old male domestic cat had progressive generalized lameness, which was preceded by a brief illness characterized by fever and lassitude. Some regional lymph nodes were palpably enlarged. Radiographs taken 1 month after onset of the clinical illness revealed periosteal new bone formation on many tarsal bones *(small arrows)*. Subchondral osteolysis is pronounced in the tarsocrural distal intertarsal articulations *(open arrow)*. Some tarsal bones show foci of osteolysis *(large arrow)*. Peritarsal soft-tissue swelling is evident. Laboratory diagnosis: feline chronic progressive polyarthritis. (Courtesy of A. K. W. Wood.)

pattern. Perichondral new bone formation is pronounced 2 to 3 months after onset of the disease.

Extensive osteophytes may bridge smaller joint spaces. More severe radiographic manifestations include perichondral bone erosion and formation of subchondral cysts. Narrowing of affected joint spaces may occur late in the disease.[86] The radiographic signs of the periosteal proliferative form of feline chronic progressive polyarthritis include periarticular soft-tissue swelling, periosteal new bone formation, perichondral osteophyte production, perichondral and subchondral erosion, subchondral cysts, osteopenia of bone adjacent to affected joints, and narrowed joint spaces (Fig. 13–11).

The Erosive Form. A second, more erosive form, has been described in three cats; it resembles human rheumatoid arthritis.[86] This form of the disease is characterized radiographically by severe subchondral bone erosion, perichondral bone erosion, subchondral cyst formation, perichondral osteophyte formation, bone destruction at points of ligamentous insertion to bone, and subluxation of small joints of the extremities.[85]

HYPERTROPHIC OSTEOPATHY

Hypertrophic osteopathy is a generalized osteoproductive disorder of the periosteum that affects the long bones of the extremities. When new bone production involves the periosteal surfaces of bony components of joints, the disorder is termed hypertrophic osteoarthropathy (Fig. 13–12).

Hypertrophic osteopathy is usually seen secondary to cardiopulmonary disease or neoplasia.[9] The majority of neoplasms are pulmonary (primary or secondary), but increasing numbers of cases are being reported in animals with primary intra-abdominal neoplasia without pulmonary involvement.[15, 74, 91]

The pathogenesis of hypertrophic osteopathy is incompletely understood. The most consistent pathologic finding in affected animals is increased blood flow to the extremities. This results in an overgrowth of vascular connective tissue with subsequent fibrochondroid metaplasia and subperiosteal new bone formation. New bone formation typically commences on the digits and progressively extends toward the axial skeleton.

Periosteal new bone formation results in cortical thickening. The periosteal surface appears nodular or spiculated when visualized radiographically. When joints are involved, the bone surfaces that are not covered with cartilage are roughened, and large perichondral osteophytes form.

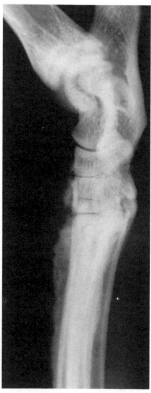

Figure 13–12. A 4-year-old female domestic cat had swollen paws and progressive lameness for 6 weeks. Radiography revealed periosteal new bone formation on the dorsal aspect of the central and fourth tarsal bones as well as on the dorsal surface of the metatarsal bones. Histologic diagnosis: hypertrophic osteoarthropathy secondary to bronchogenic carcinoma.

VILLONODULAR SYNOVITIS

Villonodular synovitis is an intracapsular joint disorder characterized by nodular synovial hyperplasia, which is thought to represent a response of the synovium to trauma. Experimentally, villonodular synovitis has been reproduced in dogs by repeated injections of whole blood intra-articularly.[114] Villonodular synovitis is an established, although uncommon, disorder of humans,[103] and it has also been reported in horses.[76] A suspected case of bilateral coxofemoral villonodular synovitis in a dog has been reported.[53]

The radiographic signs of the disease include articular soft-tissue swelling and erosion of cortical bone at the chondrosynovial junction. These cortical erosions may appear cyst-like, with slightly sclerotic borders. In severe cases of proximal femoral villonodular synovitis in

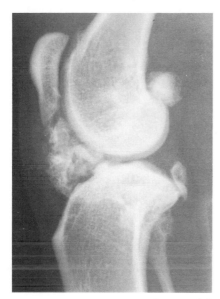

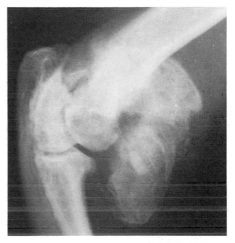

Figure 13–13. A 5-year-old female (neutered) Burmese cat had bilateral stifle enlargement. Mineralization of the infrapatellar fat pad and within the stifle joint compartment was evident radiographically. Histologic diagnosis: synovial osteochondroma.

Figure 13–14. A 6-year-old male (neutered) Burmese cat had progressive lameness of the right foreleg for 6 weeks. Radiography showed a large, well-defined, ossified mass on the craniomedial aspect of the right elbow. Histologic diagnosis: extra-articular synovial osteochondroma.

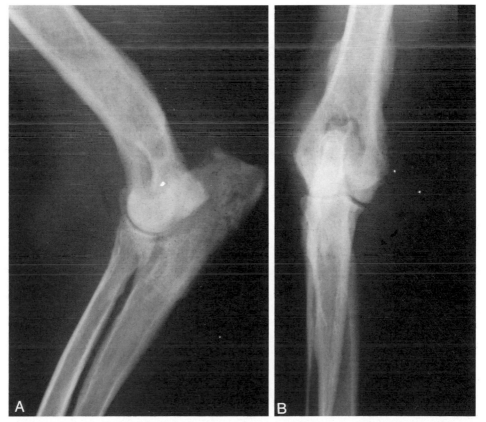

Figure 13–15. A 14-year-old female (neutered) Golden Retriever had progressive lameness of the right forelimb for 4 weeks. In addition, the elbow was swollen. *A* and *B*, active periosteal proliferation is present on the distal humerus and proximal ulna. Punctate areas of radiolucency are evident in the proximal ulna. Histologic diagnosis: synovial sarcoma.

humans, the appearance of the femoral neck has been described as an apple core. The articular cartilage and subchondral bone are not involved in the disease process.

Arthrography has been used convincingly to identify the intracapsular nodular masses of hypertrophied synovium in both humans and in horses.[4, 28, 42, 76] Arthrography also allows visualization of the expanded synovial sac. The differential diagnosis for perichondral erosive lesions, characteristic of villonodular synovitis, should include synovial osteochondromatosis, rheumatoid arthritis, and amyloidosis.[36]

SYNOVIAL OSTEOCHONDROMAS

Synovial osteochondromas have long been recognized in the joints of humans.[16, 49, 108] These lesions are described as islands of cartilage that are produced by the synovial membrane. Foci of cartilage become pedunculated and may become separated from their pedicles as loose bodies within the joint.

The radiographic appearance of mineralized synovial osteochondromas varies. These lesions are usually well-defined, rounded, often multiple intra-articular nodules of calcific opacity (Fig. 13–13). Not all osteochondromas become calcified, in which case contrast arthrography may be necessary for their diagnosis. Synovial osteochondromas may also arise from extra-articular foci of synovial tissue (Fig. 13–14).

Synovial osteochondromas have been reported in the dog[98] and in the cat.[52] Their etiology is unknown, but the theory of synovial metaplasia is generally accepted.[64, 98] These lesions have been reported to cause severe lameness in some dogs. Surgical removal of synovial osteochondromas relieves clinical signs of joint pain and lameness.

SYNOVIAL SARCOMA

Synovial sarcomas arise from synovioblastic tissue, from either inside or outside a joint. These tumors are uncommon in the dog, and are rare in the cat.[24, 64] The most commonly affected joints are the stifle and the elbow. Synovial sarcomas grow slowly, and are first noticeable as a homogeneous soft-tissue mass that involves or is near to a joint. Initially, radiographs reveal a mass of soft tissue. Portions of the tumor may be calcified, with mineral deposits appearing as hazy and punctated or as linear streaks (Fig. 13–15).

Canine synovial sarcomas are more likely to invade adjacent bone than their counterpart in humans.[13, 57] Initial bone involvement appears as a spiculated periosteal response, followed by ragged erosion of the cortical bone adjacent to the tumor. Destruction of cancellous bone can be extensive, and most commonly occurs on both sides of the joint.[57, 64, 69, 89] Distant metastasis, particularly to the lungs, occurs in up to one third of reported cases.[64, 69] Radiography of the thorax is therefore mandatory in cases of suspected synovial sarcoma.

Before the appearance of cortical and cancellous bone destruction, synovial sarcomas should be differentiated from primary tumors of soft-tissue origin, fibrosarcomas or chondrosarcomas of the periosteum, parosteal sarcoma, periosteal hematoma, ossifying myositis, and metastatic disease. The location of an osteodestructive lesion on both sides of a joint, associated with an adjacent soft-tissue mass, is strong presumptive radiographic evidence of a synovial sarcoma.[64] Primary and metastatic bone tumors occasionally invade joints (Figs. 13–16 and 13–17).

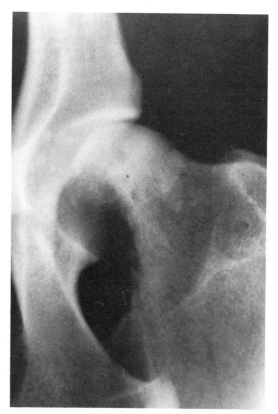

Figure 13–16. A 10-year-old female Doberman pinscher had acute onset pain and non–weight-bearing lameness referrable to the left hip. Osteolysis of the left femoral head and neck was evident radiographically. Histologic diagnosis: pancreatic adenocarcinoma metastasis to the left femoral head and neck.

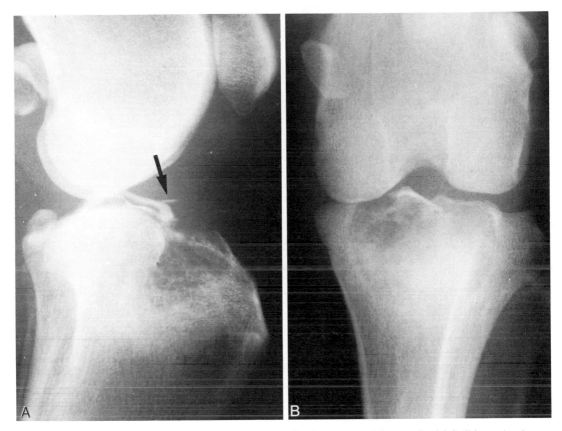

Figure 13–17. A 2-year-old female Great Dane had gradual enlargement of the proximal left tibia and subsequent acute onset of non–weight-bearing lameness of the left hind leg. A and B, a focus of osteolysis within the medial condyle of the proximal tibia extends to involve the joint space. A small bone fragment is free within the joint space (arrow). Histologic diagnosis: Hemangiosarcoma. (Courtesy of A. K. W. Wood.)

References

1. Alexander, JW: Septic arthritis: Diagnosis and treatment. J Am Anim Hosp Assoc 14:499, 1978.
2. Alexander JW: Pathogenesis and biochemical aspects of degenerative joint disease. Comp Contin Ed Pract Vet 2:961, 1980.
3. Alexander JW, Begg S, Dueland R, et al: Rheumatoid arthritis in the dog. J Am Anim Hosp Assoc 12:727, 1976.
4. Allan GS: Radiography of the equine fetlock. Equine Pract 1:40, 1979.
5. Barrett RE: Canine polyarthritis. In Kirk RW (Ed): Current Veterinary Therapy VII. Philadelphia, WB Saunders, 1980, pp. 800–802.
6. Bellah JR, and Weigel JP: Hemarthrosis secondary to suspected warfarin toxicosis in a dog. J Am Vet Med Assoc 182:1126, 1983.
7. Bennett D, Gilbertson EM, and Grennan D: Bacterial endocarditis with polyarthritis in two dogs in association with circulating autoantibodies. J Small Anim Pract 19:185, 1978.
8. Biery DW, and Newton CD: Radiographic appearance of rheumatoid arthritis in the dog. J Am Anim Hosp Assoc 11:607, 1975.
9. Brodey RS: Hypertrophic osteoarthropathy. In An-

drews EJ, et al (Eds): Spontaneous Animal Models of Human Disease. New York, Academic Press, 1980.
10. Brooymans-Schallenburg JHC: Diagnosis of hip dysplasia and selection against this trait. Vet Quart 5:8, 1983.
11. Brown SG: Infectious arthritis and wounds of joints. Vet Clin North Am 8:501, 1978.
12. Butt WP: Radiology of the infected joint. Clin Orthop 96:136, 1973.
13. Cadman NL, and Soule KPJ: Synovial sarcoma: An analysis of 134 tumors. Cancer 18:613, 1965.
14. Caywood DD, Wilson JW, and O'Leary TP: Septic polyarthritis associated with bacterial endocarditis in two dogs. J Am Vet Med Assoc 171:549, 1977.
15. Caywood DD, Osborne CA, Stevens JB, et al: Hypertrophic osteoarthropathy associated with an atypical neuroblastoma in a dog. J Am Anim Hosp Assoc 16:855, 1980.
16. Christensen JH, and Poulsen SJ: Synovial chondromatosis. Acta Orthop Scand 46:919, 1975.
17. Christman OD, Fessell JM, and Southwick WD: Experimental production of synovitis and marginal exostosis in the knee of dogs. Yale J Biol Med 37:409, 1965.
18. Cole BC, and Cassell GH: Mycoplasma infections as

models of chronic joint inflammation. Arthritis Rheum 22:1375, 1979.

19. Culvenor JA, and Howlett CR: Avulsion of the medial epicondyle of the humerus in the dog. J Small Anim Pract 23:83, 1982.

20. Culvenor JA, Hulse DA, and Patton CS: Closure after injury of the distal femoral growth plate in the dog. J Small Anim Pract 19:549, 1978.

21. Curtis PH: Cartilage damage in septic arthritis. Clin Orthop 64:87, 1969.

22. Curtis PH: The pathophysiology of joint infections. Clin Orthop 96:129, 1973.

23. Daly WR: Femoral head and neck fractures in the dog and cat: A review of 115 cases. Vet Surg 7:29, 1978.

24. Davies JD, and Little NRF: Synovial sarcoma in a cat. J Small Anim Pract 13:127, 1972.

25. Davis PE: Track injuries in racing greyhounds. Aust Vet J 43:180, 1967.

26. Denny HR: Condylar fractures of the humerus in the dog: A review of 133 cases. J Small Anim Pract 24:185, 1983.

27. Denny HR, and Minter HM: The long term results of surgery of the canine stifle. J Small Anim Pract 14:695, 1973.

28. Docken WP: Pigmented villonodular synovitis: A review with illustrated case reports. Semin Arthritis Rheum 9:1, 1979.

29. Dodds WJ: Hemostasis and coagulation. In Kaneko JJ (Ed): Clinical Biochemistry of Domestic Animals, 3rd Ed. New York, Academic Press, 1980, pp. 671–718.

30. Ellison GW, and Norrdin RW: Multicentric periarticular calcinosis in a pup. J Am Vet Med Assoc 177:542, 1980.

31. Farrow CS: Carpal sprain injuries in the dog. J Am Vet Radiol Soc 18:38, 1977.

32. Farrow CS: Stress radiography: Applications in small animal practice. J Am Vet Med Assoc 181:777, 1982.

33. Gambardella PG, and Griffiths RC: Treatment of hyperextension injuries of the canine carpus. Comp Contin Ed Pract Vet 4:127, 1982.

34. Gibson JP, and Roenigk WJ: Pseudogout in a dog. J Am Vet Med Assoc 161:912, 1972.

35. Goddard ME, and Mason TA: The genetics and early prediction of hip dysplasia. Aust Vet J 58:1, 1982.

36. Goldberg RP, Weissman BN, Naimark A, et al: Femoral neck erosions: Sign of hip joint synovial disease. AJR 141:107, 1983.

37. Grauer GF, Banks WJ, Ellison GW, et al: Incidence and mechanisms of distal femoral physeal fractures in the dog and cat. J Am Anim Hosp Assoc 17:579, 1981.

38. Grindem CB, and Johnston KH: Systemic lupus erythematosus. Literature review and report of 42 new canine cases. J Am Anim Hosp Assoc 19:489, 1983.

39. Halliwell REW, Lavelle RB, and Butt KM: Canine rheumatoid arthritis—a review and a case record. J Small Anim Pract 13:239, 1972.

40. Halliwell REW: Autoimmune disease in the dog. Adv Vet Sci Comp Med 22:221, 1978.

41. Halliwell REW: Autoimmune diseases in domestic animals. J Am Vet Med Assoc 181:1088, 1982.

42. Halpern AA, Donovan TL, Horowitz B, et al: Arthrographic demonstration of pigmented villonodular synovitis of the knee. Clin Orthop 132:193, 1978.

43. Hedhammar A, Wu F-M, Krook L, et al: Overnutrition and skeletal disease. Cornell Vet 64:9, 1974.

44. Hedhammar A, Olsson S-E, Andersson S-A, et al: Canine hip dysplasia: Study of heritability in 401 litters of German shepherd dogs. J Am Vet Med Assoc 174:1012, 1979.

45. Henricsson BE, Ljunggren G, Olsson S-E, et al.: Hip dysplasia in Sweden. Controlled breeding programmes. In Proceedings of Canine Hip Dysplasia Symposium and Workshop. St. Louis, Orthopedic Foundation for Animals, 1972, pp. 141–151.

46. Heuser W: Canine rheumatoid arthritis. Can Vet J 21:314, 1980.

47. Hoaglund FT: Experimental haemarthrosis: The response of canine knees to injection of autogenous blood. J Bone Joint Surg 49:285, 1967.

48. Hutt FB: Genetic selection to reduce the incidence of hip dysplasia in dogs. J Am Vet Med Assoc 151:1041, 1967.

49. Jeffreys TE: Synovial chondromatosis. J Bone Joint Surg [Br] 49:530, 1967.

50. Jessen CR, and Spurrell FA: Heritability of canine hip dysplasia. In Proceedings of Canine Hip Dysplasia Symposium and Workshop. St. Louis, Orthopedic Foundation for Animals, 1972, pp. 53–61.

51. Kasstrom H: Nutrition, weight gain, and the development of hip dysplasia. Acta Radiol [Suppl] (Stockh) 16:135, 1975.

52. Kealy JK: Diagnostic Radiology of the Dog and Cat. Philadelphia, WB Saunders, 1979, p. 371.

53. Kusba JK, Lipowitz AJ, Wize M, et al: Suspected villonodular synovitis in a dog. J Am Vet Med Assoc 182:390, 1983.

54. Lammerding JL, Noser GA, Brinker WO, et al: Avulsion injuries of the origin of the extensor digitorum longus muscle in three dogs. J Am Anim Hosp Assoc 12:764, 1976.

55. Larsen JS, and Corley EA: Radiographic evaluation in a canine hip dysplasia control programme. J Am Vet Med Assoc 159:989, 1971.

56. Leighton EA, Linn JM, Willham RL, et al: A genetic study of canine hip dysplasia. Am J Vet Res 38:241, 1977.

57. Lipowitz AJ, Fetter AW, and Walker MA: Synovial sarcoma in the dog. J Am Vet Med Assoc 174:76, 1978.

58. Liu S-K, Suter PF, Fischer CA, et al: Rheumatoid arthritis in a dog. J Am Vet Med Assoc 154:495, 1969.

59. Ljunggren G, and Olsson S-E: Osteoarthrosis of the shoulder and elbow joints in dogs: A pathologic and radiographic study of a necropsy material. J Am Vet Radiol Soc 16:33, 1975.

60. Lust G, and Farrell PW: Hip dysplasia in dogs: The interplay of genotype and environment. Cornell Vet 67:447, 1977.

61. Lust G, Beilman WT, Dueland DJ, et al: Intraarticular volume and hip joint instability in dogs with hip dysplasia. J Bone Joint Surg [Am] 62:576, 1980.

62. Lust G, Beilman WT, and Rendano VT: A relationship between degree of laxity and synovial fluid volume in coxofemoral joints of dogs predisposed for hip dysplasia. Am J Vet Res 41:55, 1980.

63. Lust G, and Summers BA: Early, asymptomatic stage of degenerative joint disease in canine hip joints. Am J Vet Res 42:1849, 1981.

64. Madewell BR, and Pool RR: Neoplasms of joints and related structures. Vet Clin North Am 8:511, 1978.

65. Marretta SM, and Schrader SC: Physeal injuries in the dog: A review of 135 cases. J Am Vet Med Assoc 182:708, 1983.

66. Marshall JL: Peri-articular osteophytes—initiation and formation in the knees of the dog. Clin Orthop 62:37, 1969.

67. Marshall JL, and Olsson S-E: Instability of the knee. A long-term experimental study in dogs. J Bone Joint Surg [Am] 53:1561, 1971.

68. Milgram JW: The classification of loose bodies in human joints. Clin Orthop 124:282, 1977.
69. Mitchell M, and Hurov LI: Synovial sarcoma in a dog. J Am Vet Med Assoc 175:53, 1979.
70. Moise NS, and Crissman JW: Chronic progressive polyarthritis in a cat. J Am Anim Hosp Assoc 18:965, 1982.
71. Moise NS, Crissman JW, Fairbrother JF, et al: Mycoplasma gateae arthritis and tenosynovitis in cats: Case report and experimental reproduction of the disease. Am J Vet Res 44:10, 1983.
72. Morgan JP: Radiological pathology and diagnosis of degenerative joint disease in the stifle of the dog. J Small Anim Pract 10:541, 1969.
73. Morgan JP: Radiology in Veterinary Orthopaedics. Philadelphia, Lea & Febiger, 1972, pp. 174–182.
74. Nate LA, Herron AJ, and Burk RL: Hypertrophic osteopathy in a cat associated with renal papillary adenoma. J Am Anim Hosp Assoc 17:659, 1981.
75. Newton CD, Lipowitz AJ, Halliwell RE, et al: Rheumatoid arthritis in dogs. J Am Vet Med Assoc 168:113, 1976.
76. Nickels FA, Grant BD, and Lincoln SD: Villonodular synovitis of the equine metacarpophalangeal joint. J Am Vet Med Assoc 168:1043, 1976.
77. Olsewski JM, Lust G, Rendano VT, et al: Degenerative joint disease: Multiple joint involvement in young and mature dogs. Am J Vet Res 44:1300, 1983.
78. Olsson S-E: Roentgen examination of hip joints of German shepherd dogs. Adv Small Anim Pract 3.117, 1961.
79. Olsson S-E: Degenerative joint disease: A review with special reference to the dog. J Small Anim Pract 12:333, 1971.
80. Owens JM, and Ackerman N: Roentgenology of arthritis. Vet Clin North Am 8:460, 1978.
81. Pedersen NC: Inflammatory joint diseases of the dog and cat. Proceedings of 48th Annual Meeting of American Animal Hospital Association, Atlanta, April 4–10, 1981, p. 149.
82. Pedersen NC, Pool RR, and O'Brien T: Chronic progressive polyarthritis of the cat. Feline Pract 5.42, 1975.
83. Pedersen NC, Pool RR, Castles JJ, et al: Noninfectious canine arthritis. Rheumatoid arthritis. J Am Vet Med Assoc 169:295, 1976.
84. Pedersen NC, Weisner K, Castles JJ, et al: Noninfectious canine arthritis. The inflammatory non erosive arthritides. J Am Vet Med Assoc 169:304, 1976.
85. Pedersen NC, and Pool RR: Canine joint disease. Vet Clin North Am [Small Anim Pract] 8:465, 1978.
86. Pedersen NC, Pool RR, and O'Brien T: Feline chronic progressive polyarthritis. Am J Vet Res 41:522, 1980.
87. Pedersen NC, Pool RR, and Morgan JP: Joint diseases of dogs and cats. In Ettinger SJ (Ed): Textbook of Veterinary Internal Medicine. Philadelphia, WB Saunders, 1983, pp. 2187–2235.
88. Pond MJ: Avulsion of the extensor digitorum longus muscle in the dog: A report of four cases. J Small Anim Pract 14:785, 1973.
89. Reed JR, Weller RE, and Hornoff WJ: Synovial sarcoma in a dog. Mod Vet Pract 59:605, 1978.
90. Rendano VT, Quick CB, Allan GS, et al: Radiographic evaluation of femoral head and neck fractures. The value of the flexed ventrodorsal and oblique projections in diagnosis. J Am Anim Hosp Assoc 16:485, 1980.
91. Rendano VT, and Slauson DO: Hypertrophic osteopathy in a dog with prostatic adenocarcinoma and without thoracic metastasis. J Am Anim Hosp Assoc 18:905, 1982.
92. Rhodes WH, and Jenny JA: A canine acetabular index. J Am Vet Med Assoc 137:97, 1960.
93. Riser WH: The dysplastic hip joint: Its radiographic and histologic development. J Am Vet Radiol Soc 14:35, 1973.
94. Robins GM: Some aspects of the radiographic examination of the canine elbow joint. J Small Anim Pract 21:417, 1980.
95. Roberts RE: Osteomyelitis associated with disseminated blastomycosis in nine dogs. Vet Radiol 20:124, 1979.
96. Ropes MW, Bennett GA, and Cobb S: Revision of a diagnostic criteria for rheumatoid arthritis. Bull Rheum Dis 9:175, 1958.
97. Salter RB, and Harris WR: Injuries involving the epiphyseal plate. J Bone Joint Surg 45:587, 1963.
98. Schawalder von P: Die synoviale osteochondromatose (synoviale chondrometaplasie) beim hund. Schweiz Arch Tierheilk 122:673, 1980.
99. Schrader SC: Septic arthritis and osteomyelitis of the hip of six mature dogs. J Am Vet Med Assoc 181:894, 1982.
100. Schumacher AR: Rheumatoid arthritis in dogs. J Am Vet Med Assoc 168:113, 1976.
101. Scott DW, Walton DK, Manning TO, et al: Canine lupus erythematosus. 1: Systemic lupus erythematosus. J Am Anim Hosp Assoc 19.461, 1983.
102. Shively MJ, and Van Sickle DC: Developing coxal joint of the dog: Gross morphometric and pathologic observations. Am J Vet Res 42:185, 1982.
103. Smith JH, and Pugh DE: Roentgenographic aspects of articular pigmented villonodular synovitis. AJR 87:1146, 1962.
104. Sokoloff L: The pathology of osteoarthritis and the role of ageing. In Nuki J (Ed): The Aetiopathogenesis of osteoarthritis. Tunbridge Wells, UK, Pitman Medical Publishing, 1980, pp. 1–15.
105. Suter PF, and Carb AV: Shoulder arthrography in dogs—radiographic anatomy and clinical application. J Small Anim Pract 10:407, 1969.
106. Tirgari M, and Vaughan LL: Arthritis of the canine stifle joint. Vet Rec 96:394, 1975.
107. Townsend LR, Gillette EL, and Lebel JL: Progression of hip dysplasia in military working dogs. J Am Vet Med Assoc 158:1129, 1971.
108. Trias A, and Quintana O: Synovial chondrometaplasia. Review of the world literature and a study of 18 Canadian cases. Can J Surg 19:151, 1976.
109. Trueta J: Studies in the Development and Decay of the Human Frame. Philadelphia, WB Saunders, 1968, pp. 238–240, 335–338.
110. van der Velden NA: Hip dysplasia in dogs. Vet Quart 5:3, 1983.
111. Vaughan LC: Muscle and tendon injuries in dogs. J Small Anim Pract 20:711, 1979.
112. Wilkinson GT, and Robins GM: Polyarthritis in a young cat. J Small Anim Pract 20:293, 1979.
113. Wright PJ, and Mason TA: The usefulness of palpation of joint laxity in puppies as a predictor of hip dysplasia in a guide dog breeding programme. J Small Anim Pract 18:513, 1977.
114. Young JM, and Hudacek AG: Experimental production of pigmented villonodular synovitis in the dog. Am J Pathol 30:799, 1954.

SECTION 5

APPENDICULAR SKELETON— *EQUIDAE*

CHAPTER 14

THE STIFLE AND TARSUS

MARY B. MAHAFFEY
DONALD E. THRALL

THE STIFLE

Gross Anatomy

The stifle is the largest joint in the body. It consists of three separate articulations: the femoropatellar and medial and lateral femorotibial articulations. The femoropatellar articulation is formed between the trochlea of the femur and the articular surface of the patella. The femoral trochlea consists of two oblique ridges with a deep groove between them; the medial ridge is much larger than the lateral ridge. Because of the large size of the medial trochlear ridge, the patella lies lateral to the axis of the femur.

The femorotibial articulations are formed between the condyles of the femurs and those of the tibia with the interposed menisci. Between the condyles of the tibia is a prominent intercondylar eminence consisting of medial and lateral tubercles; the medial tubercle extends further proximally than the lateral tubercle. The large medial tubercle of the intercondylar eminence of the tibia is a useful landmark when distinguishing medial from lateral in caudocranial radiographs of this joint, particularly if the patella and fibula are not visible.

The femorotibial articulations have potentially separate synovial sacs (medial and lateral), which do not communicate with each other directly. The femoropatellar synovial sac is extensive; it typically communicates with the medial femorotibial sac and occasionally (approximately 25 percent of the time) communicates with the lateral femorotibial sac.

Radiographic Technique and Anatomy

For routine evaluation, caudocranial and lateromedial projections of the stifle are made. Occasionally, craniolateral-caudomedial or caudolateral-craniomedial oblique projections are useful to project other surfaces of the joint. Because of the thickness of this area, use of a grid increases radiographic detail considerably. A grid is rarely used, however, because of the difficulty encountered in aligning the primary x-ray beam so that it strikes the grid perpendicularly. In addition, use of a grid necessitates larger exposure factors, which are often beyond the capacity of equipment available in private practice. Care must be taken when making the caudocranial projection, because personnel and equipment are in jeopardy if the horse should kick. Unruly patients should be restrained chemically.

Use of high-speed film and intensifying screens allows diagnostic radiographs of the stifle to be made with relatively low power equipment. Radiographs of the stifle of a skeletally immature and a skeletally mature horse

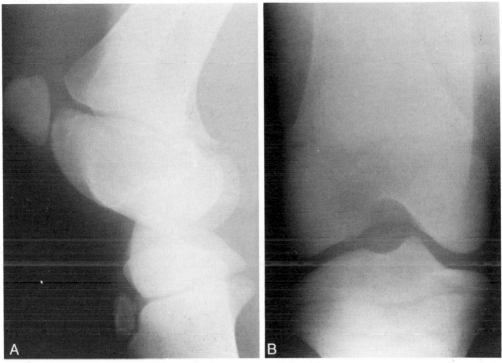

Figure 14–1. A normal, immature equine stifle, lateral *(A)* and caudocranial *(B)* views. Note distal femoral and proximal tibial physes. Also note the irregularity of the patella and cranial aspect of the condyles in the lateral view; this normal appearance should not be confused with an aggressive lesion, such as infection.

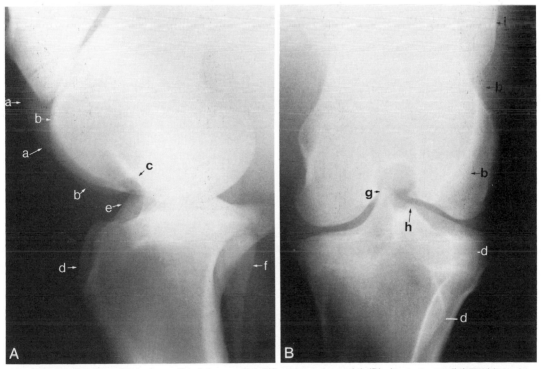

Figure 14–2. A normal, adult equine stifle, lateromedial *(A)* and caudocranial *(B)* views. a: medial trochlear ridge of femur; b: lateral trochlear ridge of femur; c: extensor fossa of femur; d: tibial tuberosity; e: intercondylar eminence of tibia; f: fibula; g: medial tubercle of tibial intercondylar eminence; h: lateral tubercle of tibial intercondylar eminence; i: patella. Note the radiolucent line in the fibula. This is a normal finding due to separate ossification centers; it is frequently misinterpreted as a fracture. Occasionally, more than one radiolucent line is seen due to the presence of more than two ossification centers.

are shown in Figures 14–1 and 14–2 respectively.[1]

Radiographic Abnormalities

Osteochondrosis and Osseous Cyst-like Lesions. Osteochondrosis is a relatively common disorder of young horses. It is a cartilage-bone maturation failure in which the proliferating cartilage model is not completely replaced by bone. The persistent cartilage appears radiographically as a radiolucent bone defect, which is usually adjacent to an articular surface. In the equine stifle, osteochondrosis may affect the lateral trochlear ridge of the femur (Fig. 14–3).[2] In this instance, the periphery of the lateral trochlear ridge has an irregular appearance due to multiple areas of cartilage that have not matured into bone. Occasionally, free or partially detached osteochondral fragments are observed adjacent to the periphery of the trochlea. Because osteochondrosis is frequently bilateral, a radiograph of the opposite stifle should be made if this condition is identified.

"Bone cysts" have been described as occurring in many locations in horses.[3] One location is in the medial femoral condyle. In some reports it has been suggested that these cystic lesions are a manifestation of osteochondrosis; such has not been proven definitively. In addition, there is still debate as to whether these lesions are true cysts. Therefore, it seems prudent to refer to them as osseous cyst-like lesions. These lesions are found primarily in the

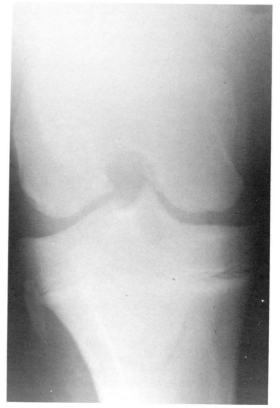

Figure 14–4. Caudocranial radiograph of an equine stifle. A small subchondral defect is present in the medial femoral condyle. This lesion can be considered as a part of the osseous cyst-like lesion syndrome. It could not be seen in the lateral view.

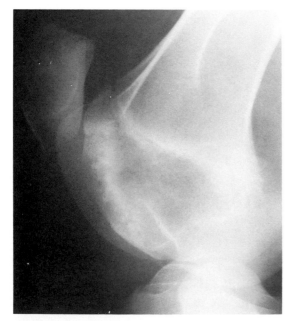

Figure 14–3. Stifle of a horse with osteochondrosis of the lateral trochlear ridge of the femur lateromedial view. The lateral trochlear ridge is irregularly marginated and subchondral bone is sclerotic.

medial condyle and may be observed at any age.[4] Radiographically, these cyst-like lesions appear as subchondral radiolucent defects (Figs. 14–4 and 14–5). Joint communication may be present; radiographic confirmation of such communication requires that the x-ray beam strike the area of joint involvement tangentially (Fig. 14–5). Thus, even if joint communication is present, it may not be identified radiographically. These osseous cyst-like lesions are frequently bilateral and if one is identified, the opposite stifle should be radiographed. Occasionally, osseous cyst-like lesions are found in the lateral condyle or the proximal tibia, but these locations are less common sites of occurrence when compared to the medial femoral condyle.

Sepsis. Septic conditions affecting the equine stifle are relatively common. One instance is in foals having disseminated bacteremia as a result of naval infection. Most of these patients develop osteomyelitis as a result of the bacter-

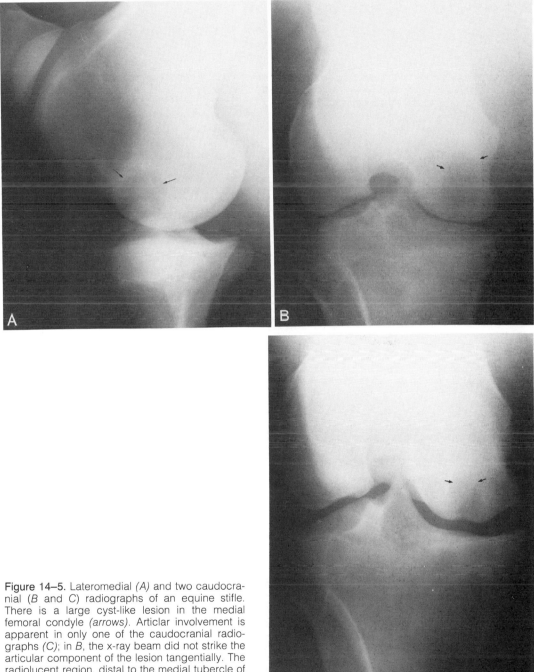

Figure 14–5. Lateromedial *(A)* and two caudocranial *(B* and *C)* radiographs of an equine stifle. There is a large cyst-like lesion in the medial femoral condyle *(arrows)*. Articlar involvement is apparent in only one of the caudocranial radiographs *(C)*; in *B*, the x-ray beam did not strike the articular component of the lesion tangentially. The radiolucent region, distal to the medial tubercle of the intercondylar eminence of the tibia in *C* is normal and should not be confused with a cyst-like lesion.

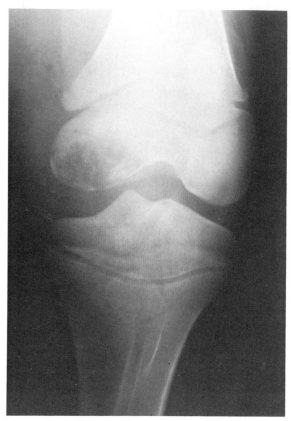

Figure 14–6. Caudocranial radiograph of the stifle of a foal with femoral osteomyelitis. There is an aggressive, primarily osteolytic lesion in the medial femoral condyle. In addition, there are focal areas of gas accumulation in soft tissues medial to the medial femoral condyle.

emia. The radiographic appearance of stifle osteomyelitis is similar to that of bone infections elsewhere in the body; the resulting bone lesion is aggressive. There is usually soft-tissue swelling, which may reflect cellulitis as well as joint effusion, and osteolytic lesions often occur in the femur, patella, or tibia (Fig. 14–6). As the disease progresses, sclerosis reflecting new bone formation may be seen and an active periosteal reaction may develop.

Skin laceration or puncture, with subsequent bacterial contamination, is another cause of septic stifle changes in horses. Changes may be limited to the soft tissue, in which instance only soft-tissue swelling is seen. If bone is involved, typical changes of osteomyelitis are seen.

Trauma. External trauma may result in various radiographic changes. These findings should be evaluated in the same manner as for traumatic changes in the stifle joint of other animals (Fig. 14–7). Degenerative joint disease may develop as a result of external trauma or may be the result of wear and tear. Signs are identical to those seen with degenerative joint disease in other joints, including periarticular osteophyte formation (Fig. 14–8), decrease in size of articular spaces, and subchondral osteolytic defects due to synovial hyperplasia. Care must be taken when evaluating articular space size, because this determination is influenced by the geometric relationship of the x-ray beam, the articular space, and the casette.

Tumoral Calcinosis. Tumoral calcinosis (calcinosis circumscripta) may appear clinically as a

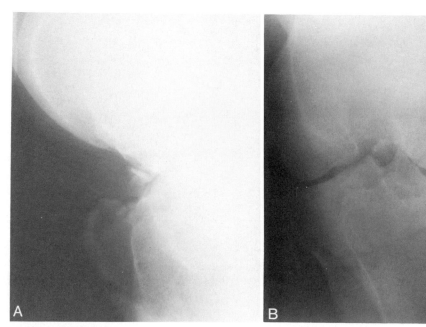

Figure 14–7. Lateromedial *(A)*, caudocranial *(B)*, and caudocranial with lateral stress *(C)* radiographs of a horse that recently had been hit by a car. There is a comminuted fracture of the proximal tibia.

Illustration continued on opposite page

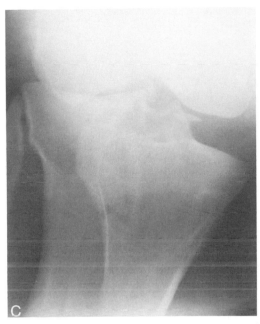

Figure 14–7 *Continued. C,* subluxation is consistent with medial collateral ligament disruption.

hard nodule on the lateral aspect of the stifle.[5] Radiographically, the nodule contains punctate areas of mineralization. The cause of tumoral calcinosis is unknown; affected horses usually are not lame as a result of this condition.

THE TARSUS

Gross Anatomy

The tarsus consists of four major articulations: the tarsocrural, the proximal and distal intertarsal, and the tarsometatarsal articulations. The tarsocrural articulation is formed by the trochlea of the talus and the corresponding cochlea of the distal tibia and fused fibula. Essentially all tarsal flexion and extension take place at the tarsocrural articulation; the intertarsal and tarsometatarsal articulations allow for only slight planar or sliding movement.

There are four synovial sacs in the tarsal complex. The tarsocrural sac is by far the largest; it communicates with the proximal intertarsal sac. The distal intertarsal and tarsometatarsal sacs are separate and distinct from each other

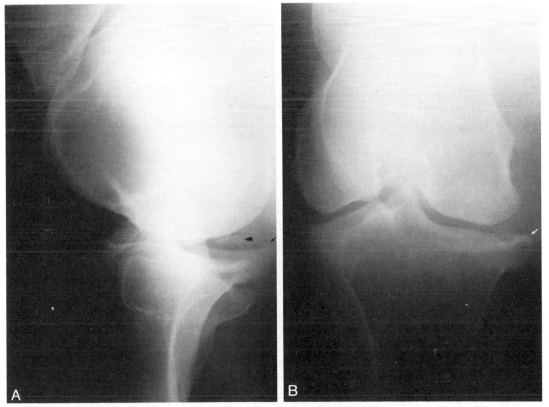

Figure 14–8. The stifle of a horse with degenerative joint disease, lateromedial *(A)* and caudocranial *(B)* views. There is a large periarticular osteophyte on the medial tibial condyle *(arrow)* and mineralization of the medial meniscus *(arrowhead).*

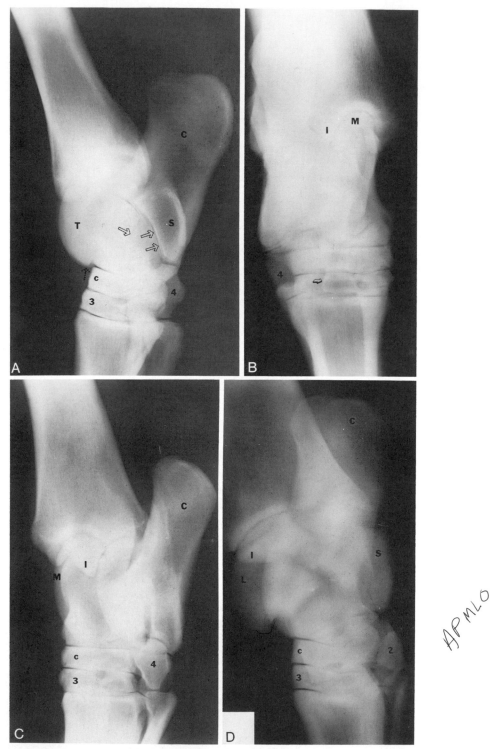

Figure 14–9. Lateromedial *(A)*, craniocaudal *(B)*, dorsolateral-plantaromedial oblique *(C)*, and dorsomedial-plantaro-lateral oblique *(D)* tarsal radiographs of a normal equine tarsus. C: calcaneus; T: talus; S: sustentaculum tali; c: central tarsal bone; 3: third tarsal bone; I: intermediate ridge of tibial cochlea; M: medial trochlea of talus; L: lateral trochlea of talus; 2: fused first and second tarsal bones; 4: fourth tarsal bone. *A, dotted arrow,* the small projection on the distal margin of the medial ridge of the trochlea tali is normal, but it is frequently misinterpreted as an osteophyte or as evidence of osteochondrosis. *A, open arrows,* radiolucent lines formed by the articulation between the calcaneus and talus are normal but are frequently misinterpreted as fracture lines. *B, open arrow,* fused first and second tarsal bones superimposed on the central and third tarsal bones.

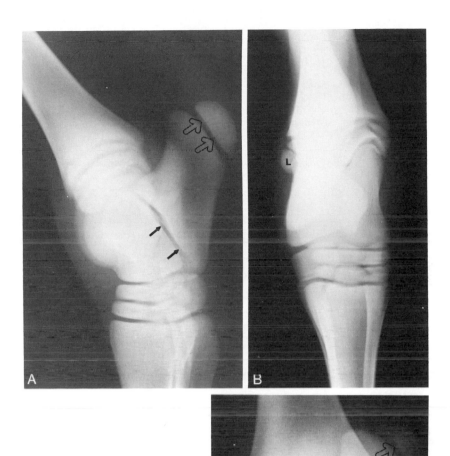

Figure 14–10. The tarsus of a foal, lateromedial *(A)*, dorsoplantar *(B)*, and dorsomedial-plantarolateral *(C)*, radiographs. The physis of the tuber calcaneus *(open arrows)*, lateral malleolus (L), and first (1) and second (2) tarsal bones are visible. *A*, the prominent radiolucent line *(closed arrow)* is the normal articulation between the talus and calcaneus; it is frequently misinterpreted as a fracture. This articulation is also visible in *C (solid arrows)*.

and do not communicate with the tarsocrural or proximal intertarsal sacs. The large calcaneus is located lateral to the axis of the tarsus and is an important radiographic landmark.[6]

Radiographic Technique and Anatomy

For routine examination of the tarsus, four radiographic projections should be made: later-omedial, dorsoplantar, dorsolateral-plantaro-medial oblique, and dorsomedial-plantarolateral oblique views (Fig. 14–9). Oblique projections are recommended as routine procedure because of the complex nature of the tarsus and the tendency for some abnormalities to remain un-detected in dorsoplantar or lateromedial projec-tions.

In young foals, physes are visible in the distal tibia and tuber calcanei. In addition, the lateral malleolus appears as a separate structure; it fuses with the tibia at approximately 100 days of age.[7] In some foals, the first and second tarsal

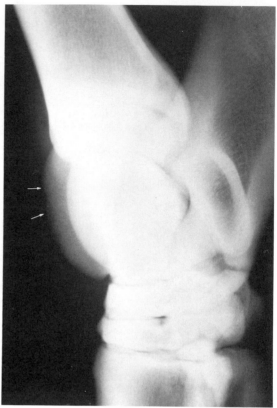

Figure 14–12. The tarsus of a horse with osteochondrosis of the medial trochlear ridge of the talus, lateromedial view. The dorsal margin of the medial trochlear ridge is irregular. Note the normal projection on the distal margin of the medial ridge of the talus.

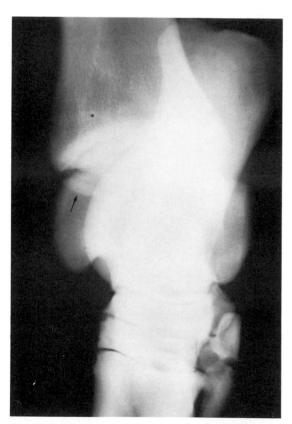

Figure 14–11. The tarsus of a horse with osteochondrosis of the tibial intermediate ridge, dorsomedial-plantarolat-eral view. There is an osteochondral fragment of the distal tibia *(arrow)*. Osteophytes are present on the dor-solateral aspects of the distal intertarsal and tarsometa-tarsal articulations, which are indicative of degenerative joint disease.

bones appear as separate structures after birth; in other horses, fusion may take place before birth (Fig. 14–10). One author estimates that the first and second tarsal bones are radiograph-ically separate in approximately 20 percent of 6-month-old foals.[7]

The use of a grid for tarsal radiography is not necessary. It is important that the horse bear weight on the joint when the radiographs are made.

Radiographic Abnormalities

Osteochondrosis and Osseous Cyst-like Le-sions. There are at least three distinct manifes-tations of these disorders in the tarsus. The first is osteochondrosis affecting the cranial aspect of the intermediate ridge of the tibial cochlea.[8] In this instance, a cleavage line may be seen in the cranial aspect of the intermediate ridge, which reflects formation of a large osteochondral fragment. This fragment can be seen in the lateromedial projection, but is more clearly seen in the dorsomedial-plantarolateral projec-

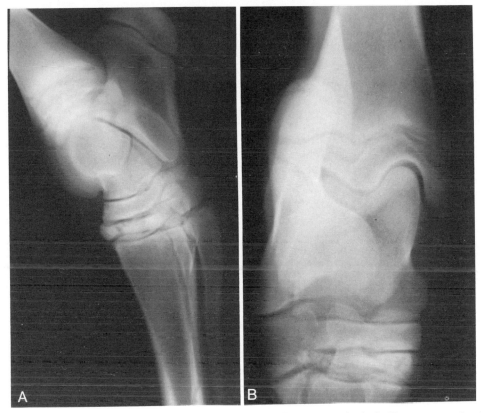

Figure 14–13. Lateromedial *(A)* and dorsoplantar *(B)* radiographs of the tarsus of a foal with a compression fraction of the third tarsal bone.

tion (Fig. 14–11). The clinical significance of this manifestation of osteochondrosis is unknown, because it has been found as an apparently incidental condition in sound horses.

The second manifestation of these conditions is osteochondrosis of the lateral or medial trochlear ridge of the talus.[8] In this condition, there is usually a radiolucent defect involving the margin of the affected talus (Fig. 14–12). Thirdly, osseous cyst-like lesions can be found in the distal tibia, the proximal aspect of the third metatarsus, the talus, or the calcaneus. All three manifestations are frequently bilateral, and if identified, radiographs of the contralateral limb should be obtained.

Another condition that has been described as a form of osteochondrosis is compression of the third tarsal bone in foals. This condition has also been described as aseptic or avascular necrosis of the third tarsal bone. To our knowledge, the exact etiology of this condition is unknown. Nevertheless, extensive compression-type fracture of the third tarsal bone is occasionally observed in foals (Fig. 14–13).[9] Many of these foals also have an associated angular limb deformity, which may be secondary to the fracture or may have been present before fracture and contributed to mechanical failure of the third tarsal bone.

Trauma. Whether the result of external trauma or joint wear and tear, degenerative joint disease of the tarsus is common. Radiographic signs are similar to degenerative joint disease in other joints. Periarticular osteophyte formation is the most frequently observed radiographic sign of tarsal degenerative joint disease in horses. It is tempting to try to evaluate tarsal joint space narrowing by radiographic means, but as in the stifle, this assessment is complicated by the difficulty associated with achieving true parallel relationship between the x-ray beam, joint surfaces, and casette. The clinical significance of radiographically detectable changes of tarsal degenerative joint disease is debatable, because there is poor clinical correlation between these changes and lameness.[10]

Periarticular osteophytes are usually best seen in the dorsolateral-plantaromedial oblique projection, because the disease seems to begin dorsomedially in many horses. Radiographic changes can frequently be seen in other tarsal projections as well (Figs. 14–11 and 14–14).

Other Conditions. Fractures and sepsis of the tarsus are relatively common. Radiographic

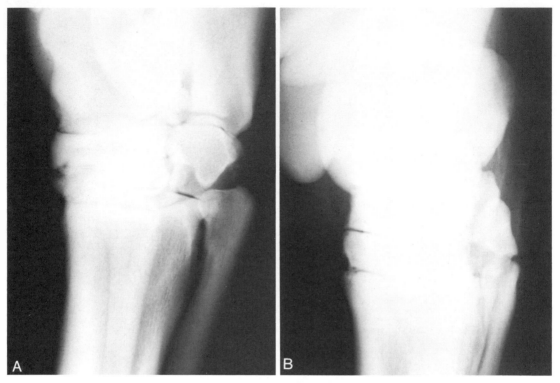

Figure 14–14. Dorsolateral-plantaromedial *(A)* and dorsomedial-plantarolateral *(B)* radiographs of horses with tarsal degenerative joint disease. Multiple periarticular osteophytes can be seen.

evaluation of these conditions is straightforward, and radiographic signs are similar to those described elsewhere in this text.

References

1. Adams WM, and Thilsted JP: Radiographic appearance of the equine stifle; birth to six months. Vet Radiol 26:126, 1985.
2. Pascoe JR, Pool RR, Wheat JD, et al: Osteochondral defects of the lateral trochlear ridge of the distal femur of the horse. Clinical, radiographic and pathologic examination and results of surgical treatment. Vet Surg 13:99, 1984.
3. Peterson H, and Reinland S: Periarticular subchondral "bone cysts" in horses. Proceedings of the 14th Annual Meeting of the American Association Equine Practitioners, Philadelphia, 1968, p. 245.
4. Stewart B, and Reid CF: Osseous cystlike lesions of the medial femoral condyle in the horse. J Am Vet Med Assoc 180:254, 1982.
5. Dodd DC, and Raker CW: Tumoral calcinosis (calcinosis circumscripta) in the horse. J Am Vet Med Assoc 157:968, 1970.
6. Shively MJ, and Smallwood JE: Radiographic and xeroradiographic anatomy of the equine tarsus. Equine Pract 2:19, 1980.
7. Smallwood JE, Auer JA, Martens RJ, et al: The developing equine tarsus from birth to six months of age. Equine Pract 6:7, 1984.
8. Stromberg B, and Rejno S: Osteochondrosis in the horse. Acta Radiol [Diagn] (Stockh) 358:139, 1978.
9. Dewes HF: The onset and consequences of tarsal bone fractures in foals. NZ Vet J 30:129, 1982.
10. Hartung K, Munzer B, and Keller H: Radiographic evaluation of spavin in young trotters. Vet Radiol 24:153, 1983.

CHAPTER 15

THE CARPUS

J. GREGG BORING

Radiographic evaluation of the carpus is essential in determining the diagnosis, treatment, and prognosis of carpal soft tissue and bone lesions. The equine carpus is composed of seven to eight cuboidal bones arranged in two rows, opposed proximally by the radius (antebrachiocarpal joint) and distally by three metacarpal bones (carpometacarpal joint). The intercarpal joint (middle carpal joint) joins the proximal and distal rows of carpal bones. All three are synovial joints, with communication of the middle and carpometacarpal spaces between the third and fourth carpal bones; the antebrachiocarpal joint cavity remains separated.[1, 2] Collectively, there are approximately 26 side-to-side and proximal-to-distal bone articulations. The irregularly curved surfaces are compounded by superimposition of the various sizes, shapes, and positions of the individual carpal bones. This superimposition justifies the use of multiple radiographic views to examine bone and soft tissue structures of this region adequately.

Five standard views have been suggested for complete radiographic evaluation of the carpus.[3] These views include the dorsopalmar (DPa), lateromedial (LM), flexed lateromedial (FLM), dorsolateral-palmaromedial oblique (DL-PaMO), and dorsomedial palmarolateral oblique (DM-PaLO) views (Fig. 15–1). In addition to the five standard views, oblique views of the dorsal surface of the carpal bones are of value in demonstrating selected carpal fractures (Fig. 15–2).[4] These views are designated as DPr-DDiO (dorsoproximal-dorsodistal oblique) when describing the dorsal aspects of the equine carpal bones (Fig. 15–2).[5]

Fractures are the most common injury in mature performance horses. Studies indicate Thoroughbreds have almost twice the incidence of carpal fractures as Quarterhorses.[6] The most common sites of carpal fractures in descending order of incidence are: radial carpal (Fig. 15–3), third carpal (Fig. 15–4), distal end of the radius (Fig. 15–5), and the intermediate carpal bone (Fig. 15–6). Fractures of the radial carpal bone account for more injuries than all other carpal bones combined.[6] The dorsodistal corner of the radial carpal bone is the most typical site (Fig. 15–3). The flexed lateromedial and dorsolateral-palmaromedial oblique projections are particularly valuable in isolating these radial carpal fractures; the former alone has been shown to isolate 89 per cent (127 of 143) of all carpal fractures.[7] This projection separates the proximal and distal borders of the radial and intermediate carpal bones by shifting the radial

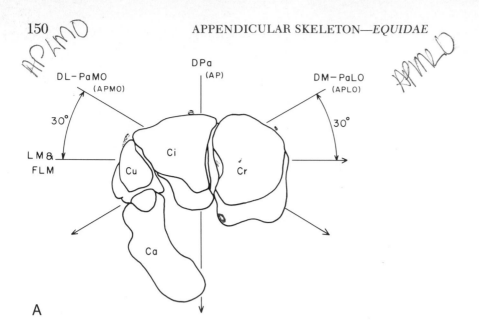

A

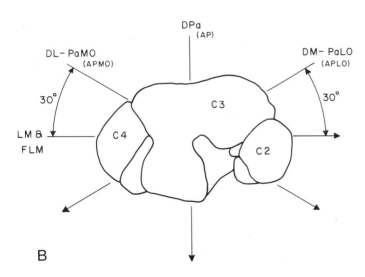

B

Figure 15–1. Five standard radiographic projections. Diagram of the proximal *(A)* and distal *(B)* rows of equine carpal bones. Directional terms describing points of entrance to point of exit of the primary x-ray beam are designated. Previously used terminology is shown in parenthesis. DL-PaMO: dorsolateral-palmaromedial oblique; DPa: dorsopalmar; DM-PaLO: dorsomedial-palmarolateral oblique; Ca: accessory carpal; Cu: ulnar carpal; Ci: intermediate carpal; Cr: radial carpal. (AP, APMO, and APLO designations are no longer in use but are included for comparative purposes.)

Figure 15–2. Dorsoproximal-dorsodistal oblique (DPr-DDiO) projections of the equine carpus. These views have been termed skyline or tangential, and are needed to project the dorsal aspects of the equine carpal bones and distal end of the radius. (PR: view to project proximal row; DR: view to project distal row.)

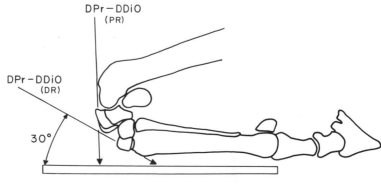

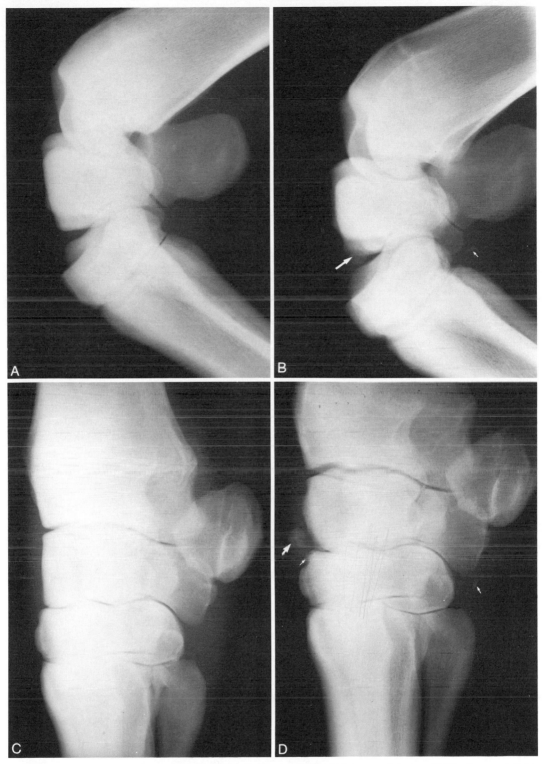

Figure 15–3. Chronic fracture of the distal radial carpal bone. *A,* flexed lateromedial view (FLM) of a normal carpus. Note the distal shift of the radial carpal bone separating the dorsoproximal and dorsodistal corners of the radial and intermediate carpal bones. *B,* a rounded (chronic) chip fracture is seen on the distal radial carpal bone *(large arrow),* and a small fragment *(small arrow)* has become displaced to the palmar aspect of the antebrachiocarpal joint. Eighty-nine percent of all carpal fractures have been reported to be visible with this view.[7] *C,* normal carpus in the dorsolateral-palmaromedial oblique (DL-PaMO) view. This view is necessary to evaluate fractures of the radial carpal bone completely. *D,* note the small periarticular osteophyte *(small dorsal arrow)* on the third carpal bone not visible on the FLM. This osteophyte is indicative of secondary joint disease. Degenerative joint disease was initiated by a long-standing radial carpal bone fracture *(large arrow).* A small piece of the chip fracture is located in the palmar aspect of the joint *(small palmar arrow).*

151

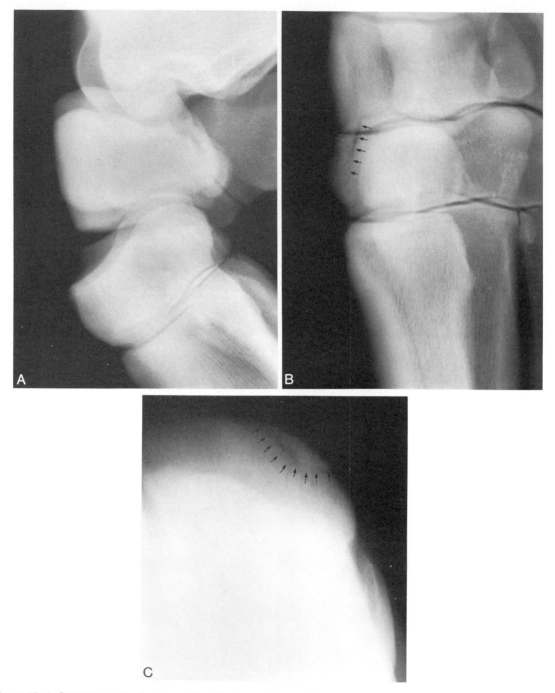

Figure 15–4. Complete corner fracture of the third carpal bone. *A,* flexed lateromedial projection does not exhibit the fracture. *B,* dorsolateral-palmaromedial oblique projection identifies the fracture line *(arrows)*. The fracture appears to be incomplete with the proximal end involving the articular cartilage. *C,* dorsoproximal-dorsodistal oblique (DPr-DDiO) view exhibits the fracture to be complete. The DL-PaMO and DP-DDiO views together identify this finding as a corner fracture *(arrows)* in contrast to a slab fracture, which would extend through the entire thickness of the bone, interrupting both articular surfaces.

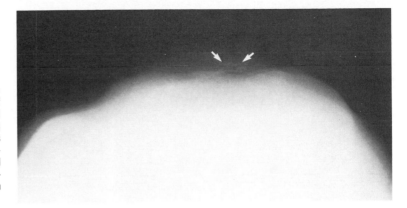

Figure 15–5. Dorsoproximal-dorso-distal projection of the distal end of the radius. Standard views exhibited only intracapsular soft-tissue swelling of the antebrachiocarpal joint. This projection highlights the dorsal aspect of the distal radius. A small periarticular subchondral bone fragment under the extensor tendon can be seen *(arrows)*.

carpal bone distally as a result of the action of the cranial aspect of the radial trochlea in the flexed position (Fig. 15–7).[1]

Dorsoproximal-dorsodistal oblique views are essential in diagnosing and morphologically describing some carpal fractures. Fractures of the third carpal bone with minimal displacement of the fracture fragment are the most difficult to evaluate.[4] Small cortical fracture fragments off the distal radius are also hidden on standard radiographic projections (Fig. 15–5). By flexing the carpus and directing an x-ray beam proximal to distal (Fig. 15–2), the dorsal aspects of the distal radius and third carpal bone can be highlighted. Fractures of the third carpal bone can appear to be simple fractures on standard views; on DPr-DDiO views, however, they are sometimes recognized as comminuted, complete instead of incomplete, and displaced versus nondisplaced.[1] The degree of subchondral sclerosis can also be evaluated, which occurs secondary to fractures of the third, radial or intermediate carpal bones (Fig. 15–4).

Presurgically, it is important for the surgeon to evaluate comminution, thickness of fracture, extent of secondary fracture lines, and the best plane for screw replacement. In the postsurgical examination, the potential for either healing or complication is assessed.[4] Severe soft-tissue swelling with acute fractures may prevent complete flexion and thus lead to poor radiographic detail in some instances.

Angular limb deformities in foals probably have a multifactorial origin; radiographic diagnosis should be correlated with the foal's morphologic and geometric appearance.[8, 9] Angular deformities involving the carpus are usually present at birth or begin to manifest themselves within the first 2 weeks of life.[9] Most foals have some angular deformity at birth but are normal by 2 weeks of age.[10] Radiographic examinations are indicated for those foals that remain angulated after 2 weeks of age. In these foals, early treatment is necessary to prevent uneven axial

compression on the growth plates, which perpetuates the existing angular deformity.[9] Joint instability may be related to flaccid or damaged periarticular structures, such as the collateral ligaments. Instability may also result from disturbances in growth of the distal radial physis,

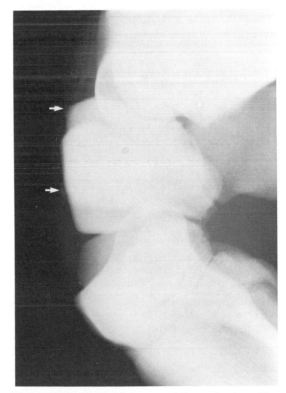

Figure 15–6. Intermediate carpal bone fracture. Two small, acute fracture fragments are marginally displaced at the proximal and distal corners of the intermediate carpal bone *(arrows)*. These small chips were vaguely visible on lateral views and could not be specifically associated with either the radial or intermediate carpal bones. Note the clear separation of the two bones in the flexed lateromedial projection, with distal displacement of the radial carpal bone.

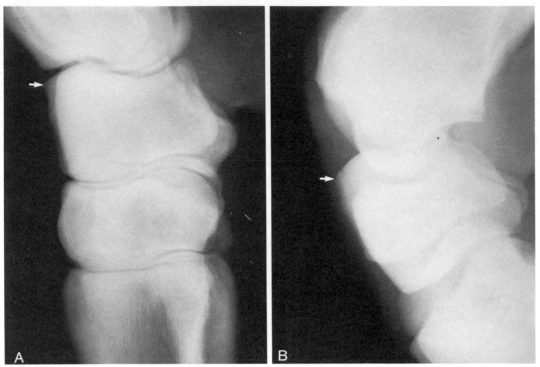

Figure 15–7. Lateromedial *(A)* and flexed lateromedial *(B)* projections identifying a nondisplaced proximal intermediate carpal bone fracture. *A,* there is periarticular new bone formation *(arrow).* *B,* fracture is clearly identified *(arrow)* on the proximal border of the intermediate carpal bone.

imbalance in longitudinal growth from the radial epiphysis, or defects in endochondral ossification of the cuboidal bones of the carpus. Direct external trauma to the physeal plate, epiphysis, or carpal bones also causes angular deformities at the carpus. These conditions may occur alone or in combination.

Radiographic analysis of carpal deformities should include an initial review of survey radiography for soft tissue and osseous abnormalities. A bisecting line should be drawn through the medullary cavity of the radius and third metacarpal bone, forming a pivot point where the lines intersect. The pivot point is usually centered at the region of osseous abnormality (Fig. 15–8). The degree of angular deformity can be measured, which is important in evaluating treatment. Joint instability from damaged or lax soft-tissue structures usually places the pivot point at the level of the distal articular cartilage of the radius with no radiographic abnormalities of the carpal bones. Growth imbalances of the metaphysis have a pivot point directly or slightly proximal to the physeal growth plate, with metaphyseal flaring and sclerosis and an irregular wave pattern to the physeal plate (Fig. 15–8B). Growth imbalances of the metaphysis have a pivot point between the joint space and the physis. Ossification defects of the cartilaginous precursors of the cuboidal

(carpal) bones have a pivot point in the row of bones where the lesion exists (Fig. 15–8A). Direct trauma may involve the growth centers, with a pivot point corresponding to the area involved. Locations of pivot points are not always reliable; therefore, secondary osseous and soft-tissue alterations should be included in the evaluation.[8, 9, 11]

Soft-tissue swelling may be the only radiographic abnormality seen on survey radiographs. This diagnosis should be accepted only after all standard and oblique views has ruled out the possibilities of fractures. Soft-tissue swelling may be extracapsular, intracapsular, or both. It is important to remember that each of the three carpal joints has a distinct joint capsule with specific origins and attachments (Fig. 15–9),[12] with communication between the middle and carpometacarpal joints.[1] Tendosynovitis, cellulitis, and bursitis produce extracapsular swelling that is diffuse and ill-defined (Figs. 15–10C and 15–11A and C) with the dorsal swelling beginning at the distal radius and extending to the proximal portion of the third metacarpal bone.[12]

Early septic arthritis may initially produce soft-tissue swelling (Fig. 15–11A and C), with or without gas shadows. It is radiographically distinguished from synovitis because of the aggressive bone and cartilage destruction. Clinical

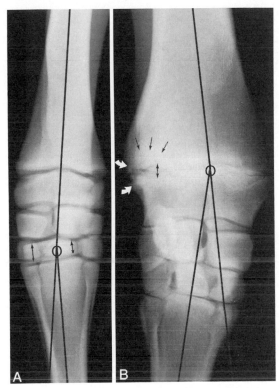

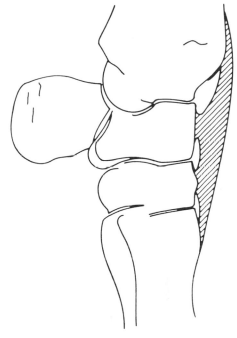

Figure 15–8. Angular limb deformities in foals. A, disecting lines through the radius and third metacarpal bones intersect and form a pivot point over the third carpal bone. An 8 degree angular deformity is present, due to a hypoplastic (ossification defect of the cartilaginous precursor) third carpal bone (short arrow) on the lateral aspect. B, bisecting lines form a pivot point at the physeal growth plate. Note the prominent bone flaring (white arrows) at the metaphyseal and epiphyseal margins. Metaphyseal sclerosis (single-pointed arrows) and the irregular wave pattern to the epiphysis (double pointed arrow) indicate growth imbalances of the metaphysis and epiphysis.

Figure 15–9. The origins and attachments of the joint capsule of the carpus. The middle carpal (intercarpal) and carpometacarpal joints communicate between the third and fourth carpal bones, but the antebrachiocarpal joint cavity remains separate.[1] (From O'Brien TR, Morgan JP, Park RD, et al: Radiography in equine carpal lameness. Cornell Vet 61:666, 1971, with permission.)

manifestation helps to diagnose septic arthritis resulting from hematogenous spread from navel ill, puncture wounds, or extension from a septic focus adjacent to a joint.[13] If bone and cartilage destruction is not evident on survey radiographs and clinical signs suggest sepsis, repeat radio-

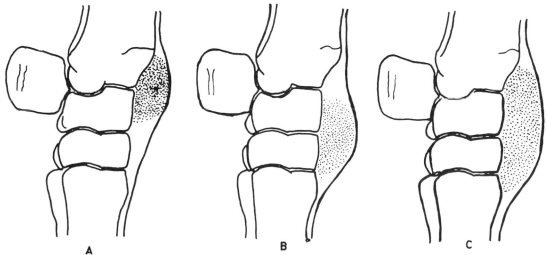

Figure 15–10. Intracapsular and extracapsular soft-tissue swelling. Intracapsular swelling of the antebrachiocarpal (A) and intercarpal and carpometacarpal joints (B). Extracapsular swelling (C) is seen with cellulitis, tendosynovitis, and bursitis. (From O'Brien TR, Morgan, JP, Park RD, et al: Radiography in equine carpal lameness. Cornell Vet 61:666, 1971, with permission.)

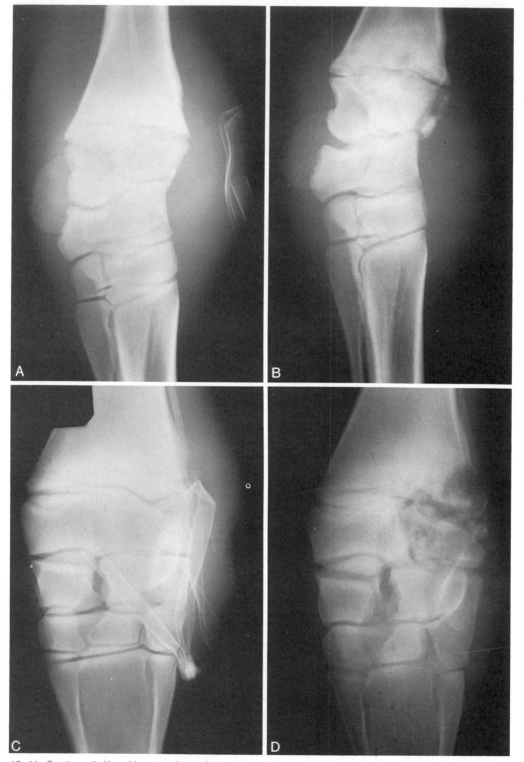

Figure 15–11. Septic arthritis with extensive soft-tissue swelling on initial examination (*A* and *C*). Initial radiographs demonstrate a dome-like soft-tissue swelling adjacent to the radial physis and epiphysis (drain tube is visible). Some gas shadows are seen on the dorsopalmar view with marginal periosteal reaction. Repeated radiographs after 10 days (*B* and *D*) delineate aggressive bone destruction of the metaphysis, physis, and epiphysis, with extension into the antebrachiocarpal joint. The dome-like soft-tissue swelling is adjacent to the antebrachiocarpal joint, but extracapsular swelling is also evident.

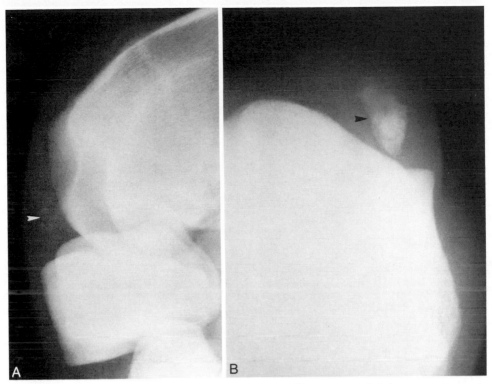

Figure 15–12. Chronic tendosynovitis with calcification of the tendon. The common digital extensor tendon *(arrows)* is visualized on the flexed lateromedial *(A)* and dorsoproximal-dorsodistal oblique *(B)* projections. Soft-tissue swelling is in the tendon sheath; the oblique view is needed to rule out the possibility of a fracture.

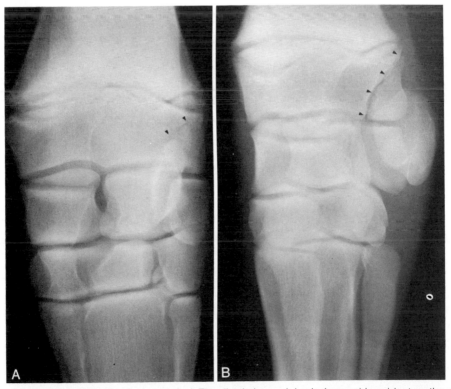

Figure 15–13. Distal radial epiphysis of a young foal. The distal ulnar epiphysis *(arrows)* is evident on the dorsopalmar *(A)* and dorsolateral-palmaromedial oblique *(B)* views. The ulnar physis fuses with the distal radial epiphysis at about 3 to 4 months of age to form the lateral styloid process of the distal radius. The epiphysis should not be diagnosed as a fracture. No soft-tissue swelling is evident.

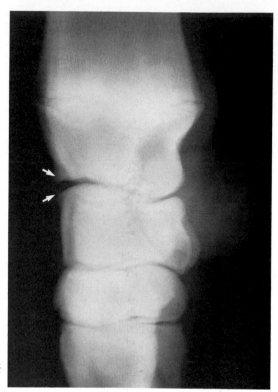

Figure 15–14. Periarticular osteophytes *(arrows)* indicate the beginning of secondary joint disease. The degree of osteophyte formation does not correlate with clinical signs.

porting soft-tissue structures, steroid injections, and other developmental disorders. Joints with the greatest range of motion are most commonly and severely involved. For this reason, it is expected that the antebrachiocarpal and middle carpal joints are the most severely and most commonly involved joints.

The radiographic signs of secondary joint disease are capsular distension (Figs. 15–10, and 15–11), periarticular osteophytes (Fig. 15–14), narrowing of joint spaces, irregular subchondral bone, and subchondral sclerosis (Fig. 15–4). A significant amount of joint production or destruction must occur before radiographic changes are visible. Therefore, the earliest visible radiographic changes should be considered significant with any clinically lame horses. Narrowing of joint spaces without other signs of secondary arthritis is usually without significance.

References

1. Smallwood JE, and Shively MJ. Radiographic and xerographic anatomy of the equine carpus. Equine Pract *1*:22, 1979.
2. Getty R (Ed): Sisson and Grossman's The Anatomy of Domestic Animals. Philadelphia, WB Saunders, 1975.
3. Morgan JP, Silverman S, and Zontine WJ. Techniques of Veterinary Radiography. Davis, CA, Veterinary Radiology Associates, 1975.
4. O'Brien TR: Radiographic diagnosis of "hidden" lesions of the third carpal bone. Proceedings of the 23rd Annual Meeting of the American Association of Equine Practitioners, Vancouver, BC, 1977.
5. Smallwood JE, Shively MJ, Rendano VT, et al: A standardized nomenclature for radiographic projections used in veterinary medicine. Vet Radiol 26:2, 1985.
6. Thrall DE, Lebel JL, and O'Brien TR: A five-year survey of the incidence and location of equine carpal chip fractures. J Am Vet Med Assoc 158:1366, 1971.
7. Park RD, Morgan JP, and O'Brien TR: Chip fractures in the carpus of the horse: A radiographic study of their incidence and location. J Am Vet Med Assoc 157:1305, 1970.
8. Pharr JW, and Fretz PB. Radiographic findings in foals with angular limb deformities. J Am Vet Med Assoc 179:812, 1981.
9. Fretz PB: Angular limb deformities in foals. Vet Clin North Am [Large Animal Pract] 2:125, 1980.
10. Adams OR: Lameness in Horses. 3rd Ed. Philadelphia, Lea & Febiger, 1974.
11. Guffy MM, and Coffman JR. The variability of angular deformity of the carpus of foals. Proceedings of the 15th Annual Meeting of the American Association of Equine Practitioners, Montreal, 1970, pp. 437–458.
12. O'Brien TR, Morgan JP, Park RD, et al: Radiography in equine carpal lameness. Cornell Vet 61:666, 1971.
13. Morgan JP: Radiographic diagnosis of bone and joint diseases in the horse. Cornell Vet 58:28, 1968.

graphs in 7 to 10 days from the onset of clinical signs are essential to re-evaluating bone involvement (Fig. 15–11*B* and *D*).

Nonseptic soft-tissue injuries producing extracapsular swelling require thorough clinical examinations for definitive diagnosis. Chronic injuries, such as tendosynovitis, produce extracapsular swelling and, in time, may calcify (Fig. 15–12). Subtle osseous radiolucencies without soft-tissue swelling should not be diagnosed as fractures. An example is the distal ulnar epiphysis of foals, which fuses to the distal radial epiphysis, forming the lateral styloid process (Fig. 15–13).

Secondary joint disease is joint degeneration, which may involve either or both the articular cartilage and bone. Such disease is named secondary because the primary etiology results from growth abnormalities (conformation), damaged articular cartilage, weak or damaged sup-

CHAPTER 16

THE METACARPUS AND METATARSUS

STEPHEN K. KNELLER

ANATOMIC CONSIDERATIONS

Third Metacarpus and Metatarsus—the Cannon Bone. Radiographically, the third metacarpus and metatarsus (MC III and MT III) are basically the same (Fig. 16–1). There is varying cortical thickness, which is often mistaken for a disease process. The midportion of the dorsal cortex is thicker than the remaining cortex, thinning gradually toward the ends. The palmar/plantar cortex is uniform in thickness and is interrupted at the junction of the proximal and middle one third by the nutrient foramen. Unlike the nutrient foramina of smaller bones, those in MC III and MT III are more like channels, which can be mistaken for lesions on lateral and oblique views, especially in the rear limb (Fig. 16–2). The palmar/plantar cortex is flattened proximally, often resulting in visualization of both medial and lateral aspects on a lateral view. There is no visible proximal physis at birth. The distal epiphysis is within the

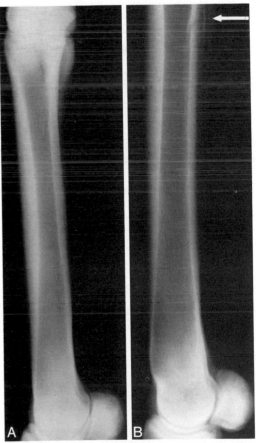

Figure 16–1. Lateral views of the metacarpus *(A)* and the metatarsus *(B)*. Note that the metacarpus is straight, whereas the metatarsus curves slightly at the distal end. The dorsal cortex in both bones is thicker, especially at the midportion. The large nutrient foramen is evident in the metatarsus *(arrow)*.

159

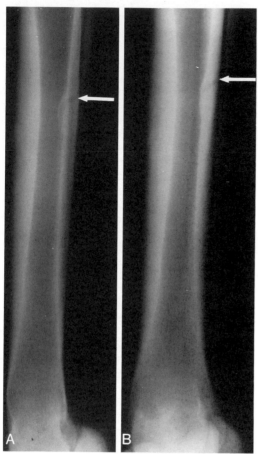

Figure 16–2. Lateral *(A)* and dorsomedial-plantarolateral *(B)* views of the left metatarsus of a 1-year-old Thoroughbred colt. The nutrient foramen is represented as a channel through the plantar cortex of MT III *(arrows)*.

pared with MT II, often extending proximally to MT III.

The proximal epiphysis, apparently present in the fetus, is fused at birth. The distal epiphysis is cartilaginous, and therefore is not visible radiographically at birth. As it ossifies, the distal epiphysis is separated from the body of the bone by cartilage until fusion occurs. Care should be taken to avoid mistaking this normal structure for a fracture (Fig. 16–3).

Mach Bands—False Fracture Lines. A visual phenomenon in radiography that causes some confusion is edge enhancement or mach bands.[2] This phenomenon is especially evident in radiographs of equine metacarpi and metatarsi. Simply stated, as one bone edge crosses another on a radiograph, a radiolucent line may appear. This line can be seen quite often on the palmar/plantar aspect of the equine metacarpus and metatarsus, resulting in erroneous diagnoses of cortical fracture of MC III or MT III, as well as fractures of the smaller metacarpal and metatarsal bones (Fig. 16–4). To guard

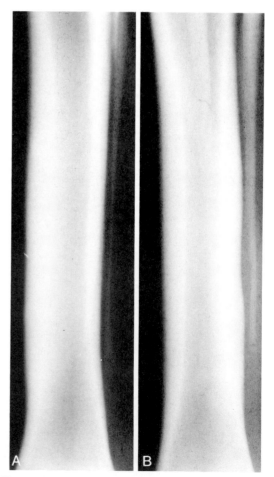

Figure 16–3. Dorsomedial-plantarolateral *(A)* and dorsolateral-plantaromedial *(B)* radiographs of the left hind limb of a 4-month-old Quarterhorse filly demonstrate MT II *(A)* and MT IV *(B)*, respectively . The distal epiphyses have not fused to the diaphyses.

metacarpo- (tarso-) phalangeal joint, and is one of the first sites to exhibit demonstrable abnormalities in metabolic bone disease, although its appearance varies in the normal animal at different ages.

On the lateral view, the metacarpus and metatarsus differ from one another at the distal end (Fig. 16–1). The metacarpus is rather straight, whereas the distal end of the metatarsus may curve slightly, giving the dorsal border a slightly convex appearance.

Second and Fourth Metacarpi and Metatarsi—the Splint Bones. These small bones articulate with the carpus or tarsus and taper distally. Size and shape are variable between animals and between limbs.[1] There is a variable degree of natural outward curvature. The distal end is usually in the form of a slight bulbous enlargement of variable size and shape, but the margins are smooth and distinct. In the forelimb, the medial metacarpus (MC II) is usually longer than the lateral (MC IV), although MC IV may be the same length or longer than MC II. In the rear limb, the MT IV is rather massive and irregular at the proximal aspect when com-

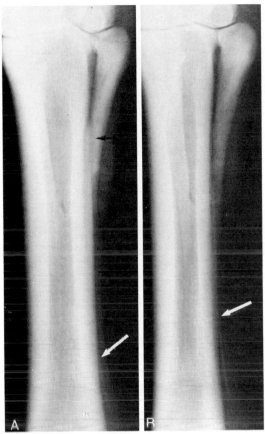

Figure 16–4. Dorsolateral-palmaromedial radiographs of the left metacarpus of a 2-year-old Standardbred gelding with a soft-tissue injury over MC IV, 10 cm distal to the carpus. The small circumscribed opacities overlying MC IV at that level are due to surface debris. *A*, there is a radiolucent line in MC IV at the site of injury *(black arrow)*; slightly different oblique view *(B)* does not show this line. The radiolucent line in *(A)* is due to overlapping margins of MC III with MC IV, which can be confirmed by tracing the margins away from the point in question. Also note the radiolucent line across the distal end of MC IV in *A* *(white arrow)*, which moves proximally in *B* as the point of overlap moves proximally. The midportion of the palmar cortex of MC III is also affected by this phenomenon. The black lines causing this confusion are called mach bands, and should not be mistaken for fracture lines.

against making erroneous diagnoses, the anatomic contour of each bone must be followed carefully, with additional radiographs obtained for clarification as needed.

CHARACTERIZATION OF LESIONS
Soft-Tissue Enlargement and Mineralization.
Shape and size changes of the soft tissues in the metacarpal and metatarsal areas may be evident on radiographs as enlargements over the dorsal surface, with early "metacarpal periostitis" (bucked shins); as generalized enlargements along the palmar/plantar surface, with suspensory desmitis and flexor tendon abnormalities;

and in localized areas along the small metacarpal/metatarsal bones (usually in the proximal portion) with interosseous ligament damage ("splints"). Soft-tissue enlargement may also be seen in random, localized areas from blunt trauma, punctures, and infection, as well as in a generalized pattern from systemic infections and circulatory disturbances. Because there is normally minimal soft tissue in these areas, such soft tissue changes should also be evident on visual inspection and palpation of the horse.

The purpose of evaluating the soft tissues for such changes is threefold. First, in a busy practice, there is a temptation to perform a quick physical examination and proceed with radiography. Finding soft-tissue enlargements radiographically should stimulate a more thorough physical examination of the area in question. Second, although thorough study of the radiographs is paramount, finding a soft-tissue abnormality should lead to in-depth review of the underlying bony structures to evaluate the extent of and to further characterize the lesion. The last purpose is correlation of abnormalities evaluating the association or lack of association of bony changes with soft-tissue enlargements in size, shape, and proximity, as well as relative activity. In many horses, tendons and ligaments can be delineated because of the loose fat-laden adventitia interposed between them. In such horses, a low degree of inflammation can sometimes be appreciated as a loss of visualization of these margins on high quality radiographs.

Soft-tissue mineralization may be identified, especially in the suspensory ligament and flexor tendon areas. Surface debris and medication should be removed to avoid confusion with mineralization within the soft tissues. Mineralization within the soft tissues is usually dystrophic, owing to injury of some duration. The injury may be from work-related stress, resulting in damaged or torn structures, or it may be caused by injection of the various medicaments used as treatment for disease of the structures in the area.

Penetrating foreign objects may also be present in the soft tissues. Therefore, it is important to be familiar with the normal appearance of soft tissue, because only then can foreign objects having an opacity similar to adjacent soft tissue be recognized as a disturbance of the normal size, shape, and opacity relationships.

Mineralization in the skin and subcutaneous tissues may result from surface injuries and must be differentiated from deeper mineralization. In the rear limb, the chestnut may contain mineral opacity that should not be mistaken for evidence of a disease process.

Mineral opacity between the small metacarpal/metatarsal bones and MC III or MT III is a common finding as a sequela to disturbance of

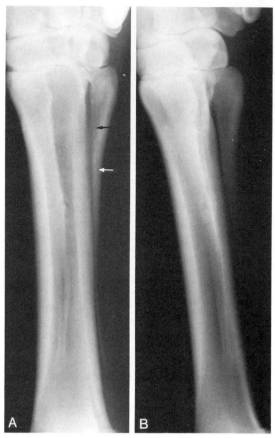

Figure 16–5. *A*, dorsolateral-palmaromedial radiograph of the metacarpal region of an 11-year-old Morgan mare demonstrates MC IV. The space between MC III and MC IV is difficult to appreciate, suggesting mineralization of the interosseous ligament *(arrows)*. *B*, Same view at a different angle. There is a clear separation of MC III and MC IV with no abnormal mineralization.

the interosseous ligament ("splint disease"). This opacity may be actual mineralization of the interosseous ligament or associated periosteal reaction. As in any dystrophic mineralization, this radiographic change would not be evident until some time after the injury. Accurate positioning is imperative when trying to evaluate mineralization of the interosseous ligament, because overlap of the bones produces a similar appearance (Fig. 16–5). In some horses, because of the bone contour, multiple views at slightly different angles must be made to separate the bones completely throughout the length of overlap. Practically speaking, when this mineralization is evident, the animal has had damage in the interosseous ligament, a finding that should have been discovered on physical examination. Splint disease is discussed more thoroughly in the subsequent section.

Periosteal Changes. On high quality radiographs, periosteal surfaces of the metacarpus and metatarsus should be smooth and well

defined. Because of the geometry of the bones, the dorsal surface of MC III or MT III may appear indistinct on overexposed radiographs, unless a high intensity illuminator (bright light) is used. Because any periosteal response is a healing response, periosteal change reflects damage differently depending on the stage of healing. If the cause is removed, the response becomes mature and smooth over time. The metacarpal/metatarsal area is subject to considerable random trauma, which may result in localized periosteal response.

The dorsal surface of the MC III may show a widespread periosteal response to microfractures, referred to as metacarpal periostitis or "bucked shins" (Fig. 16–6). This diagnosis would most likely be made after physical examination, and the injury then evaluated for severity and progress radiographically. Care should be taken to evaluate the cortex for fracture lines (see Cortical Bone Changes). Another relatively common location for periosteal response is between the second and third metacarpi/metatarsi, with changes between the fourth and third metacarpi/metatarsi occurring less often. These changes are usually associated with the proximal one half of the small bones

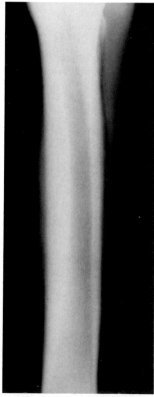

Figure 16–6. Lateral view of the left metacarpus of a 2-year-old racing Quarterhorse gelding. There is a thick layer of periosteal new bone on the dorsal aspect of the midportion of the third metacarpus. The right third metacarpus had similar changes. The horse had been stiff in the forelimbs for 3 weeks.

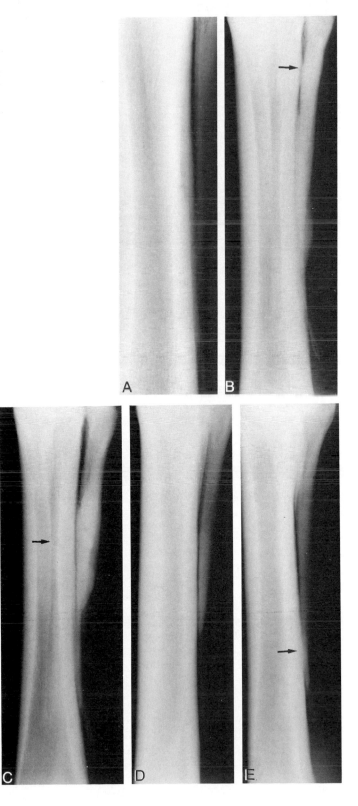

Figure 16–7. Dorsomedial-palmarolateral radiographs of the metacarpal region of several horses with different appearances of damaged interosseous ligaments ("splint lesions"). *A,* a 13-year-old Thoroughbred gelding (hunter-jumper) with a recent interosseous injury. Slight periosteal response and a small amount of cortical bone lysis are evident. This is the typical appearance of a 2- to 3-week-old lesion. *B,* a 3-year-old Standardbred gelding. The periosteal response is more organized, but still active. It involves approximately the entire attachment area of the interosseous ligament with a separate site of reaction proximally *(arrow). C,* a 2-year-old Standardbred gelding. As in *B,* this lesion is chronic, but appears active, and most likely is at least 6 weeks old. The periosteal reaction is large and opaque over a localized area, but it has not become smooth. The large mass may produce abnormal pressure on surrounding soft tissues. The nutrient foramen *(arrow)* should not be confused with the lesion. *D,* a 2-year-old Thoroughbred filly. The lesion on the midportion of MC II is small and inactive. This is typical of a 3- to 6-week-old lesion that has been protected with rest. Such a lesion would be expected to become solid with no enlargement. *E,* a 5-year-old Standardbred gelding. The lesion is near the distal end of MC II *(arrow).* It is opaque and smooth, blending together with the cortex of MC III and MC II, as a chronic inactive lesion. Lameness may result from concussion of MC II and the interosseous ligament, exaggerated by the distal fusion of MC II to MC III. The pattern at the proximal end is caused by overlap of MC II, MC III, and MC IV.

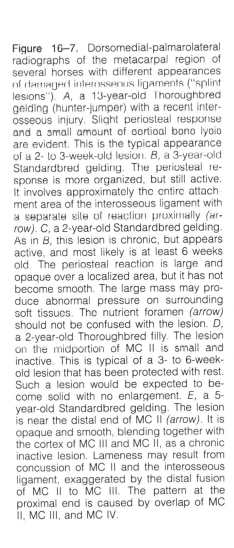

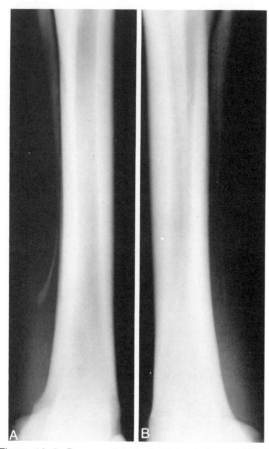

Figure 16–8. Dorsomedial-plantarolateral view of MT II *(A)* and dorsolateral-plantaromedial view of MT IV *(B)* in an 8-year-old Standardbred gelding. Soft-tissue enlargement is present on the plantar surface of the metatarsal area. MT II is deviated sharply at the distal end and MT IV is separated from MT III. Both MT II and MT IV have indistinct margins on the distal ends consistent with periosteal irritation.

(splint bones) and are secondary to interosseous ligament damage (splint disease) (Fig. 16–7). The periosteal response is variable in size; the response is ill-defined and irregular when first developed and gradually becomes smooth, opaque, and smaller as it matures, fusing the small bones to the larger bones. A large, irregular periosteal change may mimic a fracture, yet a fracture may be masked by the callus formation and appear as an active splint lesion. The periosteal reaction should be classified to facilitate staging of the lesion to aid in recommended therapy. Indistinct margins or small amounts of active periosteal reaction may be seen on the distal ends of the small metacarpal/metatarsal bones due to irritation from suspensory ligament disease (Fig. 16–8).

Cortical Bone Changes. Cortical lysis in the metacarpal and metatarsal bones is usually as-

sociated with localized trauma and puncture. Bone lysis may result from infection and degeneration in the articular surfaces, which are discussed with the appropriate joints. Because of the relatively thick cortex of the metacarpi/metatarsi, periosteal injury (especially with infection) may cause death of the outer one third, with lysis of bone leaving a sequestrum of variable size (Fig. 16–9). Soon after the interosseous ligament is damaged, multiple small lytic lesions may be seen along the opposing surfaces of the metacarpal and less often, metatarsal bones, presumably because of disruption of fibrous attachments and resultant inflammation. Random bone lysis should be evaluated and characterized as with any other

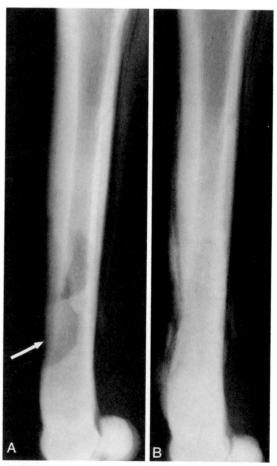

Figure 16–9. *A,* lateral view of the right metatarsal region of a 3-year-old Quarterhorse mare 10 days after the limb was injured severely in the stall, exposing a large portion of MT III. The large radiolucent areas overlying the MT III are due to missing portions of soft tissue. A faint, dark line is present within the dorsal cortex of MT III *(arrow),* indicative of fracture or impending sequestration. *B,* A lateral view, 3 weeks later. The sequestered bone can now be seen to extend proximally. Periosteal response is present around the lesion.

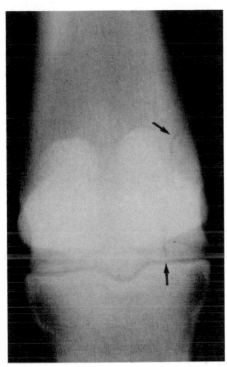

Figure 16–10. Dorsopalmar radiograph of the left front limb of a 4-year-old Thoroughbred stallion. A sagittal fracture is present in the lateral distal condyle of MC III (arrows). This lesion was not visible on lateral or oblique views.

bone, while remembering that trauma and infection are the most likely causes.

Metacarpal and metatarsal fractures are common, especially in high performance horses. The most common fracture site in these regions is the distal one half of MC and MT II and IV. As mentioned previously, care must be taken to avoid mistaking cartilaginous plates and mach bands as fractures. Fractures may also occur in the proximal one half of these structures, and may be confused with splint lesions.

Aside from complete fractures of MC III and MT III, which are obvious on first sight of the horse, fractures of MC III and MT III are rather difficult to diagnose. They do, however, occur in specific locations. These injuries are called stress fractures and are seen in high performance horses. The lesion most readily diagnosed is the distal condylar sagittal fracture (Fig. 16–10). This fracture frequently affects MC III, extending proximally from the metacarpophalangeal joint; it may or may not be significantly displaced. Often this fracture can only be visualized on the dorsopalmar or slightly oblique view; it can be easily masked on underexposed radiographs.

Stress fractures may also be found in the dorsal cortex, especially associated with meta-

carpal periostitis (Fig. 16–11). These fractures are most often on the dorsomedial aspect near the junction of the middle and distal one thirds. Because of their shape, these lesions have been called saucer fractures.

In recent years, fractures have been recognized in the palmar cortex.[3] Because of the large number of overlying bony margins and the indentation of the palmar cortex superimposed by the small metacarpal bones, fractures in this area are difficult to demonstrate. Scintigraphy has aided in proving the presence of such fractures.[4] The most common site of fracture in the palmar cortex is approximately 2 to 3 cm from the proximal articular surface (Fig. 16–12). As mentioned previously, this fracture is difficult to demonstrate on lateral and oblique views, but it can be seen on the dorsopalmar view as a crescentic decreased opacity. On the dorsopalmar view, a disturbance in the normal trabecular pattern of the bone is suggestive of a fracture. Cortical fractures have also been demonstrated more distally in the palmar cortex.

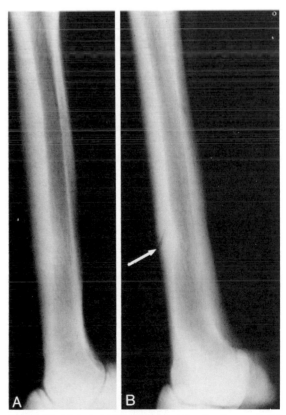

Figure 16–11. Lateral (A) and dorsolateral-palmaromedial (B) views of the left metacarpal region of a 6-year-old Thoroughbred gelding that became lame immediately after a race 2 weeks before the radiographs were made. The stress fracture (arrow) evident in B is barely visible in A.

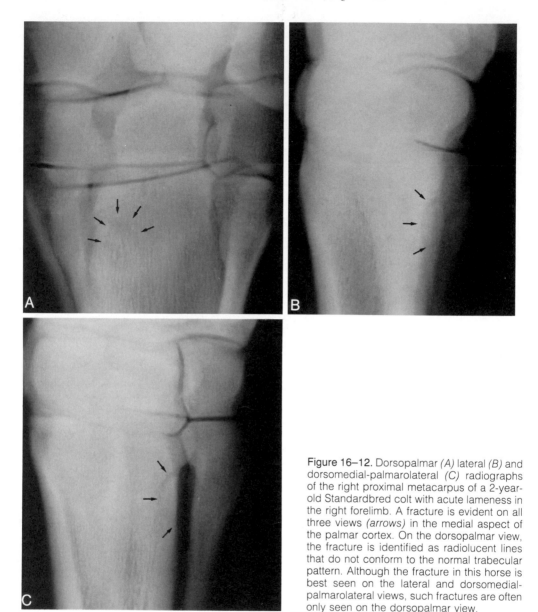

Figure 16–12. Dorsopalmar *(A)* lateral *(B)* and dorsomedial-palmarolateral *(C)* radiographs of the right proximal metacarpus of a 2-year-old Standardbred colt with acute lameness in the right forelimb. A fracture is evident on all three views *(arrows)* in the medial aspect of the palmar cortex. On the dorsopalmar view, the fracture is identified as radiolucent lines that do not conform to the normal trabecular pattern. Although the fracture in this horse is best seen on the lateral and dorsomedial-palmarolateral views, such fractures are often only seen on the dorsopalmar view.

Shape changes in MC III and MT III are most often seen at the distal end of these structures and result from growth disturbance, causing deviation of the foot. This occurrence may be seen in a single, localized problem, or in conjunction with upper limb abnormalities. Although there is considerable variety in size and shape of the small metacarpal and metatarsal bones, abaxial deviation of the distal ends is often associated with suspensory desmitis, presumably from outward pressure exerted by the enlarged ligaments (Fig. 16–8). If this outward curving is noted, the suspensory ligaments should be evaluated for inflammation and enlargement, but apparent deviation should not be considered diagnostic for suspensory desmitis.

References

1. Getty R: Sisson and Grossman's The Anatomy of the Domestic Animals, 5th Ed. Philadelphia, WB Saunders, 1975, pp. 290, 317.
2. Lane EJ, Proto AV, and Phillips TW: Mach bands and density perception. Radiology *121*:9, 1976.
3. Bramlage LE, Gabel AA, and Hackett RP: Avulsion of the origin of the suspensory ligament in the horse. J Am Vet Med Assoc *176*:1004, 1980.
4. Devous MD, and Twardock AR: Techniques and applications of nuclear medicine in the diagnosis of equine lameness. J Am Vet Med Assoc *184*:318, 1984.

CHAPTER 17

THE METACARPO-(METATARSO-)PHALANGEAL ARTICULATION

RON D. SANDE

The relative anatomic structures of the metacarpo- and metatarsophalangeal articulations are so similar that it is difficult to differentiate the right from the left or the front from the hind limb radiographically. The front articulation is most often involved with pathologic change, perhaps owing to the support function of the front limb and the characteristic difference in weight-bearing and concussion.

The metacarpophalangeal or metatarsophalangeal articulation is a ginglymus or hinge joint formed by the distal end of the metacarpal (metatarsal) and the proximal end of the proximal phalanx. The articular surface of the proximal phalanx is concave and bears a sagittal groove or depression corresponding to the sagittal ridge at the distal end of MC III or MT III. This ridge and groove divide the bearing surface into two unequal parts. The largest surface is to the medial side, where axial loading is greatest. The sagittal ridge is received into a similar depression at the palmar* surface created by the proximal sesamoids and the intersesamoidean ligament. There are two radii of articulation of the fetlock joint. The dorsal radius serves the weight-bearing portion and the palmar radius conforms to the articulation with the proximal sesamoids.[3] It is the junction of these radii of articulation that is often confused with pathologic flattening of the articular surface.

The joint capsule attachments are simple at the proximal end of the proximal phalanx and are immediately periarticular, with no redundant capsule or cul-de-sacs. The capsule attaches to the distal end of the metacarpal (metatarsal) at the periarticular margins. Dorsally, there is a cul-de-sac that extends proximally and forms a pouch that allows for full extension of the joint. There is a bursa that is interposed between extensor tendons and the dorsal joint pouch. The palmar joint capsule extends proximal to the sesamoids between the suspensory ligament and the metacarpal (metatarsal) bone.[3]

Ligaments associated with the metacarpo-(metatarso-) phalangeal articulation fetlock are important to its function and stability and, when injured, give rise to significant pathologic change. (See Figs. 18–8 to 18–10.) The origins and insertions should be committed to memory. Lateral and medial collateral ligaments arise from the fossae on either side of the distal end of the metacarpal (metatarsal) and attach to the roughened area on the medial and lateral aspect of the proximal phalanx just distal to the artic-

*"Palmar(o)" is used throughout this chapter with the understanding that "plantar(o)" should be substituted if reference is being made to the rear leg.

167

ular margin.[3] The suspensory (interosseous) ligament branches to form attachments to the abaxial surfaces of the proximal sesamoids. The annular ligament and the collateral sesamoidean ligament have fibers perpendicular to the axis of the suspensory ligament, and ultimately have some insertion at the distal ends of MC or MT II and IV.[3] The intersesamoidean ligament connects the proximal sesamoids and fills the space between them. This ligament forms one part of the fetlock articulation.[3] Distal sesamoidean ligaments are best remembered as superficial, middle, and deep. The superficial ligament attaches distally to the palmar proximal surface of the middle phalanx. The middle ligament attaches to the palmar surface of the proximal phalanx. The deep or cruciate sesamoidean ligaments originate from the basilar border of each sesamoid and attach to the opposite eminence on the proximal palmar border of the proximal phalanx.[3]

RADIOGRAPHIC EXAMINATION

This portion of the limb is usually examined radiographically in response to lameness detected distal to the carpus or tarsus and proximal to the foot. The examination should include the proximal interphalangeal joint and the distal ends of the metacarpals or metatarsals.

The intent of the examination should be to visualize the articular and periarticular skeletal structures and the adjoining soft tissues. Identification markers recorded in the emulsion are essential in radiography of the metacarpo- or metatarsophalangeal articulation; the right or left and front or hind limb should be designated. If oblique views are obtained, it is important to designate the projection. Markers are placed to the lateral surface·of all views, with the exception of the lateromedial view, when markers should be placed dorsally.[10]

Survey radiographic examination should include a lateromedial, a dorsopalmar, and two oblique projections (dorsal 45 degree lateral-palmaromedial, and dorsal 45 degree medial-palmarolateral) with the limb bearing weight if possible. The lateromedial projection should be made with the primary beam centered at the articulation and directed parallel to an imaginary line connecting the collateral fossae at the distal metacarpal or metatarsal. Palpation of the collateral ligament attachments can help to determine a true lateral projection, which is parallel to the articular surface of the joint. Since the plane of the joint is at an angle to the bearing surface of the hoof (i.e., the ground), the primary beam can be directed dorsoproximal-palmarodistal at approximately 30 to 40 degrees, i.e., dorsal 35 degree proximal-pal-

marodistal oblique. A well-performed study results in the projection of the proximal sesamoids over the background of the distal metacarpal or metatarsal and the joint space projected with maximum width.[1, 7]

The dorsal 45 degree lateral-palmaromedial and dorsal 45 degree medial-palmarolateral oblique projections are usually a routine part of the survey examination. The oblique projections should intersect the plane of the lateromedial projection so that each oblique shares a sagittal zone of common exposure with the lateromedial view. Thus, pathologic change that appears on the respective oblique and on the lateromedial projection is located in the area of common profile.

Special projections may be derived spontaneously according to the information gained from survey radiographs. Special projections should be designed to project a profile of the pathologic change. The lateromedial projection during flexion is performed while holding the foot off the ground as if inspecting the sole of the hoof. The foot should not be pulled lateral; a true lateral projection is then more difficult to obtain. Alternate positions include variations in the degree of flexion and flexed oblique views. These projections may provide better visualization of subarticular surfaces at the dorsal aspect of distal MC or MT III, the proximal part of the proximal phalanx, and the dorsal or articular margins of the sesamoids.[7]

The dorsodistal-palmaroproximal projection is made while the limb is not bearing weight. The foot is elevated on a block and the limb is extended. The primary beam direction is approximately 125 degrees to the axis of the metacarpal or metatarsal.[5] This study yields a tangential image of the articular margin of the distal metacarpal or metatarsal. The degree of flexion and the angle of the primary beam determine the tangent of the joint surface that is visualized.

The palmaroproximal-palmarodistal projection is used to visualize the palmar articular surface of MC or MT III and the proximal sesamoids. Positioning of the patient requires that the x-ray tube head be placed close to the abdominal wall. The limb is positioned as far caudal as possible and the foot is placed on a supporting tunnel containing a cassette.[7] Some magnification results from the use of this projection.

The abaxial surfaces of the proximal sesamoids may be examined by placing a cassette medial or lateral to the joint. The x-ray beam is then directed in palmaroproximolateral-dorsodistomedial or palmaroproximomedial-dorsodistolateral directions, respectively.[9]

Contrast arthrography of the joint is perhaps the most rewarding application of this special procedure in the horse. A volume of 5 to 10 ml of water-soluble contrast medium containing 300 to 400 mg iodine per ml is adequate. Injection of contrast medium should follow arthrocentesis and withdrawal of an equal volume of synovial fluid if possible. Injection is made into the lateral pouch of the joint, proximal to the lateral sesamoids and dorsal to the suspensory ligament. The joint should be vigorously manipulated before radiography.[7]

RADIOGRAPHIC INTERPRETATION OF DISEASES OF THE METACARPO- (METATARSO-) PHALANGEAL ARTICULATION

Arthrology is a complex study that requires some depth in the understanding of biomechanics. Loading, packing, shear, concussion, range of motion, limb axis, blood supply, soft-tissue supporting structures, and joint type and classification are some of the factors that must be considered when joint disease is assessed. Consideration of such factors may permit the clinician to anticipate the type of joint disease that might be present.

Radiographic examination should not be made until a thorough clinical examination has been performed. Careful anamnesis should be recorded and a tentative diagnosis should be made. Failure to complete these steps may result in a radiographic tour of the entire limb.

Joint disease in the horse is often associated with repeated trauma, and as with any species, the changes may be characteristic of the joint and of the function required of the patient. The importance of function is emphasized by pathognostic studies of joint disease. Arthritis may be anticipated in the wrists of fighters (boxers) and in the metatarsophalangeal joint of ballet dancers. The metacarpo- (metatarso-) phalangeal joint of the horse is an excellent example of diacritic arthroses.

The earliest signs of joint disease may remain obscure on radiographic examination. Wear lines in the articular cartilages or synovial hypertrophy are not recognized. Lameness and distension of a joint are clinical signs that usually precede the request for radiographic examination. A clinician is well advised to consider radiographic examination of the contralateral joint for comparison of bilateral symmetry and to preclude the presence of obvious pathologic changes in the joint that appears normal. Pathologic change is often bilateral, but is so in different stages of development. The general prognosis may be significantly changed by these findings.

Osselets. This lay term refers to swelling dorsal to the metacarpo- (metatarso-) phalangeal joint. The incorporation of this type of terminology is an unfortunate burden in equine medicine, because any degenerative joint disease of this joint may be classified with this lay terminology. This condition is usually a result of trauma, with degenerative changes in the joint capsule. Radiographic signs include soft-tissue swelling and joint distension. Dystrophic calcification of the periarticular soft tissues is considered a classic finding.[4] Despite the diacritic implication of this terminology, degenerative arthritis of the metacarpo- (metatarso-) phalangeal joint is like that of other joints.

Villonodular Synovitis. This condition is characterized by firm, nonfluctuant swelling at the dorsal aspect of the joint. The villonodular masses arise from enlargement of the proximal fibrous tabs of the joint capsule and are associated with trauma. The condition is usually diagnosed by clinical signs, history, and palpation. Radiographic signs include mild to severe erosion of the distal metacarpal (metatarsal) at a point just distal to the dorsal joint capsule attachment.[2, 8, 11] Periarticular bony proliferation may be present (Fig. 17–1). Contrast arthrography of the joint usually demonstrates a radiolucent, space-occupying mass in the dorsal cul-de-sac of the joint (Fig. 17–2)

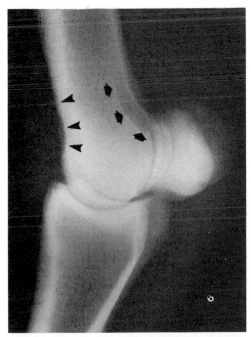

Figure 17–1. Lateromedial radiograph illustrating changes found with villonodular synovitis. Swelling was apparent dorsal to the joint. There is erosion of bone at the dorsal proximal joint capsule attachment *(arrowheads)*, and early evidence of supracondylar lysis at the palmar cortex *(arrows)*. Bony proliferation is visible at the proximal, dorsal periarticular border of the proximal phalanx.

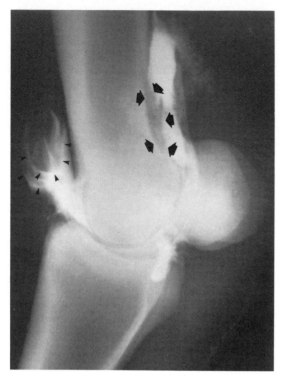

Figure 17–2. Positive-contrast arthrogram. Same horse as in Figure 17–1. There are two radiolucent, space-occupying masses in the dorsal, proximal joint space *(arrowheads)*. A space-occupying mass at the palmar surface fills the area of supracondylar lysis *(arrows)*.

Supracondylar Lysis. In the metacarpus or metatarsus, this condition is similar to the villonodular sign, except that it occurs at the palmar surface of the bone. This disease is associated with chronic proliferative synovitis. Radiographic signs are joint distension and lysis of bone at the palmar cortex of MC or MT III distal to the joint capsule attachment (Figs. 17–1 and 17–9). Contrast arthrography may be difficult to perform because of the presence of hypertrophied synovium and diminished synovial joint space. Contrast medium permeates an undulating, irregular mass filling defect. The concavity formed in the bone is clearly demonstrated (Fig. 17–2).

Degenerative Joint Disease. This disease classification is a nonspecific term describing deterioration of articular and periarticular structures. The pathologic events culminate in degenerative hypertrophic osteoarthritis regardless of the etiologies or biochemical alterations.

The first stages include cartilage degeneration and formation of wear lines that are characteristic of the ginglymoid joints. These lines are grooves in the articular surface that run parallel to the direction of joint motion. Blisters form in the surface and subsequent wear results in narrowing of the joint space. If reduction in the width of a joint space can be confirmed on two

radiographic views, there is little doubt that the articular cartilage thickness has been reduced. Progressive loss of joint width is a subjective finding and must be carefully assessed with clinical signs to determine the significance of the finding (Fig. 17–3).

Radiographic findings associated with degenerative joint disease consist of soft-tissue swelling, narrowed joint space, and skeletal changes characterized by bone remodeling with lysis or bony proliferation. These findings may occur in any combination. Joint capsule thickening may be visualized with excellent quality radiography. Soft-tissue swelling results from hypertrophy and proliferation of other periarticular tissues.

In chronic arthritis there is sclerosis or eburnation of subchondral bone with loss of trabecular architecture as a result of erosion and loss of the articular cartilage. Constant stress and tension or trauma at the joint capsule attachments result in osteophyte formation (Fig. 17–4). Similar but not identical are the bony excrescences that form at the joint margin in response to damage to the articular surface. The latter two signs are not often differentiated, in spite of their significance.

Cortisone Arthropathy. This condition must be considered in the discussion of the degenerative joint diseases. The changes associated with this disease are usually found to involve articular and periarticular structures and have variable degrees of degeneration and prolifera-

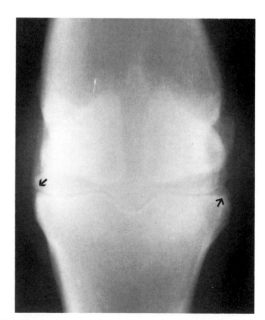

Figure 17–3. Dorsopalmar radiograph illustrating changes found with degenerative joint disease. There is narrowing of the joint space and formation of bony excrescences at joint margins *(arrows)*.

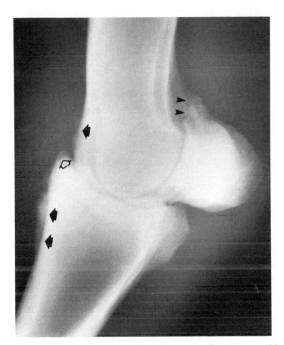

Figure 17–4. Lateromedial radiograph of a horse with chronic degenerative arthritis, sesamoiditis, and desmitis. There is generalized soft-tissue swelling and joint distension. Chronic osteochondral fractures are present at the apices of the proximal sesamoids *(arrowheads)*. Degenerative bony proliferation is present at the dorsal, proximal surface of the proximal phalanx and at the joint capsule attachment on the distal, dorsal surface of MC III *(solid arrows)*. A periarticular osteophyte is evident on the dorsal rim of the proximal phalanx *(open arrow)*. Other changes include supracondylar lysis; remodeling of bony trabeculae in the proximal sesamoids; and bony proliferation at the attachments of the deep sesamoidean ligaments at the proximal palmar aspect of the proximal phalanx.

projection of the joint may better indicate the depth of the lesion in the condyle. The shape of the defect may be a shallow concavity, a deep concavity, crescentic, oval, or circular.[6] The changes are often associated with the demarcation between the radius of articulation of the metacarpophalangeal or metatarsophalangeal joint and the metacarposesamoidean or metatarsosesamoidean articular surface (Fig. 17–6). In the normal study, one may detect this junction by the difference in the radii of articulation. This finding should not be confused with excessive flattening of this area, which indicates reduced cartilage thickness or cartilage degeneration. Contrast arthrography may demonstrate cavitation of the joint surface, although advanced degenerative subchondral bony changes may be found and the cartilage may be intact yet dimpled at the joint surface.

Septic Arthritis. This disease may be associated with hematogenous distribution of microorganisms, as occurs with omphalophlebitis or by direct contamination due to trauma or non-

tion. Radiographic changes visualized in early development are due in part to the inciting condition. Repeated steroid injections result in localized demineralization of bone and smudging of trabecular detail. Chronic changes include mineralization in the periarticular soft-tissue structures, probably associated with deposition of some steroid within those structures. A differential diagnosis of steroid-induced arthritis should be considered in the presence of degenerative change or collapse of subchondral bone with concomitant mineralization in periarticular soft tissue (Fig. 17–5).

Osteochondrosis. This disorder is associated with the distal aspect of the metacarpal or metatarsal. The radiographic findings are similar to those in other joints and have been described as well-demarcated, bulb-shaped radiolucencies that can extend several centimeters deep to the articular margins. Lateromedial

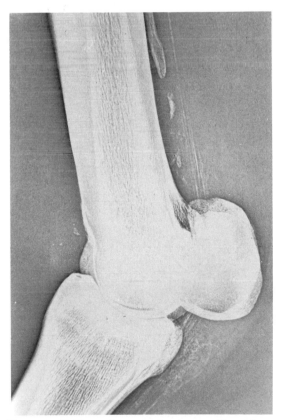

Figure 17–5. Xeroradiograph of a horse with cortisone arthropathy. There is absolute narrowing of the joint space. Coarse bone trabeculae are indicative of demineralization of bone. Mineralization in periarticular soft tissues and tendons was marginally visible when examined using conventional radiographic techniques.

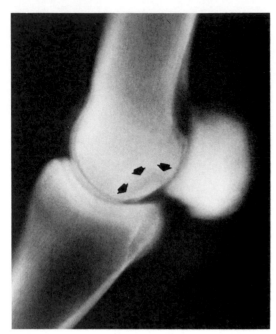

Figure 17–6. Lateromedial radiograph of a horse with distal metacarpal osteochondrosis. There is an opaque osteochondral fragment within a deep concavity of radiolucency *(arrows)*. This represents only one of several permutations of findings associated with this disease.

sterile technique. Radiographic signs of early septic arthritis are periarticular soft-tissue swelling and distension of the joint. Progression of the disease results in malalignment, subluxation, or collapse of the joint. Bony changes consist of subchondral bone lysis and periosteal proliferation at the joint margins (Fig. 17–7). The cartilage space may appear increased at areas of subchondral bone lysis. Diminished joint space is evidence of the loss of articular cartilage that precedes subchondral bony change.

The radiographic sign of an increase in the apparent joint space must be critically analyzed. Incomplete ossification of the cartilage model is present in young, developing animals and progressively diminishes with skeletal maturity. Increased thickness of the articular cartilage has not been documented in animals, but it is known to occur with acromegaly in humans. Excessive fluid or soft tissue in the joint space, as occurs with immune-mediated arthritis, results in wider joint space. These diseases have not been documented in the equine, but this clinician has studied clinical cases in which these signs were consistent with that diagnosis.

Nonseptic inflammatory joint diseases have varied etiologies and may be difficult to classify. Radiographic signs are distension of the joint and displacement of periarticular soft tissues. If

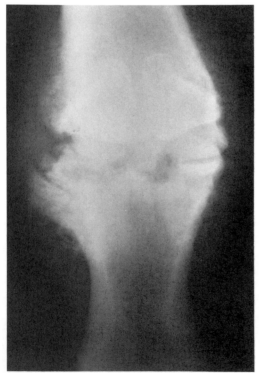

Figure 17–7. Dorsopalmar radiograph of a horse with chronic septic arthritis. There is generalized soft-tissue swelling. The joint space has collapsed and there is overt erosion of subchondral bone of the opposing joint surfaces. Bone proliferation is evident on all periarticular surfaces.

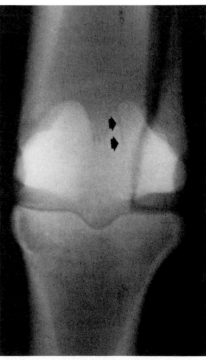

Figure 17–8. Dorsopalmar radiograph of a horse with a slab fracture of the lateral condyle of MC III. Some fracture lines may be difficult to visualize *(arrows)*. Marked displacement of a fragment such as this is often not present.

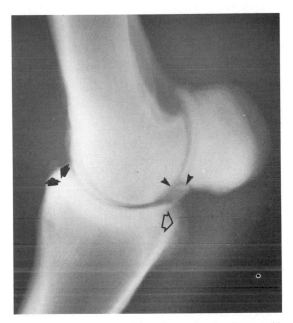

Figure 17–9. Lateromedial radiograph of a horse with chronic traumatic arthritis. An osteochondral (chip) fracture is present at the dorsal periarticular rim of the proximal phalanx *(arrows)*. A basilar osteochondral fracture of the proximal sesamoid is evident *(arrowheads)*. There is bony proliferation at the attachment of the deep sesamoidean ligaments at the proximal palmar border of the proximal phalanx *(open arrow)*. Villonodular erosion of bone and supracondylar lysis is apparent.

the condition is chronic, bony excrescences at the joint margins or periarticular osteophytes may be found.

Hypersensitivity. A cause of arthritis in the horse is hypersensitivity. Its existence would seem intuitive, although no documentation was found. If this terminology is unsatisfactory, iatrogenic synovitis may be acceptable. The occurrence of immune-mediated arthritis in the horse has been suggested. It is likely that such a disease in the horse would not develop much beyond the serous stage. Collapse of subarticular bone is seen in small animals and humans when perambulation is not essential to life.

Intermittent Hydrarthrosis. This is a recognized form of arthritis with no known etiology. Periodic effusion of a joint or bilateral joints may occur in conjunction with villous proliferation of the synovium. The radiographic sign of the latter condition is joint distension in the absence of bony change.

Traumatic Arthritis. This is likely the diagnosis made most frequently in the equine metacarpo- (metatarso-) phalangeal joint. The sequel is generally chronic degenerative hypertrophic osteoarthritis. The significance of repeated trauma was discussed in relation to chronic degenerative arthritis. Disruptive articular trauma occurs as a result of fractures through the joint surface, luxations, torn liga-

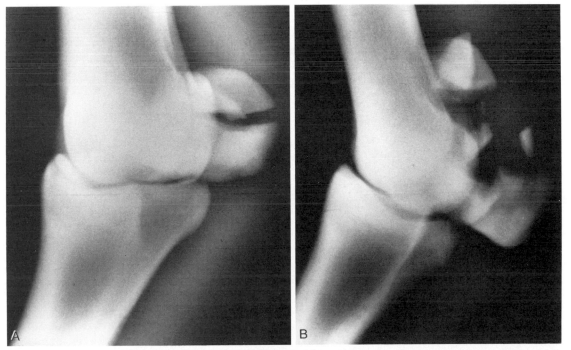

Figure 17–10. *A,* a dorsal 45 degree medial-palmarolateral oblique radiograph. Fractures through the body of the medial sesamoid are apparent. The joint is extended but separation of the fragments is minimal. The suspensory ligament remains intact. *B,* lateral radiograph of a horse with fractures of the medial and lateral proximal sesamoids. The joint is hyperextended and there is marked separation of the fragments. The suspensory ligament has separated.

ments, or penetration of foreign bodies. Structural alterations, which may be permanent or progressive, result in a decrease in the articular cartilage, instability of the joint, abnormal range of joint motion, and possible deformation of the joint.

Acute Traumatic Synovitis. This condition results in joint effusion with or without hemarthrosis. Radiographic findings are associated with soft-tissue swelling or joint distension, although osseous fractures or cartilage fibrillation may be present and not detected.

Slab Fractures. These lesions in the distal condyle of the third metacarpal (metatarsal) bone may be difficult to visualize radiographically. A complete history and the presence of hemorrhage in the joint are essential to reaching a diagnosis. The radiographic signs include uneven joint surface, interruption of the metaphyseal cortex, and the presence of a radiolucent fracture line extending from the joint surface to the cortex. These fractures usually occur at the lateral side of the joint (Fig. 17–8).

Periarticular Chip Fractures. These lesions arise from the medial or lateral eminences at the proximodorsal periarticular rim of the proximal phalanx. Acute chip fractures may have sharp borders and geometric configurations. Chronic chip fractures have smooth, rounded borders. The latter are usually attached to the joint capsule or to the joint margin as an exos-

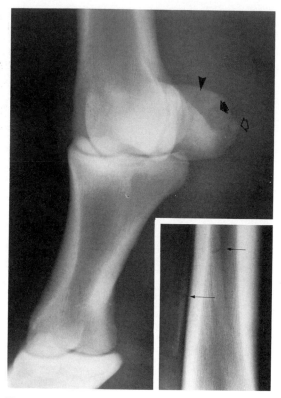

Figure 17–12. Dorsomedial-palmarolateral oblique view of a horse with chronic sesamoiditis, desmitis, and fractures of the 2nd and 4th metacarpals; the medial proximal sesamoid is projected. Degenerative remodeling is present with tunneling *(arrowhead)*, cystic change *(solid arrow)*, and an abaxial fracture *(open arrow)*. Insert: there are fractures at the distal ends of MC II and MC IV *(arrows)*.

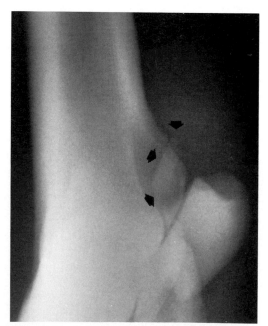

Figure 17–11. Palmaro-proximo-lateral-dorsodistolateral view of a horse with a periarticular fracture of the medial proximal sesamoid *(arrows)*. The fracture originates at an articular surface and emerges at the abaxial surface of the sesamoid.

tosis (Fig. 17–9). Free joint bodies may displace or move about within the joint.

Fractures of the Proximal Sesamoids. These fractures may be found as osteochondral fragments separated from the apex (apical fractures) (Fig. 17–4) or the base (basilar fractures) (Fig. 17–9) of the sesamoids. Fractures through the body of the sesamoid may have a narrow cleavage line, indicating that the suspensory apparatus remains intact (Fig. 17–10A). Wide separation of sesamoid fragments usually indicates bilateral sesamoid fractures and separation of the fibers of the suspensory ligament (Fig. 17–10B). Hyperextension of the fetlock is apparent if stress is applied to the joint or if the limb is bearing weight.

Abaxial fractures are detected by using special radiographic projections. These fractures result from avulsion of bone by a portion of the attachment of the branches of the suspensory ligament on the medial or lateral aspect of the respective proximal sesamoid (Fig. 17–11).

eling or fracture at the distal ends of the minor metacarpals (Fig. 17–12, insert).

Disuse Atrophy of Bone. This disorder is manifested in the proximal sesamoids as a reduction in bone opacity. Trabeculae within the bone become large and coarse. This change occurs as a result of altered stress or axial weight-bearing and does not signify primary pathologic change in the fetlock (Fig. 17–13).

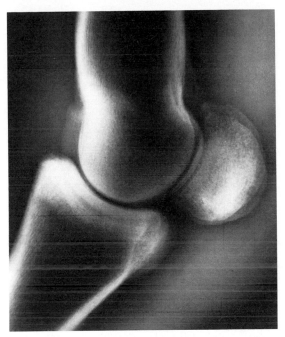

Figure 17–13. Lateromedial radiograph of a horse with chronic lameness. These is generalized remodeling of bone and cortices are thin. Osseous trabeculae are coarse and irregular with no organized pattern. The sesamoids have a sponge-like appearance.

Sesamoiditis. This condition is indicated radiographically by bony proliferation on non-articular surfaces of the proximal sesamoids. Linear or cystic lysis may appear to penetrate the sesamoid from the abaxial surface (Fig. 17–12). Sesamoiditis is usually associated with some degree of degenerative change in the suspensory ligament and degenerative remod-

References

1. Allan GS: Radiography of the equine fetlock. Equine Pract 1:40, 1979.
2. Barclay WP, White KK, and Williams A: Equine villonodular synovitis: A case survey. Cornell Vet 70:72, 1979.
3. Getty R: Sisson and Grossman's The Anatomy of the Domestic Animals. Philadelphia, WB Saunders, 1975, pp. 357–360.
4. Gillette EL, Thrall DE, and Lebel JL: Carlson's Veterinary Radiology, 3rd Ed. Philadelphia, Lea & Febiger, 1977, p. 435.
5. Hornof WJ, and O'Brien TR: Radiographic evaluation of the palmar aspect of the equine metacarpal condyles: A new projection. Vet Radiol 21:161, 1980.
6. O'Brien TR, Hornof WJ, and Meagher DM: Radiographic detection and characterization of palmar lesions in the equine fetlock joint. J Am Vet Med Assoc 178:231, 1981.
7. Morgan JP, and Silverman S: Techniques of Veterinary Radiography, 3rd Ed. Davis, CA, Veterinary Radiology Associates, 1982.
8. Nickels FA, Grant BD, and Lincoln SD: Villonodular synovitis of the equine metacarpophalangeal joint. J Am Vet Med Assoc 168:1043, 1976.
9. Palmer SE: Radiography of the abaxial surface of the proximal sesamoid bones of the horse. J Am Vet Med Assoc 181:264, 1982.
10. Rendano VT: Equine radiology: The fetlock. Mod Vet Pract 58:871, 1977.
11. van Veenendaal JC, and Moffatt RE: Soft tissue masses in the fetlock joint of horses. Aust Vet J 56:533, 1980.

CHAPTER 18

THE PHALANGES

SANDRA V. McNEEL

Radiography of the equine phalanges is most commonly performed in the diagnosis of lameness or to evaluate the cause of firm or persistent swellings. Radiographs are important because they provide information that cannot be acquired by any other diagnostic means. The *significance* of many radiographic abnormalities, however, is difficult to ascertain unless pertinent facts obtained from the patient's clinical history and physical examination are correlated with the radiographic findings. The diagnostic work-up of a lame horse should always include observation of the moving patient at a distance, close visual inspection of the lame leg, and palpation. A systematic approach to palpation should be used to examine all parts of the hoof wall, sole, frog, coronary band, and the pastern region. Careful application of hoof testers can assist in localizing the lesion if the lameness is due to abnormalities involving the distal phalanx or navicular bone. Diagnostic nerve blocks are also useful, especially in defining the location of the primary lesion in the horse with multiple abnormalities detected during the physical examination.[23] With the results of these previous procedures in mind, the veterinarian can more accurately determine the portions of the digit that should be radiographed.

TECHNICAL FACTORS

Patient Preparation
Dirt, skin lesions, and iodine-containing medications can all produce radiopaque shadows that complicate radiographic interpretation. Consequently, before the radiographic procedure begins, the patient should be examined closely to be sure that debris has been removed from the haircoat. Shoes and any additional pads used in corrective shoeing should be removed to obtain optimal diagnostic radiographs of the distal phalanx and navicular bone. The sole and sulci of the frog should be thoroughly cleaned. The sulci should be cleaned with a hoof pick, as small pieces of gravel easily become lodged in these recesses. The sulci can then be filled with a material of soft-tissue opacity (such as Play Doh, Rainbow Crafts, Cincinnati, OH) to the level of the solar surface (Fig. 18–1). Packing the central and collateral sulci eliminates the radiolucent linear shadows that are seen when the air-filled sulci become superimposed on the distal phalanx in the 65 degree dorsoproximal-palmarodistal* view (Fig. 18–2).

---

*"Palmar(o)" is used throughout this chapter with the understanding that "plantar(o)" should be substituted if reference is being made to the rear digit.

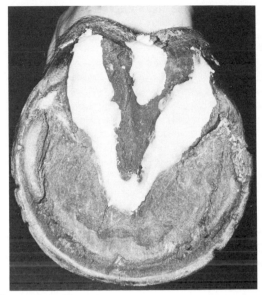

Figure 18–1. The sole of the foot after the central and collateral sulci have been filled (packed) with a pliable material that is of the same radiographic opacity as the sole.

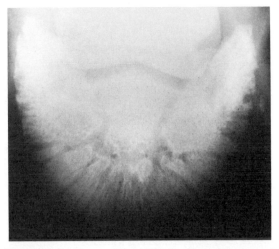

Figure 18–2. Dorsoproximal-palmarodistal (65 degree) oblique view of a normal distal phalanx with the sulci packed. Note the good definition of vascular channels without superimposed air artifacts.

Recommended Views

The equine foot is structured such that certain anatomic areas can be imaged as a group. These groupings and the projections needed to evaluate them completely are listed in Table 18–1.[21] Excellent, complete descriptions of patient positioning[1, 21, 36] and examples of normal radiographic anatomy[1, 30, 36] are available, and the reader is referred to these sources for additional technical information.

NORMAL RADIOGRAPHIC ANATOMY (INCLUDING VARIATIONS)

Osseous Structures

The foot axis (as seen on the latcromedial view of the foot) is that angle described by an imaginary line that passes through the center of the middle phalanx. This line should divide both proximal and middle phalanges equally. When the line is carried through the distal phalanx, it should create an angle of 45 to 50 degrees (front foot) or 50 to 55 degrees (hind

TABLE 18–1. VIEWS FOR EQUINE PHALANX EVALUATION

Examination	Structures Evaluated	Views
Phalangeal area	Proximal phalanx Proximal interphalangeal joint Middle phalanx	1. Dorsopalmar 2. Lateromedial 3. Dorsal 35 degree lateral-palmaromedial and/or dorsal 35 degree medial-palmarolateral obliques; as needed, especially for fracture evaluation.
Distal phalanx	Distal phalanx	1. 65 degree dorsoproximal-palmarodistal oblique with horse standing on cassette. 2. Lateromedial, with foot on block so as to include solar margin of distal phalanx and soft tissues of sole on the radiograph. 3. Dorsal 65 degree proximal 45 degree lateral-palmarodistomedial and dorsal 65 degree proximal 45 degree medial-palmaro distolateral obliques. Obliques are especially useful when distal phalanx fracture is suspected.

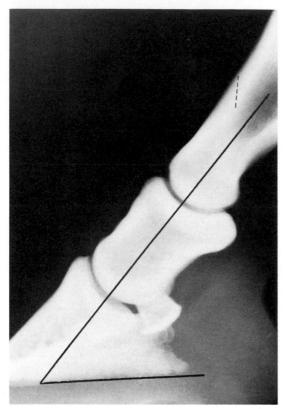

Figure 18–3. Normal lateromedial view of a front digit. The axis of the foot, measured through the plane of the middle phalanx and solar margin of the distal phalanx, is 47 degrees. *Dashed line* in the dorsal cortex of the proximal phalanx, location of a small vascular channel, which may occur at this site.

foot) with the bony solar margin.[1] Figure 18–3 illustrates the normal axis of a front foot. Minor variations in angle occur with conformational differences in individual horses.

A vascular channel may be seen in the dorsal cortex of the proximal phalanx. It appears as a radiolucent line directed obliquely through the dorsal cortex of the diaphysis, and should not be mistaken for a fracture (Fig. 18–3). Variations may also occur in the appearance of bony trabeculae in the medullary cavity of the proximal phalanx (Fig. 18–4). A prominent radiolucent center in the medullary cavity surrounded by a ring-like radiopaque shadow is illustrated in Figure 18–4B; this is a normal variation in trabeculation and does not indicate cyst formation.

The site of attachment of the oblique sesamoidean ligaments is normally seen as a roughened or thicker area of the palmar cortex of the proximal phalanx, especially in the older horse.

If the lateromedial view of the foot is slightly obliqued, the normal eminence for attachment of the collateral ligament of the distal interphalangeal joint is seen as a small bony projection along the dorsum of the middle phalanx (see Fig. 18–17).

The radiographic appearance of the normal distal phalanx varies in several respects.[28] The most obvious difference is the distribution of vascular channels. Although the pattern of vascular channel formation is unique to individual animals, the major channels identified at the solar margin should communicate with the solar canal. Figure 18–5 demonstrates some of the variations in the number of vascular channels, their distribution, and patterns of radiation from the solar canal. A smoothly rounded notch in the toe of the distal phalanx can be seen in the normal horse. This notch is referred to as the *crena marginis solearis* or toe stay.

The shape of the extensor process of the distal phalanx may also differ among individuals (Fig. 18–6).[28] The margin of the normal process, however, is smooth regardless of its shape. The palmar processes of the distal phalanx become more extensively ossified with age. Compare the palmar processes of the three horses (5 months old, 8 years old, 15 years old) in Figure 18–7.

Soft Tissue

Knowledge of the attachment sites of the joint capsules, tendons, and ligaments of the foot is imperative for accurate interpretation of the osseous changes seen in radiographs of the phalanges. Figures 18–8, 18–9, and 18–10 illustrate the attachment sites of these major structures. The ergot may create a radiopaque image when superimposed on the proximal phalanx in the dorsopalmar view (Fig. 18–4B). The lateromedial view demonstrates the ergot shadow along the palmar surface of the skin.

Articular Cartilage

In the properly positioned dorsopalmar view of the normal foot, the metacarpophalangeal, proximal interphalangeal, and distal interphalangeal joints can be visualized. The metacarpophalangeal joint is usually the narrowest of these articulations, the proximal interphalangeal joint is slightly wider, and the distal interphalangeal joint is the widest of the three joint spaces (Fig. 18–4A). If the horse is not bearing weight evenly on the leg, the asymmetric loading forces can cause an apparent narrowing of the loaded side of the joint, with subsequent apparent widening of the distracted side (see Fig. 18–24F). This artifact can be recognized because it similarly affects all three joints, seen on the dorsopalmar view.

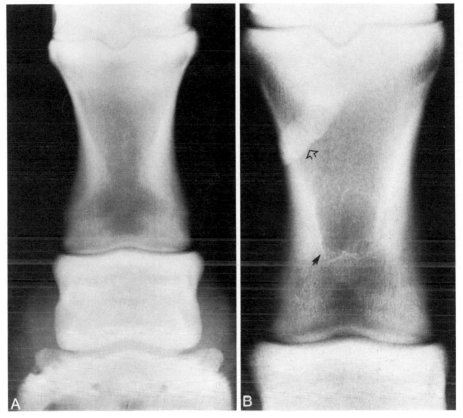

Figure 18–4. Dorsopalmar view of two normal equine proximal phalanges. *A*, note the normal thickness of the lateral and medial cortices of the proximal phalanx at the junction of the middle and distal one third of the bone. The radiolucent medullary cavity is seen between the thickest parts of the cortex. The widest joint space is usually the distal interphalangeal, with the joint spaces becoming progressively more narrow to the metacarpo- or metatarso-phalangeal joint. *B*, a thin rim of opaque trabeculae surrounds the central medullary cavity of the proximal phalanx *(solid arrow)*. The ergot is elongated in this animal and is seen due to its summation with the proximal phalanx *(open arrow)*.

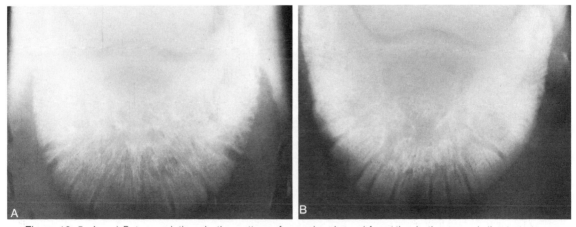

Figure 18–5. *A* and *B*, two variations in the pattern of vascular channel formation in the normal distal phalanx.

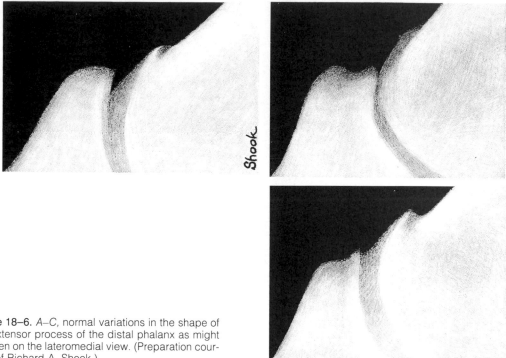

Figure 18–6. *A–C*, normal variations in the shape of the extensor process of the distal phalanx as might be seen on the lateromedial view. (Preparation courtesy of Richard A. Shook.)

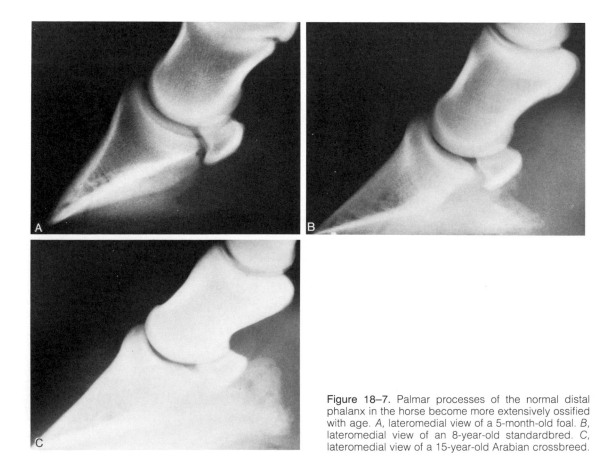

Figure 18–7. Palmar processes of the normal distal phalanx in the horse become more extensively ossified with age. *A*, lateromedial view of a 5-month-old foal. *B*, lateromedial view of an 8-year-old standardbred. *C*, lateromedial view of a 15-year-old Arabian crossbreed.

The following anatomic key is designed for Figures 18–8 to 18–10.

A. Third metacarpal bone.
B. Proximal sesamoid bone.
C. Proximal phalanx.
D. Middle phalanx.
E. Distal phalanx.
F. Distal sesamoid (navicular) bone.
1. Common digital extensor tendon.
2. Extensor branch of the interosseous (suspensory) ligament.
3. Lateral digital extensor tendon.
4. Interosseous (suspensory) ligament.
5. Superficial digital flexor tendon.
6. Deep digital flexor tendon.
7. Superficial transverse metacarpal ligament (palmar annular ligament).
8. Proximal digital annular ligament.
9. Straight sesamoidean ligament.
10. Oblique sesamoidean ligament.
11. Cruciate sesamoidean ligament.

12. Metacarpophalangeal joint capsule (fibers from the common digital extensor te
13. Distal palmar recess of the metacarp joint.
14. Dorsal recess of the proximal inter joint capsule.
15. Palmar recess of the proximal interphalangeal joint.
16. Proximal interphalangeal joint capsule (blended with fibers from the common digital extensor tendon).
17. Dorsal recess of the distal interphalangeal joint.
18. Palmar recess of the distal interphalangeal joint.
19. Collateral sesamoidean ligament.
20. Distal sesamoidean impar ligament.
21. Podotrochlear bursa.
22. Medial collateral ligament of the metacarpophalangeal joint.
23. Lateral collateral ligament of the proximal interphalangeal joint.
24. Medial collateral ligament of the distal interphalangeal joint. (Preparation courtesy of Richard M. Shook.)

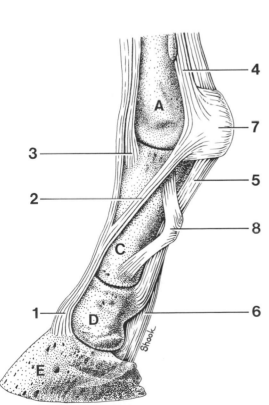

Figure 18–8. Tendon and ligament attachments of the thoracic limb digit (superficial tissues), lateral view.

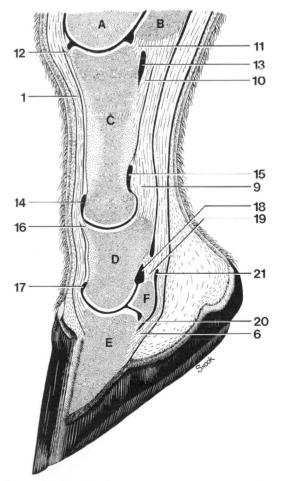

Figure 18–9. Tendon, ligament, and joint capsule attachments of the thoracic limb digit, sagittal section. (See Anatomic Key in Fig. 18–8.) (Preparation courtesy of Richard M. Shook.)

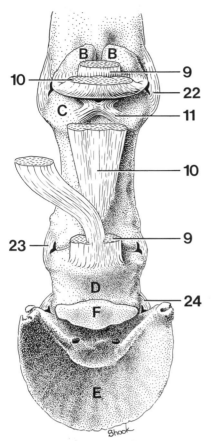

Figure 18–10. Sesamoidean and collateral ligament attachments of the digit, palmar view. (See *Anatomic Key* in Fig. 18–8.) (Preparation courtesy of Richard M. Shook.)

ROENTGEN SIGNS OF THE PROXIMAL AND MIDDLE PHALANGES

Number

Rare congenital anomalies may cause an abnormal number of digits or phalanges to be present. Polydactylism in the horse is often associated with a complete supernumerary metacarpophalangeal joint in addition to the phalanges of the digit.

Contour (Margination)—Periosteal Bone Proliferation

The underlying cause of periosteal new bone growth may be determined by evaluating the extent and the specific location of the lesion. In the case of a focal area of periosteal reaction, consider whether the lesion is at a site of attachment for a tendon, ligament, or joint capsule. Previous sprain or strain injuries of

tendons or ligaments and stretching of joint capsules due to intracapsular hemorrhage or joint effusion stimulate periosteal new bone growth at the fibro-osseous junction (Fig. 18–11). Focal periosteal proliferation that is not located at an attachment site may be due to previous direct trauma or adjacent soft-tissue inflammation or infection. Diffuse periosteal new bone formation that involves multiple phalanges in one limb is suggestive of extensive infection, especially if accompanied by inflammation. Diffuse symmetric periosteal proliferation involving multiple phalanges of all four limbs indicates a systemic process, such as hypertrophic osteopathy. The osseous lesions of this disorder are an uncommon sequela to chronic pulmonary (or rarely, abdominal) space-occupying mass lesions in the horse. Intrathoracic lesions, however, that have been reported to cause hypertrophic osteopathy include: tuberculosis, pulmonary abscesses, pulmonary neoplasms, ovarian neoplasia with pulmonary metastasis, rib fracture with adhesions, and pulmonary infarction.[20]

The smoothness of the margin and the radiopacity of the added periosteal bone can also be useful in determining the relative aggressiveness and chronicity of the lesion. The four

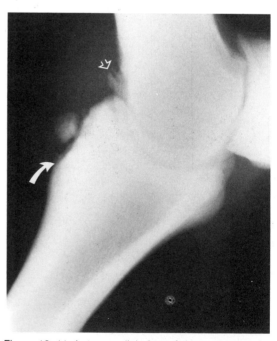

Figure 18–11. Lateromedial view of the metacarpophalangeal joint. There is periosteal proliferation and sclerosis *(curved arrow)* with avulsion fragmentation or dystrophic calcification of the insertion of the lateral digital extensor tendon. Small chip fragments from the dorsoproximal edge of the proximal phalanx are also evident *(open arrow)*.

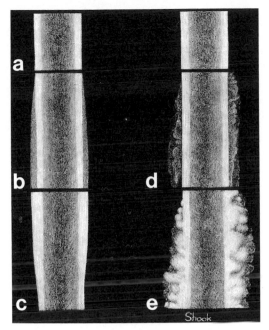

Figure 18–12. Variable appearance of contour and opacity of periosteal bone proliferation: a: normal cortex; b: smooth margin, mildly opaque periosteal bone formation; c: smooth margin, opaque bone formation; d: irregular margin, mildly opaque bone formation; e: irregular margin, opaque bone formation. Note the loss of distinction between periosteal new bone and original cortex in c and e. (Preparation courtesy of Richard M. Shook.)

appearances of periosteal proliferation commonly seen in the equine proximal and middle phalanx are illustrated in Figure 18–12. The first is a smooth margin and mildly opaque bone formation, which is indicative of recent subperiosteal hemorrhage due to trauma or elevation of the periosteum by exudate secondary to spread of infection from adjacent bone or soft tissue. Second, a smooth margin and opaque bone formation is suggestive of inactive, remodeled trauma. The third appearance is that of an irregular margin and mildly opaque bone formation. In this instance, recent, active periosteal damage due to direct trauma, avulsion injury of soft-tissue attachments or infection (acute periostitis) is likely. Finally, an irregular margin and opaque bone formation is indicative of chronic periostitis due to infection or chronic strain on soft-tissue attachments, and rarely to hypertrophic osteopathy.

Radiopacity

When alteration of expected bone radiopacity is identified, the location of the abnormality can help indicate the underlying cause. Therefore, in the following discussion the location and increase or decrease in bone opacity are considered as an integrated unit.

Increased Opacity, Subchondral Location. This finding is indicative of sclerosis due to degenerative joint disease initiated by chronic instability, previous trauma, or poor conformation (a narrowed joint space and periarticular osteophytes may also be seen, Fig. 18–13).

Increased Opacity, Periosteal Location. This alteration is usually seen with trauma, inflammation, or infection, as described previously.

Decreased Opacity of All Parts of Phalanges. If radiographic exposure factors are correct, diffuse decrease in bone opacity may be due to disuse osteoporosis. Resorption of small tertiary trabeculae can also cause the spongy components of the proximal sesamoids and the phalanges to appear abnormally coarse. Rarely does a calcium or phosphorus nutritional imbalance lead to sufficient demineralization of the appendicular skeleton to be identified radiographically.

Focal Decreased Opacity. Osteochondrosis occurs as a solitary radiolucent defect located

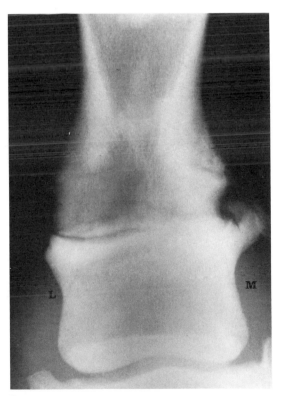

Figure 18–13. Dorsopalmar view demonstrates collapse of the medial portion of the proximal interphalangeal joint with subchondral sclerosis of the opposed surfaces of the proximal and middle phalanges. In addition, there are large osteophytes at the attachments of the medial collateral ligament (osteoarthritis secondary to trauma). L: lateral; M: medial.

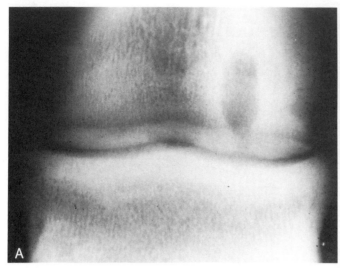

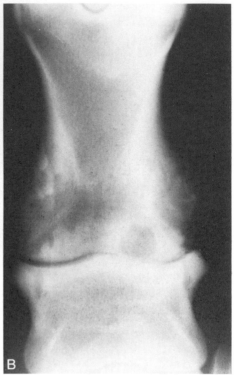

Figure 18–14. Solitary, radiolucent subchondral bone defects (osteochondrosis) of the proximal phalanx, dorsopalmar view. *A,* elliptic defect with surrounding zone of sclerosis, without osteoarthrosis, in a 1-year-old Thoroughbred. *B,* spheric defect surrounded by sclerotic subchondral bone. Collapse of contiguous joint space and periarticular osteophyte formation indicate the presence of osteoarthrosis in a 6-year-old quarterhorse that had been lame for 1 month.

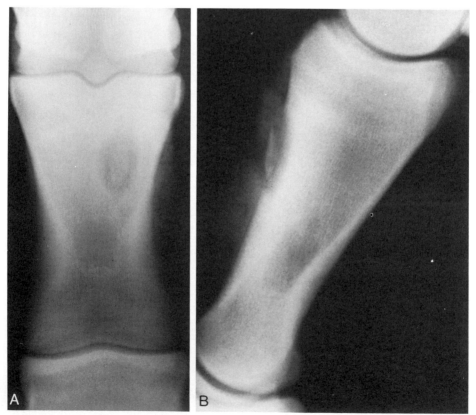

Figure 18–15. Sequestrum formation involving the proximal phalanx. *A,* dorsopalmar view indicates an ovoid radiolucent defect in the proximal part of the phalanx that surrounds a smaller oval opaque opacity. Active periosteal new bone formation is also evident. *B,* lateromedial view shows the cortical sequestrum, the defect in the underlying cortex, and the adjacent periosteal proliferation. Sequestration of bone may be caused by trauma-induced avascular necrosis or by bacterial osteomyelitis.

in the subchondral bone, which often is surrounded by a radiopaque rim or diffuse sclerosis. Figure 18–14 illustrates two examples of such a defect, one with and one without accompanying secondary joint disease. Osteochondrosis lesions are usually found in the distal portion of the proximal phalanx, and occur less commonly in the distal subchondral bone of the middle phalanx. These lesions are generally associated with joint effusion or lameness in horses of training age, that is, less than 3 years of age. One report indicated a higher incidence of occurrence in the pelvic limb in a group of Quarterhorses,[39] although either the thoracic or the pelvic limb may be affected. Osteochondrosis defects in the phalanges may lead to extensive degenerative joint disease in the proximal interphalangeal joint, as demonstrated in Figure 18–14B. In these cases, surgical arthrodesis may be warranted to allow return to useful function.[37, 38] In another series of 13 cases, in which solitary lesions of phalangeal osteochondrosis were treated by conservative management, lameness disappeared in seven horses over a period of 1 month to 2½ years.[24] In four of these animals the osteochondrosis defect could not be identified radiographically 1½ to 2½ years after the initial presentation and diagnosis. The extreme variation in outcome of phalangeal osteochondrosis may be associated with the size of the defect and the extent of associated articular cartilage fragmentation.

A solitary radiolucent defect in the body of the phalanx may be due to cortical bone necrosis and sequestrum formation (Fig. 18–15) or, rarely, to a congenital defect, such as monostotic fibrous dysplasia (nonossifying fibroma).[3] The latter anomaly can be distinguished by its thin-walled, cyst-like architecture, which may occupy the entire diaphyseal portion of the bone. Pathologic fracture through the thinned cortex of the phalanx may cause acute, severe lameness.

Multiple Radiolucent Subchondral Bone Defects. These changes are seen in septic arthritis (Fig. 18–16), some cases of degenerative osteoarthritis, and steroid arthropathy.[15, 26] The origin of joint sepsis may be a penetrating puncture wound, extension from an adjacent soft-tissue abscess or septic epiphysitis, iatrogenic (after arthrocentesis or intra-articular corticosteroid therapy), or via hematogenous route. The osseous defects represent osteomyelitis and necrosis at the subchondral bone and cartilage junction.[12] The adjacent joint space is often concomitantly narrowed owing to destruction of articular cartilage.

The pathogenesis of articular cartilage loss is multifactorial, and includes compromised nutrition due to pannus overgrowth and release of destructive lysosomal enzymes from inflamed

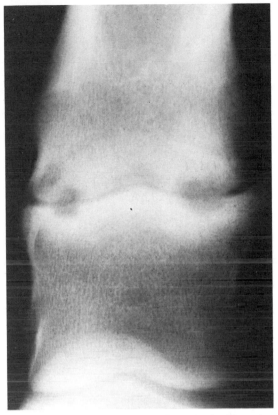

Figure 18–16. Decreased width of the proximal interphalangeal joint space with large, multiple, indistinctly marginated subchondral bone defects. The radiographic signs in this foal are due to septic arthritis with erosion of articular cartilage leading to osteomyelitis of the subchondral epiphyseal bone. The absence of the periosteal reaction, which usually accompanies lysis due to osteomyelitis, suggests a fulminating infection.

synovial membranes or neutrophils. Prostaglandins released from inflamed synovia cause loss of the proteoglycan component of the cartilage matrix. Proteoglycan and subsequent collagen depletion alters the stiffness of the cartilage, making the joint surfaces more susceptible to mechanical trauma.[17, 18]

Multiple *punctate* radiolucent subchondral defects may be seen in combination with periarticular osteophytes, uneven narrowing of the joint space, and sclerosis in some horses with chronic degenerative joint disease (osteoarthrosis). In degenerative osteoarthrosis, these small cystic defects form secondary to fissure fractures in the articular cartilage, which allow access of synovial fluid to the subchondral bone.

Decreased Opacity Adjacent to the Physis. In the proximal or middle phalanx, this is a rare radiographic sign. Physeal growth disturbances usually affect the larger long bones. Septic embolization from bacteremia could produce sites of necrosis at these physes, although the more common areas of involvement are the distal radial, distal tibial, and metacarpal/metatarsal physes.[12]

PROXIMAL PHALANX FRACTURE

Fractures of the proximal phalanx occur in different parts of the bone, depending on the type of stress applied. The most common fracture types are chip fracture at the proximal dorsal surface, spiral/longitudinal fracture of the body (diaphysis), and less frequently, avulsion fracture of the palmar proximal tuberosity.[7, 25]

The most common fracture involving the proximal phalanx is the chip fracture of the proximal dorsomedial edge of this bone (Figs. 18–11 and 18–17). Overextension of the metacarpophalangeal joint, as occurs with fatigue in racing horses, allows impaction of the dorsal edge of the proximal phalanx with the dorsal surface of the third metacarpal bone. The medial proximal margin of the proximal phalanx is larger in area than the lateral margin and therefore contacts the third metacarpal bone first during extension. The greater percentage of weight borne on the thoracic limbs results in a higher incidence of these fractures at the metacarpophalangeal joint. The size of the fragment, the amount of articular surface included, and the presence or absence of degenerative joint disease are all taken into consideration (along with clinical signs of lameness or swelling and economic factors) when determining if surgical excision of the fragment is warranted.[33]

Simple or comminuted longitudinal or spiral fractures of the proximal phalanx are commonly seen in cutting and barrel-racing horses and Standardbreds.[13] These fractures occur more frequently in the pelvic limb of cutting and barrel-racing horses, whereas Standardbreds have a significantly higher incidence in the thoracic limb. This fracture is due to the rotary force applied down through the midsagittal ridge of the third metatarsal bone as the horse makes a sharp turn with the foot bearing full weight. Thus a combination of twisting and axial compression occurs simultaneously. The rotating midsagittal ridge of the third metatarsal bone acts as a wedge driving into the more stationary proximal phalanx. In Standardbreds, the frequency of spiral fractures in the proximal phalanx is five times higher in the thoracic limb than in the pelvic limb, and twice as high in the left foreleg as in the right foreleg.[13] Oblique projections are often necessary to evaluate the extent and direction of fracture planes completely, especially if internal fixation is contemplated. Careful evaluation of the radiograph may be required for identification of the incomplete spiral or longitudinal fracture (Fig. 18–18).

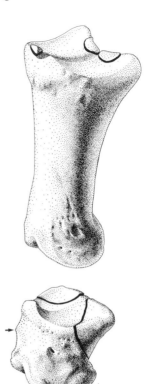

Figure 18–17. Common sites of chip or avulsion fracture involving the proximal or middle phalanx, dorsomedial view. The most common fracture is chip fracture of the dorsomedial proximal tuberosity of the proximal phalanx. Avulsion fracture of the palmar (plantar) process of the proximal phalanx may involve the weight-bearing articular surface. Torsion while the digit is under maximal axial compression can cause fragmentation of the palmar or plantar processes of the middle phalanx. *Arrow,* normal eminence for attachment of the collateral ligament of the distal interphalangeal joint. (Preparation courtesy of Richard M. Shook.)

Avulsion fractures of the proximal palmar process occur less frequently (Fig. 18–17). These fractures are identified in the pelvic limb of Standardbreds and involve the medial more often than the lateral process.[25] This fracture is usually due to avulsion of the insertion of the short sesamoidean ligament. Clinical signs of lameness may be associated with this injury if a portion of the palmar articular surface is disrupted. The lateromedial view demonstrates this lesion as a small bone fragment situated between the base of the proximal sesamoids and the palmar surface of the proximal phalanx. Oblique views may be necessary to isolate the fragment and to determine if it is from the medial or lateral palmar process.

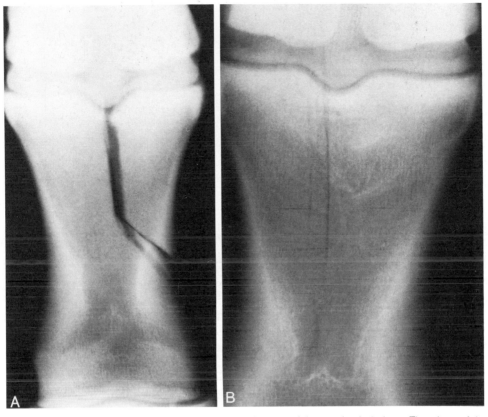

Figure 18–18. Complete (A) and incomplete (B) longitudinal fracture of the proximal phalanx. The plane of the primary beam must be parallel to the fracture plane to identify this lesion when no fragment displacement is present.

MIDDLE PHALANX FRACTURE

Fractures of the palmar processes occur in the hind leg more frequently than in the front leg. These fractures are also more common in horses that perform activities during which the bone is subject to extreme torque and compressive forces, i.e., barrel racing, calf roping, and cutting. It is unusual for only one process (lateral or medial) to fracture, and the middle phalanx usually sustains a severely comminuted fracture (Fig. 18–19). If the fracture extends into both the proximal and distal interphalangeal joints, the prognosis for return to athletic soundness is poor. Comminuted fractures are difficult to stabilize, require prolonged convalescence, and heal with a large amount of periosteal callus, which may interfere with tendon function. Prognosis is considerably improved, however, if radiographs indicate that the fracture does not enter the distal interphalangeal joint. Ankylosis of the proximal interphalangeal joint of the pelvic limb without involvement of the distal interphalangeal joint may allow limited useful function of the limb. The prognosis for return to a pretrauma level of athletic activity, however, is always guarded.[13]

ROENTGEN SIGNS OF INTERPHALANGEAL JOINT ABNORMALITIES

Alignment

Alteration in the relative position of the phalanges may occur owing to congenital, developmental, or acquired causes. Radiographs demonstrate the most common changes in alignment as overflexion or overextension of the affected joint.

Increased Flexion of the Distal Interphalangeal Joint. This developmental flexural deformity appears in foals from 6 weeks to 6 months of age. The clinical appearance of an almost vertical hoof wall indicates an underlying increased flexion of the distal phalanx with respect to the middle phalanx (Fig. 18–20). This de-

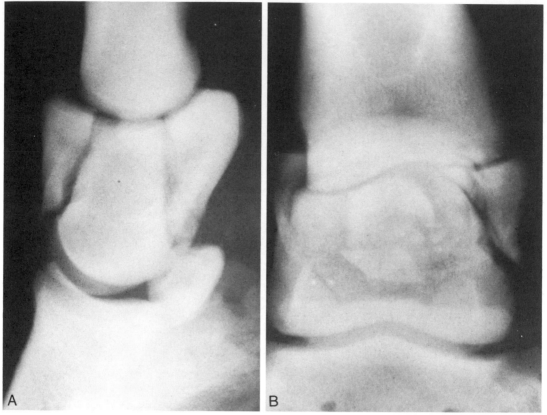

Figure 18–19. Comminuted, multiple fractures of the middle phalanx. The lateromedial view (A) shows extension of the fracture to the palmar surface into the distal interphalangeal joint in the area of the navicular bone.

formity appears to be related to overfeeding; reduction in the plane of nutrition alone may bring about resolution of the defect.[9] It has been theorized that the deformity is caused by a rapid increase in length of the third metacarpal (metatarsal) bone at its distal physis. Bone growth rate then occurs more rapidly than the rate at which the inferior check ligament (accessory ligament of the deep digital flexor tendon) can passively lengthen. The inferior check ligament or deep digital flexor tendon can be considered a functional unit running from the proximal end of the third metacarpal (metatarsal) bone to the distal phalanx.[9] Increasing tension on this unit leads to flexion of the distal interphalangeal joint, with the foal assuming a "toe dancer" stance. Secondary changes that occur if the deformity persists uncorrected include shortening of the joint capsules and suspensory ligaments of the navicular bone and pododermatitis due to abnormal wearing of the hoof wall at the toe.[10, 11] This deformity has also been seen in foals from mares that ingested locoweed, were fed goitrogenic diets, or experienced influenza during pregnancy.[19]

Increased Flexion of the Proximal Interphalangeal Joint. This abnormal alignment is uncommon and is seen as an acquired lesion (Fig. 18–21). The apparent dorsal subluxation is due to tearing of the straight sesamoidean ligament in combination with strain or disruption of the branches of the interosseous ligament. Thus, when weight is borne on the leg, the metacarpophalangeal or metatarsophalangeal joint overextends and the proximal interphalangeal joint subluxates in a dorsal direction.[22, 29]

Increased Extension of the Proximal Interphalangeal Joint. This is an unusual appearance that occurs with rupture of both the straight sesamoidean ligament and the superficial digital flexor tendon. It may also be seen in combination with overextension of the distal interphalangeal and metacarpophalangeal joints as a congenital deformity in foals.

Increased Extension of the Distal Interphalangeal Joint. This malalignment may occur in newborn foals as a congenital abnormality affecting all three joints of the foot, or it may be seen in adults owing to an acquired lesion affecting only the distal interphalangeal joint.

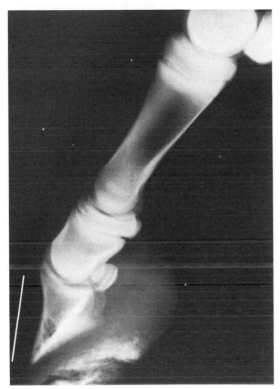

Figure 18–20. Flexural deformity of the distal interphalangeal joint in a 4-month-old foal. The dorsal surface of the distal phalanx remains parallel to the dorsal hoof wall *(white line)*, but both of these structures assume an abnormally vertical position.

In the foal, the flexor tendons may be weak at birth, thus providing inadequate support for the digit and allowing the fetlock to contact the ground. Weakened flexor tendons may also be seen secondary to poor nutrition, slow or incomplete recovery from a systemic disease, or after prolonged periods of external support (splinting or casting) of the leg.[10] Acquired overextension is seen with rupture of the deep digital flexor tendon or avulsion of its insertion (Fig. 18–22). This lesion occurs with traumatic laceration of the tendon or extension of infection from a deep sole abscess to the palmar surface of the distal phalanx.

Pericapsular Soft Tissues

Roentgen signs of abnormality include alteration of thickness or opacity of the tissues surrounding the joints. To demonstrate these changes, technical factors must allow definition of soft tissue as well as bone. Use of a relatively higher kVp and lower ma levels produces a radiograph with longer scale of contrast and better resolution of soft tissues.

Increased thickness of these tissues may be seen with intracapsular fluid accumulation, extracapsular inflammation (cellulitis), or fibrosis. If the enlargement is strictly confined to the region of the joint, then the fluid accumulation is primarily intracapsular. If the enlargement extends proximally and distally beyond the sites of joint capsule attachment, then extracapsular fluid or fibrosis is present, which obscures evaluation for intracapsular changes.

Increased opacity within pericapsular soft tissues is usually due to dystrophic calcification. Causes of this mineralization include chronic sprain or strain of supporting ligaments (Fig. 18–11), pericapsular deposition of corticosteroids, or focal necrosis secondary to neurectomy (Fig. 18–23).

Decreased opacity within the soft tissues is associated with the presence of air or gas in the subcutis or fascial planes of tendons and ligaments. Common etiologies for subcutaneous emphysema are open skin wound or infection by a gas-producing organism.

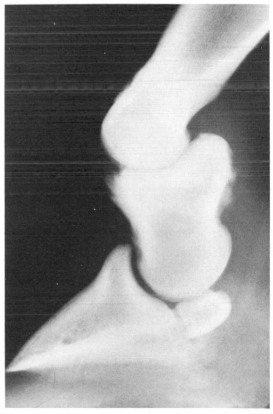

Figure 18–21. Dorsal subluxation of the proximal interphalangeal joint due to a combination of tearing of the lateral and medial branches of the interosseous ligament (allows overextension of the metacarpophalangeal joint) and strain or tearing of the straight sesamoidean ligament. Periosteal reaction at the dorsal joint capsule attachment and superficial digital flexor tendon insertion indicate chronicity of this injury.

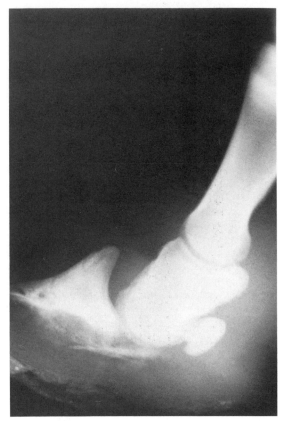

Figure 18–22. Luxation of the distal interphalangeal joint secondary to osteomyelitis and pathologic fracture of the flexor surface of the distal phalanx. Dorsal displacement of the distal phalanx is due to avulsion of the deep digital flexor tendon insertion and the subsequent unreciprocated pull of the common digital extensor tendon. The distal sesamoidean impar ligament is also ruptured, allowing proximal displacement of the navicular bone.

Joint Space Width and Subchondral Bone Opacity

These two important roentgen signs of joint disease are considered together, because the appearance of the subchondral bone affects the visualization of the joint space. Figure 18–24 illustrates normal and abnormal appearances of bone and joint space in a stylized proximal interphalangeal joint. In the normal joint (Fig. 18–24A), the subchondral bone is smooth, broader, and more opaque in the middle phalanx than in the proximal phalanx. The radiolucent zone between the adjacent bones is commonly referred to as the joint space. In the radiograph obtained during weight-bearing in a normal animal, however, this radiolucent zone is in fact the articular cartilage, and should be uniform in width across the entire surface of the joint.

Increased Width, No Change in Subchondral Bone (Fig. 18–24B). The most common cause

of this radiographic appearance is the lame horse that is non–weight-bearing at the time of x-ray exposure. Lack of axial weight compression allows slight distraction of the adjacent bones, to the limit allowed by the joint capsule and supporting collateral ligaments. This roentgen sign may also be seen in early septic arthritis, when increased synovial fluid accumulation and exudate are present in the joint cavity, but before osseous changes occur.[4] Generally, in animals evaluated for suspected joint disease, the process has progressed beyond this stage.

Increased Width, Decreased Opacity, and Irregular Contour of Subchondral Bone (Fig. 18–24C). This appearance indicates active septic arthritis that is eroding both articular cartilage and subchondral bone. Increased joint width suggests production of large amounts of exudate or cellular debris.

Decreased Width, Subchondral Bone Uniform in Opacity, With or Without Sclerosis (Fig. 18–24D). This abnormality may affect the entire width of the joint evenly, or it may occur in only part of the joint. Pathologic narrowing of the joint space is caused by loss of articular cartilage due to injury or conformational defect and subsequent abnormal wear of cartilage sur-

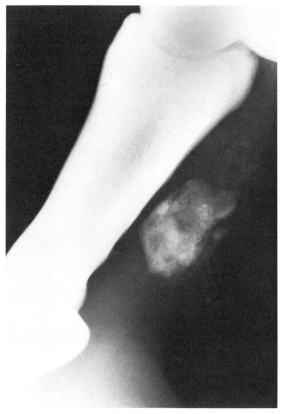

Figure 18–23. Dystrophic calcification in the palmar soft tissues secondary to previous neurectomy.

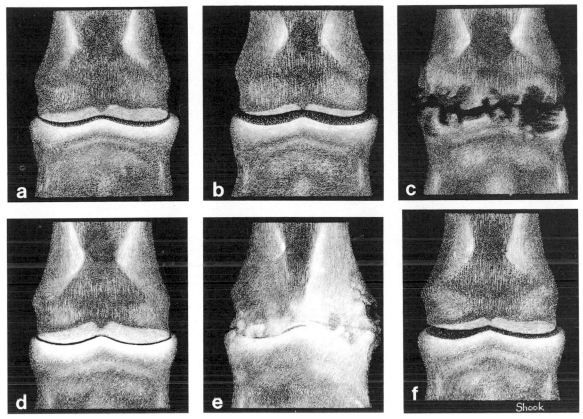

Figure 18–24. Common changes in joint space width, subchondral bone opacity or both seen in the proximal interphalangeal joint. a: normal joint space and subchondral bone. b: widened joint space, no subchondral bone changes (non–weight-bearing image)—increased intra-articular fluid volume (early infectious arthritis). c: widened joint space, lysis of subchondral bone—active septic arthritis. d: uniformly narrowed joint space, no subchondral bone changes—artifact caused by angulation of the primary x-ray beam; degenerative wearing and loss of articular cartilage. e: narrowed joint space, irregular opacity and contour of subchondral bone—chronic low-grade septic arthritis, chronic osteoarthritis due to trauma-related instability or poor conformation. f: widened joint space on the lateral or medial side, no subchondral bone changes—asymmetric weight distribution on the foot (a common artifact). (Preparation courtesy of Richard M. Shook.)

faces. Artifactual narrowing of the entire joint space may be produced by angulation of the primary beam such that the beam and joint surface are no longer parallel.

Decreased Width, Irregular Contour, and Nonuniform Opacity of Subchondral Bone. (Fig. 18–24E). This combination of abnormalities may be seen in the septic joint after erosion of articular cartilage with extension of infection to the subchondral bone (Fig. 18–16) or in chronic osteoarthrosis due to instability, in which cystic degenerative changes are occurring in the subchondral bone. Sclerosis of adjacent portions of the proximal or middle phalanx occurs with advancing chronicity of the lesion. The radiolucent defects seen in the subchondral bone due to inflammation are usually multiple, small, and have poorly defined margins when compared to lesions produced by osteochondrosis (Fig. 18–14).

Increased Width on One Side of Joint Only,

No Subchondral Bone Changes (Fig. 18–24F). If the metacarpophalangeal or metatarsophalangeal joint and both interphalangeal joints show similar narrowing, the patient is probably not bearing weight evenly on the foot. Asymmetric weight distribution causes the loaded side of the joint to be narrower than the distraction side of the joint. This is a common radiographic artifact.

Periarticular Bone Margins

New bone formation often occurs in the interphalangeal area in association with chronic joint diseases. One pattern of bone proliferation is a sharply marginated lipping of the periarticular surface in response to instability of the joint. This appearance is seen frequently in the proximal interphalangeal joint, where remodeling of the opposing bones creates a flatter, broader articular surface, with spiculated osteophytes

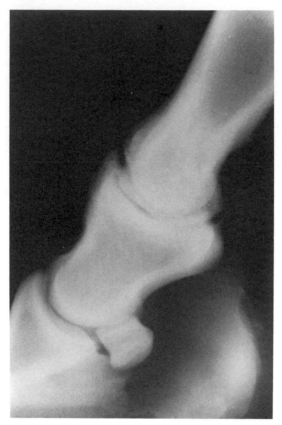

Figure 18–25. Osteoarthrosis of the proximal interphalangeal joint. The contours of the opposing surfaces of the proximal and middle phalanx are flattened. The articular surfaces are also broader due to remodeling and new bone formation at the periarticular margins. These periarticular osteophytes are often sharply spiculated in the mildly unstable joint.

along the edge of the middle phalanx (Fig. 18–25). Instability may be primary (congenital malformation of articular surfaces, poor conformation) or secondary (trauma due to overuse, laceration of supporting ligaments, sequelae after intra-articular fracture, or large osteochondrosis defect). Another common type of new bone formation is the osteophyte (spur), which forms at the attachment site of the joint capsule or collateral ligaments (Figs. 18–13 and 18–21). As previously stated, these areas of new bone growth indicate ossification of the fibro-osseous attachment or focal stimulation of underlying periosteum.

ROENTGEN SIGNS IN THE DISTAL PHALANX

Number

A supernumerary distal phalanx may be seen in the rare congenital anomaly of polydactylism, as previously described. Agenesis of the distal

phalanx has also been reported.[35] Abnormalities of this magnitude are uncommon.

Position

The normal orientation of the distal phalanx to the hoof is maintained by the interdigitating leaves of the laminar corium and the horn-like lamellae of the hoof wall. The laminar corium is attached to the dorsal surface of the distal phalanx by a modified periosteum, which contains a tightly meshed network of blood vessels.

Palmar deviation ("rotation") of the toe of the distal phalanx is a common occurrence with laminitis. A series of complex biochemical changes takes place within several body systems to cause this lesion. Research studies in which a grain overload model was used have shown that during the acute phase (up to 48 hours after initial signs of lameness), there is decreased digital capillary perfusion associated with arteriovenous shunting in the digit.[2, 6] This decrease causes local ischemia, which is responsible for the pain seen in the acute phase.[14, 16] Congestion of the laminar corium, edema of the junction between the lamina and lamellae of the hoof wall, and subsequent necrosis of these tissues result in loss of support for the dorsal surface of the distal phalanx. Ischemic necrosis of the digit may be progressive as the initial pain stimulates adrenal release of catecholamines, which cause vasoconstriction and further ischemia. With loss of the laminar or lamellar junction, the weight of the horse, the leverage force placed at the toe (as the hoof breaks over in midstride), and the pulling force of the deep digital flexor tendon combine to force the toe mechanically away from the hoof wall (Fig. 18–26).[5] A linear radiolucent shadow at the laminar or lamellar junction is another radiographic abnormality that may be seen with acute laminitis. This linear radiolucency has been attributed to air dissecting between the hoof wall and the laminar corium when necrosis has eroded through to the coronary band or "white zone" of the sole or to nitrogen that moves from the blood into the partial vacuum created by the displacement of the toe and the adjacent lamina.

Chronic laminitis may show the following radiographic changes in the distal phalanx: palmar deviation of the toe, indistinct dorsal surface, increased number of vascular channels directed to the dorsal surface, pathologic fracture of the toe due to altered weight distribution, and remodeled shape of toe to an elongated, "ski tip" appearance. These changes are demonstrated in Figure 18–26. The degree of distal phalanx deviation has been used as a prognostic sign in the evaluation of horses with laminitis. In a series of 91 horses, the degree

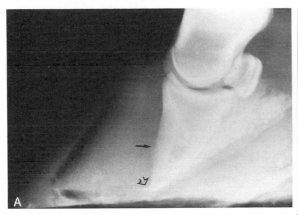

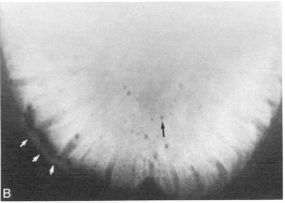

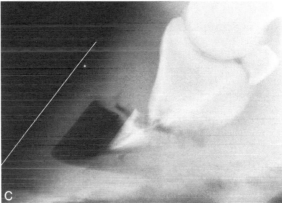

Figure 18–26. *A*, severe palmar rotation of the distal phalanx due to laminitis. Gas is seen between the hoof wall and the soft tissues of the corium. Indistinct dorsal surface *(solid arrow)* and angulation ("ski-tip" appearance) of the toe of the distal phalanx *(open arrow)* are additional changes seen in the chronic stage of laminitis. *B*, pathologic fracture of the distal phalanx secondary to laminitis. Thin bone segment is separated from the solar margin *(white arrows)*. Punctate radiolucent defects *(black arrow)* are enlarged vascular channels in cross-section. *C*, fracture of the toe with concurrent palmar rotation and large accumulation of gas between the hoof wall and the laminar corium.

of rotation was inversely correlated with return to athletic performance. Horses with less than 5.5 degrees deviation returned to their former athletic activity, whereas those horses with more than 11.5 degrees deviation were not useful as performance animals.[34]

Dorsal displacement of the distal phalanx is seen with stretching or rupture of the deep digital flexor tendon. The phalanx maintains its orientation to the hoof wall, so that the toe of the hoof is also elevated from the ground (Fig. 18–22).

Contour

Alterations in contour are those changes that affect the normal shape of the margins of the distal phalanx. The location of the radiographic

Figure 18–27. Long-standing fracture of the extensor process of the distal phalanx. The fracture extends into the articular surface of the distal interphalangeal joint and may lead to degenerative osteoarthrosis.

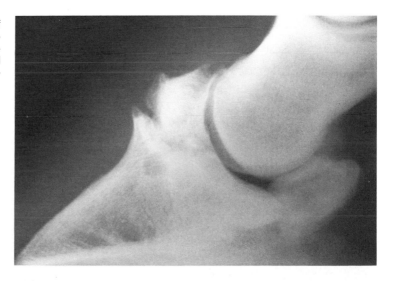

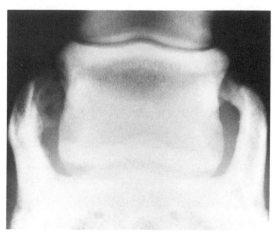

Figure 18–28. Ossification of collateral cartilage of the distal phalanx. Uniform ossification is seen in both the lateral and medial collateral cartilage. Such changes appear bizarre, but usually do not cause lameness if the foot is broad at the heel.

abnormality may provide a clue to the cause of the lesion.

Indistinct Dorsal Margin. This sign, seen on the lateromedial view, indicates chronic strain on the modified periosteum, resulting in minimal periosteal proliferation (Fig. 18–26). This appearance is one of the radiographic signs of previous chronic laminitis or other focal inflammation.

Indistinct, Irregular Solar Margin. Diffuse roughening of the solar border, creating a ragged and lacy appearance when viewed on the lateromedial or 65 degree dorsoproximal-palmarodistal oblique projection, can be an indication of chronic bruising and mild inflammatory response (pedal osteitis). Because there is considerable variation in the appearance of the solar surface of the normal distal phalanx, however, this radiographic sign may be misleading.

A positive response to hoof testers and decreased thickness of the sole are other abnormalities that, if present, increase the probability that pedal osteitis is a real finding.

Irregular Extensor Process. A defect at the base of the extensor process or fragment proximal to the process indicates fracture or incomplete ossification of this structure. Fractures may occur owing to abnormal strain on the common digital extensor tendon or to overextension of the distal interphalangeal joint. Because this abnormality can be bilateral, incomplete development from separate centers of ossification must be considered as another possible cause. Small bone opacities adjacent to the process are not considered significant if the horse is clinically sound. When the articular surface is involved, the defect is more important and can lead to secondary osteoarthritis of the distal interphalangeal joint (Fig. 18–27).[27]

Irregular Fragmentation at the Toe. These are pathologic fractures secondary to hyperemia and inflammation of the phalanx and adjacent soft tissue leading to increased number and diameter of vascular channels. Bone fragments are usually thin and may be missed if exposure factors are not optimal or if the foot is not properly cleaned before radiography. Etiologies include laminitis with ventral deviation and extension of inflammation from a sole abscess or penetrating wound.

Ossification of Collateral Cartilages (Sidebones). This is a common finding in radiographs of the distal part of the digit, especially in draft breed horses. The cartilages may become extensively ossified and project well beyond the proximal surface of the navicular bone on the dorsopalmar/plantar view (Fig. 18–28). Even an extensive degree of ossification may not be clinically significant, especially if the horse is 12 to 15 years of age, has a broad foot, and shows no pain on manipulation of the heel area.

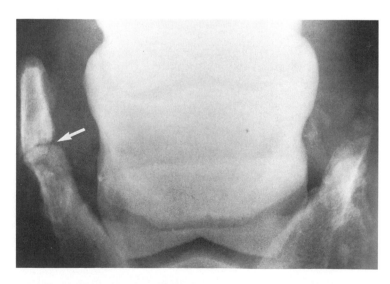

Figure 18–29. Asymmetric ossification of the collateral cartilage of the distal phalanx may indicate abnormal stress on the affected side of the foot, and warrants close examination of the heel and navicular bone for additional abnormalities. The radiolucent defect in the ossified cartilage *(arrow)* is cartilage remnants between two separate centers of ossification.

TABLE 18–2. CLASSIFICATION OF DISTAL PHALANX FRACTURES

Type	Description	Prognosis
I	Nonarticular fracture of palmar/plantar process	Most favorable outcome with corrective shoeing and 3 to 9 months stall rest
II	Articular fracture extending from the distal interphalangeal joint to the solar margin	Guarded
III	Midsagittal articular fracture that divides the phalanx into equal parts	Guarded
IV	Extensor process fracture	Poor for large fragments with articular involvement
V	Comminuted fracture or fracture due to foreign body penetration or osteomyelitis	(Insufficient data to determine)

More prominent calcification of one of the collateral cartilages than the other may indicate increased stress on the ossified portion (Fig. 18–29). Careful physical examination is warranted in such an instance to determine if localized disease is present within the foot. The appearance of the navicular bone should also be closely evaluated in the previous example, because collateral cartilage ossification may accompany a more significant degenerative lesion in the navicular bone.[27] A radiolucent linear defect or gap in the ossified cartilage usually indicates the junction between a separate, more peripheral ossification center and that part of the cartilage that is ossifying from the palmar process of the phalanx. Fracture of the ossified collateral is unusual. Response to digital pressure applied at the coronary band in the area of the suspect fracture helps to differentiate a fracture from an incomplete pattern of ossification.

Radiopacity

Abnormal opacity identified in the distal phalanx is most often radiolucent. The shape and number of abnormal opacities commonly found are subsequently described.

Solitary Linear Decreased Opacity. Traumatic fracture is the most common cause of this sign. Osteomyelitis and improper shoeing have also been suggested as possible causes for fracture of the distal phalanx. Because the hoof wall restricts displacement of a bone fragment, diagnosis of the fracture depends on visualization of the fracture line. If the plane of the primary beam is not parallel to the fracture plane, the superimposed parts of the bone obscure the fracture line and diagnosis may not be possible. Therefore, four views of the distal phalanx are recommended when a fracture is suspected— 65 degree dorsoproximal-palmarodistal oblique, lateromedial, dorsal 65 degree proximal 45 degree lateral-palmarodistomedial oblique, and dorsal 65 degree proximal 45 degree medial-palmarodistolateral oblique. A classification scheme has been devised for fractures of the distal phalanx (Table 18–2).[10]

Type II fractures were found most often in one report of 65 horses, the lesions usually involving the lateral aspect of the left front distal phalanx or the medial aspect of the right front distal phalanx (Fig. 18–30).[31,32] In that series of fractures in racehorses, the forelimb, which bore the most weight in turns, was at greatest risk (horses were raced counterclockwise).

The progression of healing of a distal phalanx fracture is difficult to determine radiographi-

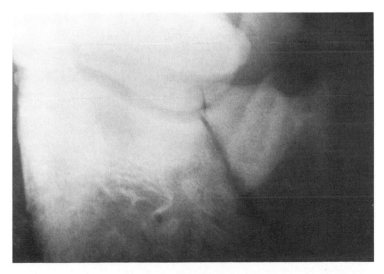

Figure 18–30. Type II fracture of the distal phalanx. Dorsal 65 degree proximal 45 degree lateral palmarodistomedial oblique view demonstrates the lesion to best advantage and is often necessary to determine whether the fracture extends into the distal interphalangeal joint, as in this horse.

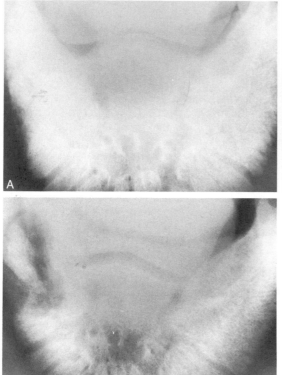

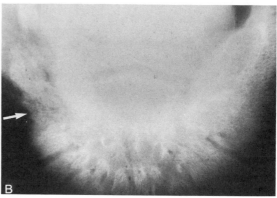

Figure 18–31. Serial 65 degree dorsoproximal-palmarodistal oblique projections of the palmar processes of the distal phalanx in an acutely lame 5-year-old Thoroughbred. *A,* initial examination shows minimal radiographic abnormality. *B,* Six days later. Radiolucent defect is evident in the medial palmar process with loss of trabecular bone detail (compare with lateral palmar process). *C,* Nine days later. More extensive lysis of bone has occurred, with separation of a sequestered fragment. Radiographic diagnosis: osteomyelitis with sequestrum formation.

cally because of the lack of or minimal formation of osseous callus. The periosteum of this phalanx is poorly developed and does not effectively respond to the stimulation of direct trauma. Therefore, it is possible to radiograph an equine foot 1 year after the original trauma and still visualize the fracture line. Consequently, refracture can occur, especially in horses returned to training after stall rest.

Multiple Linear Decreased Opacities. This appearance is usually due to increased size and number of vascular channels (hypervascularity) secondary to inflammation from laminitis (Fig. 18–27) or chronic bruising of the sole and distal phalanx (pedal osteitis).

Solitary Rounded Decreased Opacity. If the defect is sharply defined with a distinct margin between it and the rest of the phalanx, the lesion may be an aneurysmal bone cyst; a remnant of an old, currently inactive infection; osteochondrosis; or a congenital vascular malformation (uncommon).[27, 40] If the margin of the defect is indistinct and tends to fade into the surrounding bone, an infectious lesion, such as an abscess or osteomyelitis with sequestration, should be considered. Figure 18–31 illustrates serial radiographs that were made of the distal phalanx of a horse with a draining tract over a period of 15 days. This set of radiographic images indicates the degree and rapidity of osseous destruction that may occur with osteo-

myelitis. Repeat or follow-up radiographs can be useful in the work-up of the persistently lame horse in which no radiographic changes were initially noted.

RADIOGRAPHIC INTERPRETATION

Use of the roentgen sign approach can greatly assist in understanding and interpreting radiographic abnormalities in the equine phalanges. Many of the osseous or joint changes discussed in this text, however, do not completely remodel when the initial stimulus that created them is removed or the disease process reaches an inactive state. Therefore, determining the current significance of lesions seen on radiographs can be difficult, especially in the acutely lame horse with radiographic evidence of previous disease. Additionally, in some cases of acute lameness, pathologic changes occurring in the bone have not progressed to the severity that makes them radiographically detectable. Newer imaging techniques, such as nuclear medicine, appear to offer significant advantages over standard radiography in these situations. Bone scanning with a radiopharmaceutical is a sensitive test for early bone injury as it reflects changes in skeletal mineral metabolism and physiology rather than in bone density (gm/cm^3) and structure. Bone scans have also been used to determine the degree of activity of radiographically identified lesions.[8] Although bone scanning is not practical for the private practitioner, many university teaching hospitals have the capability to perform these studies, and referral for this examination is possible.

References

1. Adams OR: Lameness in Horses. Philadelphia, Lea & Febiger, 1976.
2. Ackerman N, Garner HE, Coffman JR, et al: Angiographic appearance of the normal equine foot and alterations in chronic laminitis. J Am Vet Med Assoc 166:58, 1975.
3. Attenburrow DP, and Heyse-Moore GH: Non-ossifying fibroma in phalanx of a Thoroughbred yearling. Equine Vet J 14:59, 1982.
4. Barber SM: Subluxation and sepsis of the distal interphalangeal joint of a horse. J Am Vet Med Assoc 181:491, 1982.
5. Coffman JR, Johnson JH, Finocchio EJ, et al: Biomechanics of pedal rotation in equine laminitis. J Am Vet Med Assoc 156:219, 1970.
6. Colles CM, Garner HE, and Coffman JR: The blood supply of the horse's foot. In Proceedings of the Twenty-fifth Annual Convention of the American Association of Equine Practitioners, Miami, Dec 2–5, 1979, pp. 385–389.
7. Copelan RW, and Bramlage LR: Surgery of the fetlock joint. Vet Clin North Am [Large Anim Pract] 5:221, 1983.
8. Devous MD, and Twardock AR: Techniques and applications of nuclear medicine in the diagnosis of equine lameness. J Am Vet Med Assoc 184:318, 1984.
9. Fackelman GE: Equine flexural deformities of developmental origin. In Proceedings of the Twenty-sixth Annual Convention of the American Association of Equine Practitioners, Anaheim, CA, Nov 30–Dec 3, 1980, pp. 97–105.
10. Fackelman, GE: Tendon surgery. Vet Clin North Am [Large Anim Pract] 5:381, 1983.
11. Fackelman GE, Auer JA, Orsini J, et al: Surgical treatment of severe flexural deformity of the distal interphalangeal joint in young horses. J Am Vet Med Assoc 182:949, 1983.
12. Firth EC: Current concepts of infectious polyarthritis in foals. Equine Vet J 15:5, 1983.
13. Gabel AA, and Bukowiecki CF: Fractures of the phalanges. Vet Clin North Am [Large Anim Pract] 5:233, 1983.
14. Garner HE: Update on equine laminitis. Vet Clin North Am [Large Anim Pract] 2:25, 1980.
15. Hackett, RP: Intra-articular use of corticosteroids in the horse. J Am Vet Med Assoc 181:292, 1982.
16. Hood, DM, and Stephens, KA: Physiopathology of equine laminitis. Comp Contin Ed Pract Vet 3:S454, 1981.
17. McIlwraith CW: Idiopathic synovitis, traumatic arthritis and degenerative joint disease. In Proceedings of the Twenty-seventh Annual Convention of the American Association of Equine Practitioners, New Orleans, Nov 28–Dec 2, 1981, pp. 125–139.
18. McIlwraith CW: Pathobiology and diagnosis of equine joint disease. In Proceedings of the Twenty-seventh Annual Convention of the American Association of Equine Practitioners, New Orleans, Nov 28–Dec 2, 1981, pp. 115–123.
19. McIlwraith CW, and James LF: Limb deformities in foals associated with ingestion of locoweed by mares. J Am Vet Med Assoc 181:255, 1982.
20. Messer NT, and Powers BE: Hypertrophic osteopathy associated with pulmonary infarction in a horse. Comp Contin Ed Vet Pract 5:S636, 1983.
21. Morgan P, and Silverman S: Techniques of Veterinary Radiography, 3rd Ed. Davis, CA, Veterinary Radiology Associates, 1982.
22. Moyer W: Distal sesamoidean desmitis. In Proceedings of the Twenty-eighth Annual Convention of the American Association of Equine Practitioners, Atlanta, Dec 4–8, 1982, pp. 245–251.
23. Nyrop KA, Coffman JR, DeBowes RM, et al: The role of diagnostic nerve blocks in the equine lameness examination. Comp Contin Ed Vet Pract 5:S669, 1983.
24. Pettersson H, and Reiland S: Periarticular subchondral "bone cysts" in horses. Clin Orthop Rel Res 62:95, 1969.
25. Pettersson H, and Ryden G: Avulsion fractures of the caudoproximal extremity of the first phalanx. Equine Vet J 14:333, 1982.
26. Pool RR, Wheat JD, and Ferraro GL: Corticosteroid therapy in common joint and tendon injuries of the horse. Part 1: Effects on joints. In Proceedings of the Twenty-sixth Annual Convention of the American Association of Equine Practitioners, Anaheim, CA, Nov 30–Dec 3, 1980, pp. 397–406.
27. Reid CF: Radiography and the purchase examination in the horse. Vet Clin North Am [Large Anim Pract] 2:151, 1980.
28. Rendano VT, and Grant B: The equine third phalanx: Its radiographic appearance. J Am Vet Radiol Soc 19:125, 1978.
29. Rooney JR: Biomechanics of Lameness in Horses. Baltimore, Williams & Wilkens, 1969.
30. Schebitz H, and Wilkens H: Atlas of Radiographic Anatomy of the Horse. Berlin, Paul Parey; Philadelphia, WB Saunders, 1978.
31. Scott EA, McDole M, and Shires MH: A review of third phalanx fractures in the horse: 65 cases. J Am Vet Med Assoc 174:1337, 1979.
32. Scott EA, McDole M, Shires MH, et al: Fractures of the third phalanx (P_3) in the horse at Michigan State University, 1964–1979. In Proceedings of the Twenty-fifth Annual Convention of the American Association of Equine Practitioners, Miami, Dec 2–5, 1979, pp. 439–449.
33. Speirs VC: Assessment of the economic value of orthopedic surgery in Thoroughbred racehorses. Vet Clin North Am [Large Anim Pract] 5:391, 1983.
34. Stick JA, Jann HW, Scott EA, et al: Pedal bone rotation as a prognostic sign in laminitis of horses. J Am Vet Med Assoc 180:251, 1982.
35. Taylor TS, and Morris EL: Agenesis of the distal phalanx in a mule. Vet Radiol 24:63, 1983.
36. Ticer JW: Radiographic Positioning and Technique in Veterinary Practice. Philadelphia, WB Saunders, 1984.
37. Trotter GW, and McIlwraith CW: Osteochondritis dissecans and subchondral cystic lesions and their relationship to osteochondrosis in the horse. Equine Vet Sci 5:157, 1981.
38. Trotter GW, and McIlwraith CW: Osteochondrosis in horses: Pathogenesis and clinical syndromes. In Proceedings of the Twenty-seventh Annual Convention of the American Association of Equine Practitioners, New Orleans, Nov 28–Dec 2, 1981, pp. 141–160.
39. Trotter GW, McIlwraith CW, Norrdin RW, et al: Degenerative joint disease with osteochondrosis of the proximal interphalangeal joint in young horses. J Am Vet Med Assoc 180:1312, 1982.
40. Vershooten F, and De Moor A: Subchondral cystic and related lesions affecting the equine pedal bone and stifle. Equine Vet J 14:47, 1982.

CHAPTER 19

THE NAVICULAR BONE

ROBERT L. TOAL

ANATOMY

The navicular bone is shuttle-shaped and has two surfaces (articular and flexor), two borders (proximal and distal), and two extremities (Fig. 19–1).[1] The articular surface forms the palmar (plantar) part of the distal interphalangeal joint. The flexor surface has a prominent central ridge. The deep digital flexor tendon, protected by a bursa, passes over the flexor surface. The navicular bone is held in position by three strong ligaments. The paired suspensory navicular ligament originates from the dorsolateral aspects of the proximal phalanx and attaches to the proximal navicular border and extremities. The distal sesamoidean ligament originates on the distal navicular border and inserts on the distal phalanx with the deep digital flexor tendon. Blood vessels traverse these ligaments and ramify into the navicular bone via both borders.[2]

In some horses, prominent foramina penetrate variable distances into the medulla of the navicular bone, appearing radiographically appear as radiolucent, cone-shaped invaginations contiguous with the distal border. These invaginations have been referred to as vascular channels.[2] Results of a recent histologic study suggest that when radiographically visible, these foramina are probably synovium-lined invaginations that contain a variable degree of vascular connective tissue.[3] These radiolucencies are normally seen in active horses 2 years of age or older and become larger and more numerous in heavily worked animals.[2] Their physiologic significance is not totally understood.

INDICATIONS FOR RADIOGRAPHY

Indications for navicular radiography include the assessment of bony changes in navicular disease; identification of significant bony abnormalities during prepurchase examination; check for bone or bursal involvement in foot wounds or abscesses; evaluation for suspected trauma; and to follow the morphologic progression or remission of navicular bone abnormalities.

PREPARATION FOR RADIOGRAPHIC EVALUATION

Accurate radiographic evaluation of the navicular bone depends on a radiograph that is properly positioned and properly exposed, and on a foot that is free of distracting artifacts. When possible, the shoe should be removed and the sole surface should be thoroughly cleaned and pared. The lucent shadows of the frog sulci are neutralized by using packing material of the same radiopacity as soft tissue; this

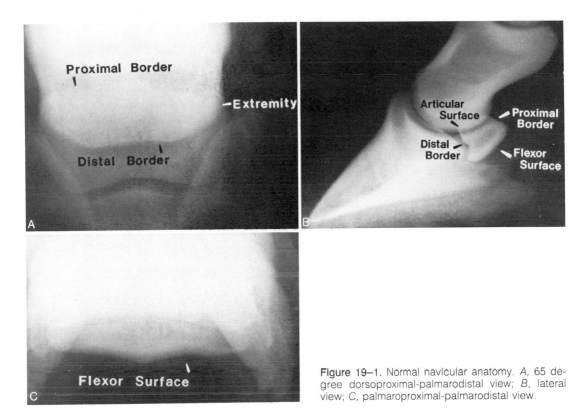

Figure 19–1. Normal navicular anatomy. *A*, 65 degree dorsoproximal-palmarodistal view; *B*, lateral view; *C*, palmaroproximal-palmarodistal view.

provides a homogeneous background opacity on the radiograph. Play Doh (Rainbow Crafts, Cincinnati, OH) works well, is inexpensive, and is reusable. Care should be taken, however, to squeeze out any air pockets that may develop while packing the frog.

Positioning aids, such as a reinforced cassette, grooved wooden blocks, and a wooden cassette tunnel, assist in radiographic evaluation of the navicular bone (Fig. 19–2). Use of a grid is optional. A grid improves radiographic detail by reducing film fog from scatter radiation. Because the grid is fragile, its use is limited to techniques during which the foot does not bear weight directly on the grid.

RADIOGRAPHIC VIEWS

The location of the navicular bone and its complex shape require that multiple views be taken for complete radiographic evaluation. Commonly used radiographic views include the an-

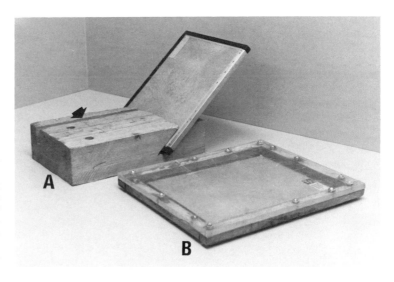

Figure 19–2. Types of positioning aids for navicular radiography. *A*, wooden block shows cassette placement for angular dorsoproximal-palmarodistal views. The longitudinally oriented slot *(arrow)* is used for lateral views. The grooves are of sufficient width to allow combined insertion of a grid and cassette. *B*, a cassette tunnel covered with plexiglass protects the cassette (and grid) during dorsoproximal-palmarodistal views.

gular dorsoproximal-palmarodistal views, the lateral-medial view, and the palmaroproximal-palmarodistal view (subsequently referred to as the flexor tangential view in this chapter). Other views, such as oblique and 0 dorsoproximal-palmarodistal projections, are valuable supplements. Special techniques, such as linear tomography, xeroradiography, and [99M]Tc bone scintigraphy, are helpful when diagnosis is difficult.[4, 5]

Dorsoproximal-Palmarodistal Views

Angular dorsoproximal-palmarodistal views of the navicular bone can be made by two different positioning techniques.[6-8] In one method (high coronary stand-on route), the horse's foot rests directly on a reinforced cassette, wooden cassette tunnel, or grooved wooden block. The x-ray beam is centered just proximal to the coronary band and angled 45 or 65 degrees from horizontal. In the other method (upright pedal route), the horse's hoof rests on the toe in tiptoe fashion with the dorsal hoof wall positioned either 80 or 90 degrees from horizontal; the x-ray beam is directed horizontally (Fig. 19–3).

Stand-on techniques are technically easier, but result in slightly more magnification of the navicular bone when compared to the upright pedal route.[7] Magnification can be minimized on the high coronary stand-on route by utilizing a grooved wooden block. A cassette and grid are placed in a precut groove behind the horse's hoof as it rests on the block. Owing to the position of the cassette, less magnification of

the navicular bone occurs when compared with other stand-on techniques (Fig. 19–3B).

Both of these dorsoproximal-palmarodistal views project the navicular bone behind the middle phalanx. The two navicular extremities and the medulla are readily seen. Visualization of the navicular borders varies, however, because the proximal and distal navicular borders are not parallel (they diverge in a palmar direction), and thus a true geometric projection of these two borders cannot be obtained in a single dorsoproximal-palmarodistal radiograph. By varying the x-ray beam angulation incident on the navicular bone in the high coronary route or by altering the position of the hoof in the upright pedal route, an accurate projection of either the proximal or distal navicular border can be obtained.

An undistorted projection of the proximal navicular border is achieved by using the 45 degree high coronary stand-on route or the 90 degree upright pedal route. Unfortunately, the distal navicular border is not well visualized by these routes because it is projected below the level of the distal interphalangeal joint. Because only the proximal navicular border can be accurately evaluated in these two projections, they are not routinely used (Fig. 19–3A and C).

A 65 degree high coronary stand-on route or an 80 degree upright pedal route projects the distal navicular border proximal to the distal interphalangeal joint and superimposes the entire navicular bone behind the middle phalanx. The distal navicular border is well visualized, and although the proximal border is slightly distorted, it is readily identified. Either one of these two positioning methods is recommended for the angular dorsoproximal-palmarodistal projection, because when done properly, the entire navicular bone is seen (Fig. 19–3B and D).

Lateral-Medial View

In the lateral view, it is important to use the best possible positioning technique so as to project both navicular extremities superimposed. If some degree of angulation occurs, this factor must be recognized and taken into account during interpretation. The horse's foot is placed on a wooden block so the x-ray tube can drop low enough to center the beam on the lateral axis of the navicular bone. A wooden block also elevates the hoof, allowing the cassette to straddle it proximally and distally. Thus, the entire hoof can be projected on the radiograph.

Flexor Tangential View

The flexor tangential view (Fig. 19–4) projects the flexor cortex, medulla, and navicular ridge.

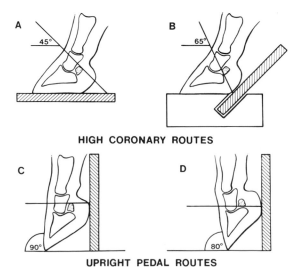

HIGH CORONARY ROUTES

UPRIGHT PEDAL ROUTES

Figure 19–3. Angular dorsoproximal-palmarodistal views. High coronary routes (*A*, direct stand-on method; *B*, wooden block technique) and upright pedal routes (*C* and *D*) are illustrated showing beam or hoof angulation relative to horizontal.

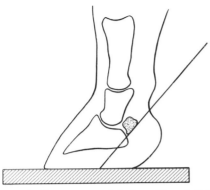

Figure 19–4. Flexor tangential view. The digit is positioned in extension, with the x-ray beam angled tangentially to the flexor surface.

The concept is to isolate the majority of the bone between the palmar processes of the distal phalanx. The horse stands on a reinforced cassette or cassette tunnel. The foot is positioned as far caudal as possible while still bearing weight.[9] Paradoxically, some individuals prefer that the foot be slightly forward than in the normal standing position.[10] Regardless of foot location, the primary beam is positioned tangential to the estimated plane of the flexor cortex and is centered between the bulbs of the heel. Too steep of a beam angle with the foot may result in superimposition of the ergot over the navicular bone. Reduced angulation alters the apparent width of the flexor cortex and results in an indistinct interface between cortical and trabecular bone.[9] Oblique flexor projections distort the navicular shape and superimpose it behind the palmar processes of the distal phalanx.

NORMAL RADIOGRAPHIC APPEARANCE

In the angular dorsoproximal-palmarodistal views, the navicular bone is of uniform radiopacity. Its spindle shape varies somewhat from horse to horse. The extremities are fairly symmetric and are bluntly pointed. The proximal border is smoothly marginated, although it may appear roughened owing to the summated opacity of the distal end of the middle phalanx over the navicular bone. The distal border has a variable number (four or five on average) of cone-shaped radiolucencies. Their size is variable, possibly being related to degree of work, although their shape should remain somewhat triangular (Figs. 19–1A and 19–5).

The lateral view offers a clear, unobstructed view of the navicular bone, but presents a foreshortened image. Both extremities should be superimposed; a well-defined medullary cavity is visualized. The flexor surface is convex palmarly and is smoothly marginated. The proximal and distal borders are smooth, as is the articular surface (Fig. 19–1B).

The flexor view shows a well-defined medullary cavity of uniform trabecular pattern with four or five small radiolucent foramina. The cortex is of homogeneous opacity and is of uniform thickness centrally, with some thinning peripherally. The flexor surface is smoothly marginated with a prominent central ridge. The ridge is positioned slightly closer to the medial extremity than to the lateral extremity. The ends of both extremities are rounded, being variably superimposed over the palmar processes of the distal phalanx. The articular surface is occasionally visualized in this view (Fig. 19–1C).[9]

NAVICULAR DISEASE

Navicular disease is primarily a bilateral fore limb lameness in the horse;[11-13] it is rarely recognized in the hindlimb.[14] Incidence data are skewed by the population characteristics of reporting institutions. In general, navicular disease is most common between 4 and 9 years of age, males are more involved than females, geldings have a greater risk than stallions, and the highest incidence is in Quarterhorses and Thoroughbreds.[15, 16]

Figure 19–5. A–D. Radiographs of navicular bones showing the normal variation in distal border fossa appearance. All fossae are considered radiographically normal except for that in A (arrow). The rounded configuration with a narrow stem suggests a lollipop shape, which is compatible with navicular disease. Note that the extremities of the navicular bone are fairly symmetric and blunt. Slight remodeling of one extremity is shown in C (arrow).

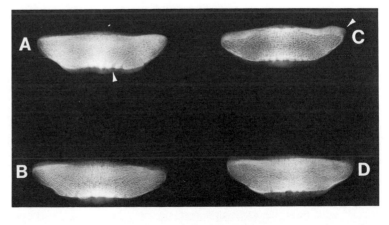

There are no clinical tests pathognomonic for navicular disease. The diagnosis is based upon a characteristic gait, localization of pain to the palmar part of the foot, and ruling out other causes of lameness.[12, 17] Radiology plays an important part in confirming the diagnosis or in excluding other disease.[15] When navicular disease is suspected, both feet should be radiographed, because changes are often bilateral even if clinical signs are not.

The pathophysiology of navicular disease is a subject that is controversial and is currently under investigation. Classically, it has been characterized as a navicular bursitis with secondary bone and tendon disease.[6, 12] More recent information suggests that navicular bone ischemia occurs owing to thromboembolism in its nutrient arteries. The ensuing bone necrosis and painful osteitis result in clinicopathologic and radiographic changes.[2, 18, 19] Histopathologic corroboration by other investigators of the infarct theory, however, is generally lacking.[20-23] Other evidence supports the concept that navicular disease is a degenerative arthrosis, albeit with a vascular component.[21, 23-25] Chronic passive venous congestion of the foot has been identified and related to navicular changes of elevated subchondral bone pressure and arterial hyperemia.[21, 26, 27] The ultimate extent and relationship of vascular pathologic processes to the complex known as navicular disease remains to be elucidated. Given the differences in opinion on the pathogenesis of navicular disease, multiple etiologies are possible.[23, 28]

Similar confusion exists concerning the significance of radiographic changes in navicular lameness. Although some individuals claim that radiographic changes are always present, it has been shown that there is a poor correlation of pathologic and radiographic findings to clinical signs and prognosis.[15, 17, 18, 20, 22] Horses without radiographic abnormalities can have clinical navicular lameness and horses with pathologic and radiographic changes can be sound. This paradox is explained in part by the fact that horses have different pain thresholds, are subjected to wide ranges of physical exercise, and are evaluated in variable stages of disease.[9] Additionally, some pathologic changes may represent insignificant wear lesions or may be located in tissues of soft-tissue opacity, and thus are not radiographically discernible.[17, 20] Several authors agree that roentgen signs of navicular disease in an otherwise clinically normal horse are significant and may warrant a cautious prognosis for future soundness.[4, 9, 29] This fact is particularly true if future vigorous activity is planned. It should be stated, however, that there is no universal agreement as to the clinical significance of all roentgen signs seen in navicular disease.

TABLE 19–1. ROENTGEN SIGNS OF NAVICULAR DISEASE

Remodeling
  Sawtooth borders
  Spurs on extremities

Osteopenia
  Lollipops on distal border
  Lollipops or cones on extremities
  Cysts in medullary cavity

Flexor Cortex Changes
  Flattened sagittal ridge
  Cortical bone lysis

Normal Findings

Roentgen Signs

Four categories of roentgen signs are seen in navicular disease (Table 19–1). Individual signs may occur separately or in combination, unilaterally or bilaterally. Their varied anatomic location warrants multiple radiographic projections. A diagram depicting roentgen signs of navicular disease is shown in Figure 19–6.

Shape and Margination Changes (Remodeling). Osteophyte formation at sites of ligamentous attachment results in margination changes that may alter the overall shape of the bone; this is termed remodeling. Osteophytes are more correctly termed enthesiophytes and represent a pathologic process at ligament, tendon, or capsular insertions.[23, 30] Many individuals believe that osteophytes are manifestations of degenerative joint disease and thus indicate navicular disease.[4, 6, 12, 23, 31, 32] There is also the contention that osteophytes of the proximal and distal border are age-related and are not always clinically significant.[18, 20, 31] This fact may be true particularly in older, heavily worked animals with bilateral remodeling of mild degree.[15] Remodeling changes in younger horses should be considered significant, particularly if accompanied by lameness.

Osteophytes are best seen in angular dorsoproximal-palmarodistal views as spur formations on the extremities or as bone proliferations along the proximal and distal borders (sawtooth borders) (Fig. 19–7A). Remodeling on the distal border is more difficult to see because of obscured visualization by the partial overlap of the distal interphalangeal joint space. In the lateral view, excessive remodeling gives the bone an elongated appearance (Fig. 19–7B). Caution should be exercised as improperly positioned lateral views may artifactually distort the bone profile. Similarly, normal variants exist that resemble remodeling laterally when angular dorsoproximal-palmarodistal images are normal.[23] In the flexor view, the summated opacities of extensive osteophytes on the proximal and distal border may result in a seemingly sclerotic medullary cavity.[9]

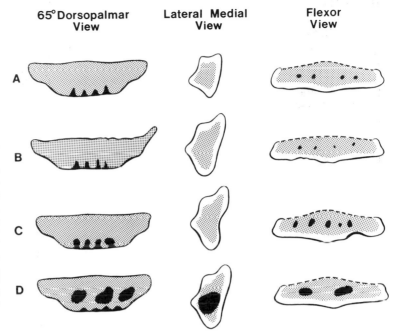

Figure 19–6. Radiographic changes seen in navicular disease: 65 degree dorsoproximal-palmarodistal view. A, normal; B, remodeling—spur on extremity and sawtooth proximal border; C, lollipop-shaped invaginations on distal border; D, cyst formation. Lateromedial view: A, normal; B, elongated navicular profile from remodeling (spur formation); C, flexor cortical erosion, D, cyst formation. Flexor tangential view: A, normal; B, flexor cortical erosions; C, enlarged fossae and flexor cortical erosions; D, cyst formation. (Modified with permission from Richard Park, Ft. Collins, CO.)

Medullary Changes of Osteopenia. Two separate manifestations of focal trabecular osteopenia may be seen. They are either abnormally shaped, radiolucent invaginations contiguous with the distal border or isolated medullary cyst-like structures.

It is generally accepted that the significance of the radiolucent invaginations of the distal navicular border seen on dorsoproximal-palmarodistal views are related to their shape and location and not to size and number.[2, 4] Increased size and number of fossae are physiologic changes related to type and frequency of work; they are considered abnormal when they change from a normal, inverted cone shape to a rounded lollipop configuration (Fig. 19–8).[4] Thus, with respect to the distal border, lollipops are bad and cones are good, regardless of number. In addition, the presence of a cone or any shape of osteopenic change that involves the extremities or proximal border is also abnormal.[4, 17]

Radiolucent changes of the distal border are not well appreciated laterally. The flexor view, however, projects them end on within the trabecular portion of the bone. Increases in size and number of visible fossae in this view are abnormal (Fig. 19–9).[9, 10] The range of normal variation of fossae appearance for this view, however, has not been established. In addition, the amount of image distortion due to variable beam angulation has not been quantitated. It is my opinion, therefore, that distal border radiolucent changes are more consistently evaluated

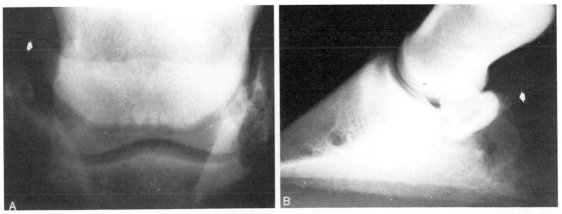

Figure 19–7. A, 65 degree dorsoproximal-palmarodistal view; B, lateral-medial view. Asymmetric mineralization of the suspensory navicular ligament resulted in a large spur on the navicular extremity (arrows).

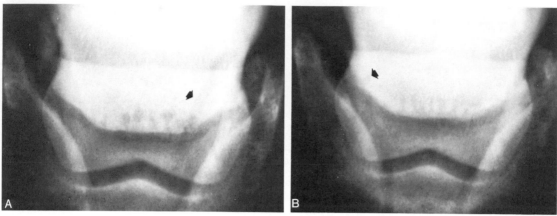

Figure 19–8. 65 degree dorsoproximal-palmarodistal views: *A,* classic lollipop-shaped fossae on the distal border and excessive spur formation on both extremities are seen. The radiolucent line superimposed over the navicular bone is the frog sulcus; this should not be mistaken for a fracture. *B,* early lollipop formation on the distal border and the extremity *(arrow)* indicates navicular disease. There is also mild spur formation on the extremities.

by using angular dorsoproximal-palmarodistal views, especially when there is only minimal enlargement.

The second medullary osteopenic change involves cyst-like radiolucencies located within the trabecular bone (Fig. 19–10). These radiolucencies can be seen on the angular dorsoproximal-palmarodistal, flexor, and occasionally lateral views. They range in size from 0.5 to 1.5 cm and are round to oval. They usually are single but may be multiple. Marginal sclerosis is variable, ranging from complete to none at all.

Lytic lesions located within the middle or distal phalanx may be superimposed over the navicular area. By evaluating other views or by repeating the dorsoproximal-palmarodistal view at a different angle, it is possible to see if the suspect lesion moves or remains associated with the navicular bone. Similarly, lucent artifacts that result from air trapped in the frog by packing material should not be misinterpreted. Air pockets usually present as linear radiolucent shadows. When in doubt, repacking the frog is helpful.

Extensive erosions of the flexor cortex are seen as osteopenic changes in angular dorsoproximal-palmarodistal views. On a flexor tangential view, the lesion can be localized to the flexor cortex.

Flexor Cortical Erosions and Rare Deep Digital Flexor Tendon Mineralization. Gross pathologic involvement of the navicular flexor fibrocartilage is varied. Lesions include yellowish discoloration, cartilage thinning, focal erosions, and cartilage ulcerations, with or without

Figure 19–9. Flexor tangential view demonstrates end-on appearance of the distal border fossae seen in Fig. 19–8*A (arrows).*

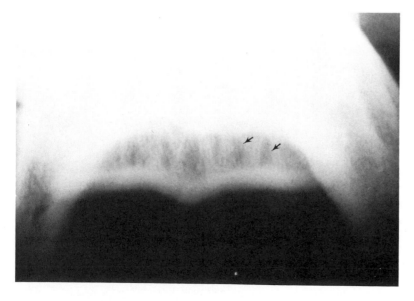

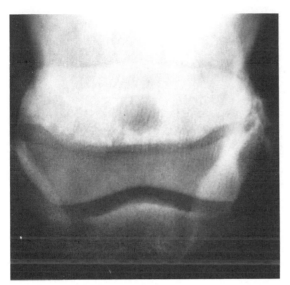

Figure 19–10. A large, round cyst-like radiolucency is seen within the medulla of the navicular bone.

subchondral bone involvement.[6, 20, 24] Some of the abnormalities may be age-related phenomena, but all have been seen in navicular disease to varying degrees.[18, 20]

Bursal, tendon, and cartilage changes are not usually seen radiographically; only subchondral bone defects are routinely detectable. Early lesions are best seen on the flexor tangential view, whereas severe defects may be recognized in other views as well. Abnormal roentgen signs consist of flattening of the central navicular ridge, cortical thinning with subchondral bone lysis (fuzzy margins of the cortex), and diffuse

to localized demineralization within the flexor compact bone (Fig. 19–11).[9] It is not unusual for large flexor cortical erosions to simulate medullary cysts in the dorsopalmar view. It is important to localize such cystic changes radiographically. Flexor cortical erosions are frequently associated with tendinous adhesions, whereas medullary cysts are not.[23, 24] This added information may be important in the overall management of the animal.

Well-positioned lateral radiographs depict the flexor cortex in profile axially. Minor dimpling of the navicular ridge in this view may be a normal variant or may be due to geometric distortion. Abrupt cavitations are abnormal. It is recommended that abnormalities of the flexor cortex observed on a lateral radiograph should be further evaluated by using the flexor tangential view.

Dystrophic mineralization of the deep digital flexor tendon may be seen in conjunction with flexor erosions. This finding is reported rarely and indicates severe tendon degeneration, rendering a poor prognosis.[23, 33] Faint visualization of the deep digital flexor tendon on the lateral view is a frequent finding normally. Diseased tendons that are sufficiently mineralized can be seen in both lateral and flexor views.

Normal Findings. Forty percent of horses with clinical navicular lameness had no radiographic abnormalities in either angular dorsoproximal-palmarodistal or the lateral view.[15] Because the flexor view was not used in this study, early lesions may have been missed, which if included would have lowered the final percentage. At any rate, it should be realized that a sizable number of horses with clinical navicular

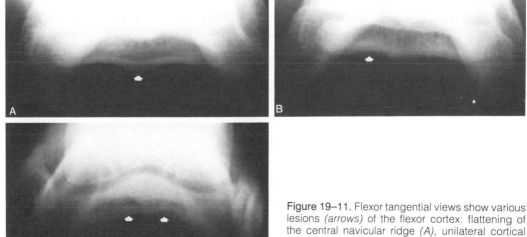

Figure 19–11. Flexor tangential views show various lesions *(arrows)* of the flexor cortex: flattening of the central navicular ridge *(A)*, unilateral cortical thinning (fuzzy margins) *(B)*, advanced subchondral bone lysis *(C)*.

lameness have normal radiographs. These animals may have disease that better falls into the category of navicular bursitis. Before arriving at this assessment, however, an adequate number of quality radiographs should be obtained. In addition, the radiographs must be viewed systematically in a quiet environment, with the use of a hot light if necessary.

FRACTURES

Navicular fractures are infrequently reported. Therefore, data are not available to draw firm conclusions about their incidence and pathophysiology. Most navicular fractures are pathologic, traumatic, or congenital in origin. Both chip and complete fracture types have been described. These lesions may be single or multiple and involve one or both forelimbs. Complete sagittal fractures have been termed multipartite sesamoids.[34] A diagram of navicular fractures is shown in Figure 19–12.

Care should be taken to avoid misinterpreting artifacts as navicular fractures. The sulci of the frog may cast overlying radiolucent shadows in the dorsoproximal-palmarodistal projection that simulate navicular fracture. This situation occurs when the foot is unpacked or when air is trapped within the sulcus by packing material. Sulcal lines typically extend above and below the navicular bone (Fig. 19–8A). Complete fractures are confined to the bone and are seen on dorsoproximal-palmarodistal and flexor views. Gravel or debris on the foot or a foot with scaly horn may simulate chip fractures. By proper hoof preparation (cleaning, paring, and packing) these artifacts can be eliminated. Lateral views or dorsoproximal-palmarodistal radiographs taken at different angles help to localize a

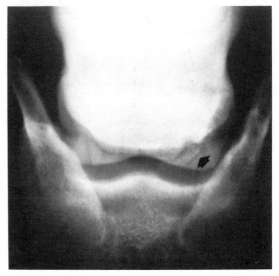

Figure 19–13. Chip fracture at the distal navicular border, the small fragment *(arrow),* and the underlying fracture "bed."

suspect opacity. When in doubt about navicular fractures, the hoof should be cleaned and repacked before more radiographs are obtained.

Chip Fractures

Small chip fractures may occur on the distal border of the navicular bone and are best seen on angular dorsoproximal-palmarodistal views when the distal border is projected proximal to the distal interphalangeal joint space. In one retrospective study, 3 percent of horses with navicular disease had roentgen signs compatible with chip fractures.[35] The lesions are seen as small, 0.2 to 1.2 cm, rectangular bone fragments separated from the distal border by a thin radiolucent zone. A fracture bed within the navicular bone corresponding in size and shape to the fragment is identified. This type of fracture has been classified as an avulsion fracture, but it is not considered a pathologic fracture.

Histopathologic characterization of chip fractures has not been available until recently. Preliminary data suggest that many chip fractures are not true fractures but rather represent dystrophic mineralization of the distal sesamoidean ligament. As such, they represent incompletely formed enthesiophytes.[23] Disarticulation of postmortem specimens reveals more of these fractures than was anticipated radiographically. Because of their small size, these "fragments" are masked by the overlying opacity of the second phalanx and distal interphalangeal joint. Whichever they represent, chip fractures do not appear to influence clinical signs or prognosis.[35] When seen, however, these lesions are

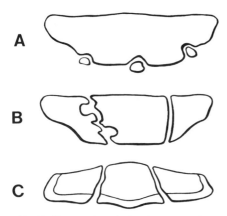

Figure 19–12. Types of navicular fractures: *A,* chip fractures of the distal navicular border, 65 degree dorsoproximal-palmarodistal projection. *B* and *C,* complete navicular fractures, 65 degree dorsoproximal-palmarodistal and flexor tangential projections, respectively.

usually associated with navicular disease (Fig. 19–13).

Complete Fractures

Complete navicular fractures can occur in normal or diseased navicular bones.[11, 36-40] Initiating causes include excess traction from flexor tendon adhesions, direct navicular trauma, sudden backward displacement of the second phalanx, and repeated concussive forces on a pathologic navicular bone in a neurectomized patient. Lameness associated with complete fractures may be acute or chronic and may be moderate to severe. In general, long-term prognosis for competitive performance is poor.[4] Postmortem studies of limited numbers of fractured navicular bones show fibrous unions between the fragments.[36] Variable instability is inherent because of the hinge-like motion allowed by the fibrous component.

Usually one or two vertical or oblique fracture lines can be seen within the body or the body-extremity junction of the navicular bone. A prominent fracture gap is usually present. Fracture fragments have irregular to smooth margins and are minimally displaced. Occasionally, fragment corners are rounded and sclerotic, as is seen in delayed union or non-union. Healing is usually not observed radiographically, regardless of fracture duration.

Bilaterally symmetric fractures are occasionally seen in minimally lame animals with otherwise normal navicular bones. This finding has fostered the belief that some multipartite sesamoids may represent multiple ossification centers that have not fused. Congenital multipartite sesamoids are occasional, incidental findings in other species. Although the navicular develops from a single ossification center, aberrant formation is theoretically possible.[1] The radiographic differentiation of potential congenital multipartite naviculars from previous traumatic or pathologic fracture is tenuous. In a recent report, the potential differences were discussed.[41] It is reported that vertically oriented radiolucent lines, especially at the body-extremity junction, suggest accessory ossification centers. Obliquely oriented radiolucent lines, particularly of the navicular body, suggest fracture. In addition, multiple ossification centers initially cause no to minimal lameness; if instability is present, however, degenerative changes resulting in lameness can occur. In either case, prognosis is guarded (Fig. 19–14).

In many cases, a fractured navicular is osteopenic or has changes compatible with advanced navicular disease. This circumstance is suggestive of the presence of a pathologic fracture of a primarily diseased bone. Another explanation

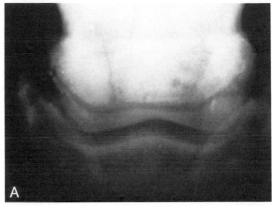

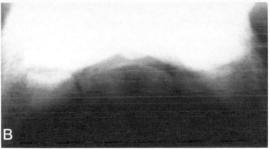

Figure 19–14. Complete navicular fractures resulting in a tripartite navicular bone. *A*, 65 degree dorsoproximal palmarodistal view; *B*, flexor tangential view.

is that fracture or multiple ossification centers are present initially. The resultant instability causes chronic secondary degenerative changes.[41] Thus, when multipartite sesamoids are seen in conjunction with degenerative navicular changes, it is not always possible to determine the sequence of events.

NAVICULAR SEPSIS

Navicular sepsis may result from penetrating puncture wounds or deep lacerations that involve the bursa or the bone itself.[42] Positive-contrast fistulograms may reveal bursal involvement in early stages. Roentgen signs depend upon the extent of the wound and the degree of bone involved. Signs include a variable amount of soft-tissue swelling and disruption, with or without soft-tissue emphysema. If osteomyelitis ensues, radiographic changes are those of an aggressive bone lesion. Flexor cortical erosions may occur and thus simulate navicular disease. Progression of osteomyelitis results in an irregular periosteal reaction in the navicular and adjacent bones. Variable amounts of sclerosis and osteoporosis alter the radiopacity of the bones chronically. Shape and size changes are associated with remodeling and pathologic fracture. Degenerative changes sim-

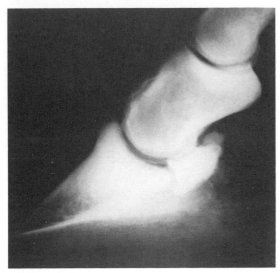

Figure 19–15. Lateral forefoot of a horse 3 years after treatment for septic navicular bursitis. Chronic proliferative and sclerotic changes involve the middle and distal phalanx as well as the navicular bone.

ilar to those seen in navicular disease have been observed as long-term sequelae in recovered patients (Fig. 19–15).

MISCELLANEOUS CONDITIONS

Congenital absence of the navicular bone (agenesis) has been reported.[43] Postmortem details were not mentioned; therefore true agenesis versus a defect in mineralization of the hyaline cartilage model cannot be resolved.

Another condition that affects the navicular bone is degenerative arthritis. The navicular bone participates in forming the distal interphalangeal joint. Reports of significant pathologic processes involving the articular cartilages in navicular disease are rare.[20, 44] It is believed, however, that changes seen in navicular disease are a form of distal interphalangeal joint arthrosis.[20, 21, 23]

References

1. Getty R: Sisson and Grossman's The Anatomy of the Domestic Animals. Philadelphia, WB Saunders, 1975, p. 317.
2. Colles CM, and Hickman J: The arterial supply of the navicular bone and its variations in navicular disease. Equine Vet J 9:150, 1977.
3. Poules P: Radiography and microangiography as a research tool. Sixth International Veterinary Radiology Conference, Davis, CA, Aug 1982.
4. Reid CF: Radiography and the purchase examination in the horse. Vet Clin North Am [Large Anim Pract] 2:173, 1980.
5. Ueltschi G: Value of technetium-99M pyrophosphate bone imaging in equine orthopedics. J Nucl Med 18:1253, 1977.
6. Oxspring GE: The radiology of navicular disease with observations on its pathology. Vet Rec 15:1434, 1985.
7. Campbell JR, and Lee R: Radiological techniques in the diagnosis of navicular disease. Equine Vet J 4:135, 1972.
8. Reid CF: Equine extremity radiography in positioning and exposure guide for veterinary radiography. Wilmington, DE, DuPont X-ray Systems.
9. O'Brien TR, Millman TM, Pool RR, et al: Navicular disease in the Thoroughbred horse: A morphologic investigation relative to a new radiographic projection. J Am Vet Radiol Soc 16:39, 1975.
10. Rose RJ, Taylor BJ, and Steel JD: Navicular disease in the horse: An analysis of seventy cases and assessment of a special radiographic view. J Equine Med Surg 2:492, 1978.
11. Johnson JH: The Foot. In Mansman RA, and McAllister ES(Eds): Equine Medicine and Surgery. Santa Barbara, CA, American Veterinary Publications, 1982, p. 1048.
12. Adams OR: Lameness in Horses. Philadelphia, Lea & Febiger, 1974, pp. 260–270.
13. Rose RJ: The treatment of navicular disease—a review and current concepts. The 29th Annual Convention of the American Association of Equine Practitioners. Las Vegas, NV, December 1983.
14. Valdez H, Adams OR, and Peyton LC: Navicular disease in the hindlimbs of the horse. J Am Vet Med Assoc 172:291, 1978.
15. Ackerman N, Johnson JH, and Dorn CR: Navicular disease in the horse: Risk factors, radiographic changes, and response to therapy. J Am Vet Med Assoc 170:183, 1977.
16. Loew JE: Sex, breed and age incidence of navicular disease. In Proceedings of the 20th Annual Convention of the American Association of Equine Practitioners, Las Vegas, NV, 1974, pp. 37–46.
17. Colles C: Navicular disease and its treatment. In Pract 4:29, 1982.
18. Colles CM: Ischaemic necrosis of the navicular bone and its treatment. Vet Rec 104:133, 1979.
19. Fricker CH, Riek W, and Hugelshofer J: Occlusion of the digital arteries—a model for pathogenesis of navicular disease. Equine Vet J 14:203, 1982.
20. Doige CE, and Hoffer MA: Pathologic changes in the navicular bone and associated structures of the horse. Can J Comp Med 47:387, 1983.
21. Svalastoga E: Navicular disease in the horse—a microangiographic investigation. Nord Vet Med 35:131, 1983.
22. Ostblom L, Lund C, and Melsen F: Histologic study of navicular bone disease. Equine Vet J 14:199, 1982.
23. Poulos PW: Correlation of radiographic signs and histological changes in navicular disease. The 29th Annual Convention of the American Association of Equine Practitioners. Las Vegas, NV, December 1983.
24. Svalastoga E, Reimann I, and Nielsen K: Changes of the fibrocartilage in navicular disease in horses. Nord Vet Med 35:373, 1983.
25. Svalastoga E, and Neilsen K: Navicular disease in the horse—the synovial membrane of bursa podotrachlearis. Nord Vet Med 35:28, 1983.
26. Svalastoga E, and Smith M: Navicular disease in the horse—the subchondral bone pressure. Nord Vet Med 35:31, 1983.
27. Colles CM: Concepts of blood flow in the aetiology and treatment of navicular disease. The 29th Annual Convention of the American Association of Equine Practitioners. Las Vegas, NV, December 1983.
28. Rooney JR: Biomechanics of lameness in horses. Baltimore, Williams & Wilkins, 1969, pp. 180–185.
29. Huskamp B, and Becker M: Diagnose und prognose der rontgenologischen Veranderungen an den Strahl-

beinen der Vordergliedma Ben der Pferde unter besonderer Berucksichtigung der Ankau fsuntersuchung. Ein Versuch zur Schematisierung der Befunde. Praktische Tierarzt *61*:858, 1980.

30. Resnick D, and Niwayama G: Entheses and enthesopathy. Radiology *146*:1985.
31. Morgan JP: Radiology in Veterinary Orthopedics. Philadelphia, Lea & Febiger, 1972, pp. 364–370.
32. Turner TA: The anatomic, pathologic, and radiographic aspects of navicular disease. Comp Contin Ed Pract Vet *4*:350, 1982.
33. Turner TA: Dystrophic calcification of the deep digital flexor tendons resulting from navicular disease. Vet Med/Small Anim Clin *77*:571, 1982.
34. Feeney DA, Booth LC, and Johnston GR: What's your diagnosis? J Am Vet Med Assoc *177*:644, 1980.
35. van De Watering CC, and Morgan JP: Chip fractures as a radiologic finding in navicular disease of the horse. J Am Vet Radiol Soc *16*:206, 1975.
36. Vaughan LC: Fracture of the navicular bone in the horse. Vet Rec *73*:895, 1961.
37. Morgan JP: Radiology in Veterinary Orthopedics. Philadelphia, Lea & Febiger, 1972, pp. 26–27.
38. Adams OR: Lameness in Horses. Philadelphia, Lea & Febiger, 1974, pp. 275–276.
39. Smythe RH: Fracture of the navicular bone in the horse—comment. Vet Rec *73*:1009, 1961.
40. Fessler JF, and Amstutz HE: Fracture repair. *In* Oehme FW (Ed.): Large Animal Surgery. Baltimore, Williams & Wilkins, 1974, p. 296.
41. Reid CF: Multipartite sesamoids in the horse. J Am Vet Med Assoc. In press.
42. Adams OR: Lameness in Horses. Philadelphia, Lea & Febiger, 1974, pp. 281–283.
43. Reid CF: Radiology panel—film interpretation session notes. The 22nd Annual Convention of the American Association of Equine Practitioners, Dallas, TX, 1976, p. 7.
44. Klessinger G: Messungen an Rontgen bilderm des Hufgelenkes und des Strahlbeines als Beitrag zur Podotrochlose des Pferdes. Inaugural Dissertation, Freie Universitat, Berlin. 1973.

SECTION 6

NECK AND THORAX— COMPANION ANIMALS

CHAPTER 20

THE LARYNX, PHARYNX, AND TRACHEA

S. K. KNELLER

LARYNX AND PHARYNX

Anatomic Considerations

Because the major function of the upper airway is to enable passage of air to the lungs, the soft-tissue structures of the pharynx and larynx are contrasted against the gas opacity of the air, providing radiographic identification. Although not outlined by air, the hyoid bones are mineral opacities in contrast to the soft-tissue surroundings. The pharynx is bordered by the base of the tongue and the retropharyngeal wall, divided into oropharynx and nasopharynx by the soft palate, which extends to the level of the epiglottis. On high-quality radiographs, most of the laryngeal structures can be identified (Fig. 20–1).[1] These structures are readily visualized on lateral radiographs but are difficult to interpret on ventrodorsal views because of the overlying bone structure of the head and neck. In lateral radiographs, the transverse basihyoid bone is usually striking because it is projected on end and may be mistaken for a foreign object.

Radiographs of brachycephalic dogs, as well as those of obese animals, are more difficult to interpret because the airway is confined by soft tissue and fat (Fig. 20–2). This results in a lower air-tissue ratio, providing less contrast as well as producing more irregular opacities overlying the structures in question.

In very young animals (2 to 3 months), laryngeal structures may not be well defined for accurate identification. Mineralization in the cartilaginous structures, including the epiglottis, is recognized as an aging change. Mineralization may be seen as early as 2 to 3 years and is expected earlier in large dogs and chondrodystrophic breeds. In one study, 96 of 99 clinically normal dogs of random breeds and random age greater than 1 year had radiographic laryngeal mineralization.[2] The cricoid cartilage is usually the first to become mineralized.

The larynx is usually ventral to the first two cervical vertebrae in a standard lateral view with the head in a normal position. It is usually just slightly farther from the vertebrae than the main portion of the trachea. If the radiograph is made with the head extended, the larynx will be drawn slightly craniad and closer to the spine, the hyoid bones tend to be at a lesser angle with one another, and the ventrodorsal diameter of the pharynx may be compressed. If the radiograph is made with the head in a flexed position, the larynx may sit as far caudad as the fourth cervical vertebra. In this position, air flow is compromised, decreasing the air:tissue ratio. This makes structures more difficult to visualize, and overlying skin folds are more likely.

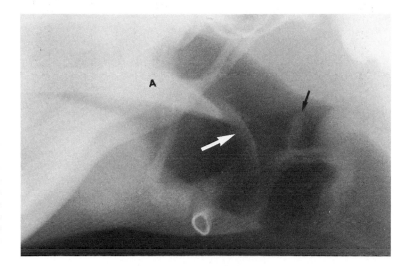

Figure 20–1. A normal lateral laryngeal radiograph of a 6-month-old mixed-breed dog. The soft palate *(A)* separates the nasopharynx from the oropharynx. The epiglottis *(large arrow)* is seen extending from the larynx to the tip of the soft palate. The cranial cornua of the thyroid cartilage *(small arrow)* should not be mistaken for a foreign object.

Depending on the phase and depth of respiration during radiography, the tip of the epiglottis may be just dorsal or ventral to the soft palate, or it may be on the ventral floor of the pharynx. This can be seen in normal animals; however, in the presence of swallowing disorders, radiography and fluoroscopy should be performed during swallowing to determine if the epiglottis moves normally as part of the swallowing reflex.

The *hyoid bones* are relatively well defined and easy to identify in the dog and cat. The key to diagnostic accuracy is simply a familiarity with the normal appearance. These bones have been mistakenly diagnosed as foreign objects. The configuration and relative position of the hyoid bones are rather uniform among small animals; however, the position of the head, tongue, and larynx during radiography will cause variation in angles between hyoid bones. Oblique views may cause significant distortion, leading to erroneous diagnosis. Few radiographic abnormalities are evident in the hyoid bones. The most common changes are fractures or dislocation.

Radiographic Signs of Disease

Changes in Size and Shape. As mentioned previously, the size and shape of the pharynx and larynx vary with breed and degree of obesity. Generalized swelling can be appreciated if it is severe.[3] However, this can be erroneously diagnosed in smaller, heavy-bodied, and obese animals. A severely elongated soft palate can be seen radiographically, although direct visual inspection is a more accurate method of evaluation. Radiography can be an aid in assessing

Figure 20–2. A normal lateral laryngeal radiograph of an obese 13-year-old German shepherd dog. Notice that nonmineralized structures are more difficult to define owing to compromise of the air space.

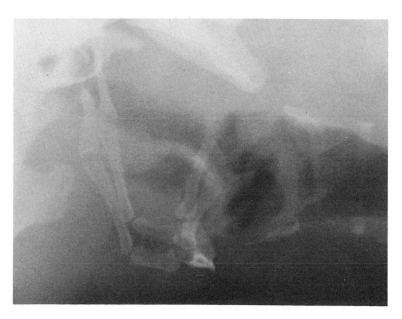

the degree of airway compromise in brachycephalic breeds before proceeding with corrective surgery of external structures. Although specific airway diameter cannot be assessed, relative size of the soft palate, epiglottis, and larynx can be evaluated.

Space-Occupying Lesions Within the Airway. Mass lesions, such as abscesses, neoplasms, and granulation tissue, can be appreciated readily with appropriate radiographic technique, accurate positioning, and knowledge of normal anatomy. When quite small, these lesions appear as variants in the normal shape of structures, and, when large, may obliterate the air-filled cavities. Such mass lesions may be found at any location from the rostral extent (Fig. 20–3) to and including the larynx. Variation in exposure technique may be necessary to demonstrate such lesions owing to the variation in overlying tissue opacity between portions of the skull and cervical region. Depending on the shape, physical density, and architecture, foreign objects lodged in the airway may be identified specifically or may appear as space-occupying tissue masses.

Space-Occupying Masses Outside the Airway. Space-occupying masses outside the airway are more difficult to identify because they are not surrounded by gas. These lesions are identified by recognizing displacement or encroachment of the air-tissue interfaces. Although masses may develop at any site, enlargement of specific structures such as lymph node and thyroid gland should be considered when determining the cause for such radiographic changes.

Functional Abnormalities. Functional abnormalities of the larynx are best evaluated by direct visual inspection. Neurogenic disorders yield mild or equivocal radiographic signs.[4]

Consistent misplacement of the epiglottis seen on radiographs should prompt visual examination. In the panting dog, the epiglottis lies on the ventral floor of the pharynx.[2] Otherwise, it is in a semi-erect position, usually with the tip just dorsal or ventral to the soft palate.

TRACHEA

Anatomic Considerations

The trachea is best visualized on the lateral view; however, the ventrodorsal view is useful to evaluate displacement of the trachea as well as displacement and compression of the stem bronchi. The trachea is a midline structure that may deviate slightly to the right in the cranial mediastinum. This deviation is more exaggerated in short-bodied breeds such as the Boston terrier and should not be mistaken for disease. On the lateral view, the trachea is nearly parallel to the cervical spine but is slightly closer to the spine in the caudal cervical region than it is cranially. Because the thoracic vertebrae angle dorsally, there is slight divergence of the trachea from the thoracic spine. The terminal trachea angles slightly ventral at the point of bifurcation into the stem bronchi. The diameter of the trachea is relatively uniform, slightly smaller than the larynx. In normal animals, the trachea does not vary significantly between phases of respiration and remains uniform in diameter from end to end. Extreme extension of the neck can cause compression and narrowing of the trachea at the thoracic inlet. Because displacement of the trachea is a sign of cervical and intrathoracic mass lesions, artifactual tracheal displacement, a common problem, must be avoided.

The trachea is a semi-rigid tube attached at

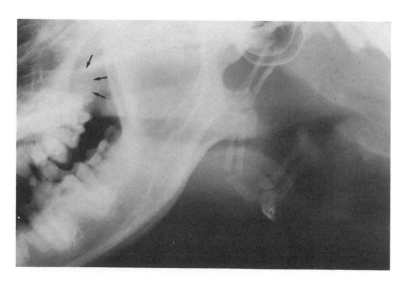

Figure 20–3. A lateral skull radiograph of a 7-year-old Labrador retriever presenting with dyspnea. A neoplastic mass 1 cm in diameter *(arrows)* was found radiographically and confirmed by endoscopy and at surgery. Lesions in this area can be easily overlooked or masked on underexposed radiographs. Notice that on this radiograph, the epiglottis is positioned in the ventral pharynx (base of tongue).

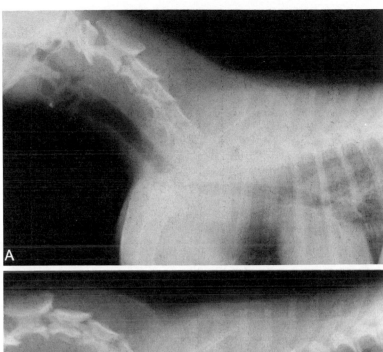

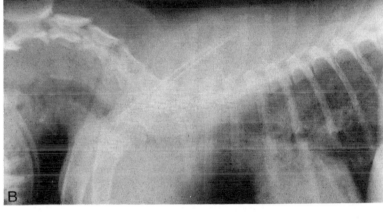

Figure 20–4. *A*, A lateral radiograph of a dog with the head and neck correctly positioned. *B*, A lateral radiograph of the same dog with the neck flexed. Notice the variation in tracheal shape compared with the well positioned view. This normal variation can become quite dramatic, leading to misdiagnosis of mass lesions. Notice also, on the flexed view, that the laryngeal region is difficult to interpret.

the larynx and the carina. It is confined in the cervical region but rather free to move in the cranial mediastinum. During radiography in the lateral view, the head and neck should be placed in an erect, but not overextended, position. If the nose is brought toward the sternum, the trachea is likely to bend in the cranial mediastinum, simulating displacement by a cranial mediastinal mass (Fig. 20–4). Mineralization of the tracheal rings may be seen as an aging process, especially in large and chondrodystrophic dogs, but is also seen in younger dogs, apparently with no significance. Diseases that stimulate metastatic mineralization may stimulate increased mineralization of the trachea along with other soft tissues.

Radiographic Signs of Disease

As mentioned earlier, displacement of the trachea is a reliable sign of mass lesions in the surrounding soft tissue if positioning artifacts and breed variation are accounted for. A common tracheal displacement is ventral displacement of the larynx and proximal trachea due to thyroid gland enlargement. Lymph node enlargement can be identified by tracheal deviation adjacent to the known location of lymph nodes. Abscesses and neoplastic masses can occur at any site. In the cervical region, mass lesions must be relatively large to cause tracheal displacement. Unless massive in size, mass lesions that compress the trachea must intimately involve the trachea. Except for tracheobronchial and cranial mediastinal lymph node involvement and gross heart enlargement, compressive masses usually involve tracheal tissue. Neoplasia and intratracheal abscesses or granulomas are the most common causes; however, compressive tracheal lesions are relatively uncommon. Localized tracheal lumen narrowing may occur without mass lesions, as the result of traumatic or congenital tracheal ring abnormalities. Mass lesions may infrequently occur within the tracheal lumen because of abscesses, neoplasia, granulomas, or foreign objects.

Overall tracheal diameter varies slightly from breed to breed; however, this variation is minimal relative to the size of the animal. English bulldogs are known to have a smaller tracheal diameter than other breeds; however, members of this breed also are more likely to have a pathologically small trachea as a congenital defect.[5] Mensuration of the trachea indicates the ratio of tracheal diameter to thoracic inlet diameter and is more reliable than comparison of tracheal diameter with the larynx.[6] In non-brachycephalic dogs, the mean ratio of tracheal diameter to thoracic inlet diameter was 0.204 ± 0.031, compared with 0.160 ± 0.034 in non-bulldog brachycephalic breeds and 0.127 ± 0.38 in bulldogs. The range in bulldogs was 0.070 to 0.206. The smallest ratio in bulldogs with no clinical signs of respiratory disease was 0.093. The ratio for dogs less than 1 year of age was slightly smaller than for older dogs. Accurate lateral positioning is necessary for accurate measurements.

Although the common infectious diseases rarely result in appreciable thickening of the tracheal wall or narrowing of the lumen, acute dyspnea may occur as the result of inflammatory tracheal disease, with significant decrease in diameter of the tracheal lumen. If the esophagus contains large or small amounts of gas, the esophageal wall may cause a silhouette sign with the dorsal tracheal wall, presenting an erroneous appearance of tracheal thickening (Fig. 20–5).

Most tracheal problems are dynamic in nature, resulting in variation in tracheal size in a region related to phase of the respiratory cycle. This is most often seen in the toy dog breeds because of weakness in the structural rigidity of the trachea. The resultant syndrome is commonly known as tracheal collapse, which because of its dynamic nature requires special attention for radiographic documentation.

Dynamic narrowing of the tracheal lumen due to tracheal instability may occur in the cervical trachea (especially at the thoracic inlet) during inspiration (Fig. 20–6) or in the thoracic trachea (especially at the carina) during expiration (Fig. 20–7), or during both. With severe loss of rigidity, the site of collapse may not match with the phase of respiration. At times, the area that collapses may actually balloon during the opposite respiratory phase if the

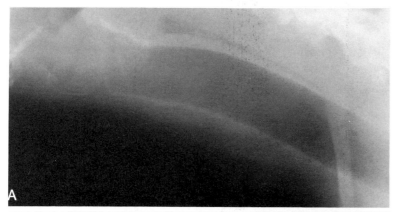

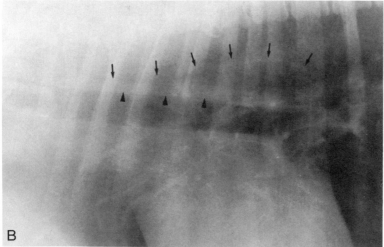

Figure 20–5. *A,* A lateral radiograph of a 9-month-old retriever. Because of the gas in the proximal esophagus, the ventral esophageal wall and the dorsal tracheal wall silhouette into one soft-tissue opacity that may be erroneously interpreted as thickening of the tracheal wall. *B,* A lateral thoracic radiograph of an 11-year-old West Highland white terrier. A barely discernible amount of gas is present in the thoracic esophagus *(arrows).* Because of this, the ventral esophageal wall is, again, silhouetted against the dorsal tracheal wall *(arrowheads).* Gas is found quite often in this location.

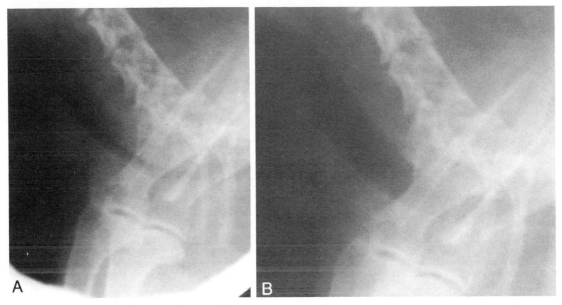

Figure 20–6. Inspiration *(A)* and expiration *(B)* radiographs of a 15-year-old poodle were made during fluoroscopy with a 105-mm spot-film camera. The cervical trachea is severely narrowed on inspiration and is larger than the thoracic trachea on expiration. This indicates that the weak trachealis muscle is being pulled into the lumen by negative pressure during inspiration, compromising air flow, and is being forced outward by positive pressure during expiration.

trachealis muscle is elongated and has very little tone. Abnormal enlargement of a portion of trachea on inspiration should lead to suspicion of obstruction of airflow cranially. This may be from disease in the trachea or larynx. It is

mentioned as a secondary radiographic sign of laryngeal paralysis.[4] Confusion may occur when tracheal rings or partial air column can be identified dorsal to the upper margin of the tracheal air column. Although some feel this is

Figure 20–7. Inspiratory *(A)* and expiratory *(B)* radiographs of an 11-year-old poodle. The entire thoracic trachea collapses nearly completely during expiration in this case. In many cases, only the caudal trachea collapses, with a characteristic end-expiratory "click" heard on auscultation.

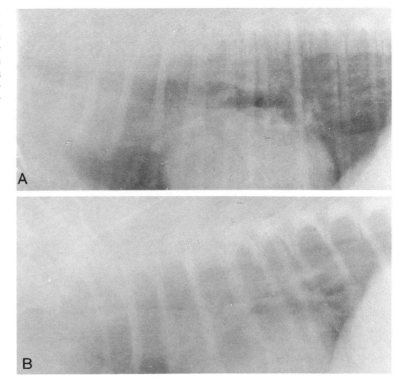

due to overlying structures, tracheography (by injecting contrast medium into the trachea) has proved narrowing of the tracheal lumen in some instances.[7] An explanation of this pattern is redundancy of the trachealis muscle folding into the dorsal trachea, narrowing the actual air space. During fluoroscopy, the soft-tissue trachealis muscle will sometimes move in and out of the lumen during respiration. The radiographic pattern can be seen in large dogs with no evidence of respiratory distress, making muscle laxity difficult to blame for the radiographic phenomenon in all dogs. Because the dorsal aspect of the trachea may normally be flattened, a similar pattern may be seen if the trachea is rotated. To fully evaluate dynamic tracheal disease, lateral radiographs should be made during both inspiration and expiration. Often, suspected abnormalities can be detected in this manner. Abnormalities in the thoracic trachea are exaggerated during coughing. At times, fluoroscopy is necessary to demonstrate the dynamic signs.

References

1. O'Brien JH, Harvey CE, Tucker JA: The larynx of the dog: its normal radiographic anatomy. J Am Vet Radiol Soc 10:38, 1969.
2. Gaskell CJ: The radiographic anatomy of the pharynx and larynx of the dog. J Small Anim Pract 14:89, 1974.
3. Carlson WD: Veterinary Radiology, 2nd ed. Philadelphia, Lea & Febiger, 1967, p. 176.
4. Reinke JD, Suter PF: Laryngeal paralysis in a dog. J Am Vet Med Assoc 172:714, 1978.
5. Suter PF, Colgrove DJ, Ewing GO: Congenital hypoplasia of the canine trachea. J Am Anim Hosp Assoc 8:120, 1972.
6. Harvey CE, Fink EA: Tracheal diameter: Analysis of radiographic measurements in brachycephalic and nonbrachycephalic dogs. J Am Anim Hosp Assoc 18:570, 1982.
7. Thrall DE: Carlson's Veterinary Radiology, 3rd ed. Philadelphia, Lea & Febiger, 1977, p. 239.

CHAPTER 21

THE ESOPHAGUS

BARBARA J. WATROUS

Disorders of the upper (pregastric) alimentary tract result in a variety of clinical signs. As a direct result of dysphagia, these signs include regurgitation, difficult swallowing, abnormal swallowing mannerisms, and gagging or retching when eating or drinking.[3] Other signs include weight loss, failure to gain or grow normally, systemic neuromuscular disorders, and chronic or recurrent respiratory problems. Aspiration pneumonia, tracheitis, and nasal discharge are frequent manifestations that overshadow the inciting cause. In several systemic neuromuscular diseases, the oropharynx, esophagus, or both may be involved because of the effect of these disorders on skeletal muscle. Indications for evaluation of the upper alimentary tract therefore include dysphagia, regurgitation, and recurrent unexplained respiratory tract infections.

Survey radiographs may provide information that can lead to a definitive diagnosis, such as the presence of radiopaque foreign bodies or mass lesions. The survey examination should include views of the cervical and thoracic areas for the entire esophagus, including the caudal pharynx and cranial esophageal sphincter, and a short segment of the cranial abdomen for the terminal esophagus and caudal esophageal sphincter. Views of the skull may be required when oropharyngeal dysphagia is suspected.

Contrast radiography is often necessary to identify lesions or to characterize further survey radiographic findings. Differentiation of functional from morphologic causes of dysphagia might be made by static contrast studies; however, specific evaluation of the functional abnormalities may be made only in dynamic studies, such as videofluorography or cinefluorography. The purpose of this chapter is to provide a gamut of distinguishing characteristics provided by static survey and contrast radiographic findings as a guide for the diagnosis of upper alimentary tract diseases.

SURVEY RADIOGRAPHIC FINDINGS

The normal esophagus is a collapsed tube bounded cranially and caudally by functional sphincters. On survey radiographs (Table 21–1), the soft tissue of the cervical esophagus is silhouetted with the surrounding vertebral hypaxial muscles and associated deep fascia of the neck. The thoracic esophagus is enveloped by the dorsal mediastinum, continuation of the deep cervical fascia, and associated loose connective tissue, and is silhouetted with these soft-tissue structures. The normal radiographic appearance of the esophagus, therefore, is the absence of a definable structure.[2]

The absence of abnormal esophageal radiographic findings does not preclude the presence

217

TABLE 21–1. **SURVEY RADIOGRAPHIC FINDINGS**

	Esophageal Status	Etiologies
Negative	Normal	—
	Abnormal	Neuromuscular disease
		Hiatal hernia
		Foreign body (nonradiopaque)
		Esophagitis
		Early strictures
		Fistulae
Radiolucency		
Regional intraluminal	Normal	Aerophagia
	Abnormal	Foreign bodies (nonradiopaque)
		Gastroesophageal intussusception
		Extraluminal masses
		Esophagitis
		Strictures
		Vascular ring anomalies
		Neoplasia
		Segmental hypomotility
Generalized intraluminal	Normal	General anesthesia
		CNS depression
	Abnormal	Megaesophagus
		Neuromuscular hypomotility
		Hypoadrenocorticism
		Autoimmune myositis
		Autoimmune neuritis
		Myasthenia gravis
		Toxicities
		Neoplasia
		Hypothyroidism
		Trauma
Periesophageal	Normal	Subcutaneous emphysema
	Abnormal	Perforation
Radiopacity		
Regional intraluminal	Abnormal	Vascular ring anomalies
		Foreign bodies (radiopaque)
		Spirocerca lupi
		Neoplasia
		Gastroesophageal intussusception
		Diverticulae
		Periesophageal masses
Generalized intraluminal	Abnormal	Megaesophagus

of esophageal disease; such is often encountered with acute esophageal disease. In addition, the presence of indirect signs of esophageal disease should be anticipated. Focal or generalized esophageal dilatation may be less apparent when the lumen is fluid-filled, creating a positive silhouette sign. The enlarged lumen, however, will affect adjacent visible structures. The weight of the dilated organ causes ventral and right lateral tracheal displacement in the cervical and cranial thoracic regions. The cranial and caudal mediastinum widens around the dilated structure. Pulmonary interstitial or alveolar infiltrates occur secondary to aspiration. Pleural effusion, pneumothorax or pneumomediastinum, and lobar consolidation are occasionally present secondary to esophageal disease.

The presence of opacity change allows for direct visualization of the normal and abnormal esophagus. Decreased radiopacity, both peri-esophageal and intraluminal, makes the esophagus visible radiographically. Pneumomediastinum or deep cervical subcutaneous gas outlines its adventitial surface (Fig. 21–1). Gas may originate from deep skin wounds, tracheal and esophageal rupture, and pulmonary leakage. Perforation of the esophagus may occur from trauma or inflammation; foreign bodies and esophageal surgical procedures are the most common causes. The radiographic sign of an acute perforation is air in the periesophageal tissues of the cervical region or pneumomediastinum. Long-standing perforation of the cervical esophagus leads to cellulitis and abscess formation with persistence of air or periesophageal mass formation. Mediastinitis and pleuritis result from a chronically perforated thoracic esophagus.

Accumulation of intraluminal gas usually indicates esophageal disease. Occasionally, how-

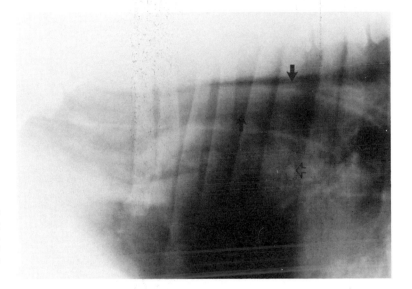

Figure 21–1. Lateral view of the dorsocranial thorax of a mature dog. Esophageal perforation by a sharp foreign body (bone) has resulted in pneumomediastinum. The outer margins of the esophagus superimposed on the tracheal lumen can be seen next to the brachiocephalic artery (*solid arrows*). A small bone fragment is visible *(open arrow)* and was present in the mediastinum. (Courtesy of New York State College of Veterinary Medicine, Ithaca, NY.)

ever, small amounts of air are seen in the normal esophagus owing to insignificant aerophagia. Common sites for this incidental occurrence on lateral radiographic views include the area immediately caudal to the cranial esophageal sphincter (Fig. 21–2), at the level of the thoracic inlet and dorsal to the heart base. Repeated views should indicate that this focal air accumulation is transient. In the dorsoventral or ventrodorsal view, this gas is often hidden because of the superimposition of the spine, sternum, and other mediastinal structures.

Abnormal luminal gas accumulation occurs in most esophageal diseases. Generalized megaesophagus with a gas-filled lumen may be visualized along all or part of its length on survey radiographs. On the lateral view, the cervical portion is apparent beginning just caudal to the cranial esophageal sphincter. When mildly dilated, the esophagus is visible dorsal to the proximal trachea, crossing somewhat lateral to the trachea at the thoracic inlet. As it dilates further, it drapes around the trachea and depresses it ventrally (Fig. 21–3). If the esophagus is fluid-filled, the lumen may not be visible because of silhouetting of the soft tissue and fluid (Fig. 21–4A). The thoracic esophagus, when gas-filled, may be inadvertently overlooked because of the relative radiolucency of the adjacent lung field. Close scrutiny, however, provides several hallmark findings characteristic of its presence. When the cranial

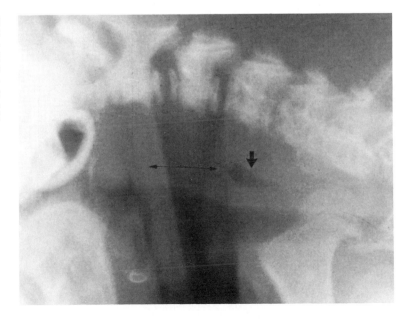

Figure 21–2. Lateral view of the neck of a normal 6-week-old puppy that struggled during radiographic examination. Air trapped in the cranial esophagus *(arrow)* just behind the cranial esophageal-sphincter *(double-headed arrow)* is commonly seen under these circumstances. (Courtesy of New York State College of Veterinary Medicine, Ithaca, NY.)

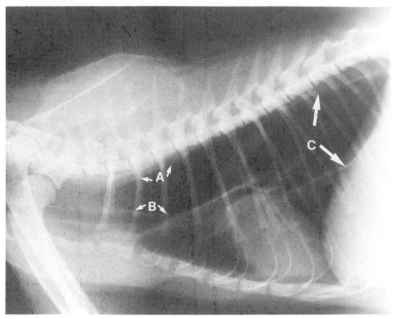

Figure 21–3. Lateral view of an aged cat with chronic upper airway obstruction secondary to a pharyngeal polyp. The entire air-filled dilated esophagus can be seen. Hallmarks of esophageal dilatation include the sharp interface between the longus colli muscles and esophageal lumen (A), the "tracheal band" sign with displacement of the trachea ventrally (B), and the paired converging soft-tissue stripes in the dorsocaudal thorax (C). (Courtesy of New York State College of Veterinary Medicine, Ithaca, NY.)

thoracic esophagus dilates, the dorsal wall abuts against the paired longus colli muscles, which can be seen as a sharp interface from the thoracic inlet to the ventral aspect of the fifth or sixth thoracic vertebra. The ventral wall projects lateral and often ventral to the trachea. The draping of the ventral wall over the dorsal tracheal wall results in summation (silhouetting) of the two walls, which creates the "tracheal band" or "tracheal stripe" sign. The caudal thoracic esophagus is seen as a pair of thin, soft-tissue stripes that converge to a point overlying the diaphragm and cranial abdomen. Absence of the ventral stripe may be due to overlap by the shadow of the caudal vena cava (Fig. 21–3).

On the dorsoventral or ventrodorsal view,

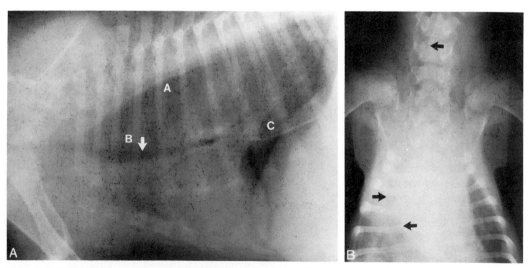

Figure 21–4. A, lateral view of a young dog with megaesophagus. The esophageal lumen is not visible in the cervical region owing to its fluid content. Some hallmark signs (see legend to Fig. 21–3) are apparent in the thoracic region. B, deviation of the cervical and thoracic portions of the trachea by the fluid-filled cranial esophagus (arrows) can be seen. (Courtesy of New York State College of Veterinary Medicine, Ithaca, NY.)

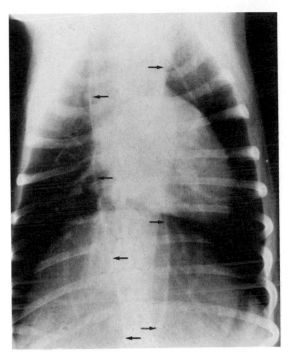

Figure 21–5. Dorsoventral view of an adult dog with megaesophagus. The lateral walls of the esophagus are seen as thin, soft-tissue bands roughly parallel to the spine *(arrows)*. They converge in the caudal thorax. (Courtesy of New York State College of Veterinary Medicine, Ithaca, NY.)

the dilated, gas-filled cervical esophagus may be hidden by the overlapping spine and radiolucent lumen of the trachea, although displacement of the trachea to the right may be seen (Fig. 21–4B). The dilated cranial thoracic esophagus produces a wide cranial mediastinum that is relatively radiolucent. The lateral margins are indented on the left and right by the descending aorta and azygous vein, respectively. The caudal thoracic esophagus converges to a "V" at the hiatus of the diaphragm (Fig. 21–5).

Abnormal regional gas accumulation may occur anywhere along the esophagus just cranial to or at the site of localized disease. Gas trapping occurs at the site of acute entrapment of intraluminal foreign bodies, esophagitis, and segmental esophageal hypomotility. Obstruction of the esophageal lumen by vascular ring anomalies (Fig. 21–6), acquired strictures, extraluminal (Fig. 21–7) and intrinsic masses, and chronic foreign bodies may or may not result in air accumulation.

Increased radiopacity associated with esophageal disease may be general or focal. Generalized radiopacity occurs when liquid, food, or foreign material accumulates in the dilated lumen in cases of megaesophagus (Fig. 21–4). The radiopacity is usually heterogeneous because of the entrapment of small gas bubbles in solid or semisolid food. Regional radiopacity may be a result of lodged radiopaque foreign bodies (Fig. 21–8), localized dilatation due to vascular ring anomalies (Fig. 21–9), diverticulae or gastroesophageal intussusceptions (Fig. 21–10) and subsequent food or foreign material accumulation (Fig. 21–9), focal soft-tissue infiltration of the esophageal wall (Fig. 21–11), or dystrophic mineralization (Fig. 21–12). The common locations of various esophageal lesions are listed in Table 21–2.

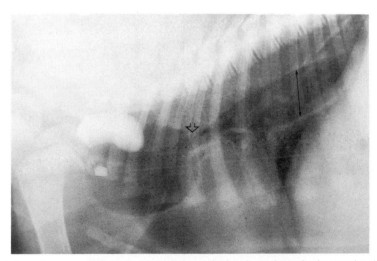

Figure 21–6. Lateral view of a young dog with a persistent right fourth aortic arch. A vascular ring anomaly entraps the midthoracic esophagus, causing dilatation of the lumen cranial to the obstruction. The characteristic site of obstruction is just cranial to the level of the tracheal bifurcation *(open arrow)*. Evaluation for possible esophageal dilatation caudal to the ring, as was present in this animal *(double-headed arrow)*, must be made. The radiopacities are foreign bodies (stones) within the prestenotic dilated lumen. Thoracic tracheal depression is evident. Rare causes for other vascular ring anomalies include double aortic arches, aberrant right subclavian artery, and dextra-aorta with left subclavian artery. (Courtesy of New York State College of Veterinary Medicine, Ithaca, NY.)

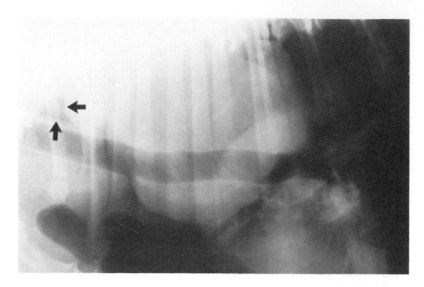

Figure 21–7. Lateral view of a dog with signs of regurgitation. A thoracic tumor encroached upon the esophagus leading to mild dilatation and focal air accumulation at the thoracic inlet *(arrows)*. (Courtesy of New York State College of Veterinary Medicine, Ithaca, NY.)

Figure 21–8. Lateral view of this mature dog reveals a radiopaque foreign body located immediately cranial to the esophageal hiatus. The sharp projection is characteristic of esophageal foreign bodies. A prominent zone of soft tissue *(arrows)* surrounds the bone indicative of esophageal wall thickening by inflammation. Four common sites of foreign body entrapment are the cranial cervical region, thoracic inlet, over the base of the heart, and cranial to the hiatus. (Courtesy of New York State College of Veterinary Medicine, Ithaca, NY.)

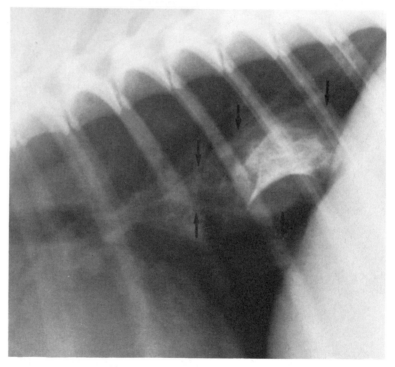

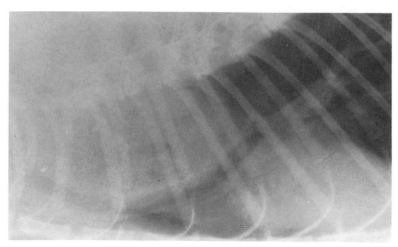

Figure 21–9. Lateral view of a young cat with a persistent right fourth aortic arch, producing a vascular ring. There is food accumulation in the dilated segment of the esophageal cranial to the obstruction. The trachea deviates ventrally. (Courtesy of New York State College of Veterinary Medicine, Ithaca, NY.)

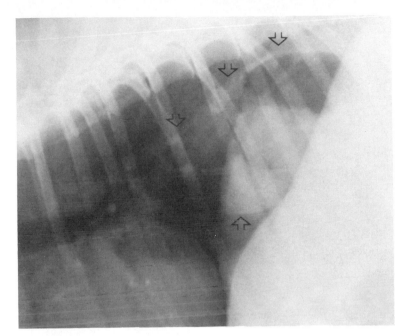

Figure 21–10. Lateral view of a mature dog with a gastroesophageal intussusception. The radiopacity of the gastric contents can be seen in the caudal thorax superimposed over the left diaphragmatic crus and dorsocaudal lung field (arrows). (Courtesy of New York State College of Veterinary Medicine, Ithaca, NY.)

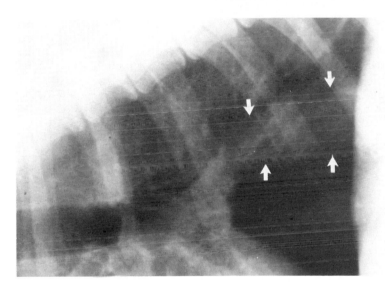

Figure 21–11. Lateral view of an old dog reveals an area of soft tissue located between the descending aorta and the caudal vena cava (arrows). This incidental finding is an esophageal leiomyoma. (Courtesy of New York State College of Veterinary Medicine, Ithaca, NY.)

Figure 21–12. Survey radiograph of an older dog reveals abnormal radiopacity in the mid to caudal portion of the dorsal thorax associated with linear to amorphous mineral opacities and increased esophageal wall thickness. Differential diagnoses include dystrophic mineralization of the esophagus associated with chronic inflammation or granuloma (Spirocerca lupi), neoplasia with mineralization, or the chronic presence of a radiolucent foreign body and coating of an eroded mucosa by an antacid or enteric coating agent. (Courtesy of New York State College of Veterinary Medicine, Ithaca, NY.)

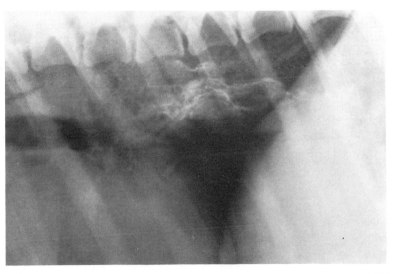

TABLE 21–2. **CHARACTERISTIC SITE OF FOCAL ESOPHAGEAL DISEASE**

Cervical Region	Cranial Thoracic Region	Caudal Thoracic/Abdominal Region
Achalasia	Vascular ring anomaly	Esophagitis (reflux) (patulent caudal esophageal sphincter)
Asynchrony	Esophagitis (reflux)	
Chalasia	Stricture	Foreign body
Foreign body	Periesophageal mass	Perforation
Esophagitis (caustic)	Redundancy	Leiomyoma
Extension of neoplasia	Diverticula	Gastroesophageal intussusception
Perforation	Foreign body	Hiatal hernia
Segmental hypomotility	Neoplasia	Esophageal fistula
	Perforation	

CONTRAST RADIOGRAPHY

Contrast Media. Many contrast media are available for esophagography, and the rationale for choosing a specific one should be based on the type of disease process suspected to be present.[1] Barium sulfate creams and pastes* have been formulated for high contrast and good adherence to the esophageal mucosa. Esophageal mucosal irregularities (esophagitis, neoplastic infiltrates) and strictures are readily evaluated with these contrast media. Because of their viscosity, however, they tend to maintain a bolus, failing to disperse well in fluid esophageal contents and to flow around intraluminal lesions. Admixture with liquid barium suspensions is also poor, resulting in clumping in the gastric lumen when an upper gastrointestinal examination follows radiography of the esophagus. In addition, aspiration of paste may lead to asphyxiation, and therefore the use of paste is not advised when aspiration is a significant clinical problem.

Liquid barium sulfate suspensions† do not adhere well to the mucosa, but a high density medium (45 to 85 percent w/w) is used for routine procedures because it is safer when aspirated, mixes well with fluid contents, and readily flows around intraluminal obstructions. Suspected motility problems of both the oropharyngeal and esophageal regions should be evaluated first with a liquid suspension. A barium-coated meal may be administered subsequently, particularly in animals with differential problems in swallowing liquids and solids. A solid meal may best demonstrate early strictures or regional motility disorders.

Oral aqueous iodine solutions‡ are considered nontoxic when accidentally spilled into body cavities. Therefore their use is indicated when esophageal perforation is suspected. These agents are hypertonic and thus, if aspirated, may induce pulmonary edema from osmosis. In addition, a volume-depleted animal may be further compromised by the fluid loss through the gastrointestinal tract from the osmotic effect. If leakage occurs into a fluid-filled pleural space, the resulting dilution may make it difficult to detect the medium and the site of leakage radiographically. The use of a barium sulfate liquid in the presence of a perforation has instigated some controversy because of the tendency of this agent to stimulate a granulomatous reaction on pleural surfaces. The use of this substance is indicated, however, when an oral iodine medium fails to define the problem. The aqueous iodine media are not recommended for routine use because of their low viscosity and thus their poor coating ability.

Other media that may be used occasionally include the bronchographic agents, such as oily suspensions of propyliodone;* they are useful for suspected esophageal-pulmonary fistulae. Because of their low level of pulmonary irritation, these media are well tolerated when extravasation into the lung parenchyma occurs.

Technique. Survey radiographs are made to establish a base technique and to identify possible definitive diagnoses. A doubling of the milliamperage-seconds for the contrast procedure increases penetration with high contrast to enhance the radiopacity of the contrast medium. Although many disorders may be adequately diagnosed with only recumbent lateral views, an orthogonal view of the esophagus is indicated. Superimposition of the spine readily obscures even the barium-coated esophageal lumen; therefore, either a right or left dorsoventral-lateral oblique position is recommended to rotate the esophagus into a more visible location. On the lateral view, by moving one thoracic limb cranially and the other caudally,

---

*Esophotrast, Barnes-Hind/Hydrocurve, Inc., Sunnyvale, CA 94086; Microtrast, Nicholas Labs Limited, Slough, England SLI4AU; HD 5000 Esophageal Cream, Lafayette Pharmacal, Inc., Lafayette, IN 47902.
†Orotrast, Barnes-Hind/Hydrocurve, Inc., Sunnyvale, CA 94086; Basosperse, Mallinckrodt, Paris, KY 40361; E-Z-paque, E-Z-EM Co., Inc., Westbury, NY 11590.
‡Gastrografin, E. R. Squibb & Sons, Inc., Princeton, NJ 08540; Oral Hypaque Sodium, Winthrop Laboratories, New York, NY 10016.

---

*Dionosil Oily, Glaxo Inc., Ft. Lauderdale, FL 33309.

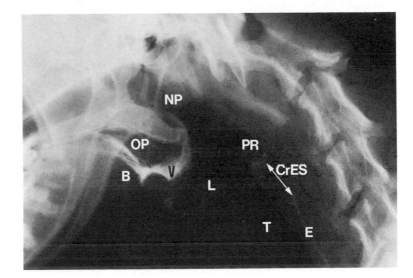

Figure 21–13. A normal oropharyngeal contrast medium examination of a mature dog (lateral view). NP: nasopharynx; OP: oropharynx; B: base of tongue; E: esophagus; V: valleculae; L: larynx; T: trachea; PR: piriform recesses; CrES: cranial esophageal sphincter. (Courtesy of New York State College of Veterinary Medicine, Ithaca, NY.)

the opacity over the thoracic inlet from the heavy musculature of the brachium is reduced.

A fractious animal may be given a nominal dose of phenothiazine tranquilizer.* The esophagus, however, is affected by most sedatives, tranquilizers, and general anesthetics, and therefore their routine use is contraindicated when motility is being evaluated.

Approximately a 5- to 20-ml amount of contrast medium is given to induce several complete swallows for coating the pharynx and esophagus. Oropharyngeal problems are best evaluated by a series of radiographs taken in the midst of a swallow and during a pause after the swallow is completed. The esophageal phase should be radiographed after a sufficient pause to ensure complete transport of the last bolus to the stomach.

The normal appearance of the oropharyngeal region after a swallow of contrast medium is coating of the mucosa without significant retention of the medium (Fig. 21–13). A small amount may occasionally remain in the valleculae and proximal esophagus immediately caudal to the cranial esophageal sphincter; none should persist in the piriform recesses or upper airway (nasopharynx, larynx, or trachea) unless laryngotracheal aspiration inadvertently occurs during contrast medium administration to a struggling patient.

The normal canine esophageal mucosa appears as a series of longitudinal folds. The lines are close together through most if its length, but may separate slightly at the thoracic inlet as the esophagus passes along the left lateral side of the trachea (Fig. 21–14). The feline esophagus has a similar appearance to the level of the heart base, but the remainder of the esophagus caudally has obliquely directed folds that correspond to the smooth muscle segment (Fig. 21–15). Oblique views of the dorsoventral or ventrodorsal position eliminate superimposition of the spine for better visualization of the esophagus (Fig. 21–16).

---

*Acepromazine maleate, 0.05 mg per pound body weight subcutaneously or intramuscularly.

Figure 21–14. Normal esophagram (lateral view) of a mature dog after the administration of a barium sulfate cream. The longitudinal folds frequently separate at the thoracic inlet.

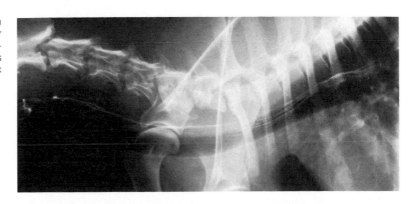

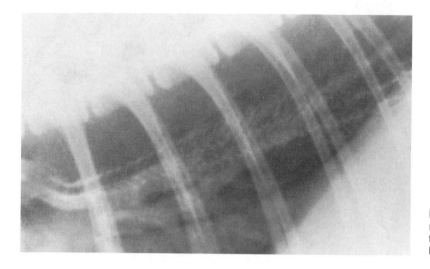

Figure 21–15. Normal caudal thoracic esophageal mucosal contour of a mature cat demonstrated by a barium swallow examination.

CONTRAST RADIOGRAPHIC FINDINGS

Diseases of the oral stage of swallowing usually involve the tongue. If an abnormality of the oral stage is present, the effect may be on prehension, caudal transport through the oral cavity, or organization of a bolus in the oro-

pharynx by the tongue. Retention of contrast medium in the oral cavity and oropharynx is present radiographically. The subsequent pharyngeal and cricopharyngeal stages are normal (Fig. 21–17).

Pharyngeal stage dysphagia is encountered with neuromuscular disease, inflammatory dis-

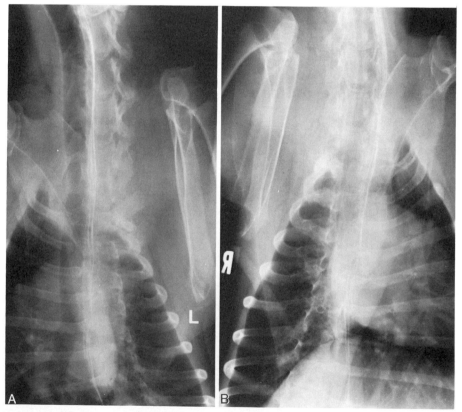

Figure 21–16. Normal esophagram (right dorsoventral oblique view) of a mature dog after administration of a barium sulfate cream. The sternum has been rolled to the right of the esophagus and the vertebral column to the left. B, same study, left dorsoventral oblique view. The sternum has been rolled to the left of the esophagus and the vertebral column to the right.

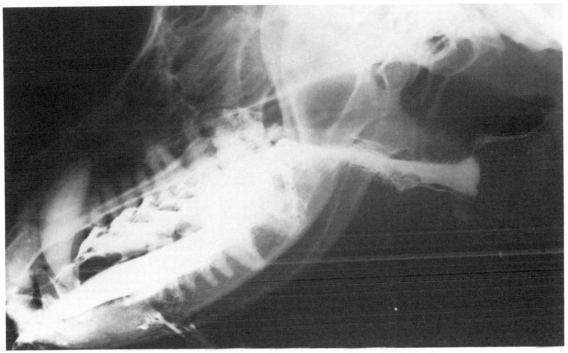

Figure 21–17. Lateral view of a mature dog with oral dysphagia. The effects of a hypoglossal deficit can be seen. Inadequate stripping action of the tongue against the hard and soft palate prevents caudal transport, and there is resulting bolus formation of contrast medium at the base of the tongue. A small amount of contrast medium has been swallowed, revealing normal pharyngeal and cricopharyngeal stages. (Courtesy of New York State College of Veterinary Medicine, Ithaca, NY.)

eases (Fig. 21–18), and trauma that may be associated with perforation (Fig. 21–19) or fracture of the hyoid apparatus (Fig. 21–20).[4,5] The oral stage is normal, but inadequate pharyngeal peristalsis leads to retention of much of the bolus. Inadequate closure of the pharyngeal egresses (nasopharynx, oral cavity, and larynx) may lead to reflux of contrast medium into these regions.

Cricopharyngeal stage dysphagia may be due

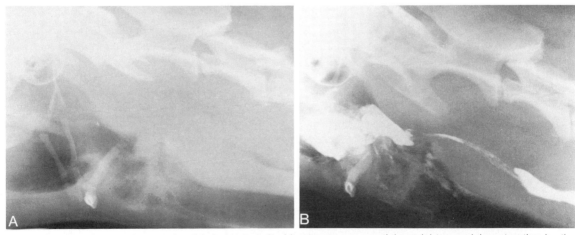

Figure 21–18. Pharyngeal stage dysphagia is a result of inadequate sequential cranial to caudal contraction by the pharyngeal constrictors. Thus, transport of a bolus through the cranial esophageal sphincter is usually incomplete. Contrast medium is retained in the pharynx and piriform recesses. This dog with chronic laryngitis and pharyngitis has retropharyngeal swelling and inflammation in addition to scarring of the larynx. A, note the short epiglottis and ventrally displaced trachea. Air is retained in the esophagus. B, contrast medium examination shows pharyngeal retention of the medium and laryngotracheal aspiration due to disturbed motility.

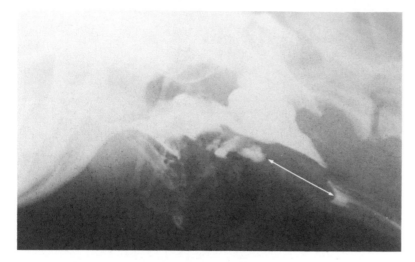

Figure 21–19. Lateral view. Pharyngeal laceration secondary to a perforating foreign body (stick) resulted in a retropharyngeal fistula and pharyngeal paresis. There is accumulation of contrast medium in the pharynx, piriform recesses, and the retropharyngeal abscess. *Double-headed arrow,* cranial esophageal sphincter. (Courtesy of New York State College of Veterinary Medicine, Ithaca, NY.)

to inappropriate opening or nonopening of the cranial esophageal sphincter (cricopharyngeal asynchrony or achalasia) or failure of closure of that sphincter (chalasia). Chalasia is recognized by the persistence of a patent passage between the pharynx and cranial esophagus (Fig. 21–21). Reflux of esophageal contrast medium results in its presence in the pharynx. Pharyngeal paresis often accompanies cricopharyngeal chalasia, which is an additional cause for pharyngeal retention of contrast medium. Dysfunction of the cranial esophageal sphincter due to asynchrony or achalasia results in interference with transport of the contrast medium. The passage may be visibly distorted, although the pattern of distribution of retained contrast medium is similar to the pattern found in pharyngeal dysphagia (Fig. 21–22). Table 21–3 is a summary

of the static contrast radiographic findings of the various oropharyngeal dysphagias.

A diffusely dilated esophagus (megaesophagus) usually produces sufficient diagnostic radiographic signs on survey radiographs to preclude the need for esophagography. On occasion, however, a partially gas- and fluid-filled lumen is difficult to detect (Fig. 21–4A), requiring identification of its presence by a contrast medium examination. In addition, esophageal dilatation may be due to causes other than primary neuromuscular abnormalities, for example, neoplasia, inflammation, or hiatal disease. Evaluation of the competency of the cranial esophageal sphincter by examination with contrast medium may be indicated to help establish a prognosis in cases of systemic neuromuscular disease.

If patency or relaxation of the caudal esoph-

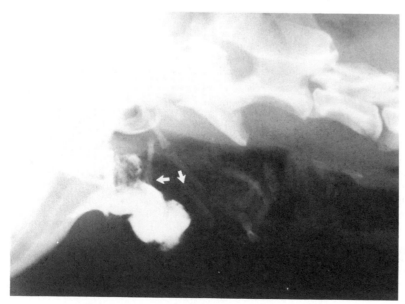

Figure 21–20. Lateral view of a mature dog. The hyoid apparatus plays an integral roll in coordinating laryngeal closure with the oral, pharyngeal, and cricopharyngeal stages of swallowing. Fracture or dislocation of the hyoid apparatus may disrupt this process, as demonstrated in this dog *(arrows).* Contrast medium has collected in the oropharynx but cannot be propelled caudally by the pharynx. (Courtesy of New York State College of Veterinary Medicine, Ithaca, NY.)

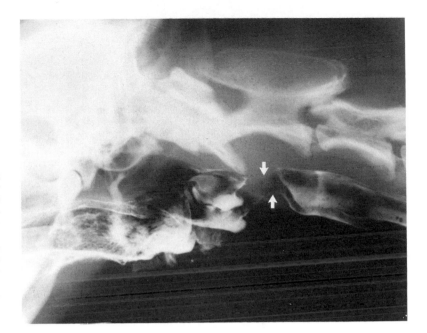

Figure 21–21. Lateral view of a mature dog affected by a systemic neuromuscular disease (tentatively diagnosed as autoimmune polymyositis). Chalasia and megaesophagus are present. Contrast medium in the valleculae and piriform recesses may be due to esophagopharyngeal reflux or to pharyngeal paresis. (Courtesy of New York State College of Veterinary Medicine, Ithaca, NY.)

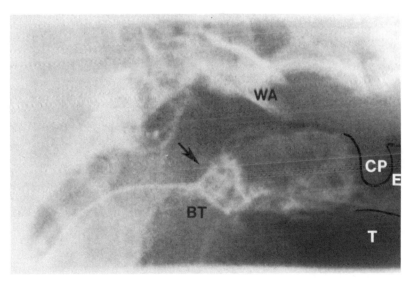

Figure 21–22. Lateral view, with contrast medium. During the pharyngeal and cricopharyngeal stages of swallowing, the pharynx is in vigorous contraction *(arrow)* against a closing cranial esophageal sphincter (CP). The floor of this passge is open, allowing air and contrast medium to outline the distorted sphincter. This asynchrony between pharyngeal and cricopharyngeal stages occurs more commonly than true cricopharyngeal achalasia. BT: base of tongue; WA: wings of atlas; E: esophagus; T: trachea. (Reprinted from Ettinger SJ (Ed): Textbook of Veterinary Internal Medicine, 2nd ed. Philadelphia, WB Saunders, 1983, with permission.)

TABLE 21–3. **SUMMARY OF LOCATION OF RETAINED CONTRAST MEDIUM RELATIVE TO TYPE OF OROPHARYNGEAL DYSPHAGIA**

	Dysphagia			
	Normal	*Oral*	*Pharyngeal*	*Cricopharyngeal*
Oral cavity	+/−	+	−	−
Nasopharynx	−	−	+/−	+/−
Oropharynx	−	+	+/−	+/−
Pharynx	−	−	+	+
Valleculae	+/−	+/−	+	+
Piriform recesses	−	−	+	+
Esophagus	−	−	+/−	+/−
Larynx/trachea	−	−	+	+

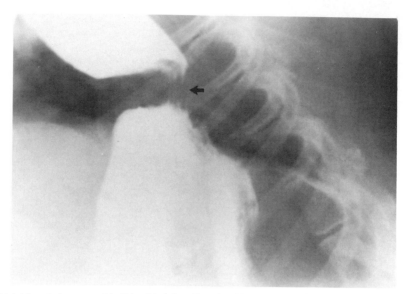

Figure 21–23. A hiatal hernia is present in this older dog. Esophagitis and caudal esophageal dilatation are associated with the gastroesophageal reflux. Caudal esophageal sphincter is well defined cranial to the diaphragm. (Courtesy of New York State College of Veterinary Medicine, Ithaca, NY.)

ageal sphincter is in doubt, liquid barium sulfate should be administered with the animal erect before contrast radiography. This procedure takes advantage of the normal transient caudal esophageal sphincter relaxation in response to the initiation of the oropharyngeal phase of swallowing. Passage of the contrast medium occurs by gravity flow during this phase. In a recumbent position, the horizontal attitude of the esophagus eliminates the gravitational influ-

ence and thus the caudal sphincter regains tone before any medium can passively flow through it. The absence of sufficient esophageal peristaltic propulsion compounds the retention of contrast medium.

Regional dilatation without obstruction may occur with primary segmental hypomotility, secondary dysmotility from inflammation, diverticulae, and redundancy. Segmental motility disturbances may affect any portion of the

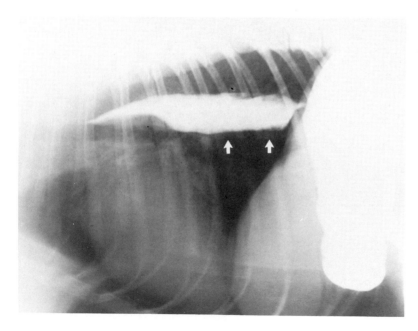

Figure 21–24. Gastroesophageal reflux is demonstrated on lateral thoracic radiographs if contrast medium is present in the caudal esophagus after clearing of this area subsequent to the initial administration of the medium. The ventral wall of the esophagus in this dog is thickened *(arrows)* by chronic inflammation, which impairs rapid clearing and further compounds the problem. (Courtesy of New York State College of Veterinary Medicine, Ithaca, NY.)

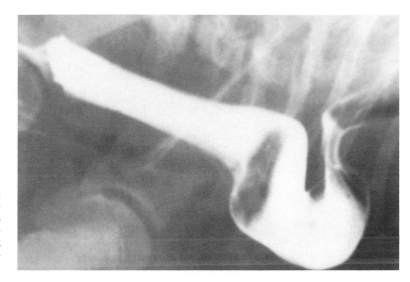

Figure 21–25. The cranial thoracic esophagus in this immature bulldog is redundant. The tortuous path may hamper peristalsis mechanically. (Courtesy of New York State College of Veterinary Medicine, Ithaca, NY.)

esophagus. Reflux esophagitis usually involves the caudal esophagus and may or may not be associated with hiatal herniation (Fig. 21–23), caudal esophageal sphincter chalasia (patulent cardia), chronic vomiting, or idiopathic reflux (Fig. 21–24). Diverticulae or sacculations of the esophagus are most often encountered cranial to strictures, including those due to vascular ring anomalies (Fig. 21–6), but also occur with esophageal or periesophageal inflammation. Esophageal redundancy is an occasional incidental finding, but this disorder may be problematic in young brachycephalic breeds. Regional dilatation can be demonstrated at the site of deviation in the thoracic inlet (Fig. 21–25).

Obstructions eventually lead to dilatation of the esophageal lumen cranial to the site, but acutely may not be apparent on survey radiographs. The source of obstruction may be intrinsic [strictures (Fig. 21–26), foreign bodies (Fig. 21–27), gastroesophageal intussusception (Fig. 21–28), and intraluminal masses (Fig. 21–29)] or extrinsic, from periesophageal masses (Fig. 21–30). Masses often cause the esophagus to deviate around them. The location of the mass determines the rapidity of onset of esophageal obstruction and degree of dilation given the limited space available in certain sites along the path of the esophagus (i.e., the thoracic inlet). Mural masses may trap small amounts of luminal contrast medium, but rarely cause obstruction until they are large (Fig. 21–31). Dysphagia is usually due to regional dysmotility.

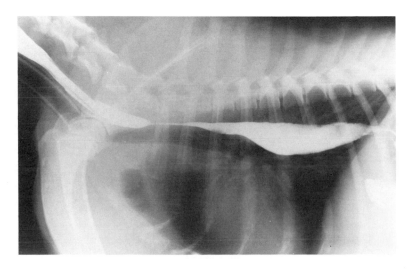

Figure 21–26. Lateral view of the thorax (with contrast medium) of a young adult female dog. There is a cranial thoracic esophageal stricture. The lesion developed after the administration of anesthesia for ovariohysterectomy. The extent of the luminal involvement was best demonstrated by placing an esophageal tube while the dog was anesthetized, and gradually administering contrast medium to fill the distensible portions of the esophagus. Inflammation of the caudal portion is shown by the small undulations in the dorsal and ventral mucosa. (Courtesy of New York State College of Veterinary Medicine, Ithaca, NY.)

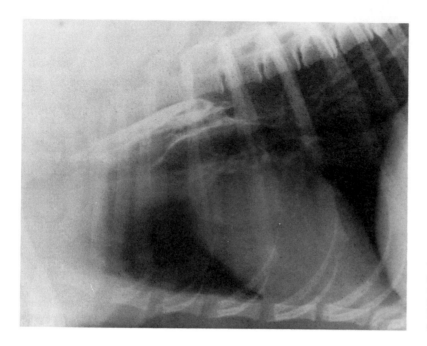

Figure 21–27. Lateral view of an immature dog. A nonradiopaque foreign body (piece of plastic) is seen as a filling defect in a pool of entrapped contrast medium. (Courtesy of New York State College of Veterinary Medicine, Ithaca, NY.)

Figure 21–28. Gastroesophageal intussusception and related obstruction of the esophagus may be intermittent or persistent depending upon the amount of stomach involvement. The signs of regurgitation and vomiting were sporadic in this cat. Gastric rugal folds can be seen projecting into the dilated caudal esophagus *(arrows)* on this lateral view. (Courtesy of New York State College of Veterinary Medicine, Ithaca, NY.)

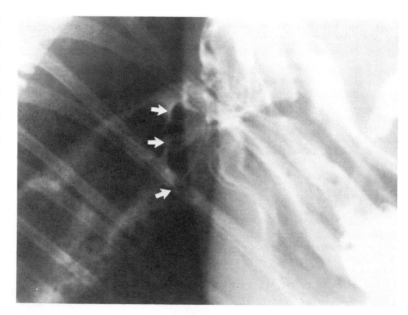

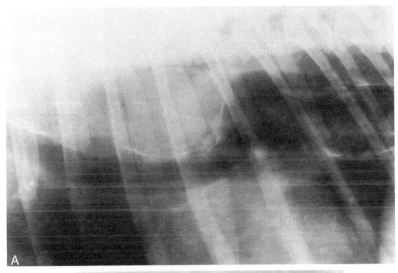

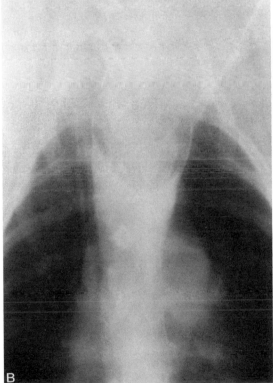

Figure 21–29. *A* and *B*, an ovoid soft-tissue filling defect is present within the esophageal lumen of an older dog. A pedunculated tumor was found at endoscopy. Although an esophageal foreign body might present a similar appearance, the round, smooth surface would not likely lodge in the esophagus. (Courtesy of New York State College of Veterinary Medicine, Ithaca, NY.)

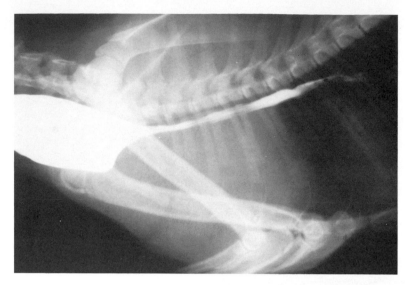

Figure 21–30. Lateral radiograph with contrast medium of an immature cat with cranial mediastinal lymphosarcoma. The periesophageal mass causes obstruction of the esophagus due to the restricted expansion capabilities at the thoracic inlet and cranial thorax and to the large mass. (Reprinted from Ettinger SJ (Ed): Textbook of Veterinary Internal Medicine, 2nd ed. Philadelphia, WB Saunders, 1983, with permission.)

Figure 21–31. Lateral view (contrast medium study) of the caudal esophagus of a puppy. The thoracic esophageal lumen is dilated. The contrast medium outlines the dilated abdominal segment, which has a markedly irregular mucosal surface *(arrows)* and a filling defect (*). The necropsy diagnosis was granulomatous esophagitis with ulceration. (Courtesy of New York State College of Veterinary Medicine, Ithaca, NY.)

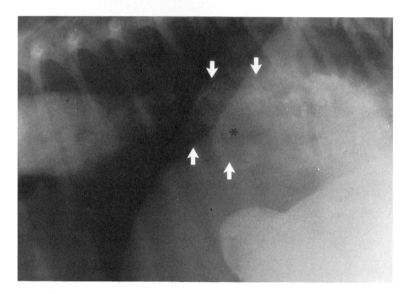

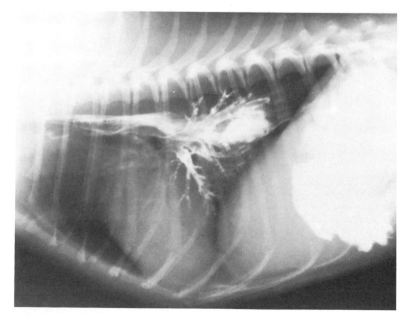

Figure 21–32. Lateral view (with contrast medium) of a young dog shows simultaneous filling of the right caudal lobe bronchus and the esophagus, indicating a bronchoesophageal fistula. (Reprinted from Ettinger SJ (Ed): Textbook of Veterinary Internal Medicine, 2nd ed. Philadelphia, WB Saunders, 1983, with permission.)

Esophageal fistulae may have extravasation of contrast medium along a tract, with dispersion of the medium into the pulmonary parenchyma via an airway (esophagotracheal or esophagobronchial) or directly (esophagopulmonary) (Fig. 21–32). Fistulae are not to be mistaken for inadvertent aspiration and subsequent alveolarization of contrast medium during a routine swallow.

An increase in esophageal wall thickness can only be identified in the thoracic region. Confirmation of a thickened wall due to inflammation or neoplasia can be made by using esophagography (Fig. 21–24). Because the periesophageal fascia and muscle in the cervical region and the liver and stomach in the cranial abdomen are silhouetted with the adjacent esophageal wall, thickening of these areas can only be presumed by the presence of concurrent changes in the mucosal contour. Infiltration by neoplasia or by inflammatory or granulation tissue usually distorts the mucosal surface, obliterating the longitudinal or oblique folds (Fig. 21–31).

References

1. Brawner WR, and Bartels JE: Contrast radiography of the digestive tract—indications, techniques and complications. Vet Clin North Am [Small Anim Pract] *13*:599, 1983.
2. Kealy JK: Diagnostic Radiology of the Dog and Cat. Philadelphia, WB Saunders, 1979, pp. 32–48.
3. O'Brien TR. Esophagus. *In* O'Brien TR (Ed): Radiographic Diagnosis of Abdominal Disorders in the Dog and Cat: Radiographic Interpretation, Clinical Signs, and Pathophysiology. Philadelphia, WB Saunders, 1978, pp. 141–203.
4. Watrous BJ: Clinical presentation and diagnosis of dysphagia. Vet Clin North Am [Small Anim Pract] *13*:437, 1983.
5. Watrous BJ: Esophageal disease. *In* Ettinger SJ (Ed): Textbook of Veterinary Internal Medicine—Diseases of the Dog and Cat. Philadelphia, WB Saunders, 1983, pp. 1191–1233.

CHAPTER 22

THE THORACIC WALL

CHARLES R. ROOT
ROBERT J. BAHR

The thoracic wall consists of skin, fat, subcutaneous muscles, ribs (or sternum ventrally), intercostal muscles, parietal pleura, and the associated vasculature and nerves[17]; normal thoracic radiographic anatomy is well described.[16, 19] Diseases involving these structures, like those in other parts of the body, may be divided into congenital, developmental, infectious, neoplastic, traumatic, metabolic, degenerative, and unknown categories. Unfortunately, the radiographic manifestations of disease of the various constituents of the thoracic wall are rarely pathognomonic. As a result, accurate differentiation may be difficult or impossible. The key to complete radiologic assessment lies in recognition of broad radiographic signs of disease; description of each in terms of abnormal size, shape, position, and opacity; application of a working knowledge of the pathogenesis of the major categories of disease; and coupling of the radiographic signs with historical, physical, and laboratory findings. Despite a systematic approach, radiographic interpretation seldom yields unequivocal conclusions; however, such an assessment frequently rules out various diseases and often suggests the specific diagnostic tools to further an understanding of the problem.

SPECIAL PROCEDURES

Routine thoracic radiography often yields enough information to permit assessment of the thoracic wall. Using high kVp–low mA technique, the contrast between subcutaneous muscles and fat may not be as striking as that produced with low kVp–high mA technique. Therefore, supplemental projections with reciprocal adjustments in mA and kVp may produce relatively better subcutaneous detail. Occasionally, oblique projections, horizontal-beam projections, or some type of contrast radiographic procedure may be helpful or necessary in differential diagnoses. Only two contrast radiographic procedures have proved to be of much value. They are *pleurography* and *fistulography*. Pleurography has been described in depth elsewhere.[1–3, 15] Fistulography has not been well described previously; it is indicated in the presence of a chronic draining lesion that either has failed to heal with rigorous symptomatic therapy or has recurred after treatment has been discontinued. Such a history is highly suggestive of the presence of a foreign body or devitalized, sequestered tissue. Fistulography is contraindicated if there are large or numerous tracts through the skin. It should be performed with care if the lesion is suspected to be infected and if it potentially communicates with a body cavity. Syringes, organic iodide contrast medium, pediatric Foley catheters, and various

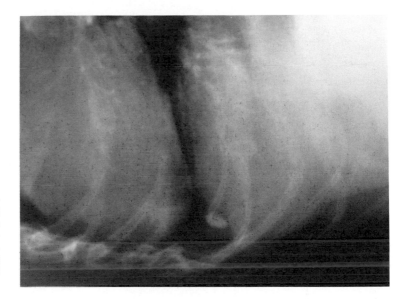

Figure 22–1. Lateral thoracic radiograph of a dog with a superimposed mammary nipple over the caudoventral thorax. Similar focal extracostal lesions may be produced by engorged ticks, pedunculated neoplasia, or scabs from superficial injuries.

catheter adapters are needed in performing fistulography. The tract is cannulated with the appropriate catheter or catheter adapter (previously filled with contrast medium to avoid introduction of air bubbles). The catheter or catheter adapter must be large enough to seal the tract against reflux of contrast medium around the device, or the cuff of the Foley catheter must be inflated for the same purpose. Undiluted contrast medium is then injected. The volume is variable, but the lesion must be filled until mild back-pressure is detected in the syringe or contrast medium refluxes around the catheter. Lateral, dorsoventral or ventrodorsal, oblique, and/or horizontal-beam projections are then made. These radiographs are carefully scrutinized for evidence of filling defects in the contrast medium or communication of contrast medium with intercostal tissues, ribs, sternum, vertebral column, or underlying body cavity.

RADIOGRAPHIC SIGNS

Radiographic lesions of each component of the thoracic wall can be grouped according to specific radiographic signs. In addition to altered size, position, opacity, and shape, it is also important to note the extent (i.e., diffuse or focal) and pattern of the lesion (homogeneous, mottled, granular, reticulated, and so forth).

Skin and Subcutaneous Tissue

Focal extracostal opacities (Fig. 22–1) may be caused by mammary nipples, engorged ticks, neoplasms, abscesses, granulomata, scabs, or metallic foreign bodies (bullet fragments, shotgun pellets, and the like). Only the last are easily identified radiographically. The others

are homogeneous fluid opacities that may or may not be well demarcated.

Diffuse extracostal opacities (Fig. 22–2) may be produced by cellulitis, contusion, edema, hypodermoclysis fluid, or neoplasia. Usually,

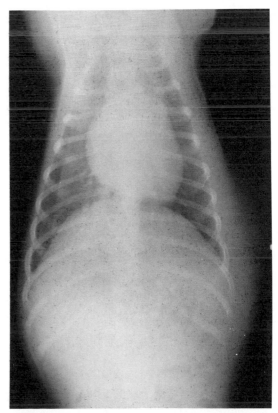

Figure 22–2. Dorsoventral thoracic radiograph of a dog with diffuse subcutaneous swelling along the left side of the thoracic wall due to hypodermoclysis. A similar radiographic finding may be produced by cellulitis.

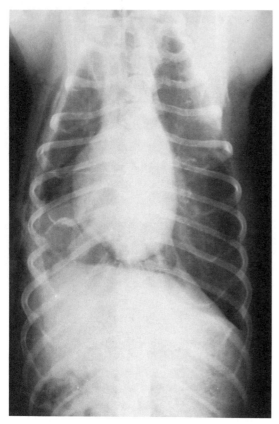

Figure 22–3. Ventrodorsal thoracic radiograph of a dog that had been attacked by a larger dog. There is focal subcutaneous gas along the right lateral thoracic wall, where the victim's skin was penetrated. There is also a fracture of the right eighth rib and adjacent pleural effusion. Abscesses, subcutaneous injections containing small air bubbles, and (occasionally) fractured ribs also may produce focal extracostal lucencies. (Courtesy of the Santa Cruz Veterinary Hospital.)

the normal subcutaneous fat striations are disturbed; they are most often locally obliterated by the aforementioned lesions but may be merely displaced if the lesion is well delineated and slowly developing (e.g., benign neoplasia).

Focal extracostal lucencies (Fig. 22–3) may be produced by laceration or punctures of skin and subcutaneous tissue, fractured ribs,[4] abscesses with gas-forming organisms, subcutaneous injections, and lipomas. The last are usually better circumscribed and less lucent than the others.

Diffuse extracostal lucencies (Fig. 22–4) may be produced by subcutaneous or intrafascial emphysema[4, 11] or by intramuscular and subcutaneous accumulation of fat due to obesity. The

former is frequently caused by external trauma but may follow pneumomediastinum.

Ribs

Focal costal opacities (Fig. 22–5) may be caused by neoplasia,[4] bacterial osteomyelitis, fungal osteomyelitis, healing fractures, foreign bodies (shotgun wounds, for example), and multiple cartilaginous exostoses.[10, 11, 17] The first three may be very difficult to differentiate radiographically, since they all may involve combinations of bone formation and bony lysis. Radiopaque foreign bodies are uncommon, but since they are usually the result of gunshot wounds, they present little diagnostic confusion. Multiple cartilaginous exostoses, as the name implies, involve many sites, including ribs,[7, 10, 11, 17] skull, and long bones. Healed rib fractures[14] generally produce local smooth bony enlargement (Fig. 22–6) at the fracture sites, as a result of exuberant callus formation in response to constant respiratory motion during healing.

Diffuse costal opacities may be caused by exuberant periosteal reaction associated with chronic bacterial osteomyelitis. In patients from the Southwest, coccidioidomycosis[6, 7, 9] may produce a diffuse sclerotic periosteal reaction (Fig. 22–7).

Focal costal lucencies (Fig. 22–8) may be caused by fractures,[7, 12] neoplasia,[7] or osteomyelitis. Of these, fractures are easiest to diagnose and usually are easily differentiated radiographically from neoplasia and osteomyelitis.

Focal intercostal fluid opacities are rare but suggest neoplasia or focal inflammation. If large, or if solid and substantive, there may be cranial and caudal displacement of the adjacent ribs. Focal intercostal metal opacities are usually due to gunshot wounds. These are often incidental findings that bear little clinical significance.

Focal intercostal lucencies (Fig. 22–9) are most often due to penetrating trauma. These lesions may or may not penetrate the pleural space and may or may not be associated with fractures or displacement of ribs. They appear as gaseous interruption of the normal homogeneous intercostal soft tissue. It is also possible for focal intercostal lucencies to develop after blunt trauma causes a fracture of a rib that lacerates adjacent lung. In this instance, there usually is pneumothorax and there may be accompanying focal or diffuse subcutaneous or intrafascial emphysema. Intercostal abscess formation may be a late sequela of external penetration of intercostal tissue. If gas-forming organisms are present, a focal intercostal lucency may develop. Such lucency, in contrast to that seen in acute injury, will be well circum-

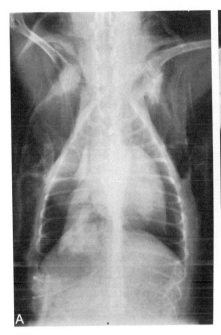

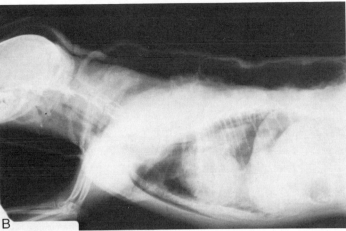

Figure 22–4. Dorsoventral *(A)* and lateral *(B)* thoracic radiographs of a dog with a common type of diffuse extracostal lucency. There is diffuse subcutaneous and intrafascial emphysema secondary to penetrating trauma of the caudal right hemithorax (fractured right ribs 8–10 with intercostal lacerations) caused by a dogfight. This type of emphysema may be initiated by pneumomediastinum, trauma near the thoracic inlet or axilla, or direct external trauma. In this dog the trauma established communication with the pleural space, resulting in bilateral pneumothorax. Gas is visible in fascial planes of the neck.

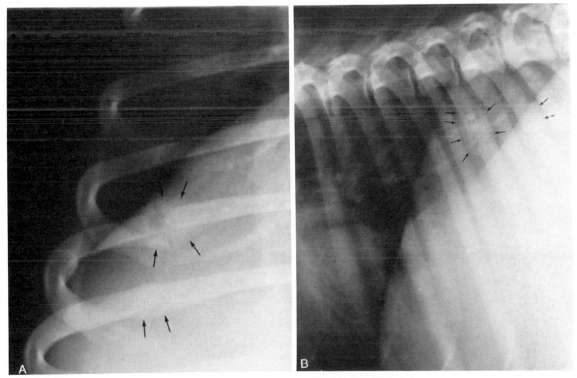

Figure 22–5. *A* and *B,* focal costal opacities resulting from healing rib fractures *(arrows).* This dog had been hit by a car several weeks prior to these radiographs. Notice the exuberant periosteal callus, which produces a focal costal opacity. Other lesions that may produce a focal costal opacity include neoplasia and focal inflammatory reaction.

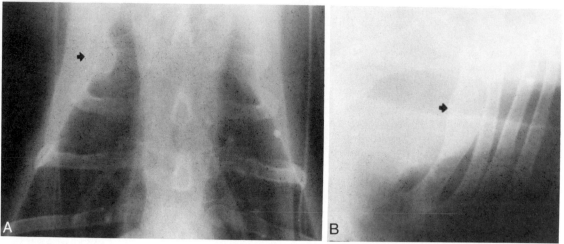

Figure 22–6. *A* and *B*, radiographs of a dog with unknown previous trauma. There is an old, healed fracture *(arrows)* of the first right rib. Its union is complete, and there is a smooth, focal costal opacity bridging the fracture site.

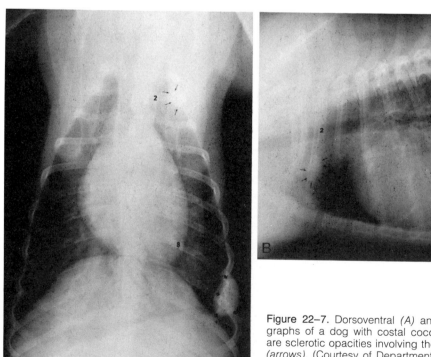

Figure 22–7. Dorsoventral *(A)* and lateral *(B)* thoracic radiographs of a dog with costal coccidioidomycosis. The lesions are sclerotic opacities involving the left second and eighth ribs *(arrows)*. (Courtesy of Department of Veterinary Medicine and Surgery, College of Veterinary Medicine, University of Missouri, Columbia, MO.)

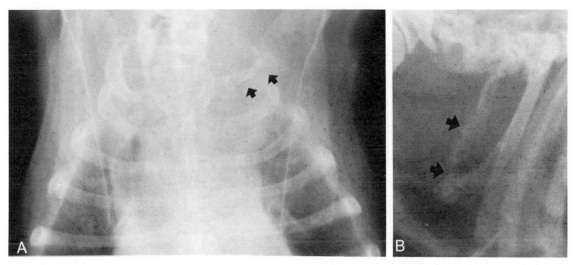

Figure 22–8. Ventrodorsal *(A)* and lateral *(B)* thoracic radiographs of a dog with lytic neoplasia *(arrows)* of the left first rib. There is dextral displacement and lateral extrinsic compression of the trachea, secondary to a cranial mediastinal mass. Histopathologic diagnosis was not obtained. Focal costal lucency may be produced by neoplasia or osteomyelitis. (Courtesy of Parkwood Pet Clinic, Woodland Hills, CA.)

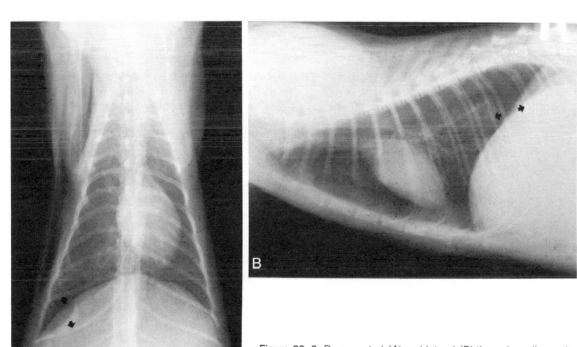

Figure 22–9. Dorsoventral *(A)* and lateral *(B)* thoracic radiographs of a cat, with intercostal lacerations *(arrows)* resulting in widening of the right tenth intercostal space. This lesion was the result of a dog bite.

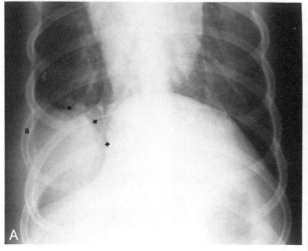

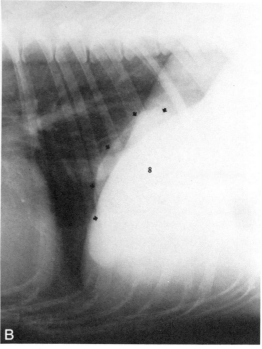

Figure 22–10. Dorsoventral (A) and lateral (B) thoracic radiographs of a dog with an extrapleural lesion adjacent to the eighth rib on the right (arrows). The diaphragm is displaced, and there is both external and internal protrusion of the mass (arrows). The concavity in the region where the internal protrusion joins the thoracic wall is characteristic of "extrapleural lesions."

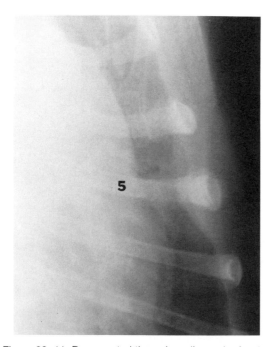

Figure 22–11. Dorsoventral thoracic radiograph of a dog with an extrapleural lesion adjacent to the fifth rib on the left. Note the concave margin of the cranial and caudal aspects of the lesion. The lesion was a subpleural hematoma resulting from blunt trauma to the lateral aspect of the thorax. Costal neoplasia is another type of lesion that can lead to the extrapleural sign. If this opacity were of pulmonary origin, it would form either a right or an acute angle with the thoracic wall rather than having a tapering junction.

scribed and confined rather than angular and poorly localized.

Expansile rib lesions,[11] regardless of their radiographic opacity, potentially cause displacement or divergence of the cranially and caudally adjacent ribs. This is usually much better appreciated in ventrodorsal or dorsoventral projections than in lateral views. The ribs, like other bony structures, do not react to pathologic insult with an either/or response. Very often, therefore, there will be *both* lysis and production of bone. Combinations of increase and decrease in opacity may have differential diagnostic significance. For instance, a focal opacity surrounded by focal lysis may suggest osteomyelitis with sequestration, whereas reactive bone surrounding a mottled lytic area may represent a neoplastic process.

Medial extension of a pathologic process from the thoracic wall, from ribs, or from intercostal tissue often causes broadly based medial displacement of parietal pleura. This is often contrasted by adjacent displaced lung and produces a characteristic "extrapleural sign" (Figs. 22–10 and 22–11).[8, 11] The extrapleural sign is best appreciated when the primary beam passes tangent to the lesion. This may require supplemental oblique projections. A characteristic of the extrapleural sign is a concavity where the intrathoracic portion joins the thoracic wall. Lesions capable of producing the extrapleural sign include any process by which tissue pro-

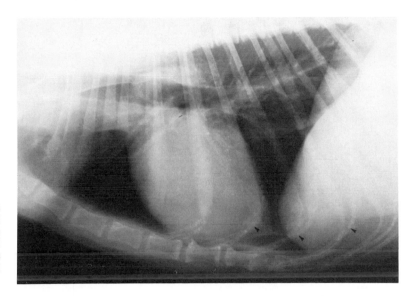

Figure 22–12. Lateral thoracic radiograph of a dog with stippled mineralization *(arrowheads)* of the costal cartilages. This is a normal finding, and usually progresses from caudal to cranial as the animal matures.

trudes inward from outside the parietal pleura. Examples are primary costal neoplasia,[11] metastatic costal neoplasia, subpleural hemorrhage,[11] primary pleural neoplasia, metastatic pleural neoplasia, and healing fractures of the ribs. Mesothelioma[18] is a good example of a lesion that should produce the extrapleural sign. Unfortunately, this lesion often produces severe pleural effusion that precludes visualization of the extrapleural sign.

Sternum

Stippled mineralization of costal cartilages[12] is probably the most frequent radiographic obser-

vation associated with the sternum. This finding (Fig. 22–12) is generally of no clinical significance,[6, 7] is most often a normal aging change, and usually progresses from caudal to cranial as the patient grows older. Pathologic changes in sternal cartilage opacity, shape, or location are very rarely observed but can be produced by neoplasia,[17] chronic inflammation,[11, 17] or trauma.[7, 14, 17] If pathologic, such changes should be expected to be accompanied by other radiographic signs, such as displacement of adjacent costal cartilages, focal or diffuse intercostal opacity, or the extrapleural sign.

Pectus excavatum (Fig. 22–13) and other ster-

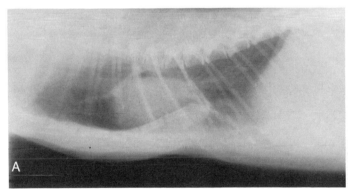

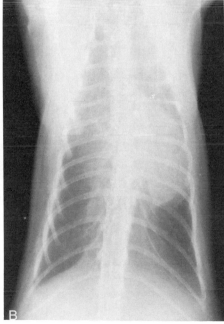

Figure 22–13. Lateral *(A)* and dorsoventral *(B)* thoracic radiographs of a cat with pectus excavatum. The heart is displaced dorsally and to the left by the sternal deformity. This cat does not have peritoneopericardial diaphragmatic hernia. Sternebra number is normal in this cat.

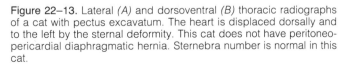

nal anomalies (including fewer than normal numbers of sternebrae and sternal dysraphism) have been seen in animals with congenital peritoneopericardial diaphragmatic hernias.[5, 17] Pectus excavatum and peritoneopericardial diaphragmatic hernia are congenital defects that occur at roughly the same time during gestational development, suggesting a more than casual relationship between sternal conformation and the other two lesions. In the lateral projection, radiographic signs of pectus excavatum include dorsal displacement of the caudal sternum and, secondarily, the cardiac silhouette. In dorsoventral or ventrodorsal views, the heart is usually displaced to the left.[7] There may be fewer than eight sternebrae, and the presence of a silhouette sign joining the ventral diaphragm and the caudal cardiac shadow is highly suggestive of concomitant congenital peritoneopericardial diaphragmatic hernia.[17]

References

1. Bhargava AK, Burt JK, Rudy RL, and Wilson GP: Diagnosis of mediastinal and heart base tumors in dogs using contrast pleurography. J Am Vet Radiol Soc, 11:56, 1970.
2. Bhargava AK, Rudy RL, and Diesem CD: Radiographic anatomy of the pleura in dogs as visualized by contrast radiography. J Am Vet Radiol Soc, 10:61, 1969.
3. Burt JK: Contrast pleurography. In Ticer JW (Ed): Radiographic Technique in Small Animal Practice. Philadelphia, WB Saunders, 1974.
4. Douglas SW, and Williamson HD: Veterinary Radiological Interpretation. Philadelphia, Lea & Febiger, 1970.
5. Evans SK, and Biery DN: Congenital peritoneoperi-cardial diaphragmatic hernia in the dog and cat: a literature review and 17 additional case histories. Vet Radiol, 21:108, 1980.
6. Gillette EL, Thrall DE, and Lebel JL: Carlson's Veterinary Radiology, 3rd ed. Philadelphia, Lea & Febiger, 1977.
7. Kealy JK: Diagnostic Radiology of the Dog and Cat. Philadelphia, WB Saunders, 1979.
8. Lord PF, Suter PF, Chan KF, Appleford M, and Root CR: Pleural, extrapleural, and pulmonary lesions in small animals: a radiographic approach to differential diagnosis. J Am Vet Radiol Soc, 13:4, 1972.
9. Morgan JP: Radiology in Veterinary Orthopedics. Philadelphia, Lea & Febiger, 1972.
10. Morgan JP, Carlson WD, and Adams OR: Hereditary multiple exostosis in the horse. J Am Vet Med Assoc, 140:1320, 1962.
11. Myer W: Radiography review: the extrapleural space. J Am Vet Radiol Soc, 14:157, 1978.
12. Owens JM: Radiographic Interpretation for the Small Animal Clinician. St Louis, Ralston Purina Co, 1982.
13. Pool RR, and Carrig CB: Multiple cartilaginous exostoses in a cat. Vet Pathol, 9:350, 1972.
14. Roenigk WJ: Injuries to the thorax. J Am Anim Hosp Assoc, 7:266, 1971.
15. Rudy RL, Bhargava AK, and Roenigk WJ: Contrast pleurography: a new technique for the radiographic visualization of the pleura and its various reflections in dogs. Radiology 91:1034, 1968.
16. Schebitz H, and Wilkens H: Atlas of Radiographic Anatomy of Dog and Cat, 3rd ed. Berlin, Paul Parey, 1977.
17. Suter PF: Thoracic Radiography: A Text Atlas of Thoracic Diseases of the Dog and Cat. Wettswil, Switzerland, Peter F Suter, 1984.
18. Thrall DE, and Goldschmidt MH: Mesothelioma in the dog: six case reports. J Am Vet Radiol Soc, 19:107, 1978.
19. Ticer JW: Radiographic Technique in Veterinary Practice, 2nd ed. Philadelphia, WB Saunders, 1984.

CHAPTER 23

THE DIAPHRAGM

RICHARD D. PARK

The diaphragm is a musculocutaneous partition between the thoracic and abdominal cavities. Embryologically, the diaphragm is formed by the septum transversum ventrally and by the mesentery of the foregut and two pleuroperitoneal folds dorsally.

The diaphragm assists with respiration. It provides approximately 50 percent of the mechanical respiratory force for inspiration.[1] The diaphragm and other skeletal muscles that assist respiration are the only skeletal muscles the continuous function of which is necessary to sustain life.

The diaphragm also acts as a mechanical partition or barrier between the thorax and abdomen; lymph vessels do penetrate and drain from subdiaphragmatic structures through the diaphragm to thoracic lymph nodes and vessels. This may be one explanation as to why an infectious peritonitis may extend through the diaphragm and develop into an infectious pleuritis. Lymph flow from the thorax to the abdomen does not occur.[2]

The diaphragm consists of a tendinous center and three thin peripheral muscles: the pars lumbalis, pars costalis, and pars sternalis. The pars lumbalis consists of the right and left crura, which attach to the cranial ventral part of L_4 and the body of L_3. The pars costalis attaches in an oblique direction to the 13th through 8th ribs, and the pars sternalis attaches to the xyphoid cartilage.[3] The diaphragm is convex and extends into the thorax from its attachments. In doing so, the phrenicocostalis and phrenicolumbalis recesses are created. There are three openings through the diaphragm: the aortic and esophageal hiatuses and the caudal caval foramen.

NORMAL RADIOGRAPHIC ANATOMY

Radiographically, only a small portion of the diaphragm can be visualized on any one view. It appears as a thin, convex structure of water opacity extending in a cranial and ventral direction. Radiographic visualization of the diaphragm is dependent on adjacent structures being of different opacity. Most of the thoracic surface is visible because of the adjacent gas-filled lungs. Parts of the thoracic surface are not visualized where lung is not in contact with the diaphragm, i.e., the phrenicocostalis and phrenicolumbalis recesses. A large portion of the abdominal surface is not seen because of the adjacent liver. The ventral abdominal diaphragmatic surface is visible on the lateral view when fat is present within the falciform ligament, and the dorsal abdominal surface can be seen if gas is present within the gastric fundus.

245

Diaphragmatic structures that may be distinctly visualized radiographically are the right and left crura, the intercrural cleft, and the cupula (body) (Figs. 23–1 to 23–4). Associated structures that may also be seen are the phrenic origin of the caudal vena cava and the caudal ventral mediastinum. On the lateral view, the right crus of the diaphragm blends with the caudal vena caval border and the gastric fundus may be seen adjacent to the abdominal surface of the left crus. The intercrural cleft is a shorter, convex, opaque line caudal and ventral to the crura (Figs. 23–1 and 23–2). The cupula is the most cranial, convex portion of the diaphragm on both the lateral and the dorsoventral/ventrodorsal view. Also, on this view, the thoracic surface of the diaphragm may be visualized as one, two, or three convex projections into the thoracic cavity (Figs. 23–3 and 23–4).

Several normal variations of diaphragmatic position and shape may be seen radiographically. Factors that cause this variable appearance are both real and apparent. Real factors consist of breed, age, obesity, respiration, and gravity. Apparent factors are x-ray beam centering and animal positioning during radiography. When all permutations of these variables are considered, over 51,000 combinations are possible.[4] Obviously, most of these variables are not radiographically significant; however,

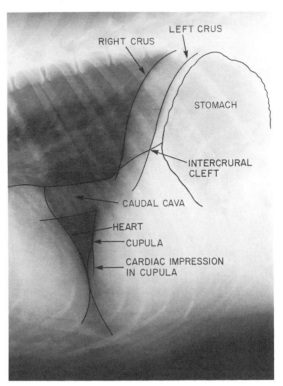

Figure 23–2. Right lateral recumbent view of a normal diaphragm in a dog.

some must be recognized and understood. Changes that are most apparent radiographically are the position, shape, and visualization of the cupula and crura. The relative position of the crura is most dependent on position and size of the animal and primary x-ray beam centering.

The most dependent crus is displaced cranially when an animal is in lateral recumbency. In right lateral recumbency, the crura appear to be parallel (Fig. 23–2); in left lateral recumbency, they sometimes appear to cross (Fig. 23–1). The crura also appear to be more extensively separated, i.e., up to 2.5 vertebral lengths, if the animal is slightly rotated or if the x-ray beam is centered over the mid or cranial thorax.[4]

The radiographic appearance of the diaphragm varies with the x-ray beam centering in the ventrodorsal/dorsoventral projections. The diaphragm may appear as a single, dome-shaped structure (Fig. 23–4) or as two or three separate domed structures (Fig. 23–3). The three structures represent the cupula and two crura. A single, domed diaphragm may be seen on a ventrodorsal or dorsoventral view when the x-ray beam is centered on the midabdomen or midthorax, respectively. Two or three separate domed structures are seen when the animal is in the ventrodorsal position and the x-ray beam

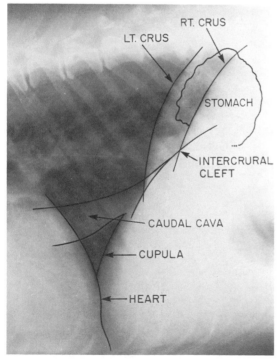

Figure 23–1. Left lateral recumbent radiograph of a normal diaphragm in a dog.

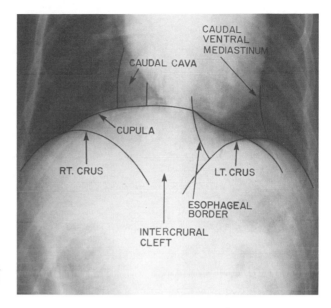

Figure 23–3. Ventrodorsal/dorsoventral view of a normal diaphragm in a dog with the cupula and both crura projecting into the thorax

is centered on the midthorax or on a dorsoventral view with the x-ray beam centered on the midabdomen.[4]

The diaphragmatic position and shape vary with respiration and intra-abdominal pressure. The normal intersection point of the diaphragm and spine is between T_{11} and T_{13} but may vary between T_9 and L_1. The diaphragm changes position with normal respiration from one half to two vertebral lengths. On extreme inspiration, the diaphragm changes position and shape. On a lateral thoracic view, the diaphragm is more caudal and lies horizontally; the shape changes from convex to straight. The diaphragm is displaced cranially by increased intra-abdominal pressure, which in turn may be produced by obesity, ascites, gastric or intestinal distension, abdominal pain, and abdominal masses.

Separate diaphragmatic structures are not seen as distinctly in a cat, probably because of the small relative thoracic size (Fig. 23–5). On extreme inspiration, particularly if the animal is in respiratory distress, small symmetric muscle projections are noted from the thoracic diaphragmatic surface in the ventrodorsal/dorsoventral view (Fig. 23–6).

Figure 23–4. Ventrodorsal/dorsoventral view of a normal diaphragm in a dog with only one convex shape projecting into the thorax.

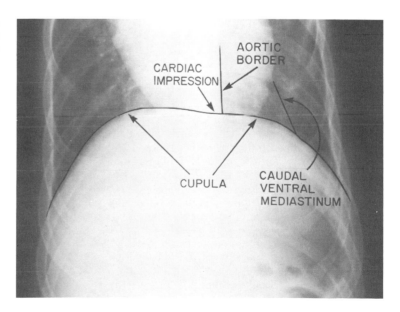

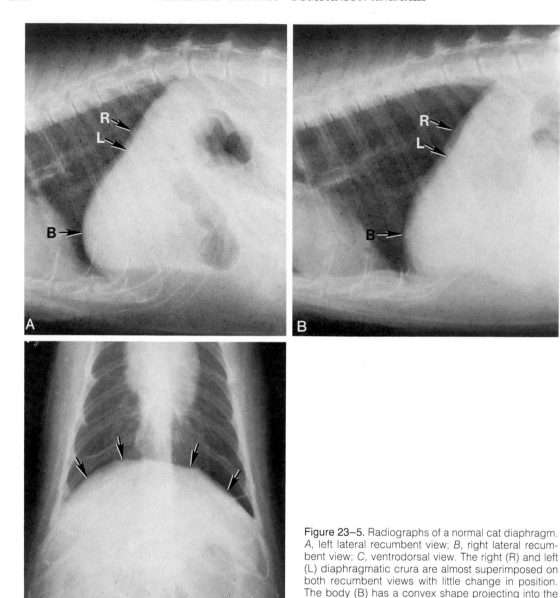

Figure 23–5. Radiographs of a normal cat diaphragm. *A,* left lateral recumbent view; *B,* right lateral recumbent view; *C,* ventrodorsal view. The right (R) and left (L) diaphragmatic crura are almost superimposed on both recumbent views with little change in position. The body (B) has a convex shape projecting into the thorax. In *C,* the diaphragm projects as a single convex shadow into the caudal thorax *(arrows).*

RADIOGRAPHIC SIGNS OF DIAPHRAGMATIC DISEASE

The signs associated directly with the diaphragm are not as numerous and specific as are found in many other organs. Radiographic changes observed most frequently with diaphragmatic disease are general or local outline loss of the thoracic diaphragmatic surface and changes in diaphragmatic shape and position (Table 23–1).

The thoracic diaphragmatic surface outline may be obliterated or not visualized radiographically if anything of the same opacity, i.e., organs of water opacity or fluid, is adjacent to the surface. Changes in the diaphragm shape occur most frequently on the cupula; they are

often normal and are caused by contact with the heart (Fig. 23–7) or the position of the animal during radiography. Thoracic masses adjacent to the diaphragm, hiatal and small traumatic diaphragmatic hernias, and chronic pleural inflammatory reactions are the most frequent causes of shape changes. An asymmetric diaphragmatic shape may occur with unilateral tension pneumothorax or hemiparalysis. Suspected hemiparalysis should be confirmed by observing respiration under fluoroscopy.

Positional changes consist of cranial and caudal displacement. Because the position of the diaphragm varies with the respiratory cycle, marginal changes are difficult to diagnose and in most instances not clinically significant. Se-

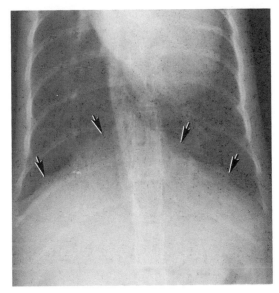

Figure 23–6. Ventrodorsal view of a normal cat diaphragm on deep inspiration. Small, regularly spaced projections *(arrows)* are evident along the thoracic diaphragmatic surface. These reflect pulling against the costal attachments of the diaphragm.

vere positional changes may be significant and indicative of thoracic or abdominal disease. Cranial diaphragmatic displacement is usually associated with abdominal disease (Table 23–1) or generalized diaphragmatic paralysis, which should be confirmed with fluoroscopic observation. In some cases, pleural fluid between the lungs and diaphragm produces a pseudodiaphragm. This occurrence should not be mistaken for the actual diaphragmatic outline. Caudal diaphragmatic displacement is usually associated with severe respiratory disease (Fig. 23–8). The caudally positioned diaphragm is an attempt by the animal to increase the level of systemic PO_2, which may be low because of ventilation or perfusion deficiencies in the lungs. Bilateral tension pneumothorax may also

TABLE 23–1. RADIOGRAPHIC SIGNS OF DIAPHRAGMATIC DISEASES

Radiographic Signs	Causes
General loss of thoracic surface outline	Bilateral pleural fluid Generalized pulmonary disease in caudal lung lobes
Localized or partial loss of the thoracic surface outline	Thoracic masses adjacent to the diaphragm Diaphragmatic hernias Focal pulmonary disease in caudal lung lobes
Shape changes	Displacement of the cupula caused by contact with the heart Thoracic masses adjacent to the diaphragm Hiatal hernias Small diaphragmatic hernias Pleural reaction on the diaphragmatic surface Neoplasia Hemiparalysis of the diaphragm Unilateral tension pneumothorax
Position changes—cranial displacement	Obesity Peritoneal fluid Abdominal pain Abdominal masses or organ enlargement; liver enlargement and masses frequently cause cranial displacement Generalized diaphragmatic paralysis
Position changes—caudal displacement	Severe respiratory distress—ventilation or perfusion problems Tension pneumothorax

Figure 23–7. Ventrodorsal view of a normal diaphragm in a dog. A cardiac impression *(solid arrows)* is present on the diaphragmatic body (cupula). The left diaphragmatic crus *(open arrows)* is distinctly visible. The right crus cannot be visualized as a separate structure.

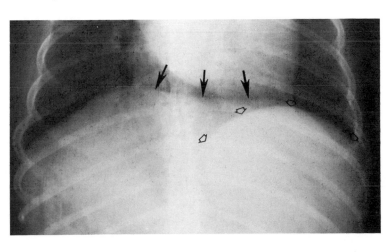

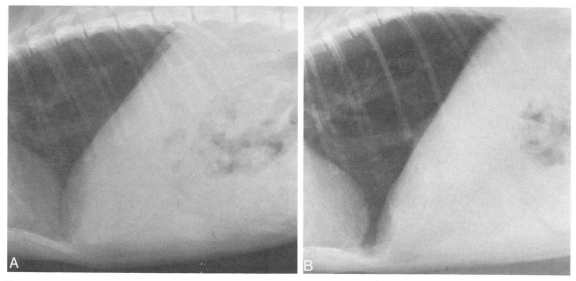

Figure 23–8. Lateral views of the diaphragm in a cat. *A*, on expiration; *B*, on extreme inspiration. The entire diaphragm is displaced caudally with inspiration and has a more flat contour when compared with the expiratory radiograph.

cause a caudally displaced diaphragm from increased pleural pressure. In most instances of pneumothorax, however, the caudally displaced diaphragm is probably an attempt to increase respiratory ventilation.

Although many of the general radiographic signs of diaphragmatic disease are not specific, they should be observed and their cause should be determined. In some instances, additional radiographic studies, i.e., positional views or contrast medium studies, may be indicated to determine the cause of the radiographic signs observed.

DIAPHRAGMATIC DISEASES

Diseases of the diaphragm include traumatic and congenitally predisposed hernias and motor or innervation disturbances. Diaphragmatic hernias are the most frequent diaphragmatic diseases diagnosed in the dog and cat.

Diaphragmatic Hernias

A diaphragmatic hernia is a protrusion of abdominal viscera through the diaphragm into the thorax. Diaphragmatic hernias that can be recognized radiographically include traumatic, peritoneal-pericardial, hiatal, mediastinal, and congenital diaphragmatic defects.

Abdominal trauma is the key etiologic factor with most types of diaphragmatic hernias. A high momentary increase in abdominal pressure when the glottis is open produces a high pleuroperitoneal pressure gradient that may result in a diaphragmatic hernia. The high pleuroperitoneal gradient may produce a rent in the muscular portion of the diaphragm or herniate abdominal viscera through congenitally weak or defective areas. Clinical signs that may be observed with diaphragmatic hernias are pain, vomiting, regurgitation, muffled heart sounds, and a weak femoral pulse.[5, 6] Some diaphragmatic hernias may be clinically silent and are detected incidentally on thoracic radiographs.

Radiology plays an important role in confirming a diagnosis of diaphragmatic hernia, and may provide information about location, extent, contents, and secondary complications associated with the hernia.[7] If a diagnosis cannot be confirmed from survey radiographic signs (Table 23–2), additional radiographic procedures may be performed to add further information. These procedures consist of administering barium sulfate per os, positional radiographic views, removing pleural fluid and re-examining the thorax, and peritoneography.

A small amount (20 to 40 ml) of barium sulfate (30 percent w/v) can be given per os and radiographs may be obtained in 15 to 20 minutes. The barium outlines the position of the stomach and proximal small bowel (Fig. 23–9). Positional radiographs made with a horizontal x-ray beam

TABLE 23–2. RADIOGRAPHIC SIGNS ASSOCIATED WITH TRAUMATIC DIAPHRAGMATIC HERNIA

Abdominal viscera within the thorax
Displacement of abdominal structures
Displacement of thoracic structures
Partial or complete loss of the thoracic
    diaphragmatic surface outline
Pleural fluid

help to identify solid organ structures that are not easily gravitated within the thorax (Fig. 23–10). Thoracocentesis and pleural fluid removal followed by another radiographic examination provide better radiographic visualization of thoracic structures. Peritoneography with positive (tri-iodinated) contrast medium may be used to identify a communication between the abdomen and thorax through the diaphragm.[8, 9] Any or all of these procedures may be used, but the most simple procedures should be used first. Peritoneography with tri-iodinated contrast medium should be used after other diagnostic procedures have failed to provide the needed information.

Traumatic Diaphragmatic Hernias

Traumatic diaphragmatic hernias usually involve the muscular part of the diaphragm.[6, 10] In one report, it is suggested that there is equal incidence on right and left sides;[10] another states there is a higher incidence on the right side in the dog.[6] The organs that herniate through the diaphragm most frequently, in order, are:

liver, small bowel, stomach, spleen, and omentum.[6, 10, 11]

The most consistent radiographic signs with traumatic diaphragmatic hernias are: abdominal viscera within the thorax, displacement of abdominal or thoracic organs, or both, partial or complete loss of the thoracic diaphragmatic surface outline, and pleural fluid (Fig. 23–11).

Identification of abdominal structures in the thorax is a conclusive sign of a diaphragmatic hernia. Small bowel is easily identified when it is gas-filled; when fluid-filled, it appears as a tubular structure. The stomach may be filled with gas, fluid, or ingested material. Ingested material usually has a granular appearance and is easily identified radiographically. In addition, gastric rugal folds may provide a marker for identifying the stomach within the thorax. A herniated, gas-distended stomach may appear as a unilateral left pneumothorax and should be corrected immediately by surgical intervention (Fig. 23–12).[6] Such instances are life-threatening because of potential or actual cardiovascular tamponade.

Herniated solid abdominal parenchymal or-

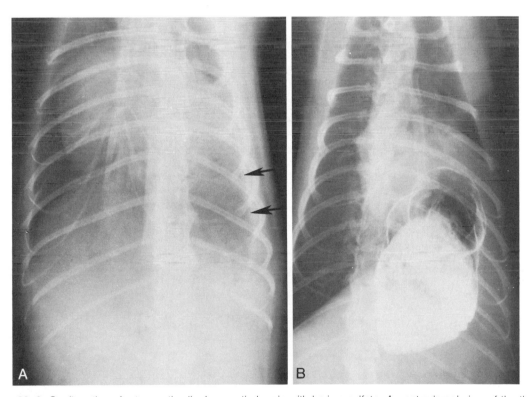

Figure 23–9. Confirmation of a traumatic diaphragmatic hernia with barium sulfate. *A,* ventrodorsal view of the thorax of a cat. There is increased soft-tissue opacity in the left caudal thorax with obliteration of the left diaphragmatic outline. There is displacement of the left caudal lung lobe away from the thoracic wall *(arrows)* by pleural fluid. The heart is displaced toward the right thoracic wall, which may be accentuated by the slightly oblique position of the animal. *B,* the stomach is easily identified in the left caudal thorax opacified with barium sulfate, thus confirming a left-sided diaphragmatic hernia.

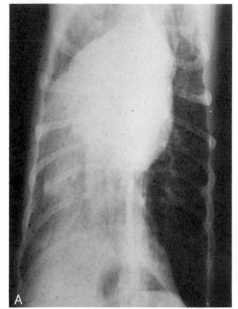

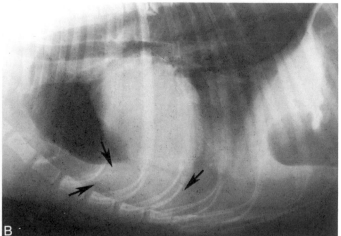

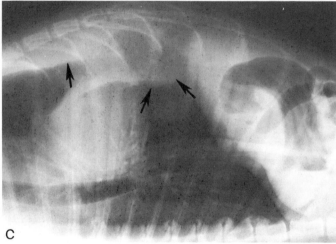

Figure 23–10. Ventrodorsal *(A),* lateral *(B),* and dorsal *(C)* recumbent, horizontal-beam lateral views of a traumatic diaphragmatic hernia. *A,* there is an increased soft-tissue opacity in the caudal right thorax with loss of the thoracic diaphragmatic surface outline over the cupula. *B,* the heart is displaced dorsally and a soft-tissue opacity is between the heart and the sternum *(arrows).* The thoracic diaphragmatic outline is indistinct over the cupula. *C,* the soft tissue opacity *(arrows)* remains in the same position, which would indicate that the opacity is a solid structure and is not free pleural fluid. This finding could be compatible with a diaphragmatic hernia.

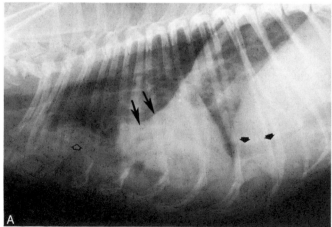

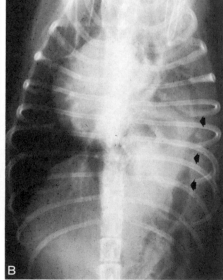

Figure 23–11. Lateral *(A)* and ventrodorsal *(B)* views of the thorax of a dog with a traumatic diaphragmatic hernia. Radiographic signs compatible with a diaphragmatic hernia in *A* are: gas and ingesta-filled bowel *(open arrow)* within the thorax, cranial displacement of abdominal structures, i.e., small bowel *(small solid arrows),* and a cranially displaced diaphragmatic segment *(large solid arrows).* Radiographic signs in *B* are: a heart displaced away from the herniated viscera; gas-filled small bowel within the thorax *(arrows);* cranially displaced abdominal structures, i.e., small bowel, stomach, and liver; and loss of the left diaphragmatic surface outline.

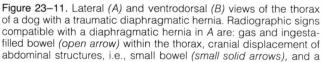

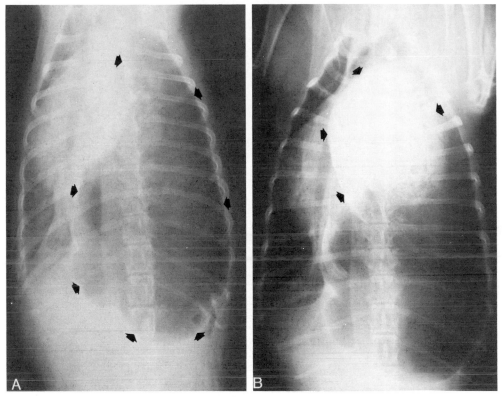

Figure 23–12. Ventrodorsal views of the thorax without (A) and with (B) barium in the stomach. A, the gas-filled stomach (arrows) is herniated into the left hemithorax simulating a unilateral tension pneumothorax; it displaces the heart and lungs to the right side. The normal gastric and left diaphragmatic outlines are not present. B, barium is present in the cranial stomach (arrows), with severe gaseous gastric distension.

gans are difficult to distinguish from localized pleural fluid, pulmonary opacity, or both. Omentum is the most difficult to detect unless it is herniated in association with other abdominal organs. In such instances, it provides a fat opacity and helps to outline other abdominal visceral organs.

In the absence of identifying abdominal organs in the thorax, cranial abdominal organ displacement or absence of organs from their normal location serves as an excellent radiographic sign for identifying diaphragmatic hernias. The liver, spleen, and stomach are organs to check most closely for displacement. Including the cranial abdomen on the thoracic radiograph when diaphragmatic hernia is suspected is helpful to evaluate abdominal organ displacement. Barium sulfate may also be administered to mark the stomach and to help detect mild to moderate gastric displacement not observed on survey radiographs.

Thoracic structures may also be displaced, depending on the amount and position of abdominal organs within the thorax. The heart, mediastinum, and lungs may be displaced. The heart and lungs are usually displaced cranially and to one side by herniated abdominal viscera, and the mediastinum is usually displaced laterally from its normal midline position.

A localized, diaphragmatic surface outline loss usually indicates the area through which the diaphragmatic hernia has occurred. Abdominal viscera and pleural fluid adjacent to the thoracic diaphragmatic surface cause the outline loss. This occurrence must be distinguished from the many other thoracic conditions that produce a water opacity adjacent to the diaphragm. Occasionally, the torn diaphragmatic segment or muscle may be displaced in a cranial direction from the diaphragm, producing an almost horizontal diaphragm outline in one area. When present, this is a reliable radiographic sign of diaphragmatic hernia.

Pleural fluid is consistently present with chronic diaphragmatic hernias or if a herniated abdominal organ is strangulated through a small diaphragmatic opening. Pleural fluid is a nonspecific sign of a diaphragmatic hernia and often masks other more important radiographic signs. Thoracocentesis and aspiration of the pleural fluid is often necessary before a diagnostic examination can be made.

Congenitally Predisposed Diaphragmatic Hernias

Included in this group are peritoneal-pericardial diaphragmatic hernias, hiatal hernias, and diaphragmatic defects. Defects in diaphragmatic development may be present and yet never result in a hernia or may occur in an animal of any age after some form of abdominal trauma or transitory increase in intra-abdominal pressure.

Peritoneal-Pericardial Diaphragmatic Hernias. A peritoneal-pericardial diaphragmatic hernia is produced when abdominal viscera herniate into the pericardial sac through a congenital hiatus formed between the tendinous portion of the diaphragm and the pericardial sac. They have been reported in litter mates,[12] and it has been suggested that this trait is carried on a simple autosomal recessive gene in cats, with a 1:500 to 1:1500 rate of incidence.[13] The hernia may have been present from birth or it may have been caused by increased intra-abdominal pressure. Even mild increases in intra-abdominal pressure may cause abdominal organs to herniate through a congenital hiatus.

Peritoneal-pericardial hernias may produce clinical signs or they may be an incidental finding on radiographs of the thorax. These hernias may be present in old and in young animals,[5, 14-18] with the liver, stomach, omentum, and small bowel most frequently herniated.

Radiographic signs associated with peritoneal-pericardial hernias are listed in Table 23–3. Herniated abdominal organs in the pericardial sac are usually caudal or caudal and lateral to the heart. Gas- or ingesta-filled hollow visceral organs are usually not difficult to identify within the pericardial sac. Radiographically, a gas opacity within the bowel is in abrupt contrast to the adjacent structures of water opacity. As stated previously, ingested material usually has a granular appearance radiographically. Solid parenchymal organs, unless surrounded by omentum, are difficult to distinguish as separate structures within the pericardium. When abdominal organs are herniated into the pericardial sac,

TABLE 23–3. RADIOGRAPHIC SIGNS ASSOCIATED WITH PERITONEAL-PERICARDIAL DIAPHRAGMATIC HERNIAS

Abdominal organs identified in the pericardial sac. Gas, ingested material, or structures of soft-tissue opacity may be present
Large, round cardiac silhouette
Convex projection of the caudal cardiac silhouette
Indistinguishable border of the ventral thoracic diaphragmatic surface and the caudal ventral cardiac silhouette
Confluent silhouette between the diaphragm and the heart

cranial and ventral organ displacement within the abdomen may be seen, but the displacement is usually not as pronounced as that noted with traumatic diaphragmatic hernias.

The large, round cardiac silhouette and a cardiac silhouette with an abnormal convex projection on the caudal border are signs consistent with peritoneal-pericardial diaphragmatic hernias. These two signs are dependent on the amount of abdominal viscera within the pericardial sac. Large amounts of viscera produce a large, round cardiac silhouette, whereas smaller amounts, such as a portion of the liver or stomach, may produce an abnormal convex caudal cardiac border. A large, round silhouette must be differentiated from pericardial effusion, generalized heart enlargement, or both. An abnormally convex caudal cardiac border must be differentiated from neoplasia, pleural granulomas, or localized pleural fluid.

An indistinguishable outline to the ventral diaphragmatic surface and the caudal ventral cardiac silhouette is produced by the communication between the two structures. This finding must be differentiated from normal contact between the heart and diaphragm, pleural fluid, localized pleuritis, and pleural granulomas.

An apparently confluent silhouette between the heart and diaphragm may appear as a wide caudal mediastinum; depending on the size of the communication, it may or may not be seen radiographically. This confluent silhouette must also be differentiated from other pathologic conditions that have been listed. Additional radiographic studies that may be performed to confirm a diagnosis are barium sulfate per os, nonselective angiography,[19] peritoneography, and pericardiography. Barium sulfate may be used to demonstrate gastrointestinal structures within the pericardial sac or cranial ventral displacement of abdominal structures (Fig. 23–13).

Nonselective angiography is easy to perform. The procedure results in heart chamber opacification, thus differentiating the heart from other possible structures in the pericardial sac. Peritoneography with negative or positive contrast medium may be used. For this study, the animal is positioned to gravitate contrast medium from the peritoneum into the pericardial sac. This positioning may not be successful because of the inability to gravitate contrast medium through a small or obstructed hiatus. As a result, false-negative results may be seen.

Pericardiography is an acceptable technique if used properly and with extreme caution. Pericardiography may produce external pressure on the heart and may increase or create a cardiac tamponade. A small amount (5 ml) of tri-iodinated contrast medium is used for pericardiography in suspected instances of perito-

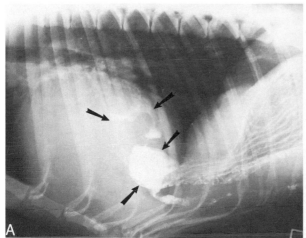

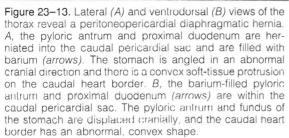

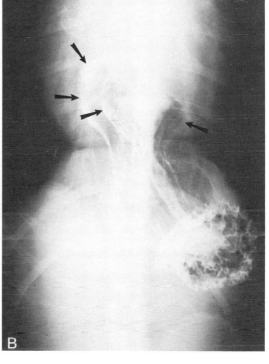

Figure 23–13. Lateral *(A)* and ventrodorsal *(B)* views of the thorax reveal a peritoneopericardial diaphragmatic hernia. *A,* the pyloric antrum and proximal duodenum are herniated into the caudal pericardial sac and are filled with barium *(arrows).* The stomach is angled in an abnormal cranial direction and there is a convex soft-tissue protrusion on the caudal heart border. *B,* the barium-filled pyloric antrum and proximal duodenum *(arrows)* are within the caudal pericardial sac. The pyloric antrum and fundus of the stomach are displaced cranially, and the caudal heart border has an abnormal, convex shape.

neal pericardial diaphragmatic hernias. A negative-contrast study may require larger quantities of gas and would therefore have a greater potential to produce a serious cardiac tamponade. Negative-contrast pericardiography is not recommended as a diagnostic procedure to confirm the diagnosis of a peritoneal pericardial diaphragmatic hernia.

Hiatal Hernias. Hiatal hernias are produced when a portion of stomach enters the thorax through the esophageal hiatus. These hernias are reported to occur through a congenitally or traumatically enlarged esophageal hiatus, and also can result from contraction of the longitudinal esophageal muscle.[20, 21]

There are three types of hiatal hernias: sliding, paraesophageal, and gastroesophageal intussusceptions. The caudal esophageal sphincter and a portion of the stomach, usually the cardia, are herniated into the thorax with sliding hiatal hernias.[22] Sliding hiatal hernias are usually also associated with esophagitis from gastroesophageal reflux. As the name implies, the caudal esophagus and cardia slide intermittently from the abdomen into the thorax. Because the hernia is dynamic, it may not be seen on any one static radiograph; fluoroscopy is sometimes necessary to make a diagnosis. The number of reported cases of sliding hiatal hernia in animals is not high.[23-25] The low incidence may be a reflection of the subtle clinical signs and intermittent manifestations on static radiographs.

Paraesophageal hiatal hernia is the herniation of the cardia and fundus through the esophageal hiatus lying adjacent to the distal esophagus. They are usually static and do not slide between the thorax and abdomen, and the caudal esophageal sphincter is in a normal position.[21, 22] The herniated stomach may cause esophageal obstruction from external pressure on the caudal esophagus. Gastroesophageal intussusceptions occur when the stomach invaginates through the esophageal hiatus into the caudal esophagus;[21, 26] it also causes esophageal obstruction.

The most consistent clinical sign observed with hiatal hernias is regurgitation. This condition may be suspected from the clinical signs and survey radiographic findings, but it must be confirmed with an esophagram. Paraesophageal hiatal hernias and gastroesophageal intussusceptions cause esophageal obstruction and must be corrected surgically.

Radiographic signs consist of survey findings and those observed with an esophagram (Table 23–4). The most consistent survey radiographic sign is stomach displacement. The cardia appears to be stretched toward the diaphragm or may extend into the thorax. This displacement produces an abnormal shape to the cardia and fundus remaining in the abdomen. The caudal esophagus may or may not be distended and a soft-tissue opacity (mass) may be seen adjacent to the left diaphragmatic crura. The size and visibility of this mass depends on the amount

TABLE 23–4. RADIOGRAPHIC SIGNS ASSOCIATED WITH HIATAL HERNIAS

Survey Radiographs

Soft-tissue opacity (mass) adjacent to the left diaphragmatic crura
Moderately dilated caudal thoracic esophagus
Cranially displaced stomach, cardia, or cardia and fundus

Esophagram

Dilated esophagus
Cardia and caudal esophageal sphincter cranial to the diaphragm—sliding hiatal hernia
External pressure on and displacement of the distal esophagus by a barium-filled cardia and fundus—paraesophageal hiatal hernia
Intraluminal filling defect in the caudal esophagus and the outline of rugal folds—gastroesophageal intussusception

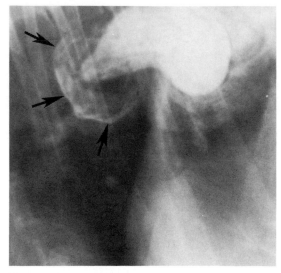

Figure 23–15. Lateral view of the thorax shows barium outlining a paraesophageal hiatal hernia. The barium outlines the gastric cardia *(arrows)*, which is cranial to the diaphragm. The cardia has herniated through the esophageal hiatus beside the caudal esophagus, which is not opacified.

of stomach that has actually herniated in the thorax.

A dilated caudal esophagus is usually best seen on an esophagram. An esophagram is also helpful to differentiate the types of hiatal hernia. The caudal esophageal sphincter and a portion of the cardia are seen cranial to the diaphragm with a sliding hiatal hernia.[27] The caudal esophageal sphincter can be identified as a concentric, smooth 1 to 2-cm narrowing in the caudal esophagus (Fig. 23–14). Displacement and narrowing of the caudal esophagus by the cardia and fundus is seen with paraesophageal hiatal hernias, along with barium opacification of the herniated stomach (Fig. 23–15).

Gastroesophageal intussusceptions produce a large intraluminal filling defect within the caudal esophagus, and rugal folds may be outlined when coated with barium (Fig. 23–16).

Diaphragmatic Defects. Congenital diaphragmatic defects in the dog and cat have been reported rarely.[28-31] The defects are created

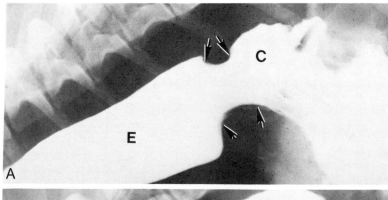

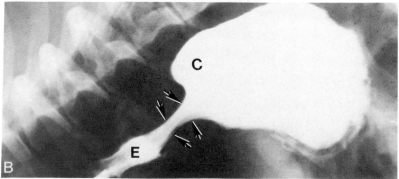

Figure 23–14. Lateral views of barium esophagram demonstrate a sliding hiatal hernia. *A,* contrast medium distends the distal esophagus (E), the caudal esophageal sphincter *(arrows)*, and the cardia (C). The caudal esophageal sphincter and gastric cardia are displaced cranial to the diaphragm through the esophageal hiatus. *B,* the esophagus (E) and caudal esophageal sphincter *(arrows)* are outlined, but are not distended with barium; most of the barium has passed into the stomach. The caudal esophageal sphincter and gastric cardia are herniated through the esophageal hiatus and are cranial to the diaphragm.

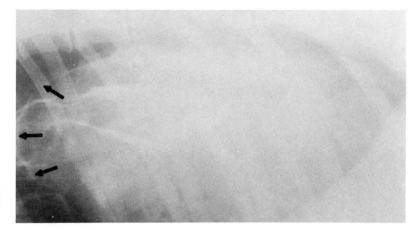

Figure 23–16. Lateral radiograph of the thorax reveals a gastroesophageal intussusception. Barium outlines its cranial aspect *(arrows)*. The large soft-tissue mass in the caudal dorsal thorax is the stomach intussuscepted into the caudal esophageal lumen.

when the septum transfers or the pleural peritoneal folds do not develop and fuse to form a complete diaphragm. The diaphragmatic defect allows abdominal viscera to enter the thoracic cavity and may produce clinical signs consistent with a traumatic diaphragmatic hernia.

In humans, diaphragmatic defects have a familial incidence with a multifactorial mode of inheritance.[32] Congenital defects in dogs have been reported in the muscular diaphragm, dorsolateral in position,[28] and in the membranous diaphragm associated with umbilical hernias.[29-31]

The radiographic signs of congenital diaphragmatic defects are the same as those listed for traumatic diaphragmatic hernias. With membranous defects, however, the liver is displaced cranially, while remaining in the caudal ventral thorax, often confined to the mediastinum (Fig. 23–17).

MOTOR DISTURBANCES OF THE DIAPHRAGM

The diaphragm is the principle muscle of respiration and is innervated by the phrenic nerve. Motor disturbances in most instances are clinically asymptomatic and as a result have not been well documented in animals.

Motor disturbances of the diaphragm consist of unilateral paralysis, bilateral paralysis, and diaphragmatic flutter.[1] Diaphragmatic paralysis may be produced by pneumonia, trauma, myopathies, and neuropathies, or the cause may be unidentified.[1] Diaphragmatic paralysis may be suspected from survey radiographs, i.e., cranial displacement of one or both diaphragmatic crura (Fig. 23–18). Confirmation of paralysis is best achieved with fluoroscopy. Unequal movement between the crura is seen with unilateral paralysis, and minimal or no diaphragmatic movement is noted with bilateral paralysis. Bi-

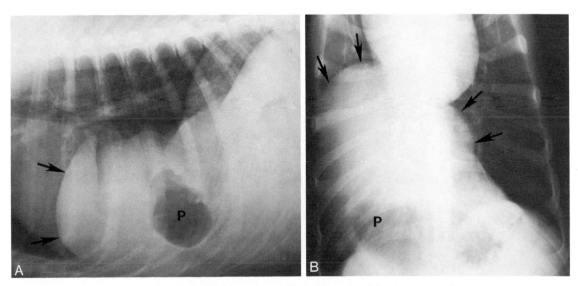

Figure 23–17. Recumbent left lateral *(A)* and ventrodorsal *(B)* radiographs of the thorax reveal a diaphragmatic defect. The defect was in the cupula, and the liver and stomach herniated into the thorax. The liver *(arrows)* and gas-filled pyloric antrum (P) are within the thorax. The stomach and liver are displaced cranially.

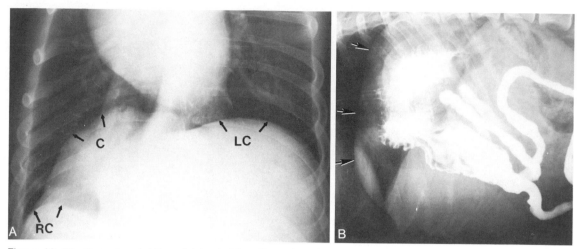

Figure 23–18. Ventrodorsal *(A)* and lateral *(B)* radiographs of the diaphragm. There is hemiparalysis of the left diaphragm. *A,* the left diaphragmatic crus is cranial to the right (LC). The cupula (C) and right crus (RC) are in a normal inspiratory position. *B,* the cranial position of the left diaphragmatic crus *(arrows)* causes the gastric cardia and fundus to be displaced cranially.

lateral paralysis may be more difficult to confirm with fluoroscopy, because diaphragmatic movement is sometimes produced by compensatory abdominal muscle contraction during respiration.

References

1. Shim C: Motor disturbances of the diaphragm. Clin Chest Med *1*:125, 1980.
2. Rivero O, and del Castillo H: Lymphatics of the diaphragm in the dog. Acta Radiol [Diagn] (Stockh) *17*:663, 1976.
3. Miller ME, Christensen GC, and Evans HE: Anatomy of the Dog. Philadelphia, WB Saunders, 1964, p. 178.
4. Grandage J: The radiology of the dog's diaphragm. J Small Anim Pract *15*:1, 1974.
5. Schulman J: Peritoneopericardial diaphragmatic hernia in a dog. Mod Vet Pract *60*:306, 1979.
6. Garson HL, Dodman NH, and Baker GJ: Diaphragmatic hernia. Analysis of fifty-six cases in dogs and cats. J Small Anim Pract *21*:469, 1980.
7. Silverman S, and Ackerman N: Radiographic evaluation of abdominal hernias. Mod Vet Pract *58*:781, 1977.
8. Rendano VT: Positive contrast peritoneography: An aid in the radiographic diagnosis of diaphragmatic hernia. J Am Vet Radiol Soc *20*:67, 1979.
9. Stickle RL: Positive contrast celiography (peritoneography) for the diagnosis of diaphragmatic hernia in dogs and cats. J Am Vet Med Assoc *185*:295, 1984.
10. Carb A: Diaphragmatic hernia in the dog and cat. Vet Clin North Am [Small Anim Pract] *5*:477, 1975.
11. Wilson GP, Newton CD, and Burt JK: A review of 116 diaphragmatic hernias in dogs and cats. J Am Vet Med Assoc *159*:1142, 1971.
12. Feldman DB, Bree MM, Cohen BJ: Congenital diaphragmatic hernia in neonatal dogs. J Am Vet Med Assoc *153*:942, 1968.
13. Saperstein G, Harris S, and Leipold HW: Congenital defects in domestic cats. Feline Pract *6*:18, 1976.
14. Bjorck GR, and Tigerschiold A: Peritoneopericardial diaphragmatic hernia in a dog. J Small Anim Pract *11*:585, 1970.
15. Gourley IM, Popp JA, and Park RD: Myelolipomas of the liver in a domestic cat. J Am Vet Med Assoc *158*:2053, 1971.
16. Rendano VT, and Parker RB: Polycystic kidneys and peritoneopericardial diaphragmatic hernia in the cat: A case report. J Small Anim Pract *17*:479, 1976.
17. Weitz J, Tilley LP, and Moldoff D: Pericardiodiaphragmatic hernia in a dog. J Am Vet Med Assoc *173*:1336, 1978.
18. Evans SM, and Biery DN: Congenital peritoneopericardial diaphragmatic hernia in the dog and cat. Vet Radiol *21*:108, 1980.
19. Willard MD, and Aronson E: Peritoneopericardial diaphragmatic hernia in a cat. J Am Vet Med Assoc *178*:481, 1981.
20. Edwards MH: Selective vagotomy of the canine oesophagus—a model for the treatment of hiatal hernia. Thorax *31*:185, 1976.
21. Teunissen GHB, Happé RP, Van Toorenburg J, et al: Esophageal hiatal hernia; case report of a dog and a cheetah. Tijdschr. Diergeneesk *103*:742, 1978.
22. Ellis Jr FH: Controversies regarding the management of hiatus hernia. Am J Surg *139*:782, 1980.
23. Rogers WA, and Donovan EF: Peptic esophagitis in a dog. J Am Vet Med Assoc *163*:462, 1973.
24. Gaskell CJ, Gibbs C, and Pearson H: Sliding hiatus hernia with reflex oesophagitis in two dogs. J Small Anim Pract *15*:503, 1974.
25. Iwasaki M, DeMartin BW, DeAlvarenga J, et al.: Congenital hiatal hernia in a dog. Mod Vet Pract *58*:1018, 1977.
26. Pollock S, and Rhodes WH: Gastroesophageal intussusception in an Afghan hound. J Am Vet Radiol Soc *11*:5, 1970.
27. Steiner GM: Gastro-oesophageal reflux, hiatus hernia and the radiologist with special reference to children. Br J Radiol *50*:164, 1977.
28. Bath GF: Congenital diaphragmatic hiatus in a dog. Case report. J S Afr Vet Assoc *47*:55, 1976.
29. Nicholson C: Defective diaphragm associated with umbilical hernia. Vet Rec *98*:433, 1976.
30. Sawyer SL: Defective diaphragm associated with umbilical hernia. Vet Rec *98*:490, 1976.
31. Swift BJ: Defective diaphragm associated with umbilical hernia. Vet Rec *98*:511, 1976.
32. Wolff G: Familial congenital diaphragmatic defect: Review and conclusions. Hum Genet *54*:1, 1980.

CHAPTER 24

THE MEDIASTINUM

DONALD E. THRALL

NORMAL ANATOMY

The term mediastinum is defined collectively as the two layers of mediastinal pleura and the space between them. The two mediastinal pleural layers are part of the right and left pleural sacs and are continuous with diaphragmatic, costal, and pulmonary pleura (see Fig. 25–1). The mediastinum extends from the diaphragm to the thoracic inlet and is essentially located in the median plane of the thorax, thus dividing the thoracic cavity into the right and left halves (Fig. 24–1).

The mediastinum can be classified into a cranial portion, cranial to the heart; a middle portion, containing the heart; and a caudal portion, caudal to the heart. The mediastinum can also be divided into dorsal and ventral portions by a dorsal plane through the carina. Organs present in the mediastinum are listed in Table 24–1.

In dogs and cats, the ventral part of the caudal mediastinum is fenestrated, providing potential communication between the two pleural cavities.[1] Unilateral pleural space disease or pleural space disease with asymmetric distribution can occur, however, if: (1) the mediastinum happens not to be fenestrated; (2) the fenestrations have been closed by inflammatory disease; or (3) the pleural space contents are too large or viscid to pass through the fenestrations.

The mediastinum, unlike the pleural space, is not a closed cavity. Cranially, it communicates with the fascial planes of the neck via the thoracic inlet; caudally, it communicates with the retroperitoneal space via the aortic hiatus. These communications provide the means for the spread of mediastinal disease to the neck and abdomen and vice versa.

Of the mediastinal organs listed in Table 24–1, only a few can be seen in normal thoracic radiographs: the heart, trachea, caudal vena cava, aorta, and, in young animals, the thymus. Other mediastinal organs are not seen because either they are not large enough to absorb a sufficient number of x rays or they are in contact with other mediastinal structures of the same radiopacity. This latter phenomenon is evident when the cranial mediastinum is viewed in a lateral thoracic radiograph. A distinct opacity can usually be seen in the cranial mediastinum ventral to the trachea, but individual organs can not be discerned (Fig. 24–2). The opacity is due to the absorption of x rays by cranial mediastinal organs, e.g., left subclavian artery, cranial vena cava, and mediastinal lymph nodes. These organs are not seen individually, however, because they are in contact with each other, and thus their margin is obliterated. On the lateral projection, the cranial mediastinum ventral to the trachea is more radiopaque dor-

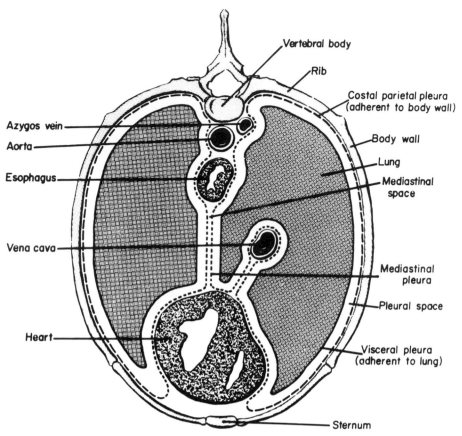

Figure 24–1. Cross-section of the canine thorax in a transverse plane. The mediastinum divides the thorax into right and left halves. Note that the mediastinum does not communicate with the pleural space. (From Feline Pract. *8*(6), 1978, with permission.)

TABLE 24–1. MEDIASTINAL ORGANS

Organ	Cranial Mediastinum	Middle Mediastinum	Caudal Mediastinum
Cranial vena cava	X		
Thymus	X		
Sternal lymph nodes	X		
Aortic arch	X		
Brachiocephalic artery	X		
Left subclavian artery	X		
Mediastinal lymph nodes	X		
Trachea	X	X	
Right and left vagosympathetic trunk	X	X	
Dorsal intercostal abdominal arteries and veins	X	X	X
Internal thoracic abdominal arteries and veins	X	X	X
Esophagus	X	X	X
Thoracic duct	X	X	X
Right and left sympathetic trunks	X	X	X
Right and left phrenic nerves	X	X	X
Descending aorta		X	X
Bronchoesophageal arteries and veins		X	X
Azygous vein		X	X
Heart		X	
Tracheobronchial lymph nodes		X	
Main pulmonary artery		X	
Main pulmonary veins		X	
Principal bronchi		X	
Caudal vena cava			X
Right and left vagus nerves			X

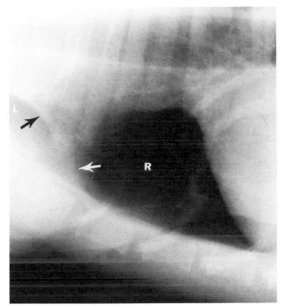

Figure 24–2. Lateral view of the thorax of a normal dog. The opacity ventral to the trachea is the cranial mediastinum. Although there are several different organs in this part of the mediastinum, e g , left subclavian artery, brachiocephalic trunk, and cranial vena cava, they cannot be discerned because they are in contact with each other and there is insufficient surrounding fat to provide contrast. It is important to realize that the mediastinum extends from the vertebrae to the sternebrae, but is most radiopaque ventral to the trachea because its thickness is greatest in this location. Note also the mediastinal reflection *(arrows)* between the cranial portion of the left cranial lobe (L) and the right cranial lobe (R), which appears as a curving line of soft-tissue opacity that extends from the end of the first rib in a caudoventral direction to the second sternebra.

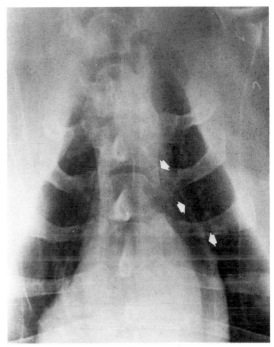

Figure 24–3. Ventrodorsal view of the thorax of a normal dog. The cranial mediastinum is superimposed on the thoracic spine; it is relatively indistinct. As an approximation, the thickness of the cranial mediastinum should not be wider than twice the diameter of the cranial thoracic spine in normal dogs. Note the mediastinal reflection between the right cranial lobe and the cranial part of the left cranial lobe *(arrows);* it appears as a curving line of soft-tissue opacity that extends from the C_7-T_1 junction in a left caudolateral direction to the cardiac silhouette in the region of the main pulmonary artery. See Figure 24–2 for the appearance of this reflection in the lateral view.

sally than ventrally because of the greater thickness of the mediastinum just below the trachea.

In ventrodorsal or dorsoventral thoracic radiographs, most of the cranial mediastinum is superimposed on the cranial thoracic spine; its normal thickness is usually less than approximately two times the transverse width of the cranial thoracic spine (Fig. 24–3). In obese patients, the cranial mediastinum may be widened by fat accumulation and can be confused with an abnormal mediastinal mass (Fig. 24–4).

There are three mediastinal reflections that can frequently be identified in normal thoracic radiographs. The first is a reflection of the cranioventral mediastinum to the left. This reflection accommodates extension of the right cranial lobe across the midline to the left. On the ventrodorsal or dorsoventral projection, this reflection appears as a curving radiopaque line, with the concave surface on the right, extending from the approximate region of T_1-T_2 to the vicinity of the main pulmonary artery (Fig. 24–3). The thickness of this reflection is affected

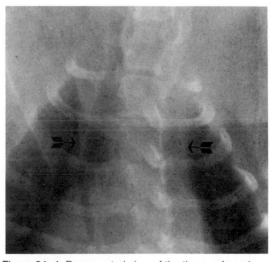

Figure 24–4. Dorsoventral view of the thorax of an obese dog. The cranial mediastinum contains a large amount of fat and therefore appears wide *(arrows)*. It is wider than twice the diameter of the thoracic spine. Care should be taken to avoid misinterpreting this finding as an abnormal mediastinal mass.

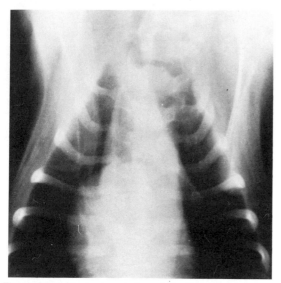

Figure 24–5. Ventrodorsal view of the thorax of a young dog before involution of the thymus. The thymus appears as a sail-shaped area of soft-tissue opacity cranial and to the left of the cardiac base.

by the amount of fat that it contains. On the lateral view, this reflection, and the margin of the right cranial lobe, can frequently be identified immediately cranial to the heart (Fig. 24–2). The cranioventral mediastinal reflection is not visible in every radiograph of the thorax. The thymus lies in this mediastinal reflection and can be identified on ventrodorsal or dorsoventral radiographs of many young animals (Fig. 24–5 and 24–6). The thymus is not readily visualized on lateral views of the thorax because of its thinness, but it may obscure the cranial margin of the heart before involution.

The second mediastinal reflection is one of the caudoventral mediastinum to the left. This reflection is seen only on dorsoventral or ventrodorsal radiographs and accommodates extension of the accessory lobe across the midline to the left. It appears as a relatively straight radiopaque line extending from the region of the cardiac apex in a caudolateral direction toward the gastric fundus (Fig. 24–7). The thickness of the reflection depends on the amount of fat it

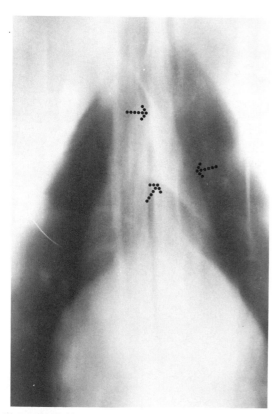

Figure 24–6. Ventrodorsal linear tomogram of the cranial thorax of a dog before involution of the thymus. The thymus, which appears as a sail-shaped area of soft-tissue *(arrows)*, lies in the mediastinum between the right cranial and cranial part of the left cranial lobes.

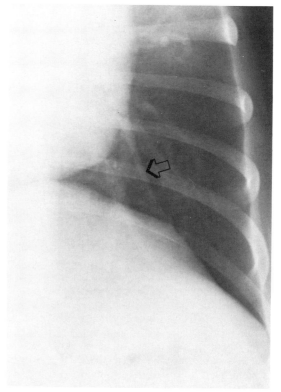

Figure 24–7. Ventrodorsal view of the caudal thorax of a normal dog. The caudoventral mediastinal reflection appears as a line of soft-tissue opacity that extends from the region of the cardiac apex in a left caudolateral direction to the diaphragm *(arrow)*.

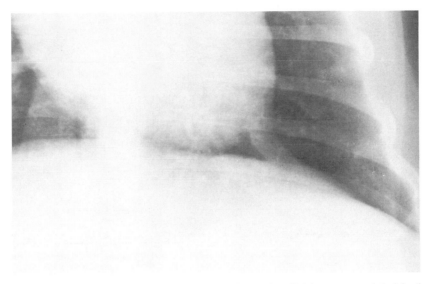

Figure 24–8. Ventrodorsal view of the caudal thorax of an obese dog. Fat has accumulated in the caudoventral mediastinum, resulting in its increased thickness. Compare its appearance in this radiograph to that in Figure 24–7.

contains (Fig. 24–8); it cannot be seen on every dorsoventral or ventrodorsal radiograph.

The third mediastinal reflection is one associated with the caudal vena cava (Fig. 24–1). This reflection is not visible per se in radiographs of the thorax, but its presence as an extension of the mediastinum to the right must be recognized.

MEDIASTINAL PATHOLOGY

There are four general classifications of mediastinal disease: mediastinal shift, mediastinal masses, mediastinal fluid, and mediastinal air or gas.

Mediastinal Shift. Shifting of mediastinal position can occur as a result of a unilateral decrease in lung volume, a unilateral increase in lung volume, or the presence of an intrathoracic mass. A mediastinal shift cannot be readily identified from the lateral projection; thus, the position of the mediastinum should always be evaluated on ventrodorsal or dorsoventral radiographs of the thorax. Mediastinal position can be evaluated by noting the position of visible mediastinal organs, such as the trachea, heart, aorta, and caudal vena cava, or the previously described mediastinal reflections. A shift of the mediastinum cannot occur without a change in position of one of the previously mentioned structures (Fig. 24–9). Improper patient positioning due to rotation creates a false impression of a mediastinal shift.

Mediastinal Masses. Mediastinal mass lesions are common. Localization to the mediastinum

of a mass lesion seen on the lateral radiograph of the thorax is difficult because its position relative to the mediastinum cannot be determined. In a ventrodorsal or dorsoventral radiograph, however, the mediastinal location of a

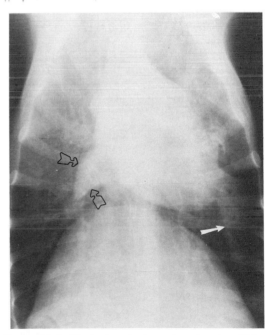

Figure 24–9. Ventrodorsal view of a dog in which a mediastinal shift has occurred. The heart and caudoventral mediastinal reflection (solid arrow) are displaced to the left because of decreased volume of the left caudal lung lobe. The right middle lobe is collapsed (open arrows), and there is alveolar disease in the left caudal lobe.

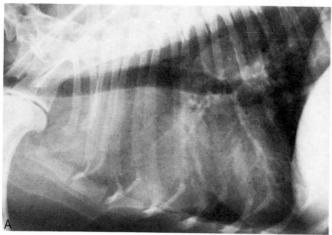

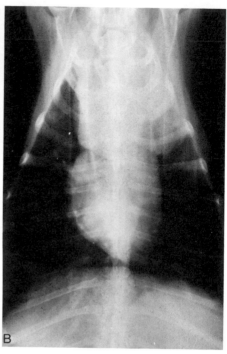

Figure 24–10. Lateral *(A)* and ventrodorsal *(B)* views of the thorax of a dog with lymphosarcoma. *A,* a large mass can be seen cranial to the heart. Although its position is consistent with mediastinal mass, and there is dorsal displacement of the trachea, this mass cannot be localized by examination of this projection alone. *B,* the mass is centered about the midline, suggesting a mediastinal location. Diagnosis: thymic lymphosarcoma.

mass should be considered if it lies on or adjacent to the midline or in one of the three previously described mediastinal reflections (Fig. 24–10). Definitive localization of a mass as mediastinal in origin from radiographs may be difficult, because such things as juxtamediastinal pleural fluid or lung disease can mimic a mediastinal mass.

Mediastinal masses can result in lung displacement, displacement of other mediastinal organs, or both. Of particular importance is tracheal elevation. Tracheal elevation can result from a cranioventral mediastinal mass, but it can also be seen in animals with pleural fluid but no mediastinal mass (Fig. 24–11). If pleural effusion and tracheal elevation are present, a concurrent mediastinal mass may not be apparent unless there is a contact indentation of the trachea. If pleural fluid obscures mediastinal evaluation and mediastinal mass is being considered, the fluid should be removed and the radiographs should be repeated. Causes of mediastinal masses are listed in Table 24–2.

Mediastinal Fluid. Free mediastinal fluid occurs occasionally. The fluid is usually of soft-tissue opacity; thus, it may assume the radiographic appearance of a mediastinal mass, cardiomegaly, or both (Fig. 24–12). If mediastinal fluid is considered, its presence can be detected, unless it is trapped or loculated, by

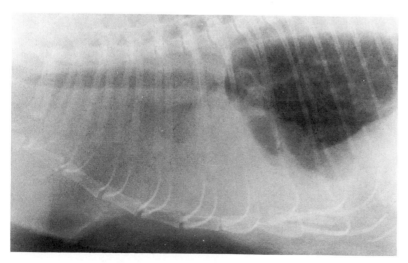

Figure 24–11. Lateral view of the thorax of a cat with pleural effusion. The trachea is displaced dorsally, but the presence of a mediastinal mass cannot be confirmed because (1) pleural fluid can be accompanied by tracheal elevation when no mediastinal mass is present; (2) a mass cannot be seen; and (3) there is no contact indentation of the trachea.

TABLE 24–2. **CAUSES OF MEDIASTINAL MASSES**

Cause of Mass	Mediastinal Location	Cause of Mass	Mediastinal Location
Lymphosarcoma—cat	Cranioventral	Generalized megaesophagus	Dorsal
Lymphosarcoma—dog	Perihilar, cranioventral	*Spirocerca lupi*	Caudodorsal
Inflammatory lymphadenopathy	Perihilar, cranioventral	Mediastinal diaphragmatic hernia	Caudoventral
Neoplastic lymphadenopathy— metastatic	Perihilar, cranioventral	Ectopic thyroid or parathyroid tumor	Cranioventral, perihilar
Periesophageal vascular ring	Craniodorsal*	Thymoma	Cranioventral
Neurogenic tumor	Dorsal	Heartbase tumor	Craniodorsal, perihilar
Paraspinal tumor	Dorsal	Hiatal hernia	Caudodorsal
Mediastinal abscess— usually secondary to esophageal perforation	Cranioventral, caudoventral, caudal	Diaphragmatic eventration	Caudodorsal
		Hematoma	Variable

*Severe esophagomegaly may appear cranioventrally.

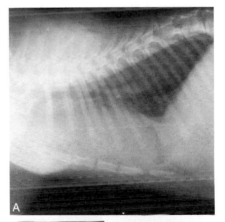

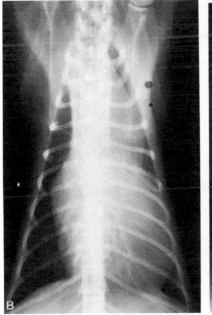
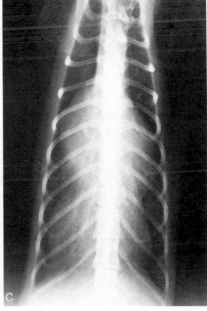

Figure 24–12. Lateral *(A)*, ventrodorsal *(B)*, and horizontal beam, ventrodorsal *(C)* views of the thorax of a cat with free mediastinal fluid. *A*, the cardiac silhouette is obscured by homogeneous opacification of the thorax. *B*, the cranial mediastinum is wide and the cardiac silhouette is enlarged with an unusual, seemingly rectangular right margin. *C*, the heart is clearly seen in the middle of the thorax and the caudal mediastinum is increased in width due to the caudal gravitation of free mediastinal fluid. (From Feline Pract. *8*(6), 1978, with permission.)

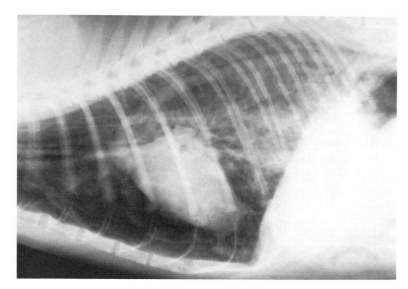

Figure 24–13. Lateral view of the thorax of a cat with pneumomediastinum. There is enhanced visualization of mediastinal structures, namely the esophagus, adventitial surface of the trachea, cranial vena cava, and major branches of the aortic arch, because of contrast provided by the mediastinal gas. The lung is also opacified caudally. (Courtesy of Dr. Mary Mahaffey, University of Georgia, Athens, GA.)

horizontal-beam radiography. Causes of mediastinal fluid are feline infectious peritonitis, coagulopathy, esophageal perforation, and trauma.

Pneumomediastinum. Free mediastinal gas is called pneumomediastinum. In most instances, gas in the mediastinum results in enhanced visualization of mediastinal organs because of the contrast it provides (Fig. 24–13). If only a small amount of mediastinal gas is present, the only apparent abnormality may be a patchy decrease in radiopacity of the cranioventral mediastinum (Fig. 25–13). The size of the mediastinum is not greatly increased when pneumomediastinum is present; thus, pneumomediastinum is more easily detected on the lateral radiograph than on ventrodorsal or dorsoventral radiographs (Fig. 24–14). Pneumomediastinum may progress to pneumothorax if mediastinal pressure results in rupture of mediastinal pleura, establishing communication between the mediastinum and the pleural space. Signs of respiratory embarrassment are usually not seen with pneumomediastinum unless it progresses to pneumothorax. It would be extremely uncommon for pneumothorax to result in pneumomediastinum. Pneumomediastinum may result in extensive subcutaneous emphysema because of the communication between the mediastinum and the fascial planes of the neck. Pneumomediastinum may also result in pneumoretroperitoneum, because of the communication between the mediastinum and the retroperitoneal space via the aortic hiatus (Fig. 24–15). Pneumoretroperitoneum resulting from pneumomediastinum is usually not apparent clinically.

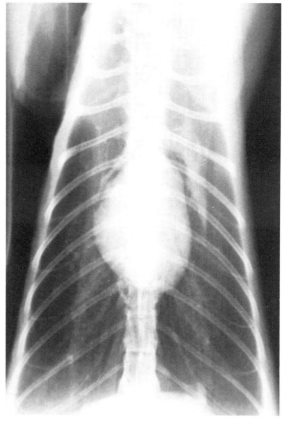

Figure 24–14. Ventrodorsal view of a cat with pneumomediastinum. Note the inability to identify the mediastinal gas. The opacity craniolateral to the cardiac base on the cat's left side is probably the thymus, which was displaced laterally by the emphysematous mediastinum. There is subcutaneous emphysema on the right side. Mediastinal gas has migrated to the subcutaneous tissues through the thoracic inlet.

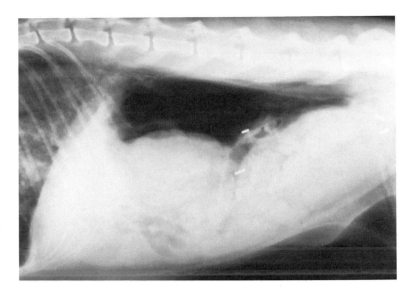

Figure 24–15. Abdominal radiograph of the same cat as depicted in Figure 24–13. There is a large volume of gas in the retroperitoneal space as a result of dissection of mediastinal gas caudally through the aortic hiatus. (Courtesy of Dr. Mary Mahaffey, University of Georgia, Athens, GA.)

There are six causes of pneumomediastinum. Firstly, air escaping from sites of alveolar rupture can dissect in a retrograde direction in loose connective tissue adjacent to bronchi and vessels into the mediastinum. This dissection occurs commonly after trauma and is also the source of pneumomediastinum that occurs secondary to iatrogenic pulmonary hyperinflation during anesthesia or resuscitation. Pneumothorax is not present when pneumomediastinum results from the above mechanism, unless the lung trauma causes tearing of the pulmonary pleura or the mediastinal air build-up results in rupture of mediastinal pleura, thereby establishing communication between the mediastinum and pleural space. Secondly, a tracheal wall defect from trauma or erosion associated with neoplasia or inflammatory disease can result in pneumomediastinum. If the defect is intrathoracic, air enters the mediastinum directly. If the defect is in the neck, air can dissect along the trachea into the medias-

tinum. Thirdly, an esophageal defect resulting from trauma, inflammation, or neoplasia is an uncommon cause of pneumomediastinum. The fourth cause is caudal extension of cervical emphysema along fascial planes into the mediastinum, which is common. Cervical emphysema is a common sequela to neck or oral cavity trauma, and may also result from tracheal or esophageal rupture. Fifthly, cranial extension of air from the retroperitoneal space into the mediastinum is an uncommon cause of pneumomediastinum. The usual direction of air flow is from the mediastinum into the retroperitoneal space. Finally, emphysematous mediastinitis, with a gas-forming organism, is a rare cause of pneumomediastinum.

Reference

1. Schummer A, Nickel R, and Sack WO: The Viscera of the Domestic Mammals, 2nd Ed. New York, Springer-Verlag, 1979.

CHAPTER 25

THE PLEURAL SPACE

DONALD E. THRALL

BASIC ANATOMY

Pleura is divided into two types, parietal and pulmonary, depending on its location. Parietal pleura is subdivided into costal, diaphragmatic, and mediastinal parts; costal parietal pleura lines the intrathoracic side of the thoracic wall, diaphragmatic parietal pleura covers the diaphragm, and mediastinal parietal pleura forms the boundaries of the mediastinum. Pulmonary pleura covers the lung parenchyma. There are two distinct pleural sacs in the thorax, right and left. Both have costal, diaphragmatic, mediastinal, and pulmonary parts, which are continuous (Fig. 25–1). The pleural space is a potential space between parietal and pulmonary pleural layers and between pulmonary pleural layers in interlobar fissures. The pleural space normally contains a small volume of fluid, which serves as a lubricant.

NORMAL RADIOGRAPHIC APPEARANCE AND PLEURAL THICKENING

For all practical purposes, normal pleura is not visible radiographically. Pleura outside of interlobar fissures cannot be seen because it silhouettes with adjacent soft tissue. Pleura within

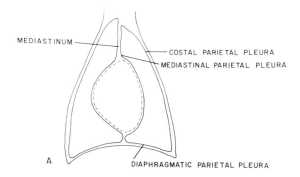

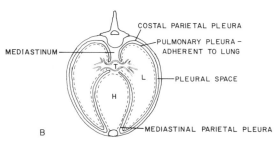

Figure 25–1. Line drawings of cross sections of the thorax in dorsal *(A)* and transverse *(B)* planes in which the relationship of the pleural layers can be seen. *A,* Note the continuity of the costal, mediastinal, and diaphragmatic parts of the parietal pleura. (Lungs have not been included in *A*.) *B,* Note how the mediastinal pleura is reflected onto the lung as pulmonary pleura. Note also that the pleural space is not continuous with the mediastinum. T: trachea; L: lung; H: heart.

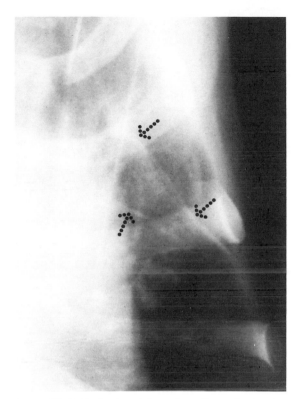

Figure 25–2. Ventrodorsal thoracic radiograph of a dog in which a radiopaque interlobar fissure *(arrows)* can be seen between the cranial and caudal parts of the left cranial lobe. This fissure visualization is more prominent than the occasionally seen normal fissure, and it may be due either to pleural thickening or to a small pleural effusion. In this dog, pleural effusion was not identified by horizontal-beam radiography.

intralobar fissures is surrounded by intrapulmonary air, which provides contrast, but the pleura is so thin that it generally does not absorb a sufficient number of x rays to be seen. Occasionally, thin pleural lines are noted between lobes. Thickened pleura could assume this appearance.[7] On occasion, however, the x-ray beam strikes normal pleura in an interlobar fissure exactly tangentially, resulting in absorption of a sufficient number of x rays for the pleura to be visible. It is impossible to determine radiographically whether isolated thin pleural lines are normal or represent evidence of pleural thickening. In either instance, minimal or no clinical significance is attached. When pleural thickening is advanced, more prominent pleural lines may be seen (Fig. 25–2). Only interlobar pleura can be seen when thickened, however, because thickened pleura outside of fissures silhouettes with adjacent soft tissue. In pleural thickening, the interlobar fissures seen radiographically depend on the position of the animal and the direction of the x-ray beam, because the abnormal fissure must be struck tangentially by the x-ray beam.

TABLE 25–1. CAUSES OF PLEURAL FLUID

Cause	Fluid Type*
Congestive heart failure	M
Idiopathic	M
Infection	E
Malignancy	M
Pneumonia	M,E
Trauma	M
Coagulation defect	M
Hypoproteinemia	T
Pericardial effusion	M
Mediastinitis	M,E
Chylothorax	M
Diaphragmatic hernia	M
Foreign body	M,E

*M: modified transudate; E: exudate; T: transudate.

PLEURAL EFFUSION

Pleural effusion is defined as the presence of fluid in the pleural space. Pleural fluid can be an exudate, transudate, or modified transudate, depending on its cause (Table 25–1). When pleural effusion is present, radiographically detectable changes result. The character of these changes depends on the volume of fluid, the relative position of the animal and the x-ray beam, the distribution of the fluid, and whether it is free or loculated.

Free Pleural Effusion. Typical radiographic changes associated with free pleural effusion are basically the same regardless of fluid type. Intuitively, one might expect the distribution of free pleural fluid to be related to its nature, but such is not true in people[2] and is probably not true in animals. In general, free fluid distributes itself in the pleural space according to gravity and the ability of the lung to expand, i.e., compliance. Thus, the appearance of free pleural effusion in lateral, ventrodorsal, and dorsoventral vertical-beam radiographs is different.[3] Typical roentgen signs of free pleural fluid are listed in Table 25–2.

TABLE 25–2. TYPICAL ROENTGEN SIGNS OF FREE PLEURAL FLUID

Visualization of widened interlobar fissures. Fissure is of soft-tissue opacity

Retraction of pleural surface of lung away from pleural surface of thoracic wall. Space between lung and thoracic wall is of soft-tissue opacity

Increased soft-tissue opacity dorsal to sternum on lateral radiographs. Opacity frequently has scalloped margins

Blunting of costophrenic sulci in ventrodorsal radiographs

Decreased visualization of the heart in dorsoventral radiographs

Obscured diaphragmatic outline in dorsoventral and lateral radiographs

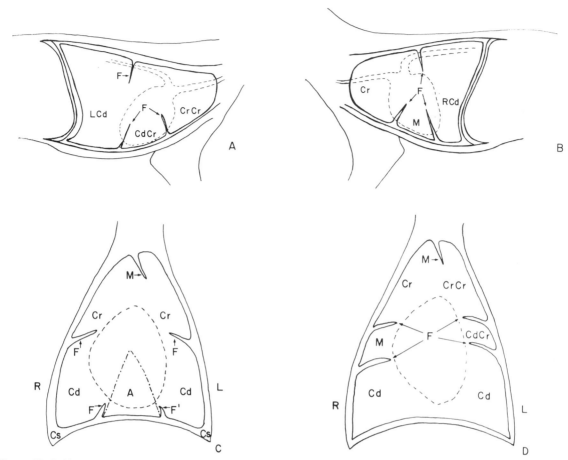

Figure 25–3. Line drawings of the thorax indicating the location of interlobar fissures. The exact fissures visible when pleural effusion is present depend on the position of the patient, on the volume of fluid, and on whether the x-ray beam strikes the fissure tangentially. Only fluid-filled fissures struck tangentially will be seen. *A*, Fissures of the lateral aspect of the left lung (looking medial to lateral). These fissures are more likely to be seen when the patient is in left lateral recumbency. *B*, Fissures of the lateral aspect of the right lung (looking medial to lateral). These fissures are more likely to be seen when the patient is in right lateral recumbency. *C*, Fissures on the dorsal aspect of the lungs. These fissures are more likely to be seen when the patient is in dorsal recumbency. Note that the costophrenic sulcus becomes rounded when patients with pleural effusion are placed in dorsal recumbency. *D*, Fissures on the ventral aspect of the lungs. These fissures are more likely to be seen when the patient is in ventral recumbency. F: Interlobar fissure; F': mediastinal reflection between the left caudal lobe and the accessory lobe (pleural fluid can accumulate adjacent to this reflection); CrCr: cranial part of left cranial lobe; CdCr: caudal part of left cranial lobe; Cd: caudal lobe; Cr: right cranial lobe; Md: middle lobe; A: accessory lobe; Cs: costophrenic sulcus; M: mediastinal reflection; L: left; R: right.

Interlobar Fissures. The appearance and number of interlobar fissures seen with free pleural fluid depend on the amount of fluid present and the relative position of the patient and x-ray beam (Fig. 25–3). Approximately 100 ml of fluid must be present in the pleural space of a medium-sized dog before widened interlobar fissures are visible.[4] Visualization of widened interlobar fissures due to accumulated fluid within results from the x-ray beam striking the fluid-containing fissure tangentially. It must be noted that other fluid-containing fissures may not be seen because their relationship to the x-ray beam is not tangential. With small effusions, interlobar fissures are most likely seen on ventrodorsal rather than dorsoventral radiographs, because when the patient is placed in ventral recumbency small effusions collect dorsal to the sternum and may not enter fissures to a sufficient degree that they may be seen.[4] In lateral radiographs, small effusions may result in visualization of fissures. As the volume of fluid increases, more interlobar fissures become apparent in each radiograph, and their thickness may increase secondary to the increasing volume of fluid in the fissure (Figs. 25–4 and 25–5).

Horizontal Beam Radiography. It may not be possible to identify small effusions on survey radiographs if the x-ray beam fails to strike a fluid accumulation tangentially. To enhance fluid detection, a horizontally directed x-ray beam can be used to assure a tangential relationship between the x-ray beam and the fluid collection. The patient can be placed in lateral recumbency and then be examined with a horizontal x-ray beam. If free pleural fluid is present, it will gravitate into the dependent portion of the dependent hemithorax, where the x-ray beam will intersect it tangentially (Fig. 25–6). It is important to remember that a sharply demarcated fluid line is not seen in patients with pleural fluid when radiographed with a horizontal x-ray beam unless free gas is also present in the pleural space. Sharp fluid lines are not seen in horizontal beam radiographs of patients with free pleural fluid but without pneumothorax, because the configuration of the fluid is altered by the adjacent lung, which retracts because of elastic recoil. Sharp fluid

lines are seen in horizontal beam radiographs only when there is a free fluid–free air interface.

Retraction of Lung Margin. Pleural fluid also results in retraction of the pleural surface of the lung away from the pleural surface of the thoracic wall. The magnitude of this separation depends on the volume of fluid present and the compliance of the lung. With normal lungs or with lungs of uniformly decreased compliance, retraction of the lungs away from the thoracic wall is relatively uniform and its degree is a function of fluid volume. Retraction of lung from the thoracic wall can be seen on lateral, dorsoventral, and ventrodorsal projections (Fig. 25–5). It is important to remember that fluid surrounds the lung, but the fluid is most apparent radiographically when the x-ray beam is tangential to the fluid (Fig. 25–7).[5]

Vascular markings cannot be identified in the portion of fluid that is viewed tangentially. Vascular markings can be seen, assuming good radiographic technique is used, through the portion of fluid that is traversed perpendicularly by the x-ray beam (Fig. 25–7). Lung displacement, however, cannot be detected if the x-ray beam does not traverse the fluid tangentially

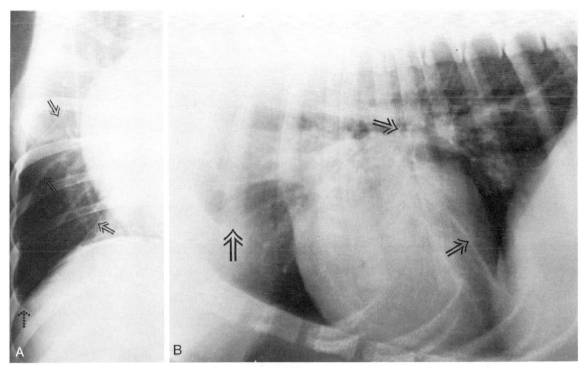

Figure 25–4. Ventrodorsal *(A)* and left lateral *(B)* thoracic radiographs of a dog with a moderate-volume pleural effusion. *A,* A number of interlobar fissures can be seen; some have more fluid within than others (double open arrows). The costophrenic sulci are blunt *(dotted arrows)*. *B,* Fewer interlobar fissures can be seen *(small double arrows)*. The cranial part of the left cranial lobe has been displaced *(large double arrow)* by surrounding fluid. (Courtesy of the University of Georgia.)

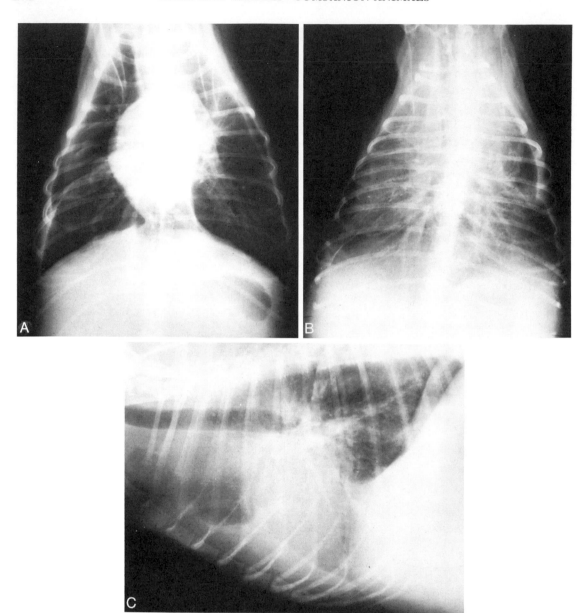

Figure 25–5. Ventrodorsal (A), dorsoventral (B), and left lateral (C) views of the thorax of a dog with a large-volume pleural effusion. A, There are numerous interlobar fissures and the right caudal lobe is separated from the thoracic wall by an area of soft-tissue opacity. The cardiac silhouette can be seen. Note the appearance of the costal cartilages; they should not be mistaken for interlobar fissures. B, Interlobar fissures and lung displacement away from the thoracic wall are again evident. The cardiac silhouette, however, is not visible, the diaphragm is obscured, and the overall radiopacity of the thorax is increased. Vascular markings are apparent. (See Fig. 25–10 for explanation.) C, There are interlobar fissures, the cardiac silhouette is partially obscured by surrounding fluid, and the overall radiopacity of the thorax is increased. In addition, there is an area of radiopacity just dorsal to the sternum, the margins of which are scalloped due to fluid accumulation in the ventral thorax.

(Fig. 25–7). Visualization of vascular markings in an intrathoracic opacity is evidence that the opacity is not due to consolidation. In consolidation, vascular markings cannot be identified in any view. In rare instances, massive effusions may result in total atelectasis of a lung, and no vascular markings are visible.

Retrosternal Opacification. In lateral radiographs, free pleural fluid frequently results in an increased radiopacity dorsal to the sternum (Fig. 25–5C). This finding is because of fluid having collected in the ventral thorax, possibly layered against the ventral mediastinum in the nondependent hemithorax. If the patient has a

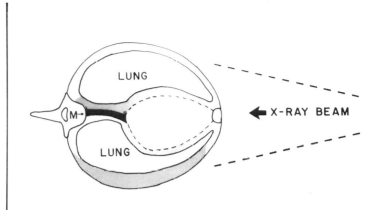

Figure 25–6. The demonstration of pleural fluid by horizontal beam radiography. Fluid is represented by dotted areas. Fluid in the nondependent hemithorax "layers" against the mediastinum unless there is a large opening in the mediastinal pleura that allows it to enter the dependent hemithorax. Fluid in the dependent hemithorax gravitates to the area between the lung and the thoracic wall where the horizontally directed x-ray beam will strike it tangentially. M: mediastinum.

unilateral effusion and the fluid is in the dependent hemithorax, this opacity may not be present. Frequently, the margin of the opacity is scalloped because of adjacent, partially collapsed lung, which alters the configuration of the fluid.

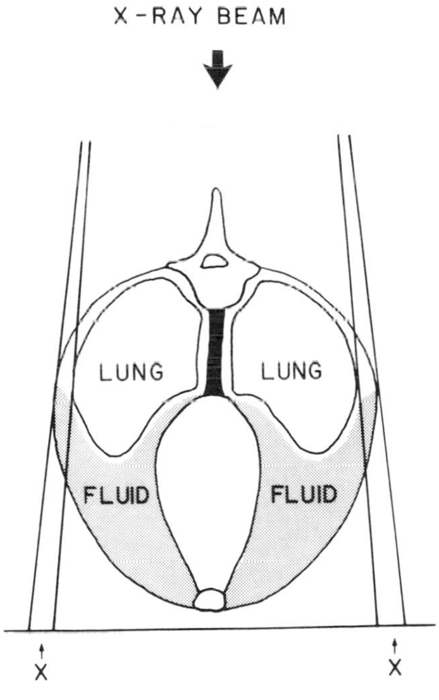

Figure 25–7. Principle of lung retraction and visibility of pulmonary vessels through pleural effusion. This patient, with a large pleural effusion, is radiographed in ventral recumbency. Fluid, therefore, has gravitated ventrally, resulting in dorsal displacement of lung. The most lung displacement occurred ventrally, but is not apparent radiographically because this part of the retracted lung has not been struck tangentially by the x-ray beam. The only lung retraction that is apparent is in the regions indicated by "x," because it is here that the fluid between the lung and the thoracic wall is struck tangentially by the x-ray beam. In the region between the x's, thoracic radiopacity is increased, the heart is obscured, and the pulmonary vessels are visible. (Compare to Fig. 25–5B.)

Blunting of Costophrenic Sulci. Whether or not the costophrenic sulci become blunted by pleural fluid depends on the position of the patient during radiography. In dorsoventral radiographs, the fluid gravitates ventrally and the costophrenic sulci may appear normal. In ventrodorsal radiographs, fluid gravitates into the dorsal portion of the thorax, resulting in alteration of the costophrenic sulci. There are other differences between dorsoventral and ventrodorsal radiographs when free pleural fluid is present.[3] In dorsoventral radiographs, the fluid that has gravitated ventrally frequently obscures visualization of the heart and ventral part of the diaphragm (dome) because of the silhouette sign. In ventrodorsal radiographs, pleural fluid does not as readily obscure the heart and diaphragm, because the fluid is distributed over a larger area in the dorsal thorax where it does not contact the heart or dome of the diaphragm (Figs. 25–5 and 25–8). Also, fluid does not tend to obscure the heart as readily in ventrodorsal radiographs because the fluid is located dorsally, "above" the heart, and does not silhouette with it (Fig. 25–8).

Atypical Distribution of Free Pleural Fluid. An atypical distribution of free pleural fluid most often results from parts of the lung having different compliance. When a portion of a lung has decreased compliance because of intrinsic disease or extrinsic compression, fluid present in the pleural space tends to accumulate around it because it is less expansile than other parts of the lung. Thus, atypical fluid distribution can be a clue to an underlying pulmonary lesion. These atypical collections result in an intrathoracic radiopacity that is usually irregularly marginated and shaped when compared to opacities typically seen with pleural effusion. These collections may be confused with thoracic wall or

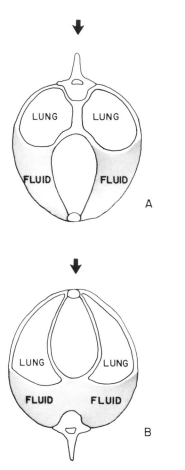

Figure 25–8. Effect of dorsal versus ventral recumbency on the radiographic appearance of pleural effusion. In A, the patient is in ventral recumbency and fluid gravitates ventrally. The fluid is in contact with the heart, thus obscuring the heart from view. When the patient is placed in dorsal recumbency (B), the fluid gravitates dorsally and is not in contact with the heart; thus the cardiac silhouette is visible. The absolute depth of the fluid is greater when the patient is in ventral recumbency (A) because the ventral part of the thoracic cavity is narrower and the fluid rises to a higher level because of the space occupied by the heart. Thus, overall thoracic radiopacity is greater when the patient is in ventral recumbency.

pulmonary lesions. Because the fluid is free, it changes position with gravity. Thus, horizontal beam radiographs are helpful in evaluating atypical collections of pleural fluid.

In most instances, free pleural fluid is approximately equally distributed between the two pleural spaces. In some patients, however, there is more fluid in one pleural space or the effusion is totally unilateral. Causes of unilateral pleural effusion or an effusion more voluminous in one pleural space are: a difference in compliance between lungs; closing of mediastinal fenestrations from herniated organ, mass, adhesions, or exudate; and an anatomically complete

mediastinum. In extensive unilateral effusion, it may be difficult to identify whether the resultant opacity is due to a pathologic process in the pleural space, thoracic wall, or lung.

Loculated Pleural Fluid. The position of loculated pleural fluid is unaffected by gravity. Loculation can result from the formation of pleural fluid in a closed pleural cavity, one possibly formed by pleural adhesions; the incitement of pleural adhesions by the fluid, which subsequently wall off the fluid; or the concurrent formation of pleural fluid and adhesions.[5] Loculated effusion can occur anywhere within the thorax. The resultant opacity is homogeneous and may be easily confused with a thoracic wall, pulmonary, or mediastinal mass. Loculated effusion in animals is less common than free pleural fluid; when present, however, its diagnosis can be difficult and may have to be made by invasive means.

Pitfalls in Pleural Fluid Diagnosis. Under certain circumstances, an erroneous radiographic diagnosis of pleural fluid may be made. Thickened pleura, having resulted from previous surgery or infection for example, may have an identical appearance to a fluid-containing fissure (Fig. 25–2). A distinction can be made, if the pleural fluid is free, by using a horizontally directed x-ray beam and a patient position, such as lateral recumbency, whereby the x-ray beam transects a greater thickness of pleural fluid.

Mineralized costal cartilages can be confused with fluid-containing interlobar fissures. Their position is similar, but the concave surface of costal cartilages is directed cranially, whereas the concave surface of fluid-filled fissures is directed caudally (Fig. 25–5C). Thoracic wall deformities, such as those present in chondrodystrophic breeds, may result in increased radiopacity at the margin of the lung field. Without knowledge of this fact, the opacity may be incorrectly misinterpreted as retraction of the lung from the thoracic wall because of pleural fluid (Fig. 25–9).

Significance of Pleural Fluid. Pleural fluid can result from a primary pleural disorder, but most often it is a sign of disease elsewhere. It is frequently impossible to determine the cause of pleural effusion from survey radiographs. When pleural fluid is present, structures are obscured, making them increasingly difficult to evaluate radiographically, especially as fluid volume increases. Extremely large lesions can be obscured by pleural fluid. When pleural fluid is identified radiographically, careful scrutiny of the radiograph is necessary. Occasionally, subtle radiographic findings, such as a rib lesion or an asymmetric distribution of free fluid, are noted, which can be of great help in the overall evaluation of the patient. In patients with a

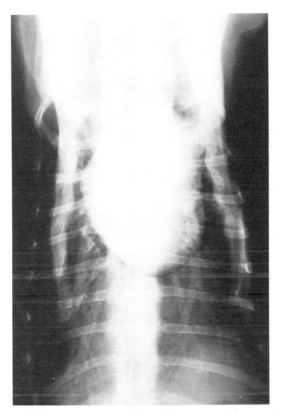

Figure 25–9. Ventrodorsal view of the thorax of a normal basset hound. The sternum is displaced slightly to the left side. There is an area of soft tissue opacity adjacent to the thoracic wall on the dog's left side and an area of radiolucency adjacent to the thoracic wall on the right side. These are artifacts created by the irregular thoracic wall configuration of this chondrodystrophic dog. The opacity on the left side is due to the prominent costochondral region; rotation of the patient resulted in it being located at the periphery of the thorax. The location and appearance of this opacity could result in it being confused with pleural effusion; interlobar fissures are not seen, however. On the right side, the opacity created by the costochondral deformity is located closer to the midline because of patient rotation. Lateral to this opacity is normal lung, which appears radiolucent because of the sharp contrast provided by the costochondral opacity. The radiolucency of this lung could be confused with pneumothorax. A horizontal beam radiograph was normal.

large pleural effusion, one can attempt to gain more information by using a horizontally directed x-ray beam with various patient positions to obtain unobstructed views of portions of the thorax. In most instances, this indiscriminate approach is unrewarding and should only be used to evaluate regions of suspected abnormalities. In addition, the patient may be so dyspneic from the secondary lung collapse or lung disease that such maneuvers are impossible. A more rewarding approach is to refrain from additional radiographs until some or all of

TABLE 25–3. CAUSES OF PNEUMOTHORAX

Iatrogenic
Extension of Pneumomediastinum
Trauma
  Lung rupture
  Chest wall rent
Bulla Rupture
  Pneumatocele
  Abscess
  Paragonimiasis
  Cavitary tumor
Complication of Pneumonia

the fluid has been removed by invasive means or medical treatment.

All pleural effusions are significant and it is important to attempt to reach a definitive diagnosis. In small effusions, there may be no abnormal clinical signs, whereas large effusions usually result in dyspnea. It should not be assumed, however, that small effusions are less significant than large ones. Thoracocentesis with appropriate fluid analysis should be done when pleural fluid is identified.[1, 7]

PNEUMOTHORAX

Gas or air in the pleural space is called pneumothorax. Air can enter the pleural space from the outside or from the lung or mediastinum (Table 25–3). It is unusual for gas to be produced in the pleural space by bacteria. The presence of pleural air or gas usually results in radiographically detectable changes that depend on the volume of air present and the relative position of the patient and the x-ray beam. Typical roentgen signs of pneumothorax are listed in Table 25–4.

Retraction of the lung from the thoracic wall can be seen on lateral, ventrodorsal, and dorsoventral radiographs. In a small pneumothorax, this separation is small and may appear as a fine radiolucent line (Fig. 25–10). As in pleural effusion, air surrounds the lung, but is most apparent radiographically when the air is struck tangentially by the x-ray beam (Fig. 25–10). Visualization of interlobar fissures is not as frequent with pneumothorax as with pleural effusion.

TABLE 25–4. TYPICAL ROENTGEN SIGNS OF PNEUMOTHORAX

Retraction of pleural surface of lung away from pleural surface of thoracic wall. Space between lung and thoracic wall is radiolucent
Lung markings do not extend all the way to thoracic wall
Lung has increased opacity because of collapse
Appearance of dorsal displacement of the heart on the lateral view

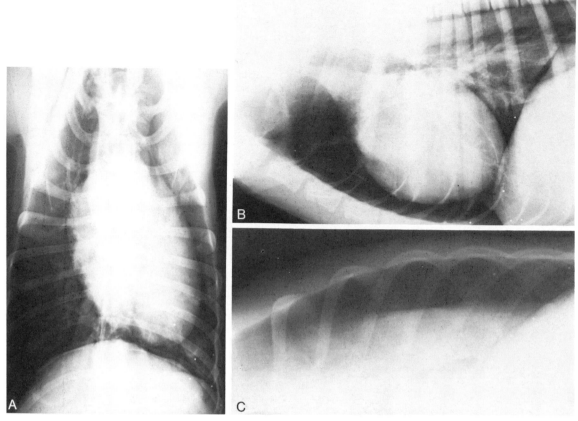

Figure 25–10. Ventrodorsal *(A)*, left lateral *(B)*, and right lateral recumbency, horizontal beam *(C)* radiographs of a dog with pneumothorax. *A,* The heart is shifted to the left, but evidence of pneumothorax is not seen because the air has risen and accumulated ventral to the sternum; in this region, it is not struck tangentially by the x-ray beam. There is emphysema medial to the right scapula and an area of hemorrhage in the left caudal lobe. *B,* There is a thin radiolucent line between the diaphragm and a caudal lobe resulting from air in the pleural space. The heart is separated from the sternum and there is a radiolucent area between the sternum and the heart. There is an interlobar fissure that extends caudoventrally from the carina, suggestive of pleural thickening or concurrent pleural effusion. *C,* The extent of pneumothorax is readily apparent. By placing the patient in right lateral recumbency and by using a horizontally directed x-ray beam, air in the left hemithorax was struck tangentially by the x-ray beam. Radiographic technique was decreased by 50 per cent to facilitate air visualization by rendering the lung more radiopaque.

As air enters the pleural space, the lung collapses because of its elasticity, and pleural space pressure increases. As lung volume decreases because of collapse, it contains less air and becomes more radiopaque (Fig. 25–11). The degree of increased opacity is directly related to the degree of collapse, and it may interfere with detection of pre-existing or concurrent lung disease. The pulmonary collapse is also responsible for obscuring lung markings that extend to the periphery of the thoracic cavity. Pulmonary collapse may be incomplete or asymmetric if compliance is decreased.

If the pneumothorax is open, i.e., no valve at the site of air entrance, air may continue to enter the pleural space until pleural pressure equals atmospheric pressure. At this point, the lung is maximally collapsed but still maintains roughly the shape of a normal lung, assuming compliance is uniform, because of its elasticity.

Separation of the heart from the sternum is commonly seen in lateral radiographs of patients with pneumothorax (Fig. 25–10). The heart appears elevated from the floor of the thorax, but actually it is displaced into the dependent hemithorax because of lack of underlying inflated lung to support it in its normal midline position. As the heart falls into the dependent hemithorax, it slides dorsally, creating the appearance of "elevation" when seen on a lateral radiograph (Fig. 25–12). Thus, "cardiac elevation" seen in the lateral projection is not pathognomonic for pneumothorax; it is a sign of lateral cardiac displacement.

As with pleural effusion, diagnosis of pneumothorax may not be possible from survey radiographs. The likelihood of diagnosis can be increased by using a horizontally directed x-ray beam and placing the patient in a position such that the x-ray beam is tangent to the area of air accumulation, e.g., lateral recumbency. Decreasing radiographic technique by 50 percent enhances visualization of the air by rendering the lung more opaque (Fig. 25–10C).

Justification for use of horizontal beam radiography to detect pneumothorax should be based on the suspected underlying cause. It is not as important to detect each small pneumothorax as it is each small pleural effusion. For example, small pneumothorax after trauma is insignificant in many patients, whereas small spontaneous pneumothorax that is the result of lung disease is potentially more serious.[6, 8]

In most animals, pneumothorax is bilateral; however, asymmetry of pleural space air volume or unilateral pneumothorax can occur for the same reasons as in pleural effusion. Appearance of unilateral pneumothorax in lateral radiographs depends on whether the affected

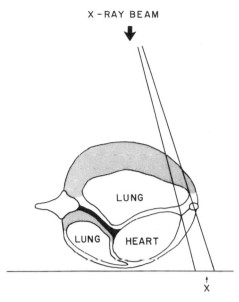

Figure 25–12. Principle of separation of the heart from the sternum in lateral radiographs of patients with pneumothorax. When the patient is placed in lateral recumbency, the lack of a fully inflated lung in the dependent hemithorax allows the heart to gravitate into the dependent hemithorax. As the heart falls into the dependent hemithorax, it slides dorsally because of the shape of the thoracic wall, thus creating a space between the heart and the sternum. As x rays pass through this space, the heart appears separated from the sternum (lateral view) by the distance "x".

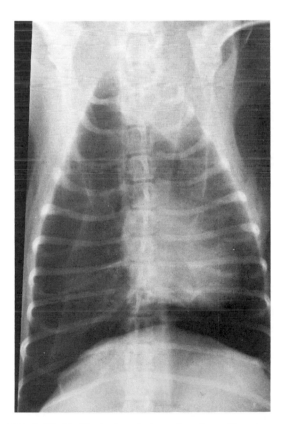

Figure 25–11. Ventrodorsal view of a dog with a large right pneumothorax. The right lung is partially collapsed and therefore is of increased radiopacity. The radiolucent area lateral to the right lung is due to gas in the pleural space. The heart has shifted to the left.

side is dependent or nondependent. The pleural space air is more apparent if the affected side is nondependent, because the air collects around the dorsocaudal portion of the caudal lobe. In this situation, the air collection is struck tangentially by the x-ray beam. If the affected side is dependent, the air collects against the mediastinum and is struck en face by the x-ray beam (Fig. 25–13).

Tension Pneumothorax. Tension pneumothorax occurs when pleural space pressure exceeds atmospheric pressure during both phases of respiration.[5] Tension pneumothorax results from a check-valve mechanism at the origin of pleural space air. In tension pneumothorax, the increased pleural pressure causes the lung to collapse to a greater degree than its maximal collapse in an open pneumothorax. Thus, it may no longer maintain the shape of a lung, but can assume the appearance of a relatively amorphous opacity on the midline. The increased pleural pressure also results in caudal displacement of the diaphragm and a shift of the mediastinum to the contralateral side during inspiration and expiration. Caudal displacement of the diaphragm may be to the degree that its

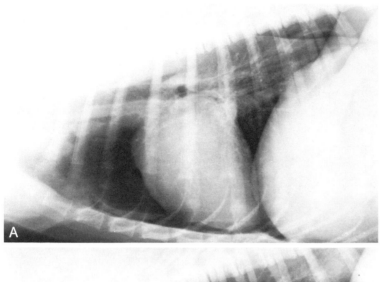

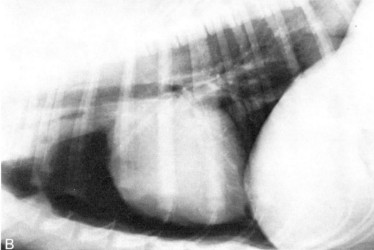

Figure 25–13. Right *(A)* and left *(B)* lateral views of a dog with a large left and a small right pneumothorax. *A*, The large pneumothorax collects around the left caudal lobe, resulting in clear visualization of collapse of the lobe. There is a small area of radiolucency ventral to the heart due to a slight shift in cardiac position to the right. Note the lack of heart displacement because of the almost fully inflated dependent right lung, which supports the heart on or near the midline. *B*, The large pneumothorax is now dependent. Rather than being located between the lung and the thoracic wall, where it can be struck tangentially by the x-ray beam, air is layered against the dependent side of the mediastinum. There is increased separation between the heart and the sternum due to atelectasis of the dependent left lung, which permits the heart to fall into the dependent hemihorax. A bullous lesion in the right caudal lung lobe and pneumomediastinum are also present.

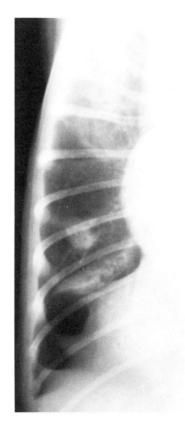

Figure 25–14. Ventrodorsal view of the thorax of a dog with tension pneumothorax. The increased pleural space pressure has displaced the diaphragm caudally to the extent that its costal attachments appear as tent-like projections from its surface.

tent-like costal attachments become visible (Fig. 25–14). It is important to recognize tension pneumothorax because it requires immediate thoracocentesis.

Pitfalls in Pneumothorax Diagnosis. In certain circumstances, erroneous diagnosis of pneumothorax may be made. Radiolucent areas frequently appear lateral to skin folds. Usually, it is possible to identify lung markings in the radiolucent area or to identify the opacity of the fold extending beyond the limits of the thorax. In chondrodystrophoid breeds, the configuration of the costochondral region frequently results in it appearing opaque radiographically. If the dog's sternum is rotated slightly to one side during radiography for the ventrodorsal or dorsoventral view, the area peripheral to the opacity appears radiolucent and can be convincing evidence for pneumothorax. Lung markings may be difficult to identify in this radiolucent region, and it may be necessary to resort to the use of horizontal beam radiography (Fig. 25–9).

Pleural Effusion with Pneumothorax. The combination of pleural effusion and pneumothorax is sometimes observed in animals as a result of trauma. The radiographic signs may be any combination of those already listed for pleural effusion (Table 25–2) and pneumothorax (Table 25–4). Definitive diagnosis can be made from horizontal beam radiographs in which a sharp air-fluid interface is seen.

References

1. Cantwell HD, Rebar AH, and Allen AR: Pleural effusion in the dog: Principles for diagnosis. J Am Anim Hosp Assoc 19:227, 1983.
2. Felson B: Chest Roentgenology. Philadelphia, WB Saunders, 1973, p. 351.
3. Groves TF, and Ticer JW: Pleural fluid movement: Its effect on appearance of ventrodorsal and dorsoventral radiographic projections. Vet Radiol 24:99, 1983.
4. Lord PF, Suter PF, Chan KF, et al: Pleural, extrapleural and pulmonary lesions in small animals. J Am Vet Radiol Soc 8:4, 1972.
5. Rabin CB, and Baron MG: Goldern's Diagnostic Radiology. Section 3: Radiology of the Chest, 2nd Ed. Baltimore, Williams & Wilkins, 1980, pp. 641, 652, 670.
6. Schaer M, Gamble D, and Spencer C: Spontaneous pneumothorax associated with bacterial pneumonia in the dog—two case reports. J Am Anim Hosp Assoc 17:783, 1981.
7. Suter PF, and Zinkl JG: Mediastinal, pleural and extrapleural thoracic diseases. In Ettinger SJ (Ed): Textbook of Veterinary Internal Medicine, 2nd Ed. Philadelphia, WB Saunders, 1983, pp. 840–883.
8. Yoshioka M: Management of spontaneous pneumothorax in 12 dogs. J Am Anim Hosp Assoc 18:57, 1982.

CHAPTER 26

THE HEART AND GREAT VESSELS

CHARLES R. ROOT
ROBERT J. BAHR

Normal radiographic anatomy of the thorax (Fig. 26–1) has been well documented.[2, 3, 5, 8, 14, 17, 21] Recommended routine radiographic projections vary.[3, 5, 8, 17, 18, 21] Some prefer dorsoventral as opposed to ventrodorsal projections, and others recommend right lateral rather than left lateral views. Most seem to offer logical justification for their preferences, depending upon suspected clinical diagnoses and the organs or structures of interest. The dorsoventral projection seems to be preferred to the ventrodorsal view for assessment of the cardiac silhouette,[3, 11, 21] whereas the opposite projection seems to be preferred for assessment of the lung.[11] In the opinion of the authors, the lateral projection with the left side down results in less distortion in position of the cardiac shadow than right lateral dependency, although this point is subject to some equivocation.[3, 8, 17] Fast exposure times are vital, if blurring due to patient motion is to be avoided.[8, 13, 17]

SPECIAL PROCEDURES

Critical radiographic assessment of diseases of the heart and great vessels requires rapid-sequence contrast radiography of the various cardiac chambers (angiocardiography) or portions of one or more of the great vessels (angiography) after selective opacification via a suitable catheter. Such special radiographic procedures are familiar to most veterinarians, but most are rarely employed in practice owing to the expense of the equipment and the infrequent indications for use. Patent ductus arteriosus (PDA) is a condition for which contrast radiography of a portion of the cardiovascular system is indicated. Fortunately, with adequate forethought and preparation, this condition is one of several that can be satisfactorily assessed with contrast radiography using a simple cassette changer.[12] Many other conditions can be evaluated by nonselective intravenous angiocardiography. The technique for radiographic demonstration and characterization of PDA is fairly straightforward and has been described elsewhere.[21] Angiocardiographic signs of cardiovascular diseases have been discussed.[3, 17, 21]

NORMAL RADIOGRAPHIC ANATOMY

Normal cardiovascular radiographic anatomy has been very well described by several authors[3, 5, 8, 11, 13, 17] and the description need not be augmented here. Several points are worthy of discussion, however. The external and internal boundaries of the individual chambers of the heart cannot be directly visualized on routine radiographs. Rather, their external margins

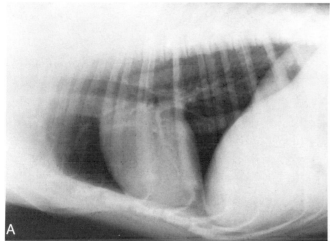
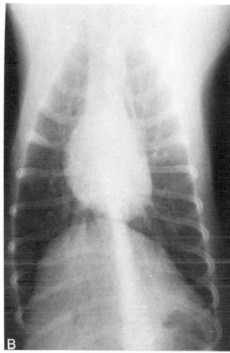

Figure 26–1. Lateral *(A)* and dorsoventral *(B)* thoracic radiographs of a normal 3-year-old, male mixed-breed dog.

merge with those of adjacent chambers because they are all contained within the pericardial sac and surrounded by a small amount of fluid. The coronary arteries cannot be seen, although pulmonary vessels superimposed upon the cardiac silhouette in the lateral projection are often confused with such. Similarly, the junctions of the left atrium and left ventricle can only be inferred radiographically, as can the point at which the right ventricle and atrium join. The internal features of the cardiac chambers are completely invisible unless contrasted by an opaque medium during angiocardiography.

RADIOGRAPHIC SIGNS

Individual Cardiac Chamber Enlargement

Unfortunately, there are no reliable mensuration techniques that can be used to assess cardiomegaly. Although such a technique has been reported,[7] its routine clinical application is equivocal[3, 11, 16, 17] and inaccurate for several reasons. First, the range of patient sizes is great, and there is considerable breed and individual variation in normal thoracic conformation. Second, it is impossible to routinely correlate radiographic exposure with respiration, heart cycle, and precise positioning of the thorax. Therefore, assessment of cardiac size is subjective at best. There are certain radiographic signs, however,

that seem to correlate well with specific cardiac lesions, especially when considered in light of clinical history, physical findings, and other radiographic observations. Differential diagnoses of cardiomegaly in dogs and cats has been especially well discussed in a recent text.[17]

Left Atrium. The left atrium is situated immediately ventral to the left main stem bronchus. Therefore, left atrial enlargement causes dorsal deviation of the left main stem bronchus, as viewed in the lateral projection (Fig. 26–2). Furthermore, in the same view, there is increase in size of the caudodorsal border of the heart. Viewed dorsally, the normal left atrium is roughly between the left and right main stem bronchi. Therefore, in the ventrodorsal projection, left atrial enlargement causes the left and right main stem bronchi to separate or diverge (Fig. 26–2). Distension or enlargement of the left atrial appendage (auricle) is rarely recognized radiographically; even when massive, it is recognized only in the ventrodorsal or dorsoventral projection and produces focal bulging of the left cardiac border between the main pulmonary artery and the apex of the heart (Fig. 26–3).

Left Ventricle. Since the left ventricle is relatively thick-walled, hypertrophy causes little distortion of its contour in the lateral projection; rather, it tends to elongate, causing dorsal displacement of the trachea (Fig. 26–4).[5, 17] This dorsal displacement involves the entire intra-

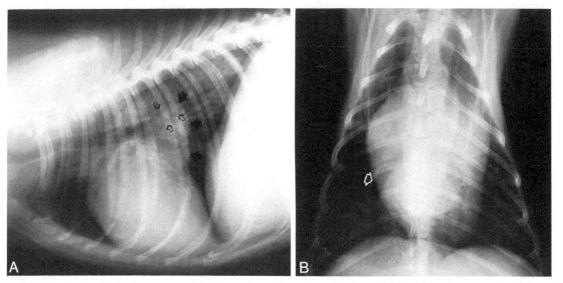

Figure 26–2. Lateral *(A)* and dorsoventral *(B)* thoracic radiographs of a dog with left atrial enlargment *(solid arrows)*. There is dorsal deviation of the left main stem bronchus *(open arrows)* in the lateral projection. In the dorsoventral projection, there is divergence of the left and right caudal lobar bronchi, the right caudal lobar bronchus (arrow) is bowed around the enlarged left atrium, and the caudal portion of the base of the heart is increased in opacity. (Courtesy of Grand Avenue Pet Hospital, Santa Ana, CA.)

thoracic portion of the trachea, from the thoracic inlet to the carina, resulting in decrease in the angle between the trachea and the thoracic vertebral bodies. The caudal margin of the left ventricular wall may become convex. In ventrodorsal or dorsoventral projections, there is rounding and levad displacement of the normally straight left side of the cardiac silhouette

(Fig. 26–4), and the apex of the heart may become rounded at its point of contact with the diaphragm.

Right Atrium. In the ventrodorsal or dorsoventral view, there is little of a reliable nature that can be attributed to right atrial enlargement. In the lateral projection, however, enlargement of the right atrium may cause dorsal

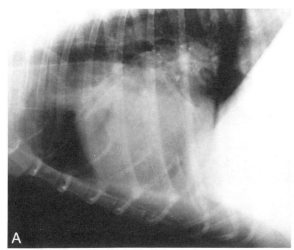

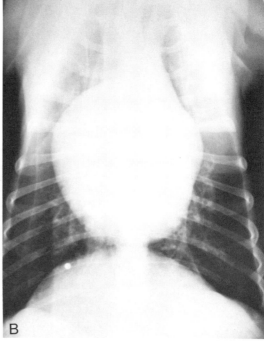

Figure 26–3. Lateral *(A)* and ventrodorsal *(B)* thoracic radiographs of a dog with enlargement of the left atrium and auricle. Notice the bulging auricle along the left side of the cardiac silhouette in the ventrodorsal view and elevation of the left main stem bronchus in the lateral projection.

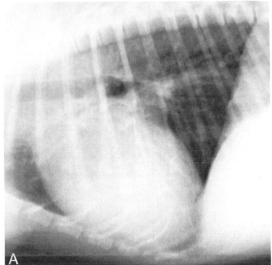

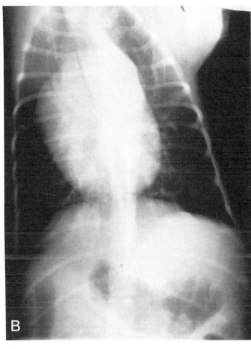

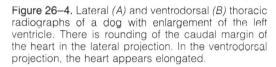

Figure 26–4. Lateral *(A)* and ventrodorsal *(B)* thoracic radiographs of a dog with enlargement of the left ventricle. There is rounding of the caudal margin of the heart in the lateral projection. In the ventrodorsal projection, the heart appears elongated.

bowing of the terminal portion of the trachea (Fig. 26–5). This finding may cause the caudal trachea (over the cranial portion of the heart base) to assume a distinct hook shape. It should be noted that the carina remains in its normal location unless there is concomitant left atrial or ventricular enlargement. In other words, in instances of selective right atrial enlargement, a line drawn from the middle of the tracheal lumen at the thoracic inlet through the midportion of the carina should duplicate the normal angle of the trachea with the vertebral column.

Right Ventricle. Rounding and enlargement of the right ventricle causes increased cardiosternal contact in the lateral projection and bulging of the right ventricular component of the cardiac silhouette in the ventrodorsal or dorsoventral view (Fig. 26–6). The latter lesion has been described as the "reversed D" sign.[5] In some instances, presumably because of hypertrophy rather than dilation of the right ventricular wall, the apex of the heart is markedly elevated from the sternum (Fig. 26–7). In most instances, right ventricular enlargement has little obvious effect upon the positions of the structures at the base of the heart.

Figure 26–5. Lateral thoracic radiograph of dog with enlargement of the right atrium. Notice that the caudal portion of the intrathoracic trachea is deviated (bowed) dorsally *(arrow)*. Yet the carina is not elevated, ruling out left atrial or ventricular enlargement.

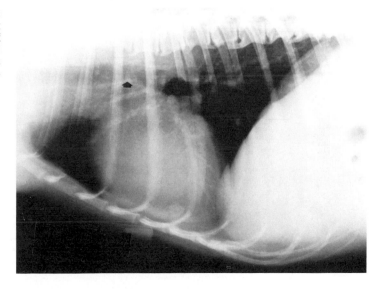

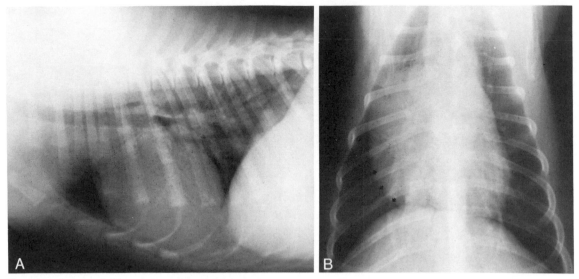

Figure 26–6. Lateral *(A)* and dorsoventral *(B)* thoracic radiographs of a dog with right ventricular enlargement. In the lateral projection there is extensive cardiosternal contact, while in the dorsoventral projection the right ventricle is rounded and projects into the right hemithorax *(arrows)*. The latter observation has been referred to as the reversed D sign.

Changes in the Great Vessels

There are several notable alterations in the radiographic appearances of the aorta, the caudal vena cava, and the main pulmonary artery.[17] Some of these are quite specific, whereas others may have several possible causes.

Caudal Vena Cava. The caudal vena cava is variable in diameter, depending upon the stage of the cardiac cycle and upon various disease states. Therefore, there is no specific ratio of measurements between the width of the caudal vena cava and other thoracic structures. Because of its normal variation in size it is not a very sensitive indicator of the existence of cardiac disease. If it is persistently large, right-sided congestive heart failure should be considered. If it is small in both projections or in repeated radiographs, hypovolemia should be considered.

Aorta. The aortic arch may be segmentally enlarged, as might occur as the result of PDA (Fig. 26–8). The entire aortic arch may also be dilated. In this instance, the result is widening of the caudal portion of the cranial mediastinum (Fig. 26–10) or a bulge on the cranial aspect of the heart on the lateral view.

Main Pulmonary Artery. Enlargement of the main pulmonary artery appears in the ventrodorsal or dorsoventral view as a bulge on the left cranial part of the cardiac silhouette in the 12:30–2 o'clock position (Fig. 26–9).

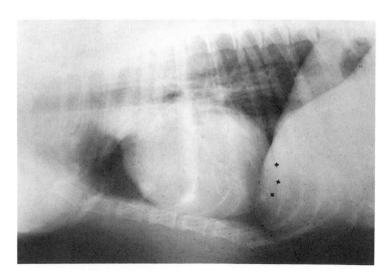

Figure 26–7. Lateral thoracic radiograph of a dog with marked rounding of the right ventricle. Notice that the apex *(arrows)* of the heart no longer contacts the ventral floor of the thorax. This radiographic sign is suggestive of hypertrophy, rather than dilation, of the right ventricle.

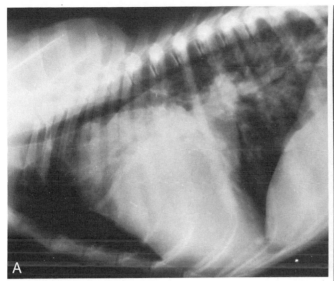
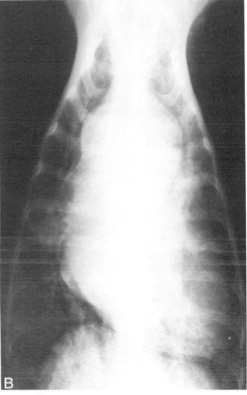

Figure 26–8. Lateral (A) and dorsoventral (B) thoracic radiographs of a dog with patent ductus arteriosus. In the dorsoventral projection, aortic enlargement has resulted in the caudal part of the cranial mediastinum becoming wide. Aortic enlargement is also seen in the lateral projection cranial to the heart base, which has resulted in elevated of the trachea. The heart is elongated in both projections, indicating left ventricular enlargement. The pulmonary vessels are prominent, and the left atrium is enlarged. Note the bowing of the right caudal lobe bronchus in the dorsoventral view owing to the enlarged left atrium. The main pulmonary artery is enlarged and can be seen in the dorsoventral view on the left just caudal to the enlarged aorta.

Congenital Lesions

Patent Ductus Arteriosus. There is segmental enlargement of the descending aortic arch (Fig. 26–8). This radiographic sign is theoretically caused by local aortic mural weakness adjacent to the patent ductus arteriosus.[17] The left ventricle is usually enlarged, as is the left atrium because of pulmonary overcirculation and/or distortion of the mitral annulus with secondary mitral insufficiency. Furthermore, the pulmo-

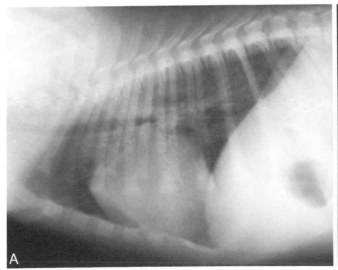
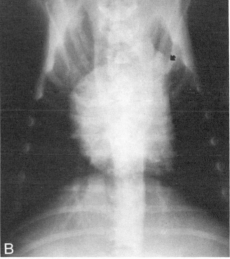

Figure 26–9. Lateral (A) and ventrodorsal (B) thoracic radiographs of a dog with pulmonic stenosis. There is right ventricular enlargement in both projections, and there is bulging of the main pulmonary artery (arrow) in the ventrodorsal projection. The latter radiographic sign is due to poststenotic dilation.

nary vascular pattern is enhanced because of pulmonary overcirculation and hypertension.

Pulmonic Stenosis. The main pulmonary artery is dilated. Turbulent blood flow creates nonlaminar vector forces that theoretically result in dilation of the affected segment of the pulmonary artery or right ventricular outflow tract through a mechanism that is, at best, poorly understood.[17] This poststenotic dilation results in distinct bulging of the left craniolateral aspect of the cardiac silhouette in the ventrodorsal or dorsoventral projection (Fig. 26–9). The pulmonary vascular pattern is usually normal unless right heart failure has developed. In both projections, the right ventricle is usually enlarged.

Aortic Stenosis. There is widening of the caudal aspect of the cranial mediastinum to accommodate poststenotic dilation of the aortic arch. This is usually obvious in both projections (Fig. 26–10). Also, there is usually elongation of the left ventricle owing to hypertrophy, since the heart has had to work against a partially obstructed left ventricular outflow tract. Pulmonary changes are generally absent, unless left ventricular enlargement has caused stretching of the mitral annulus leading to mitral insufficiency and secondary pulmonary edema.

Ventricular Septal Defect. There is usually slight biventricular enlargement (Fig. 26–11). The lung fields may be hypervascular but usually not to the same extent as in PDA.

Tetralogy of Fallot. This complex anomaly is classically described as the existence of four lesions: pulmonic stenosis, right ventricular hypertrophy, ventricular septal defect, and overriding aorta. Actually, this disorder can be thought of as two primary lesions, each with a secondary lesion. Pulmonary stenosis leads to right ventricular enlargement, and overriding aorta automatically creates a high ventricular septal defect. Radiographically, there may be no abnormalities, but in most instances there is biventricular enlargement, and hypovascular lung fields (Fig. 26–12).

Eisenmenger's Complex. This disorder is

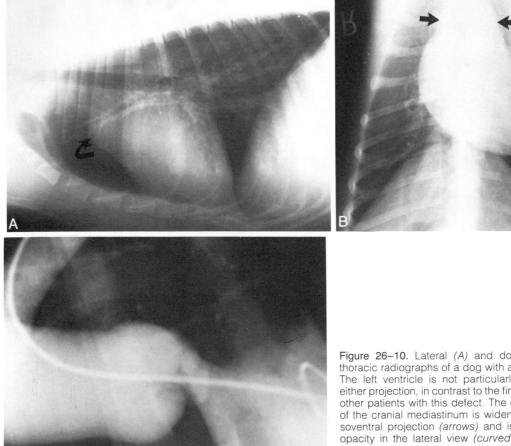

Figure 26–10. Lateral *(A)* and dorsoventral *(B)* thoracic radiographs of a dog with aortic stenosis. The left ventricle is not particularly enlarged in either projection, in contrast to the findings in many other patients with this defect. The caudal portion of the cranial mediastinum is widened in the dorsoventral projection *(arrows)* and is increased in opacity in the lateral view *(curved arrow);* these radiographic signs are produced by poststenotic dilation of the root of the aorta. *C,* note narrow subvalvular region and dilatation of aorta distal to the aortic sinus in the angiogram.

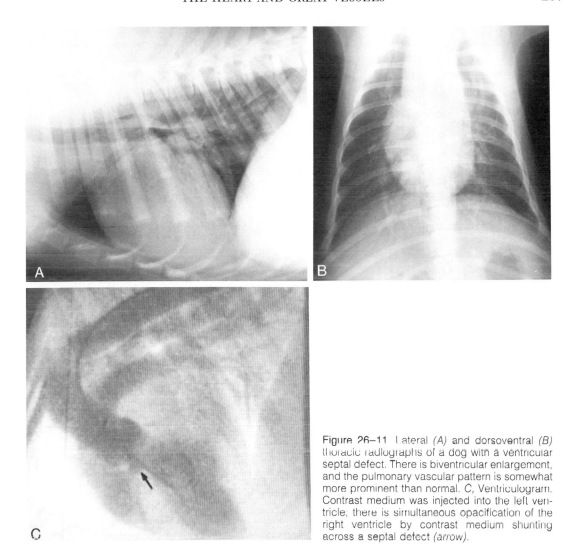

Figure 26-11 Lateral *(A)* and dorsoventral *(B)* thoracic radiographs of a dog with a ventricular septal defect. There is biventricular enlargement, and the pulmonary vascular pattern is somewhat more prominent than normal. *C,* Ventriculogram. Contrast medium was injected into the left ventricle; there is simultaneous opacification of the right ventricle by contrast medium shunting across a septal defect *(arrow).*

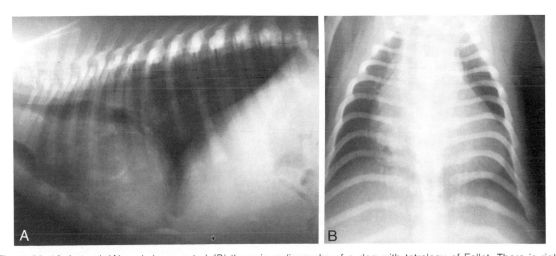

Figure 26-12. Lateral *(A)* and dorsoventral *(B)* thoracic radiographs of a dog with tetralogy of Fallot. There is right ventricular enlargement with displacement of the apex to the left. The pulmonary vascular pattern is markedly diminished. In some dogs there is biventricular enlargement and enlargement of the main pulmonary artery.

morphologically described as consisting of over-riding aorta, high ventricular septal defect, and right ventricular hypertrophy.[4] Radiographically, as in tetralogy of Fallot, the right ventricle may be enlarged. The lung markings may not be abnormal, but (in contrast with the findings expected in tetralogy of Fallot) pulmonary hypervascularity is sometimes seen, since there is left-to-right shunting.

Situs Inversus. This is an extremely rare congenital malformation in which the thoracic and abdominal viscera are reversed in laterality as mirror images of their normal location. It is usually associated with sinusitis and bronchitis, in which instance the condition is known as Kartagener's syndrome.[1, 15, 17] Radiographically (Fig. 26–13), the cardiac apex is on the right, the caudal vena cava is on the left, the accessory lobe of the lungs originates on the left side, the pylorus and fundus of the stomach are reversed, the right kidney is farther caudad than the left, the liver lobes are reversed, and so forth. Other than the associated respiratory problems, this condition has little significance beyond humbling veterinarians who are abusively critical of

their technical assistants for allegedly mismarking radiographs. Kartagener's syndrome is but one of several possible congenital diseases resulting in malorientation of the thoracic and abdominal viscera.[17]

Acquired Cardiovascular Lesions

Mitral Insufficiency. Insufficiency of the mitral valve produces left atrial enlargement, which, as previously discussed, often causes dorsal deviation of the left main stem bronchus and bowing and lateral divergence of the left and right main stem bronchi (Fig. 26–14). Additionally, by the time the patient is examined clinically, the left ventricle is usually also enlarged, causing dorsal elevation of the axis of the trachea and possible rounding of the normally straight caudal and levad borders of the cardiac silhouette. As left-sided heart failure occurs, the pulmonary veins become distended and possibly tortuous and pulmonary edema occurs, causing alveolar infiltrate.

Tricuspid Insufficiency. Although much less common as a single lesion than mitral insufficiency, tricuspid insufficiency occasionally exists without other cardiac lesions. Often, however, tricuspid insufficiency is secondary to distortion of the right atrioventricular annulus as a result of mitral insufficiency. Radiographic signs of this disorder, without concomitant left-sided changes,[3, 17] include right atrial enlargement and possible secondary right ventricular enlargement. The right atrium is enlarged, possibly causing dorsal bowing of the trachea over the cranial aspect of the base of the heart. Also, the right ventricle is enlarged, causing greater than normal sternal contact or elevation of the apex of the heart from the caudoventral floor of the thorax in the lateral projection. In the ventrodorsal or dorsoventral projection, the right ventricle is rounded, bulging into the right hemithorax and causing the "reversed D" sign.[5] If the right side of the heart is in failure, there may be hepatomegaly, splenomegaly, ascites, and pleural effusion.

Heartworm Disease. Heartworm disease is probably the most common cause for acquired *cor pulmonale* in dogs. The adult parasites most commonly reside in the right ventricle or the pulmonary arteries, occupying space in the respective lumina, causing physical obstruction of the outflow tract, and destroying normal laminar blood flow in the pulmonary arteries. Typically, as the disease progresses, the vascular intima becomes roughened, irregular, and hypertrophic, further compromising laminar flow. The pulmonary arteries dilate and become tortuous. Perivascular fibrosis follows pulmonary hypertension, and the disease becomes self-

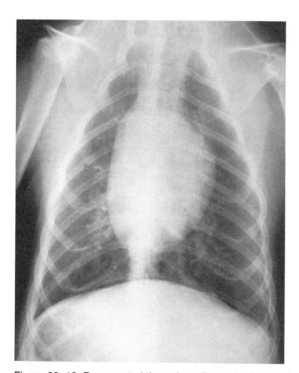

Figure 26–13. Dorsoventral thoracic radiograph of a dog with Kartagener's syndrome. The dorsoventral radiograph is positioned correctly with respect to right and left. There is complete situs inversus, resulting in mirror-image positioning of the thoracic and abdominal viscera. The apex of the heart is on the right, the caudal vena cava is on the left, the trachea is on the right, the ventral portion of the caudal mediastinum is on the right, and so forth. Notice also that the bronchial pattern is quite prominent.

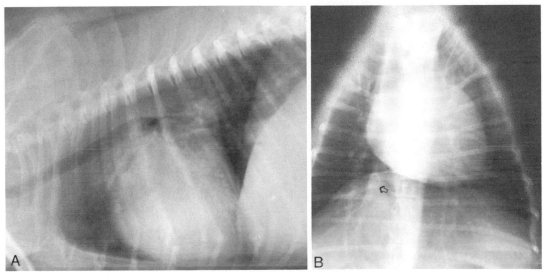

Figure 26–14. Lateral *(A)* and dorsoventral *(B)* thoracic radiographs of a dog with mitral insufficiency. There is left atrial and left ventricular enlargement. The trachea is elevated, and the left ventricular contour is rounded in both projections. An enlarged right caudal lobar pulmonary vein can be seen *(arrow)*.

perpetuating to the extent that progressive cardiovascular changes may occur even after the parasites are no longer present. Typical radiographic signs[11, 17, 21] of heartworm disease (Fig. 26–15) include right ventricular enlargement, dilation of the main pulmonary artery at the cranial left border of the ventrodorsal or dorsoventral cardiac silhouette, dilation and tortuosity of the lobar arteries, truncation or "pruning" of pulmonary arterial shadows, and pulmonary parenchymal infiltrate. As a general

rule, the diameter of the left and right pulmonary arteries at the base of the heart should not exceed the width of the ribs. Also, the cranial lobar arteries should be about the same size as the respective lobar veins. If right heart failure occurs, the radiographic signs may include ascites, splenomegaly, and hepatomegaly. Occasionally, adult heartworms may obstruct the caudal vena cava, producing dramatic clinical signs of central hypovolemia and caudal congestion.

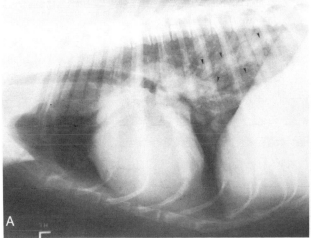

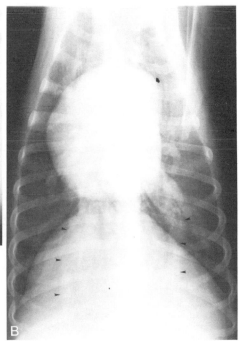

Figure 26–15. Lateral *(A)* and dorsoventral *(B)* thoracic radiographs of a dog with heartworm disease. There is right ventricular enlargement in both projections. The main pulmonary artery *(arrow)* is distended in the dorsoventral projection, and the left and right caudal lobar pulmonary arteries *(arrowheads)* are dilated and tortuous in both projections. The right cranial lobar pulmonary artery is also enlarged.

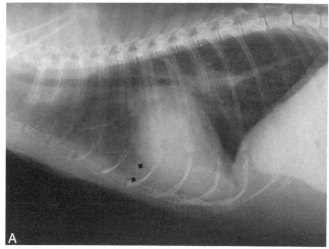

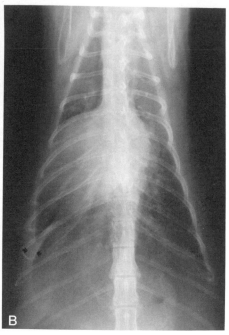

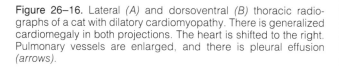

Figure 26–16. Lateral *(A)* and dorsoventral *(B)* thoracic radiographs of a cat with dilatory cardiomyopathy. There is generalized cardiomegaly in both projections. The heart is shifted to the right. Pulmonary vessels are enlarged, and there is pleural effusion *(arrows)*.

Cardiomyopathy. Dilatory cardiomyopathy in cats[9, 10, 17] (Fig. 26–16) and dogs (Fig. 26–17) produces generalized cardiomegaly[11, 17] and various radiographic signs of heart failure. In cats, right ventricular enlargement predominates, whereas in dogs both left- and right-sided failure often occur simultaneously. Therefore,

there may be ascites, hepatomegaly, splenomegaly, and pleural effusion associated with right ventricular failure in congestive cardiomyopathy in cats. In dogs, dilatory cardiomyopathy is often associated with pulmonary edema secondary to left ventricular failure, in addition to radiographic signs of right heart

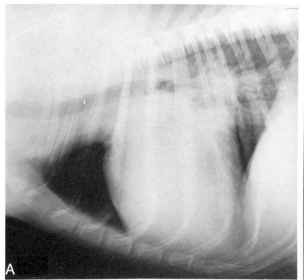

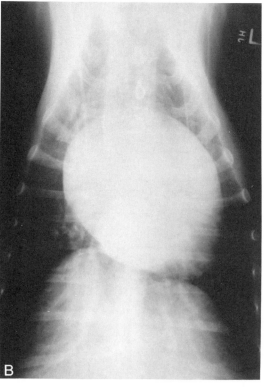

Figure 26–17. Lateral *(A)* and dorsoventral *(B)* thoracic radiographs of a dog with dilatory cardiomyopathy. There is generalized cardiomegaly, and the cardiac silhouette (in addition to being generally enlarged) is somewhat angular in shape.

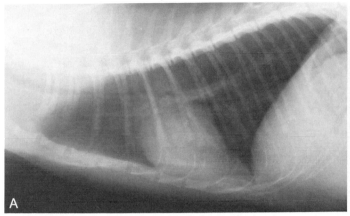

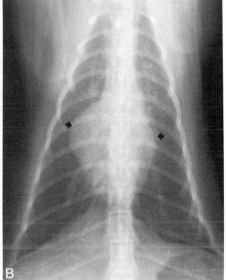

Figure 26–18. Lateral *(A)* and dorsoventral *(B)* thoracic radiographs of a cat with hypertrophic cardiomyopathy. There is no enlargement of the ventricles, but the atria *(arrows)* are enlarged. This is best appreciated in the dorsoventral projection.

failure. These clinical observations are consistent with the pathologic findings in this syndrome in dogs.[20] Hypertrophic cardiomyopathy in the cat (Fig. 26–18) produces biatrial enlargement[6, 17] but little external change in the ventricles. Secondarily, there may be extracardiac radiographic signs of heart failure, such as ascites, pleural effusion, pulmonary edema, and so forth. Differentiation of the feline cardiomyopathies has been greatly improved by the use of M-mode diagnostic ultrasound. This is now the imaging method of choice for clinical assessment of feline cardiomegaly.

Pericardial Effusion. As described earlier, the epicardial edges of the heart are normally not visualized, because of the presence of a small amount of free fluid in the pericardial sac. This fluid, between the pericardial sac and the epicardium, forms a silhouette sign between, and obliterates, the inside aspect of the pericardial sac and the outside aspect of the heart. Distension of the pericardial sac with large amounts of fluid causes the cardiac silhouette to be enlarged and globoid. Its distinctive radiographic outline (Fig. 26–19) has led to its description as globular. In the ventrodorsal or dorsoventral projection, the edge of the pericardial sac may touch the costal margins on both sides. Furthermore, the edge of the distended pericardial sac is often very distinct, since it undergoes little, if any, motion during systole and diastole. If the efficiency of the cardiac cycle is disrupted by the presence of the pericardial fluid, radiographic signs of congestive heart failure may also be present in the thorax or abdomen. The causes of hydropericardium may be neoplastic, inflammatory, congenital, or idiopathic. Among the possible neoplastic

causes for hydropericardium are heart-base tumors (chemodectomas) and metastatic or primary hemangiosarcomas. Of course, chemodectomas and other neoplasms at the base of the heart do not necessarily involve the pericardial sac. Pericardiocentesis and pneumopericardiography[17] have been recommended for the purpose of differential diagnosis of pericardial diseases. Diagnostic ultrasound is now the method of choice for imaging such lesions.

Cardiac Neoplasia. Neoplasms of the heart, whether primary or metastatic, are extremely rare and afford few reliable radiographic signs.[17] Cardiac hemangiosarcomas most commonly involve the right atrium and may produce selective enlargement of that chamber. Metastic or primary lesions in the myocardium may produce focal irregularity of the border of the cardiac silhouette.

Microcardia. Decrease in size of the cardiac silhouette may be absolute or relative.[17] If relative, the thorax has been overinflated by one of several possible conditions, such as emphysema or simple hyperventilation. If absolute, the causes include hypovolemia (due to blood loss or shock) and hypoadrenocorticism (Addison's disease). The pathogenesis of hypovolemia in Addison's disease is apparently equivocal. Hypovolemia appears to be the major reason for the decrease in size of the heart in the more acute form of the disease. In the chronically afflicted patient, however, decrease in cardiac size appears to be due, at least in part, to electrolyte imbalance, which theoretically results in decrease in myocardial mass owing to chronically weak contractions (disuse atrophy). Further discussion of the pathogenesis of microcardia is not within the scope of this text;

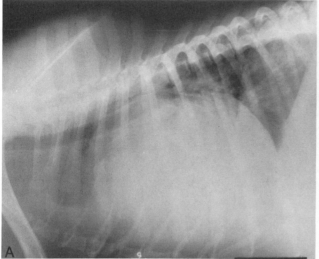

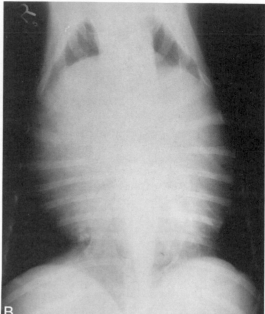

Figure 26–19. Lateral *(A)* and ventrodorsal *(B)* thoracic radiographs of a 5-year-old male mixed-breed dog with pericardial effusion due to a right atrial neoplasm. In the ventrodorsal projection, the cardiac silhouette is markedly enlarged and globoid. The edge of the pericardium is distinct in this view, since it underwent little motion during the radiographic exposure, but it is partially obliterated in the lateral projection owing to free pleural fluid secondary to right heart failure.

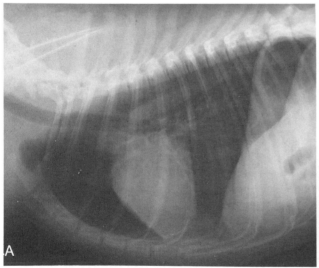

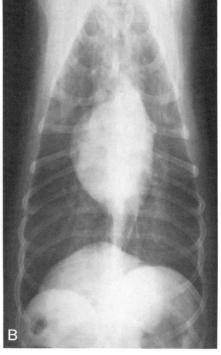

Figure 26–20. Lateral *(A)* and dorsoventral *(B)* thoracic radiographs of a dog with microcardia due to hypoadrenocorticism. The heart is markedly smaller than expected relative to the size of the chest cavity. Acute hypovolemic shock produces similar radiographic signs. (Courtesy of the Santa Cruz Veterinary Hospital.)

the interested reader is referred to existing physiology and internal medicine texts for more information. The radiographic sign associated with microcardia (Fig. 26–20) is, as the term suggests, the appearance of a smaller than normal cardiac silhouette relative to the size of the thoracic cavity. There are no objective measurements that can be made for assistance in borderline or equivocal situations, but the heart should generally occupy space in the thorax between the fifth and ninth ribs in the lateral projection exposed at maximum inspiration. It should not be widely separated from the diaphragm and the sternum, and its height should be sufficient to create an angle of approximately 10 to 15 degrees between the trachea and the cranial thoracic vertebral column in the dog. In the cat, this angulation may be less obvious and more difficult to measure than in the dog because of the natural lordosis that exists in the feline cranial thoracic spine.

References

1. Carrig CB, Suter PF, Ewing GO, and Dungworth DL: Primary dextrocardia with situs inversus, associated with sinusitis and brochitis in a dog. J Am Vet Med Assoc, 164:1127, 1974.
2. Douglas SW, and Williamson HD: Veterinary Radiological Interpretation. Philadelphia, Lea & Febiger, 1970.
3. Ettinger SJ, and Suter PF: Canine Cardiology. Philadelphia, WB Saunders, 1970.
4. Feldman EC, Nimmo-Wilkie JS, and Pharr JW: Eisenmenger's syndrome in the dog: case reports. J Am Anim Hosp Assoc, 17:477, 1981.
5. Gillette EL, Thrall DE, and Lebel JL: Carlson's Veterinary Radiology, 3rd ed. Philadelphia, Lea & Febiger, 1977.
6. Lord PF, Wood A, Tilley LP, and Liu S-K: Radiographic and hemodynamic evaluation of cardiomyopathy and thromboembolism in the cat. J Am Vet Med Assoc, 164:154, 1974.
7. Hamlin RL: Analysis of the cardiac silhouette in dorsoventral radiographs from dogs with heart disease. J Am Vet Med Assoc, 153:1446, 1968.
8. Kealy JK: Diagnostic Radiology of the Dog and Cat. Philadelphia, WB Saunders, 1979.
9. Liu S-K: Acquired cardiac lesions leading to congestive heart failure in the cat. Am J Vet Res, 31:2071, 1970.
10. Liu S-K, Tashjian RJ, and Patnaik AK: Congestive heart failure in the cat. J Am Vet Med Assoc, 156:1319, 1970.
11. Owens JM: Radiographic Interpretation for the Small Animal Clinician. St Louis, Ralston Purina Co, 1982.
12. Patterson DF, and Botts RP: A simple cassette changer. Small Anim Clinician, 1:1, 1960.
13. Roenigk WJ: Injuries to the thorax. J Am Anim Hosp Assoc, 7:266, 1971.
14. Schebitz H, and Wilkens H: Atlas of Radiographic Anatomy of Dog and Cat, 3rd ed. Berlin, Paul Parey, 1977.
15. Stowater JL: Kartagener's syndrome in a dog. J Am Vet Radiol Soc, 17:174, 1976.
16. Suter PF, and Lord PF: A critical evaluation of the findings in canine cardiovascular disease. J Am Vet Med Assoc, 158:358, 1970.
17. Suter PF: Thoracic Radiography: A Text Atlas of Thoracic Diseases of the Dog and Cat. Wettswil, Switzerland, Peter F Suter, 1984.
18. Ticer JW: Radiographic Technique in Veterinary Practice, 2nd ed. Philadelphia, WB Saunders, 1984.
19. van den Engh TSGAM, and van der Linde–Sipman JS: Vascular rings in the dog. J Am Vet Med Assoc, 164:939, 1974.
20. Van Vleet JF, Ferrans VJ, and Weirich WE: Pathologic alterations in congestive cardiomyopathy of dogs. Am J Vet Res, 42:416, 1981.
21. Watters JW: Radiographic signs of cardiovascular disease. Comp Contin Ed Pract Vet, 1:766, 1979.

CHAPTER 27

THE PULMONARY VASCULATURE

JOHN M. LOSONSKY

Diseases of the cardiovascular and pulmonary systems may exhibit similar clinical signs.[2] Thoracic radiographs can assist in differentiating pulmonary and cardiac diseases. In some diseases, both the pulmonary and cardiovascular systems can be affected. Lateral and dorsoventral or ventrodorsal survey radiographs can be used to evaluate the pulmonary vasculature. An attempt should be made to differentiate pulmonary arteries from veins, because cardiopulmonary diseases can result in radiographic changes involving pulmonary arteries, pulmonary veins, or a combination of the two types of vessels.

ANATOMY OF THE PULMONARY VASCULATURE

The pulmonary trunk arises from the pulmonary fibrous ring at the conus arteriosus.[4] After coursing for 3 to 4 cm, there is a division into the left and right pulmonary arteries. The left pulmonary artery divides into two or more branches. One of two smaller branches enters the cranial portion of the left cranial lobe (cranial lobar artery of the left cranial lobe). The larger branch subdivides and enters the caudal portion of the left cranial lobe (caudal lobar artery of the left cranial lobe) and the left caudal lobe (left caudal lobar artery).

The right pulmonary artery leaves the pulmonary trunk at almost a right angle and courses to the right. The first branch is the right cranial lobar artery. The vessel then divides into the right middle lobar, accessory lobar, and right caudal lobar arteries.

Commonly, there is one main vein from each lung lobe, but there can be two from the right cranial lobe.[4] The right middle lobar and right cranial lobar veins merge, as do the right caudal lobar and accessory lobar veins, before entering the left atrium. All lobar pulmonary veins from the left lung open individually into the left atrium.

RADIOGRAPHIC ANATOMY OF THE PULMONARY VASCULATURE

If radiographs are of diagnostic quality, the pulmonary vasculature of the central (hilar) and middle thirds of the lung parenchyma can be seen. In the peripheral one third of the lung, the vasculature may be seen only in larger dogs.

The large left and right pulmonary arteries may be seen on the lateral view from their origin cranial to the tracheal bifurcation (Fig. 27–1). The large left pulmonary artery lies dorsal to the trachea, whereas the large right pulmonary artery is ventral to the trachea. On the ventrodorsal or dorsoventral radiograph, the

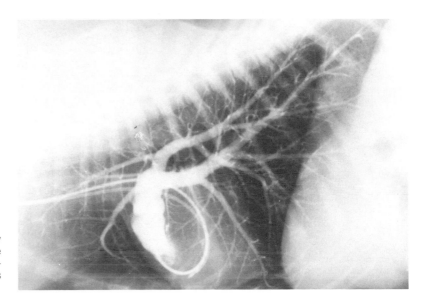

Figure 27–1. Lateral pulmonary angiogram of a 2-year-old male mixed-breed canine. The distribution of pulmonary arteries is normal.

left and right pulmonary arteries can be seen extending caudolaterally from the midcardiac region.

Large pulmonary veins may be seen on the dorsoventral view coursing medially to the caudal cardiac region as they merge near the left atrium. Pulmonary arteries and veins are better visualized on a dorsoventral radiograph as opposed to a ventrodorsal radiograph; this may be due to a greater degree of lung inflation on the dorsoventral view and also the more perpendicular relationship of these vessels relative to the primary x-ray beam.[16]

When an artery, bronchus, and vein to a corresponding lobe are seen on a lateral radiograph, the artery is dorsal to the bronchus and the vein is ventral.[4, 17] The right cranial lobar artery, bronchus, and vein can be seen most frequently (Fig. 27–2). The right cranial lobar artery is most commonly visualized when the animal is radiographed in left lateral recumbency (Fig. 27–3), a position in which the right cranial lobe can inflate to a greater extent, resulting in greater separation between these vessels. The right cranial lobar vessels are also located slightly ventral to the mediastinum,

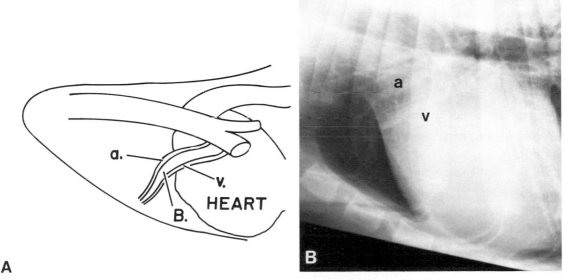

A

B

Figure 27–2. *A,* The lateral canine thorax. Location of the right cranial lobar artery (a), right cranial lobar vein (v), and right cranial lobar bronchus (B) can be seen. *B,* lateral view of the thorax of a normal 6-month-old male St. Bernard. Note the right cranial lobar artery (a) and the right cranial lobar vein (v). The right cranial lobar bronchus is located between the artery and vein. (From Thrall DE, and Losonsky JM: J Am Anim Hosp Assoc *12*:457, 1976, with permission.)

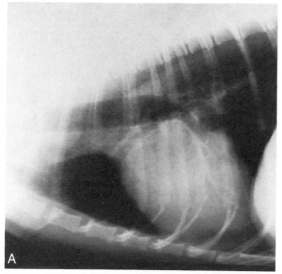

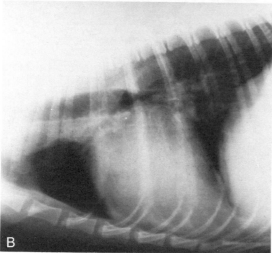

Figure 27–3. Lateral views of the thorax of a 12-year-old male beagle. A, with the dog in left lateral recumbency and on inspiration. B, with the dog in right lateral recumbency on expiration. Note the enhancement of visualization of the right cranial lobar vessels in A.

whereas the paired left cranial lobar vessels are superimposed over the mediastinum. The paired artery and vein to remaining lobes are not usually seen on lateral views.

When a lobar artery, vein, and bronchus can be seen on a dorsoventral radiograph, the artery is lateral to the vein with the bronchus located between the two vessels.[4, 17] The paired arteries and veins of the left and right caudal lung lobes can be identified more frequently on a dorsoventral view than on a ventrodorsal view (Fig. 27–4).[16] Paired arteries and veins are seen less frequently in the remaining lung lobes.

It has been stated that pulmonary arteries are more opaque, are better delineated, have a greater number of branches, and curve cranially and laterally relative to pulmonary veins.[2, 17] Pulmonary arteries and veins should have uniform tapering toward the periphery.

ROENTGEN SIGNS OF THE PULMONARY VASCULATURE

Geometric Changes

Size. On the left lateral recumbent radiograph, the right cranial lobar artery and vein should be approximately equal in size. The relative size of these two vessels at the level of the fourth intercostal space should be compared, and the size of each should be compared to the right fourth rib just ventral to the spine.[20] The diameter of each vessel should not exceed the smallest diameter of the right fourth rib.

On the dorsoventral radiograph, the size of caudal lobar arteries and veins should be compared to each other and to the diameter of the ninth rib at the point of intersection of the ninth rib and the corresponding vessel. The artery and vein of each caudal lobe should be similar in size. The diameter of the artery and vein caudal to the ninth rib should not exceed the diameter of that rib.

Table 27–1 is a list of some common diseases in which there can be an increase in size of pulmonary arteries and veins.[20] History, physical examination, electrocardiogram, survey thoracic radiographs, angiocardiogram, and clinical pathology results can be used to differentiate these conditions. The radiographic changes depend on the severity and duration of the disease (Fig. 27–5). Associated cardiac abnormalities are described in Chapter 26. Opacity changes in the lung parenchyma may also occur with vascular enlargement.

Pulmonary arterial enlargement can occur with diseases listed in Table 27–2.[5, 11, 12, 18, 20] Heartworm disease in the dog is the most common cause of pulmonary arterial enlargement. In heartworm disease, vessel enlargement occurs because of lesions in the tunica intima and tunica media, or thromboembolic disease, or both. Thoracic radiographic abnormalities seen in spontaneous dirofilariasis are documented.[3, 7, 13, 14] The percentage of dogs with right heart enlargement, main pulmonary artery enlargement, and right cranial lobar pulmonary artery enlargement has been reported.[10] The percentage of right cranial lobar pulmonary artery enlargement was only 47 percent (Fig. 27–6). In that study, caudal lobar pulmonary arteries were not measured because the animals were in dorsal recumbency as opposed to sternal recumbency. In the author's experience, the lobar arteries that enlarge most

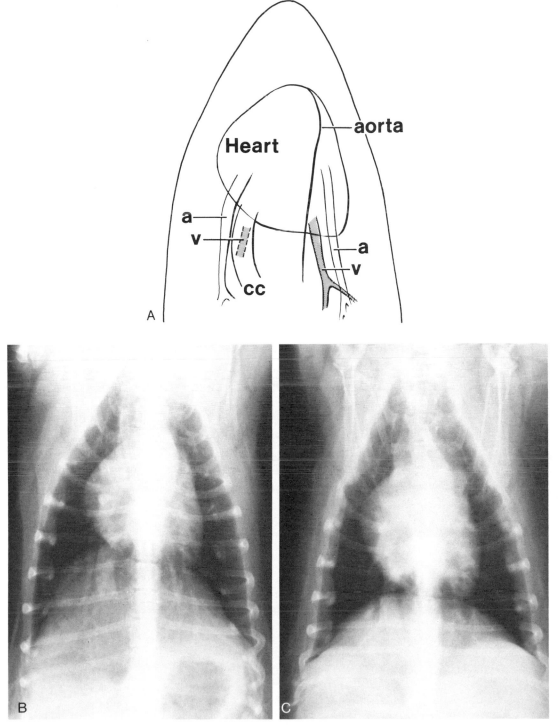

Figure 27–4. *A*, dorsoventral canine thorax. The location of pulmonary arteries and pulmonary veins to caudal lung lobes is illustrated. Dorsoventral *(B)* and ventrodorsal *(C)* views of a 12-year-old female Dachshund. Note the caudal lobar arteries and veins are better seen in *B* (sternal recumbency).

TABLE 27–1. DISEASES THAT MAY INCREASE THE SIZE OF PULMONARY ARTERIES AND PULMONARY VEINS

Left to right shunts
    Patent ductus arteriosus
    Ventricular septal defect
    Atrial septal defect
    Peripheral arteriovenous fistula
Iatrogenic fluid overload
Mitral insufficiency and heartworm disease
Feline cardiomyopathy
Right heart failure secondary to chronic left
    heart failure

TABLE 27–2. DISEASES THAT MAY INCREASE THE SIZE OF PULMONARY ARTERIES

Tunica intimal proliferation or tunica medial
    hypertrophy
    Dirofilariasis
    Angiostrongyliasis
    Aelurostrongylus (feline)
Thromboembolic disease or primary
    thromboses
    Dirofilariasis
    Disseminated intravascular coagulation
    Trauma
Secondary to cardiac diseases
    Angiostrongyliasis
    Active pulmonary congestion
Renal disease—amyloidosis,
    glomerulonephritis
Systemic venous thrombosis
Septicemia
Necrotic pancreatitis
Hyperadrenocorticism
Severe chronic lung disease

frequently in spontaneous heartworm disease are the caudal lobar arteries, with a predilection for the right over the left (Fig. 27–7). Experimentally, the right caudal lobar artery was the first to enlarge and did so most frequently. The

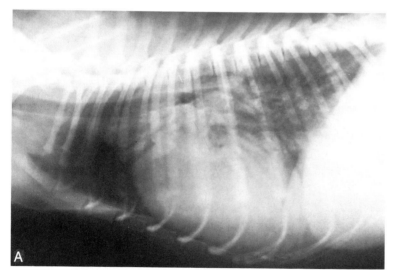

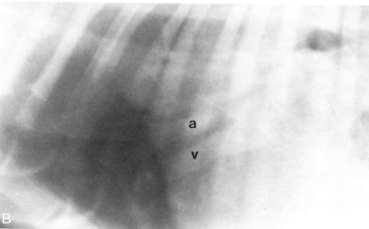

Figure 27–5. Lateral view of the thorax *(A)* is of a 6-month-old male cocker spaniel with a continuous heart murmur. Note the increase in size of the right cranial lobar artery and vein due to a left to right shunt. There is also heart enlargement. Note the increased opacity in the caudal lobes due to hypervascularity. Diagnosis, confirmed angiograpically, was patent ductus arteriosus. *B,* a close-up view in which the right cranial lobar artery (a) and right cranial lobar vein (v) can be seen. (From Thrall DE, and Losonsky JM: J Am Anim Hosp Assoc *12*:457, 1976, with permission.)

left caudal lobar artery was the next most frequently enlarged vessel.[9, 14, 19, 21] It is common in canine heartworm disease to see main pulmonary artery enlargement in association with peripheral pulmonary arterial enlargement (Fig. 27–7).[10] In feline heartworm disease, it is unusual to see main pulmonary artery enlargement on survey radiographs. With angiography, however, it is possible to see that the main pulmonary artery is enlarged, as are peripheral pulmonary arteries (Fig. 27–8).[1]

Other changes with canine heartworm disease that can be used to differentiate this disease from other diseases are pulmonary artery tortuosity (Figs. 27–7 and 27–9), loss of normal tapering (pruning) (Figs. 27–7 to 27–9), and foci of increased lung opacity seen on the lateral view along the course of the caudal lobar arteries (Fig. 27–10).[13, 14] The foci of increased opacity in the caudal lobes were present 6 months after experimental infection with L_3 larvae, and were still evident 12 months after treatment (Fig. 27–11). These lesions represent peripheral pulmonary arteries with dilatation, diverticulations, and residual tortuosity.[14] Fibrous connective tissue and chronic inflammatory cells can also persist in the arterial wall and perivascular tissue.

Heartworm disease is also the most common cause of thromboembolic disease in that there is arterial occlusion by worm emboli (Fig. 27–12).[13] Pulmonary emboli in heartworm disease have been described as round, irregular, semiopaque pulmonary infiltrates with hazy borders.[7] Pulmonary infarction in heartworm disease is rare.[9, 22]

One author has described normal-sized or enlarged hilar pulmonary arteries in dogs with pulmonary thrombosis or thromboembolism that was not due to dirofilariasis.[19] Also de-

Figure 27–6. Lateral view of the thorax *(A)* of a 7-year-old male English setter. Note the enlarged right cranial lobar artery relative to the right cranial lobar vein. Diagnosis: heartworm disease. *B,* a close-up view illustrates the size differential between the artery (a) and the vein (v).

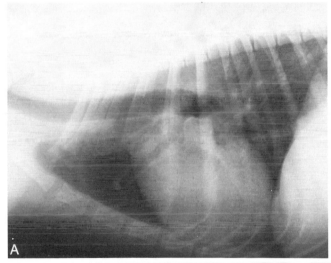

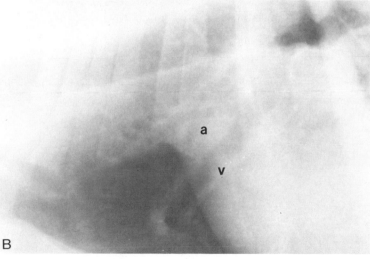

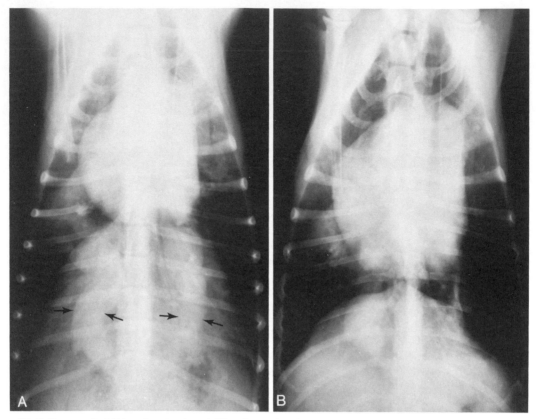

Figure 27–7. Dorsoventral *(A)* and ventrodorsal *(B)* radiographs of a 4-year-old male German shepherd with heartworm disease. The right and left caudal lobar pulmonary arteries are severely enlarged *(arrows),* lack the normal uniform tapering (pruning), and are blunted (truncated) at their most distal aspect. Both views show main pulmonary artery enlargement. There is severe tortuosity of the right caudal lobar artery. Note the enhanced visualization of these vessels in the dorsoventral view *(A).*

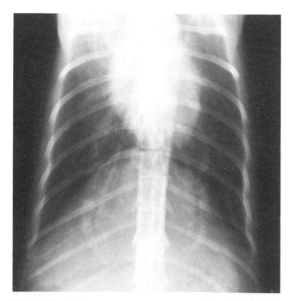

Figure 27–8. Dorsoventral view of the thorax of a 3-year-old castrated male domestic shorthair cat. Note the increase in size of the caudal lobar arteries and abrupt tapering of the distal portions of the caudal lobar arteries. Six adult heartworms were found at necropsy.

scribed were normal to reduced lung volume with lobar hyperlucency, reduced size of peripheral lung vessels in affected areas, small pleural effusion, right ventricular enlargement, and absence of consolidations, atelectasis, or edema commensurate with the severity of the clinical signs. In another report, 21 dogs with pulmonary thrombosis or thromboembolism not associated with dirofilariasis or disseminated intravascular coagulation were described.[5] Radiographic changes included some of the following: alveolar disease, hyperlucency of a lung lobe or lung region (hypovascular), and pleural effusion especially with infarction or cardiac disease. In those instances with hyperlucency of a lung lobe or lung region, the major artery (11 cases) or major vein (14 cases) could not be identified or was abruptly attenuated. Seven dogs had pulmonary arterial occlusion, seven dogs had pulmonary arterial occlusion with hemorrhage, and seven dogs had pulmonary arterial occlusion with infarction. The most definitive procedure to diagnose pulmonary thrombosis or embolism is pulmonary angiography.

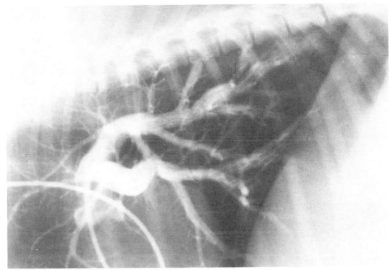

Figure 27–9. Lateral arteriogram of a mixed-breed dog 12 months after experimental infection with third-stage heartworm larvae. Note the tortuosity of the pulmonary arteries, linear filling defects (adult heartworms), nonuniform arterial tapering, and saccular dilatations of the smaller intralobar arteries. Contrast medium was not seen more distally in the caudal lobar arteries on subsequent radiographic examinations, indicative of pulmonary arterial obstruction. (From Rawlings CA, et al: J Am Anim Hosp Assoc 16:17, 1980, with permission.)

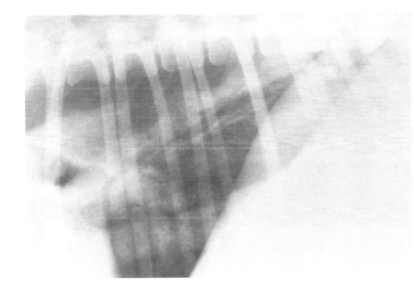

Figure 27–10. Close-up lateral radiograph of the dorsocaudal lung lobes of a 4-year-old mixed, spayed female dog. Note the increased lung parenchymal opacity in the dorsocaudal lung region. This change is due to caudal lobar pulmonary arterial enlargement, saccular diverticulations of small arteries, and associated lung disease. The dorsoventral view can be used to confirm that this opacity represents abnormal caudal lobar arteries.

Figure 27–11. Lateral arteriogram of a mixed-breed, male canine 12 months after treatment for heartworm disease. Slight arterial enlargement, saccular dilatations of the intralobar arteries, and minimal tortuosity remain. (From Rawlings CA, et al: J Am Anim Hosp Assoc 16:17, 1980, with permission.)

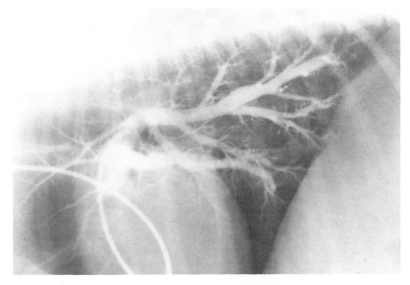

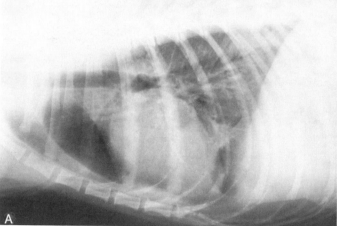

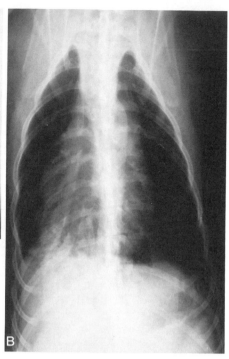

Figure 27–12. Lateral *(A)* and dorsoventral *(B)* radiographs of a 3-year-old male Siberian husky 1 week after heartworm treatment. The dog was depressed, febrile, and dyspneic. There is alveolar lung disease and partial atelectasis of the right caudal lung lobe. The heart is displaced slightly to the right due to lung atelectasis. Pleural effusion is present. These radiographic changes represent thromboembolic disease secondary to heartworm therapy.

Table 27–3 outlines the differential diagnoses for pulmonary venous enlargement (Fig. 27–13).[8, 20] The majority of the diseases are associated with congenital or acquired cardiac disease. The radiographic changes associated with cardiac disease are described in Chapter 26.

Table 27–4 is a list of diseases with a decrease in size of pulmonary arteries and pulmonary veins.[2] The lung field appears hyperlucent, which results from the pulmonary arteries and veins contributing less soft-tissue opacity to the

lung parenchyma because of their reduction in size (Fig. 27–14).

Shape. Shape changes are most commonly seen in dogs with heartworm disease. With dirofilariasis, in addition to an increase in size of the pulmonary arteries, there can be vascular tortuosity (Figs. 27–7, 27–9, 27–11), nonuniform tapering from the midportion of the artery distally (Figs. 27–7 and 27–8), and dilatation of smaller arterial branches. Changes can be seen on survey thoracic radiographs, but they are best documented by pulmonary arteriography. On survey radiographs of 200 dogs with spontaneous heartworm disease, only 16.5 percent were identified as having tortuous arteries (J. Losonsky, unpublished data). In this study, radiographs of dogs in left lateral recumbency and dorsal recumbency were evaluated. In radiographs made with the animal in ventral recumbency, the caudal lobar arteries are better visualized (Fig. 27–7).[16] Shape changes with heartworm disease are seen early in the disease, and frequently involve caudal lobar arteries, although they can also be seen in the remaining peripheral arteries.[10, 13, 14, 21] Rapid peripheral arterial tapering and focal saccular dilatations can occur with any disease that produces pulmonary arterial thrombosis or thromboembolism, but the rate of occurrence is greater in heartworm disease.

Margination. Loss of pulmonary vessel margins can be focal, multifocal, diffuse, symmetric, or asymmetric (Fig. 27–15). Soft-tissue opaque material (fluid, cells, or debris) in the intersti-

TABLE 27–3. DISEASES THAT MAY INCREASE THE SIZE OF PULMONARY VEINS

Cardiac
Volume overload
Mitral insufficiency
Early left to right shunts—thinner wall of vein
  dilated more easily
  Patent ductus arteriosus
  Ventricular septal defect
  Atrial septal defect
Pressure overload
Aortic stenosis
Primary myocardial disease
Myocardial failure
  Dilatory cardiomyopathy
Diastolic compliance failure
  Hypertrophic cardiomyopathy
  Restrictive cardiomyopathy
Noncardiac
Left atrial obstruction
Neoplasm
Thrombosis

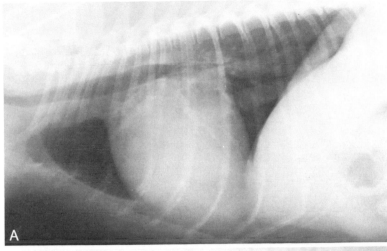

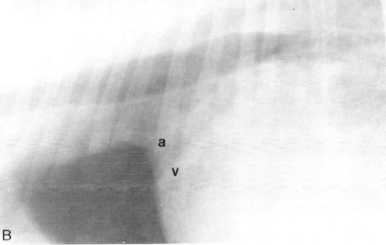

Figure 27–13. Lateral view of the thorax (A) of an 8-year-old male poodle. Note the slight pulmonary venous distension as the right cranial lobar vein is larger than the right cranial lobar artery. There is severe left atrial enlargement. Diagnosis: mitral insufficiency. B, a close-up view of A shows the large right cranial lobar pulmonary artery (a) relative to the vein (v).

tium or alveoli adjacent to a pulmonary vessel silhouette with the vessel and obscure its margins.

Radiopacity Changes

The pulmonary arteries and veins are the most prominent structures of the lungs.[2] Therefore, these vessels contribute more opacity to the

TABLE 27–4. DISEASES THAT MAY DECREASE THE SIZE OF PULMONARY ARTERIES AND VEINS

Right to left shunts
  Tetralogy of Fallot
  Ventricular septal defect with pulmonic
    stenosis
  Atrial septal defect with pulmonic stenosis
  Severe pulmonic stenosis
Hypovolemia
  Shock
  Dehydration
Adrenocortical hypofunction

normal lung parenchyma than any other structures. It is difficult to describe what normal lung opacity should be. Incorrect technical exposures present problems in that underexposed radiographs may create artificial lung opacities, whereas overexposed radiographs may mask increases in lung opacity. Phase of respiration can also alter the opacity of the lung parenchyma. Radiographs made during expiration increase the background lung opacity, whereas those made during inspiration reveal less background opacity. Frequently, there is more lung opacity in older animals because of interstitial accentuation.[15] Experience in viewing radiographs facilitates the differentiation of diseases from technical errors.

All diseases that produce an increase in size of pulmonary arteries, pulmonary veins, or both increase the opacity of the lung (Figs. 27–5, 27–10, 27–15). Those abnormalities listed in Table 27–4, which result in a decrease in size of pulmonary arteries and veins, also decrease lung opacity (Fig. 27–14). Lobar or sublobar

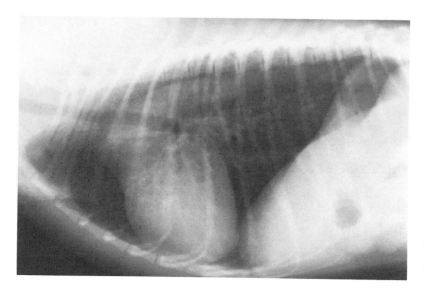

Figure 27–14. Lateral view of the thorax of a female spayed 9-month-old poodle. Note the lack of opacity in the lung lobes due to hypovascularity and lung hyperinflation. Tetralogy of Fallot was confirmed at necropsy.

Figure 27–15. Lateral view of the thorax (A) of a 6-year-old male Doberman pinscher. Note the discrepancy between the right cranial lobar vein and artery. There is loss of margination of the vasculature and increased lung parenchymal opacity due to heart failure with pulmonary edema. B, a close-up view shows the enlarged cranial lobar pulmonary vein (arrows) with loss of distinct margination. Diagnosis: dilatory cardiomyopathy.

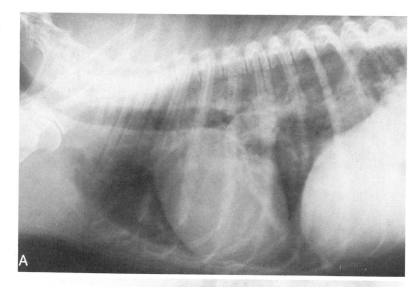

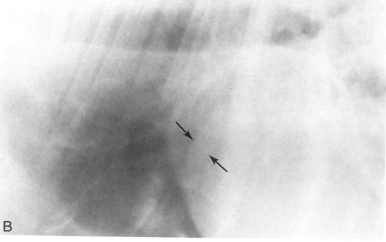

hyperlucency due to the reduced size of lung vessels (hypoperfusion) has been reported in pulmonary thromboembolism.[18] In another report, loss of visualization of a lobar artery or vein in a lung lobe with pulmonary thrombosis or embolism was mentioned.[5]

Functional Changes

Functional changes involving the pulmonary vasculature can be documented by pulmonary angiography. Pulmonary thromboembolic disease occurs when the pulmonary arterial blood flow to a portion of the lung is interrupted by thrombosis or embolism.[6] The occlusion of a pulmonary artery can result in ischemia, hemorrhage, or infarction.[5] Loss of surfactant in the occluded lung may result in atelectasis and edema, but hemorrhage, edema, and infarction may have identical radiographic patterns.[5] Pulmonary infarction implies lung parenchymal necrosis resulting from pulmonary vascular obstruction.[6]

Thromboembolic or primary thrombotic etiologies listed in Table 27–2 are capable of producing functional pulmonary arterial occlusive diseases. The pulmonary angiogram may show intraluminal filling defects in the artery with compromised blood flow, or total obstruction may be revealed (Fig. 27–9). Pulmonary thromboembolism occurs most frequently in canine heartworm disease (Fig. 27–12). Pulmonary infarction is unusual in dogs and cats.

References

1. Donahoe JM, Kneller SK, and Lewis RE: In vivo pulmonary arteriography in cats infected with Dirofilaria immitis. Pulmonary arteriography in cats infected with Dirofilaria immitis. J Am Vet Radiol Soc 17:147, 1976.
2. Ettinger SJ, and Suter PF: Radiographic examination. In Canine Cardiology. Philadelphia, WB Saunders, 1970, pp. 40–101.
3. Ettinger SJ, and Suter PF: Cor pulmonale. In Canine Cardiology. Philadelphia, WB Saunders, 1970, pp. 425–428.
4. Evans HE, and Christensen GC: The respiratory apparatus. In Miller's Anatomy of the Dog. Philadelphia, WB Saunders, 1979, p. 541.
5. Fluckiger MA, and Gomez JA: Radiographic findings in dogs with spontaneous pulmonary thrombosis or embolism (PTE). Vet Radiol 25:124, 1984.
6. Fraser RG, and Paré JP: Diagnosis of Diseases of the Chest. Philadelphia, WB Saunders, 1970.
7. Jackson WF: Radiographic examination of the heartworm-infected patient. J Am Vet Med Assoc 154:380, 1969.
8. Kittleson M: Concepts and therapeutic strategies in the management of heart failure. In Kirk RW (Ed): Current Veterinary Therapy VIII. Philadelphia, WB Saunders, 1983, pp. 279–284.
9. Liu SK, Yarns DA, Carmichael JA, et al: Pulmonary collateral circulation in canine dirofilariasis. Am J Vet Res 30:1723, 1969.
10. Losonsky JM, Thrall DE, and Lewis RE: Thoracic radiographic abnormalities in 200 dogs with spontaneous heartworm infestation. Vet Radiol 24:120, 1983.
11. Losonsky JM, Thrall DE, and Prestwood AK: Radiographic evaluation of pulmonary abnormalities after Aelurostrongylus inoculation in cats. Am J Vet Res 44:478, 1983.
12. Prestwood AK, Green CE, Mahaffey EA, et al: Experimental canine angiostrongylosis. I. Pathological manifestations. J Am Anim Hosp Assoc 17:491, 1981.
13. Rawlings CA, Lewis RE, and McCall JW: Development and resolution of pulmonary arteriographic lesions in heartworm disease. J Am Anim Hosp Assoc 16:17, 1980.
14. Rawlings CA, Losonsky JM, Lewis RE, et al: Development and resolution of radiographic lesions in canine heartworm disease. J Am Vet Med Assoc 178:1172, 1981.
15. Reif JS, and Rhodes WH: The lungs of aged dogs: A radiographic-morphologic correlation. J Am Vet Radiol Soc 7:5, 1966.
16. Ruehl WW, and Thrall DE: The effect of dorsal versus ventral recumbency on the radiographic appearance of the canine thorax. Vet Radiol 22:10, 1981.
17. Suter PF: Principles of respiratory function and disease: Normal radiographic anatomy as a basis for a systemic interpretation of diseases of the thorax. In Scientific Presentations and Seminar Synopses. 41st Annual Meeting of the American Animal Hospital Association, San Francisco, CA, 1974, pp. 707–715.
18. Suter PF: Miscellaneous diseases of the thorax. In Ettinger SJ (Ed): Textbook of Veterinary Internal Medicine. Diseases of the Dog and Cat. Philadelphia, WB Saunders, 1983, pp. 887–890.
19. Tashjian RJ, Liu SK, Yarns DA, et al: Angiocardiography in canine heartworm disease. J Vet Res 31:415, 1970.
20. Thrall DE, and Losonsky JM: A method for evaluating canine pulmonary circulatory dynamics from survey radiographs. J Am Anim Hosp Assoc 12:457, 1976.
21. Thrall DE, Badertscher RR, Lewis RE, et al: Radiographic changes associated with developing dirofilariasis in experimentally infected dogs. Am J Vet Res 41:81, 1980.
22. Thrall DE, Badertscher RR, Lewis RE, et al: Collateral pulmonary circulation in dogs experimentally infected with Dirofilaria immitis. Vet Radiol 21:131, 1980.

CHAPTER 28

THE LUNGS

JOHN W. WATTERS

There are a limited number of ways in which the lungs can respond to disease. By using a method of pattern recognition of radiographic signs, it is easier to arrive at a list of differential diagnoses. The lungs become more opaque or more radiolucent depending on the disease, trauma, or other insult. These changes can be divided into localized or generalized areas of involvement. It is difficult if not impossible to make a definitive diagnosis on the basis of radiographic signs alone. Therefore, all the information should be used, including the results of laboratory analysis, physical findings, history, and any other data that might be available to reach a final diagnosis.

Pattern recognition helps to categorize lung changes according to alveolar, interstitial, bronchial, and vascular changes.[8] When it is known how the lungs respond to various insults, the correct list of differential diagnoses can be formulated. The lungs are composed of only two radiographic opacities—water and air. Also, it is not possible to determine if an increased radiopacity is the result of free fluid, exudate, blood, or any other material of fluid opacity. Once an abnormality has been determined to be of a certain pattern, the appropriate list of differential diagnoses can be consulted.

RADIOGRAPHIC TECHNIQUE

The quality and size of the x-ray machine is probably more important for radiography of the thorax than for any other body part. It is necessary to have high milliamperage (preferably 300 mA) and a timer capable of short exposure times (less than 1/30 second) to reduce cardiac and respiratory movement. Use of a high kVp technique is desirable, to reduce the contrast of the ribs and other osseous structures. Because air and soft tissue are contrasted in the lungs, it is not necessary to increase patient contrast by using a low kVp technique. Use of a low mA, high kVp technique for the thorax also permits the use of shorter exposure time. The high kVp technique produces a long gray scale (low contrast), which provides a larger amount of information than is seen with a short gray scale (high contrast). It is recommended that rare-earth screens be used for large-breed dogs and in facilities that do not have a 300 milliamperage x-ray machine. There is a great deal of variation between rare-earth screens; those screens that do not have a great deal of quantum mottle should be purchased. At one time, it was necessary to compromise detail for speed, but there are rare-earth screens now available that have good detail and high speed.

Some individuals recommend that a grid be used for thoracic radiography of large dogs and a non-grid technique be used for smaller dogs.

It is not necessary, however, that two different procedures be used. Fewer mistakes are made if all thoracic radiographs are made with a grid. There is some scatter produced even with small dogs and this can be reduced with a grid. The type of grid is optional, although it is suggested that a grid with at least 103 lines/in be used without a Bucky diaphragm. The noise produced by the reciprocating grid mechanism often causes the patient to move during the exposure. The grid ratio should be at least 8:1; 10:1 is better for large patients. It is also recommended that an aluminum interspaced grid be used instead of a fiber, paper, or plastic interspaced grid. This type of grid is more critical for radiography of the thorax than for other body parts. The fiber interspaced grids often produce a mottled pattern in the lung, which may be confused with lung disease.

The lungs cannot be used as a criterion for evaluating radiographic technique; this must be determined by relative opacities between bone and soft tissue outside the lung field.

It is not possible to obtain a maximal amount of radiographic information about the cardiovascular and pulmonary systems with the same exposure technique. To evaluate the lungs, it is necessary to use about one half the exposure factors required for the heart and vessels. It is a compromise to use the same technique for assessment of both systems. It is suggested that the lesser technique be used first, the exposure may then be doubled if the cardiovascular system cannot be adequately evaluated.

PATIENT POSITIONING

The patient should be consistently positioned so that the same relationship of the heart, mediastinum, lungs, diaphragm, and rib cage is always seen. The number of variables should be kept to a minimum so that more attention can be paid to the radiographic signs. Good quality radiographs of the lungs depend to a great extent on the amount of air that is within the lungs. Therefore, it is imperative to try and make the radiographic exposure during maximum inspiration for most conditions. It is essential that two views be taken at 90 degrees to each other. Occasionally, it is also necessary to take oblique views to see portions of the lungs that otherwise might be superimposed on the heart, mediastinum, sternum, or spine.

It is recommended that ventrodorsal views be obtained for pulmonary evaluation.[4] The central x-ray beam should be positioned over the heart with the animal in dorsal recumbency. The patient should be aligned so that the sternum is superimposed on the spine. The front legs should be extended cranially with the scapulae rotated away from the cranial thoracic

region. It is possible to remove the scapulae completely from the thoracic field by pulling the legs caudally along the body wall. This position allows an end-on view of the scapulae, which are outside of the thoracic area.

Either the right lateral or the left lateral recumbent view is satisfactory for evaluation of the lungs. More information, however, is seen in the nondependent lung (Fig. 28–1). The nondependent lung contains more air and therefore there is more contrast with any pathologic process that might be present.[6] Radiography is contraindicated for patients that have been in lateral recumbency under general anesthesia for even a few minutes. Atelectasis of the dependent lung causes increased lung field opacity and may obliterate pathologic lung changes. Because it is usually not feasible to routinely make both the right and left lateral projections, it is suggested that the left lateral recumbent view be taken first. If there are suspicious areas on the ventrodorsal view, the right lateral recumbent view can then be taken. If it is necessary that animals be radiographed under general anesthesia, it is recommended that the patient's lungs be inflated several times before the radiographs are taken. It may also be helpful to roll the animal periodically from one side to the other to help prevent hypostatic congestion.[9]

LUNG MODEL

A lung model was prepared to illustrate different types of pulmonary changes that occur with disease processes. A thin section of sponge was used to represent the pulmonary parenchyma. Straws filled with air and water were used to represent bronchi and pulmonary vessels. Figure 28–2A represents normal lung parenchyma. Figure 28–2B was made by soaking the sponge in water. The water-filled sponge was used to illustrate a generalized interstitial infiltrate, which results in generalized increased lung opacity, as compared with the normal lung. Figure 28–3A represents a longitudinal and a cross-sectional view of a pulmonary vessel contained within normal pulmonary parenchyma. Figure 28–3B is a syringe case filled with water that represents a pulmonary vessel. The syringe case was radiographed end-on and in lateral recumbency. As can be seen, end-on vessels are more radiopaque than are the same-sized vessels seen longitudinally because of greater thickness.

The lung model in Figure 28–4A illustrates radiographic signs seen with severe interstitial infiltrate. The vertical radiolucent area represents a bronchus. Smaller circular radiolucent areas represent smaller airways, or groups of

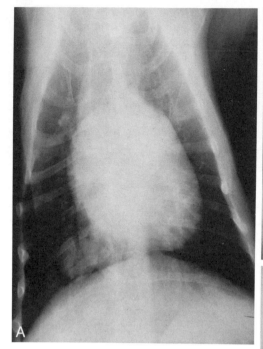

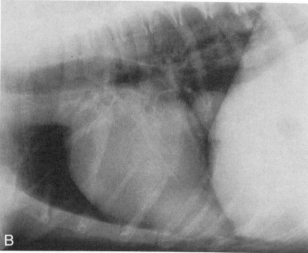

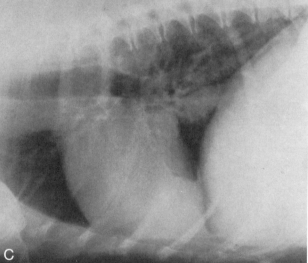

Figure 28–1. *A,* ventrodorsal thoracic radiograph of a dog with a mass in the right caudal lobe. *B,* left lateral thoracic radiograph. The right caudal lobe mass is clearly visible because it is in the well-inflated nondependent lung. *C,* right lateral thoracic radiograph. The right caudal lobe mass is not visible because it silhouettes with the partially collapsed dependent lung.

alveoli, seen in cross section. In severe interstitial infiltrate, airways and groups of alveoli appear more prominent because of adjacent increased lung opacity. The large, black tubular structure running longitudinally in Figure 23–4*B* represents an air-filled bronchus. The bronchus is surrounded by more homogeneously opacified lung than is seen in interstitial lung diseases. This pattern is that of an air bronchogram, representative of alveolar disease.

Perivascular and peribronchial infiltrates are illustrated in Figure 28–5. There are longitudinal and cross-sectional views of vessels and bronchi surrounded by increased opacity. This portion of the model was accomplished by filling the sponge that immediately surrounded the areas of interest with diluted contrast medium.

Figure 28–2. *A,* lung model that represents the radiographic opacity of normal lung. The support structure does not stand out sharply against the air-filled spaces. *B,* the support structure is highly contrasted to the air-filled spaces. Compare with *A. B* represents a generalized interstitial infiltrate.

Figure 28–3. *A,* radiopaque circular and tubular objects represent longitudinal and cross-sectional views of vessels surrounded by lung tissue. The vessels appear more opaque than adjacent lung. Cross and oblique sections of airways are present in the surrounding portions of the model. *B,* this model was made by filling a syringe case with water and examining it radiographically end on and in lateral recumbency. End-on vessels appear more radiopaque than the same sized vessels seen end on.

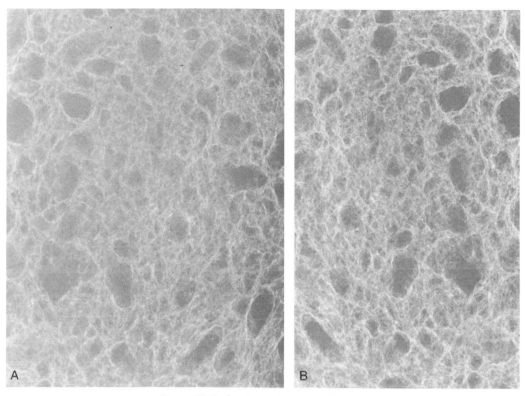

Figure 28–2. *See legend on opposite page*

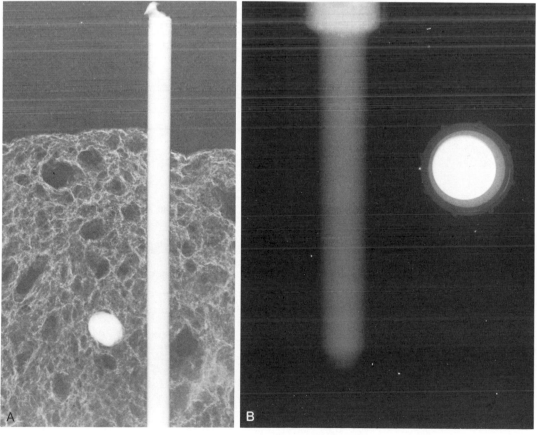

Figure 28–3. *See legend on opposite page*

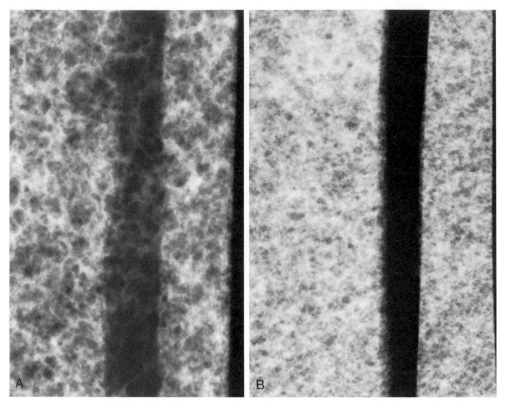

Figure 28–4. *A*, major bronchi, illustrated by the vertical radiolucent region, can be enhanced radiographically by severe interstitial infiltration. In this illustration, luminal margins are not sharp enough to be representative nor is lung radiopaque enough for this model of alveolar disease. *B*, air bronchograms, which are a sign of alveolar disease, appear as sharply demarcated radiolucent areas surrounded by lung tissue that is fluid-filled or collapsed and thereby more homogeneously opaque than in interstitial disease.

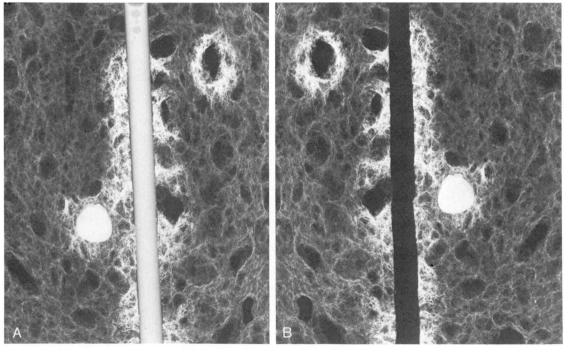

Figure 28–5. *See legend on opposite page*

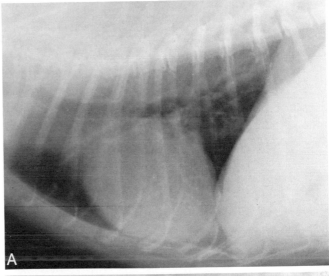

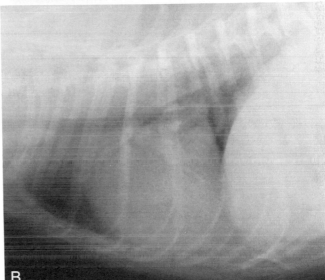

Figure 28–6. Radiographs made during inspiration (A) and expiration (B). Note the increased lung capacity in B. Unless it was known that this was an expiratory radiograph, the lung opacity would probably be interpreted as abnormal.

NORMAL LUNG ANATOMY

The normal lungs are composed primarily of air. The remaining portion of the lungs is the interstitium, which contains bronchi, bronchioles, alveoli, alveolar connections, lymphatics, nerves, and muscle. The two radiographic opacities present in the lungs are air and soft tissue. The lungs are divided into three areas for descriptive purposes: the central, middle, and peripheral zones. The major vessels and bronchi are seen in the central zone. Usually only the vessels are observed in the middle zone, and only fine vasculature is seen in the peripheral zone. The vessels and bronchi that are observed should be smooth-walled and tapered. The lung tissue should appear uniform in opacity without any abrupt change.

The normal appearance of lungs can be changed readily if the radiograph is obtained during expiration. Just a small change in the

Figure 28–5. A, perivascular infiltrate is a specific category of the broad classification of interstitial infiltration. Increased opacity is seen to surround the vessel in both views. The infiltrate gives the vessel margins a fuzzy, indistinct appearance. B, infiltration around the air-filled bronchus is contrasted with the lumen. It is thus seen easily when compared to the perivascular infiltration. Visualization of a bronchial lumen because of peribronchial or bronchial wall opacification is not referred to as an air bronchogram because adjacent lung tissue is not opacified except in the immediate vicinity of the bronchus, i.e., alveolar disease is not present.

TABLE 28–1. GAMUT OF SOLITARY CAVITARY INTERSTITIAL NODULE OR MASS

Primary lung tumor
Abscess
Traumatic lung bulla
Granuloma
Secondary lung tumor

TABLE 28–2. GAMUT OF MULTIPLE CAVITARY INTERSTITIAL NODULES OR MASSES

Traumatic lung bullae
Metastatic lung disease
Paragonimiasis
Bronchiectasis
Granuloma
Abscess

TABLE 28–3. GAMUT OF GENERALIZED HYPERLUCENCY

Bronchiolitis with secondary air trapping
Upper airway obstruction
Iatrogenic hyperinflation (intubation)
Generalized oligemia
Compensatory hyperinflation

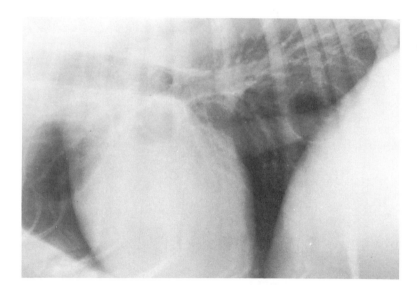

Figure 28–7. Several thin-walled radiolucent cavities are present in the lungs. The walls are smooth and uniform in thickness. These cavities are representative of traumatic lung bullae.

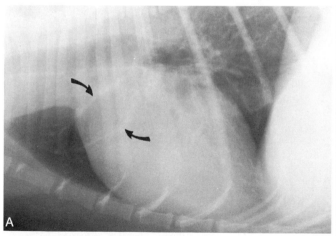

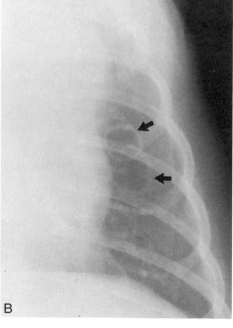

Figure 28–8. *A*, lateral view. There is separation of the right cranial lobar pulmonary artery and vein *(arrows)* by an enlarged right cranial lobe. *B*, two cross-sections of enlarged bronchus are present in the left lung *(arrows)*. These radiographic signs are representative of bronchiectasis.

TABLE 28–4. GAMUT OF DIFFUSE INTERSTITIAL MILIARY NODULES

Secondary lung tumor
Mycoses
Primary lung tumor
Parasitism
Interstitial fibrosis

TABLE 28–6. GAMUT OF SOLITARY PULMONARY NONCAVITARY INTERSTITIAL NODULE OR MASS

Chest wall lesion or artifact (nipple)
Primary lung tumor
Abscess
Secondary lung tumor

volume of air can produce a large increase in lung opacity (Fig. 28–6). There must also be an acceptable range of normalcy when evaluating different breeds and species. The feline thorax, for example, is more lucent than that of the dog. Bulldogs have more opaque pulmonary patterns than most other breeds of dogs. Deep-chested dogs have an extremely radiolucent lung pattern on the ventrodorsal view when compared to more shallow-chested dogs. Extremely obese patients have difficulty in attaining full inspiration and therefore do not have the same degree of radiolucency as dogs of normal weight. The heart and vessels of young dogs occupy a greater proportion of the thorax in contrast to mature dogs, and therefore the lung pattern is, slightly more opaque. Patients that are breathing more rapidly cannot be radiographed during maximum inspiration and therefore their lungs appear more radiopaque. The relationship of the heart and diaphragm should be evaluated when determining the degree of inspiration. Aged animals usually have chronic pulmonary fibrosis and a loss of elasticity of the lungs, which produce a more opaque pattern and possibly a nodular interstitial opacity. Patients that live in a polluted atmosphere also have an increased interstitial pattern. All of these factors of increased pulmonary opacity cannot be considered normal. They should be recognized, however, and it should be understood that what is seen is not a disease process that can be cured. These factors should be considered in the prognosis of the patient as well as identified on follow-up radiographic studies.

LUNG CHANGES

To understand how the lungs respond to specific insults, it is necessary to understand the pathologic response of the lung to various types of insults. Many pulmonary diseases cause the lung to respond in exactly the same way, and it is therefore not possible to differentiate the etiologic factors. By categorizing the pulmonary patterns, it is possible to make a list of differential diagnoses based on the radiographic patterns; this list is called a gamut. Because the lungs consist only of two radiographic opacities, air and soft tissue, it is important to consider the limited number of patterns possible as they involve the interstitium and the alveoli.

Increased Radiolucency. Increased lucencies are classified as localized or generalized and single or multiple (Tables 28–1 to 28–3).[5] The radiographic signs of localized radiolucent lesions are localized areas of decreased pulmonary opacity with thin surrounding walls (Fig. 28–7).

Another form of localized increased radiolucency is bronchiectasis (Fig. 28–8). Bronchi are enlarged and filled with air which results in a decreased lung opacity. In bronchiectasis, there may be increased opacity of the pulmonary tissue surrounding the enlarged bronchi.

Generalized lung hyperlucency can be associated with iatrogenic causes, such as iatrogenic hyperinflation under anesthesia. It may also be secondary to hypovolemia. The radiographic appearance of generalized increased lucency is a darker than expected shade of gray to the entire lung fields when compared to the surrounding soft tissue and bone. The diaphragm may be flattened and the thorax may take on a rounded appearance, as evidenced by changes in the alignment of the ribs and sternum.

Interstitial Infiltration. Interstitial infiltration can be categorized as generalized or localized.[2] The generalized form can be further classified into nodular and linear patterns (Tables 28–4 to 28–7). The linear form of interstitial infiltration has been reported as having a reticulated pattern in some instances (Fig. 28–9 and Table 28–5).[7]

TABLE 28–5. GAMUT OF UNSTRUCTURED LINEAR INTERSTITIAL PATTERNS

Expiratory radiograph
Improper radiographic technique
Interstitial fibrosis
Low-grade inflammatory lung disease
Primary lung tumor
Secondary lung tumor
Allergy
Interstitial edema
Parasite

TABLE 28–7. GAMUT OF MULTIPLE NONCAVITARY INTERSTITIAL NODULES OR MASSES

Secondary lung tumor
Granulomas
Septic pulmonary embolism
Primary lung tumor

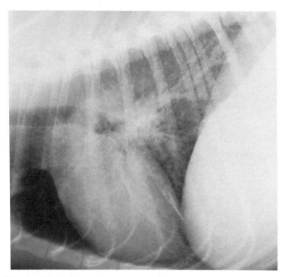

Figure 28–9. Lateral radiograph of a dog with a linear (non-mass) type of interstitial lung infiltrate due to blastomycosis.

A subclassification of interstitial infiltrate is peribronchial infiltration (Table 28–8). Peribronchial infiltration viewed longitudinally may appear as converging linear tracks; in cross-sectional views, it appears as peribronchial cuffing, as shown in Figure 28–10. These signs have been referred to as railroad tracks and doughnuts, although these are metonyms that should probably be discarded. The term doughnut does not differentiate between bronchial

TABLE 28–8. GAMUT OF ABNORMAL BRONCHIAL OPACITY

Chronic bronchial inflammation
Allergy
Infection

wall thickening, peribronchial infiltration, and mucosal thickening. A bronchial pattern is quite often sharp and well delineated when due to calcification of bronchial cartilages. Calcification of pulmonary tissue allows visualization of small lesions that would not otherwise be seen. Severe interstitial disease usually results in scar formation that will remain for the life of the patient. This is one of the causes of the old-age change of increased interstitial pattern.

Another form of interstitial infiltration is a nodular pattern (Figs. 28–11 and 28–12; Tables 28–4, 28–6, and 28–7). Interstitial nodules may range from a miliary type (Fig. 28–11), which are uniformly distributed throughout the lung fields, to isolated areas of nodule formation.

Alveolar Infiltration. The radiographic signs of alveolar infiltration are a relatively homogeneous opacity to the lung with air bronchogram visualization, as seen in Figure 28–13.[1] Alveolar infiltration can be classified as localized areas of patchy infiltrate, entire lobar involvement, or regional, such as hilar, involvement (Fig. 28–14; Tables 28–9 and 28–10). It is possible to have alveolar disease and not have air bronchograms if the bronchioles and bronchi are filled with fluid opacity, as shown in Figure 28–15.

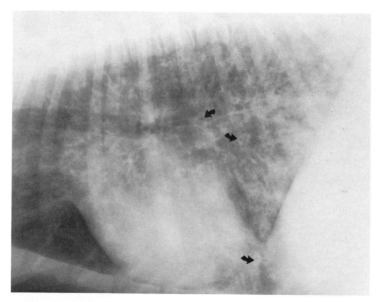

Figure 28–10. There is severe peribronchial infiltration throughout the lungs. Many airways are seen end on surrounded by soft-tissue opacity *(arrows)*. Several parallel linear opacities are present, which represent longitudinal views of airways with surrounding interstitial infiltration.

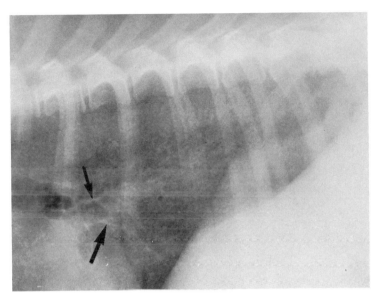

Figure 28–11. *A*, a miliary pattern is present in the caudal lung lobes. There are some small (1 mm)-sized granules that are prominent. There is also some bronchial mineralization *(arrows)*.

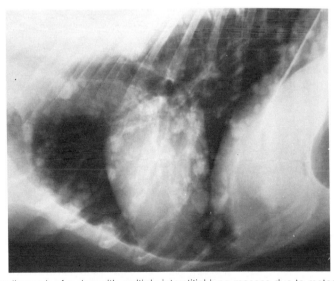

Figure 28–12. Lateral radiograph of a dog with multiple interstitial lung masses due to metastatic chondrosarcoma.

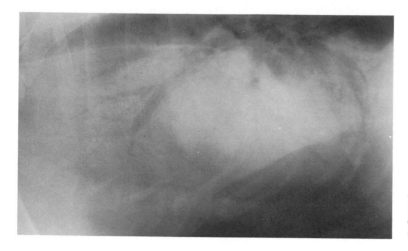

Figure 28–13. Air bronchograms are visible in the ventral portion of the lungs. The lungs have a homogeneous, soft-tissue opacity. These findings are typical of alveolar disease.

TABLE 28–9. **GAMUT OF LOCALIZED ALVEOLAR DISEASE, SOLITARY OR MULTIPLE LOBES**

Pneumonia
Pulmonary hemorrhage
Atelectasis
Pulmonary edema
Thromboembolic disease
Primary lung tumor
Secondary lung tumor

TABLE 28–10. **GAMUT OF GENERALIZED ALVEOLAR DISEASE**

Pulmonary hemorrhage
Pneumonia
Pulmonary edema
Allergic lung disease
Thromboembolic disease
Primary lung tumor
Secondary lung tumor
Toxicosis

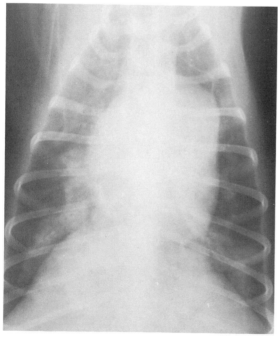

Figure 28–14. Patchy, ill-defined areas of alveolar infiltration in the caudal lung lobes represent pulmonary infarction after heartworm therapy.

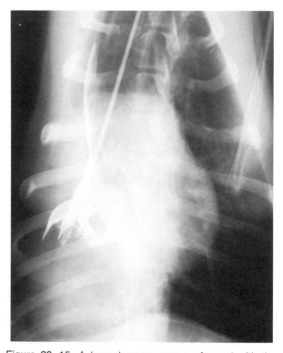

Figure 28–15. A bronchogram was performed with the use of 100 percent barium sulfate suspension. The contrast medium stopped abruptly and did not enter secondary bronchi. Note that there is no evidence of air bronchograms. The lung is of a homogeneous opacity. The study was performed to determine if there was dorsion of the right middle lung lobe; this possibility was ruled out. The findings are representative of atelectasis.

References

1. Myer W: Radiography review: The alveolar pattern of pulmonary disease. J Am Vet Radiol Soc 20:10, 1979.
2. Myer W: Radiography review: The interstitial pattern of pulmonary disease. J Am Vet Radiol Soc 21:18, 1980.
3. Reif JS, and Rhodes WH: The lungs of aged dogs. J Am Vet Radiol Soc 7:7, 1976.
4. Ruehl WW, and Thrall DE. The effect of dorsal versus ventral recumbency on the radiographic appearance of the canine thorax. J Am Vet Radiol Soc 22:10, 1981.
5. Silverman S, Poulos PW, and Suter PF: Cavitary pulmonary lesions in animals. J Am Vet Radiol Soc 17:134, 1976.
6. Spencer CP, Ackerman N, and Burt JK: The canine lateral thoracic radiograph. J Am Vet Radiol Soc 22:262, 1981.
7. Suter PF, and Lord PF: Radiographic differentiation of disseminated pulmonary parenchymal disease in dogs and cats. Vet Clin North Am [Small Anim Pract] 4:687, 1974.
8. Suter PF, and Chan KF: Disseminated pulmonary diseases in small animals: A radiographic approach to diagnosis. J Am Vet Radiol Soc 9:67, 1968.
9. Walker MA: Thoracic blastomycosis: A review of its radiographic manifestations in 40 dogs. Vet Radiol 22:22, 1981.

SECTION 7

NECK AND THORAX—
EQUIDAE

CHAPTER 29

THE LARYNX, PHARYNX, AND TRACHEA

CHARLES S. FARROW

RADIOGRAPHY AND RELATED ANATOMY

The larynx, pharynx and guttural pouches of the horse may be imaged completely by using a single 14 by 17 in x-ray film (Fig. 29–1). The exposure is made typically with the animal in the standing position, with the head held normally (neither extended nor flexed) and with the x-ray beam centered just rostral and slightly above the mandibular angle. The position of the cassette relative to the right or left side of the head does not influence the appearance of the radiographic image significantly. Likewise, the image is altered only slightly as a function of respiratory phase (inspiration or expiration). A ventrodorsal or dorsoventral view is useful when evaluating disorders of the guttural pouch in which it may be difficult to differentiate right from left side and unilateral from bilateral involvement. The inherent drawback of this projection is that the use of general anesthesia is required. Oblique projections rarely provide additional information.

Head position of the patient is critical to accurate radiographic assessment. Not only must the head be parallel to the cassette and perpendicular to the primary beam, but the head must be in the neutral (natural, resting) position. Extremes of head position, such as dorsoflexion and ventroflexion, substantially change the absolute and relative positions of the larynx, pharynx, and guttural pouch. In some instances this mimics disease and usually makes normal comparison difficult and objective measurement impossible.

The cervical trachea requires at least two 14 by 17 or 7 by 17 in films to be imaged completely. The exposures are made with the horse in the standing position, right side to the cassette. With the exception of obstructive lesions, there is little difference in the relative appearance of inspiratory and expiratory radiographs. The intrathoracic trachea may be imaged using thoracic techniques (see Chapter 31).

DIAGNOSTIC STRATEGY

Quality Assessment. Because of the physical and functional relationships of the larynx, pharynx, and guttural pouches, these structures are best imaged collectively on a single 14 by 17 in film. In so doing, these parts can be assessed completely in the context of important surrounding structures, such as the hyoid bones, mandible, cranium, and cranial cervical spine. It must be remembered, however, that the primary target tissues, the larynx, pharynx and trachea, are soft in nature—a fact that should be reflected in the chosen radiographic technique. As mentioned previously, the organs of

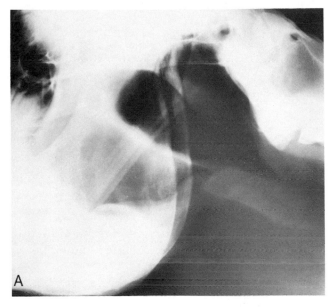

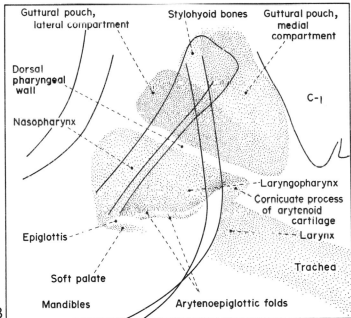

Figure 29–1. *A*, Right lateral projection. The normal equine larynx, pharynx, and guttural pouches. *B*, companion line drawing.

interest must be projected laterally with a minimum of obliquity, with the head in a natural, semiflexed position.

Radiographic Examination. As mentioned elsewhere in this text, it is imperative to analyze the entire radiograph or radiographic series before rendering a diagnostic judgment. Thoroughness is paramount; the order of assessment is unimportant.

SPECIAL PROCEDURES

Fluoroscopy. This technique is immensely useful in establishing dynamic events and relation-

ships, something not possible with a single radiograph or only partially obtainable with a series of radiographs. Fluoroscopy is most effective when combined with the use of other special procedures, such as a barium swallow. The image may then be recorded on video tape for immediate and future viewing. Cinefluorography may also be used, but the immediate playback capacity of video tape recording is not possible. Unfortunately, most large animal facilities lack fluoroscopy.

Barium Swallow. A barium swallow may be performed to assess suspected soft palate and epiglottic dysfunction in addition to swallowing

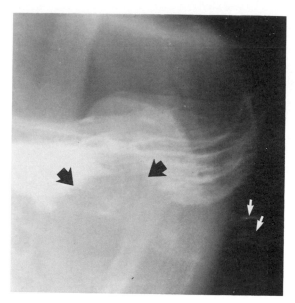

Figure 29–2. Laryngogram. There is a large mass ventral to the epiglottis *(large arrows)* and contrast medium within the laryngeal body *(small arrows).*

laterality of the involved pouch. Opacification may then be used to establish drainage capacity in cases of suspected obstruction and to detect leakage or fistula formation.

Arteriography. Hemorrhage into a guttural pouch arising from necrosis of the internal carotid artery secondary to guttural pouch infection may require angiographic verification, especially if arterial occlusion therapy is being considered. A normal comparison study can greatly facilitate examination (Fig. 29–3A and B).

Tracheography. Only rarely performed in our hospital, contrast examination of the trachea can provide information concerning the size, shape, and position of the trachea, in addition to assessment of deformities, stenosis, masses, foreign bodies, and postoperative status or complications. We have used a technique similar to that described for transtracheal aspiration, employing either barium or an iodinated contrast medium.

disorders in general. Pharyngeal and laryngeal mass lesions may often be differentiated from one another by using this technique, as can the protective function of the epiglottis (Fig. 29–2).

Contrast Examination of the Guttural Pouch. Iodinated contrast media are sometimes useful in delineating the luminal surface of the guttural pouches. This technique may be helpful in outlining mass lesions or solid content, as well as establishing the size, shape, position, and

ROENTGEN SIGNS OF LARYNGEAL DISEASE

In terms of what may be specifically identified in a radiographic image, the larynx consists of the epiglottis, the arytenoepiglottic folds, the corniculate process of the arytenoid cartilage, the lateral ventricles, and the body of the larynx. Architectural or spacial alterations to these structures constitute the basis for the roentgen signs of laryngeal disease. These signs

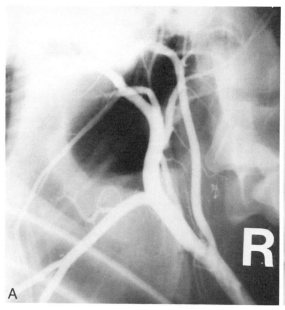
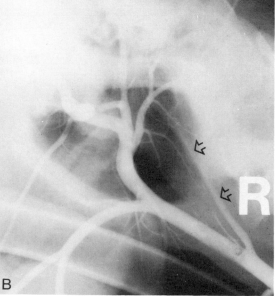

Figure 29–3. *A,* normal carotid arteriogram. *B,* abnormal carotid arteriogram shows incomplete filling of the internal carotid artery *(arrows).*

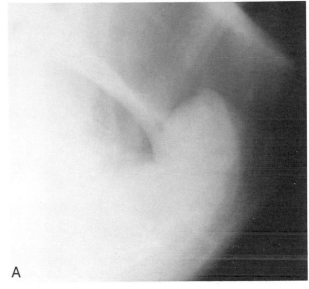

A

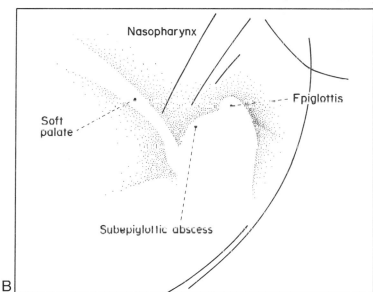

B

Figure 29–4. *A,* example of a sub-epiglottic mass, lateral view. Diagnosis: subepiglottic abscess. *B,* companion line drawing.

include abnormal epiglottic position relative to the soft palate; epiglottic thickening or marginal irregularity; decreased epiglottic size (includes length if measurable); displaced, deformed, indistinct arytenoepiglottic folds or corniculate processes; and laryngeal or paralaryngeal mineralization.

Examples of laryngeal disease in the horse include subepiglottic, epiglottic, and paraepiglottic masses. These lesions, particularly if of the subepiglottic type, may displace the epiglottis in a dorsocaudal direction, effectively increasing the distance between the epiglottis and the soft palate. Unfortunately, it is often not possible to establish the etiology of such lesions, because they closely resemble one another physically. Some diagnostic possibilities include subepiglottic cyst, granuloma, and abscess (Fig.

29–4). Inflammation (especially if chronic), surgical manipulation, and congenital disorders may distort or otherwise alter the appearance of the epiglotticarytenoid tissues (Figs. 29–5 and 29–6). Likewise, a paraepiglottic mass or mass effect may similarly distort or obscure the rostral part of the larynx (Fig. 29–7).

Mineralization, a pathologic footprint of sorts, is encountered with frequency in laryngeal examinations. Usually dystrophic in nature, mineralization is usually associated with chronic inflammation or surgery. With respect to surgery, it appears that dystrophic mineralization is most apt to occur after laryngoplasty. The presence of laryngeal mineralization is personally regarded as a significant finding in that it indicates not only damaged tissue, but may imply functional disturbance as well (Fig. 29–6).

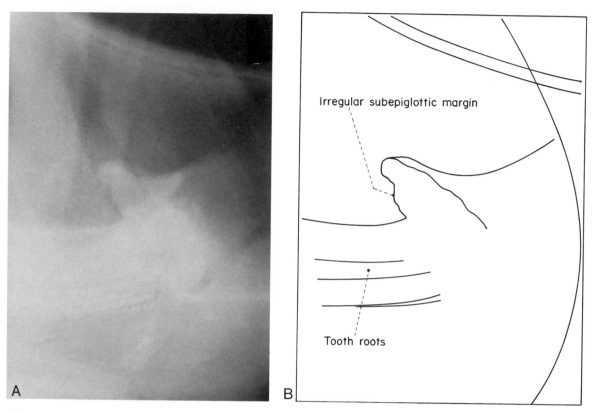

Figure 29–5. *A*, lateral view. Chronic laryngeal inflammation has resulted in epiglottic deformity and restricted motion. *B*, companion line drawing.

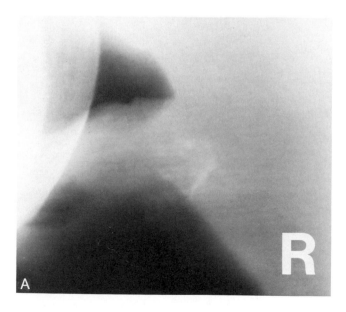

Figure 29–6. *A*, deformity of arytenoid cartilage and associated laryngeal mineralization resulting from surgical failure, lateral view.

Illustration continued on opposite page

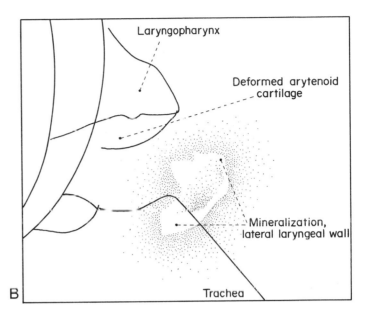

Figure 29–6 *Continued. B,* companion line drawing.

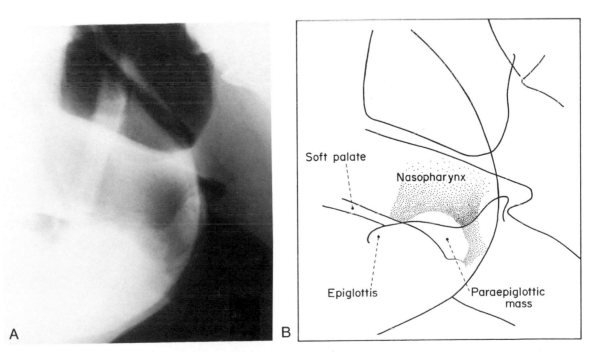

Figure 29–7. *A,* para-epiglottic mass resulting in secondary epiglottic immobilization, lateral view. *B,* companion line drawing.

ROENTGEN SIGNS OF PHARYNGEAL DISEASE

The pharynx, as viewed in a lateral radiographic projection, consists of a large, roughly rectangular, air-filled chamber that is subdivided into three regions: the nasopharynx, which constitutes the major part of the cavity; the laryngopharynx (the area immediately dorsal to the arytenoepiglottic folds), and the oropharynx (the area ventral to the caudal aspect of the soft palate, which is typically not visualized radiographically because of insufficient contrast).

Dorsally, the pharynx is bounded by the paired guttural pouches, readily identifiable by their large gas content. The larynx, discussed previously, forms the caudal pharyngeal margin

as well as a portion of the ventral border. The soft palate completes the remainder of the ventral pharynx. The rostral aspect of the pharynx is radiographically nonspecific, being a composite image of multiple contiguous and overlapping structures or cavities (Fig. 29–1). (For the purposes of organizational simplicity, the pharyngeal cavity and guttural pouches will be considered separately.)

The Pharyngeal Cavity. Roentgen signs of pharyngeal disease include decreased gas content, alterations in size or contour, and alterations in size, shape, or position of the soft palate. Reduction in pharyngeal gas content is usually of an extrinsic nature, stemming from disease-induced enlargement of surrounding

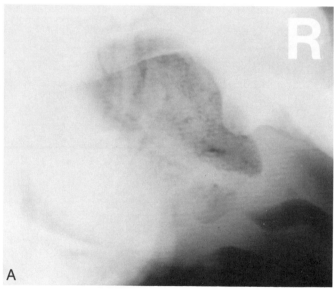

A

Figure 29–8. *A,* guttural pouch infection resulting in marked compression of the pharynx, larynx, and trachea, lateral view. *B,* companion line drawing.

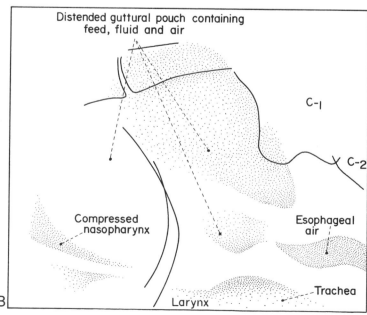

Distended guttural pouch containing feed, fluid and air

C-1

C-2

Compressed nasopharynx

Esophageal air

Trachea

Larynx

B

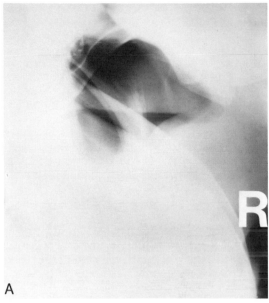

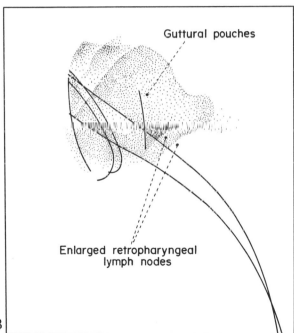

Figure 29–9. *A,* localized adenopathy producing altered contours in the guttural pouches, lateral view. *B,* companion line drawing.

structures, such as the guttural pouches and retropharyngeal lymph nodes (Fig. 29–8). These lymph nodes often produce a distinctive convexity in the caudoventral margin of one or both guttural pouches (Fig. 29–9).

Dorsal displacement of the soft palate may be associated with organic or functional disorders of the larynx or pharynx (Fig. 29–10). Occasionally, normal horses may have dorsal palatal displacement; however, this is usually only an intermittent finding. When present radiographically, dorsal displacement should be considered abnormal until proved otherwise.

Possible laryngeal etiologies include: epiglottic hypoplasia, persistent eipglottic frenulum, epiglottic cicatrix, and epiglottic entrapment by diseased or malformed arytenoepiglottic folds. Pharyngeal causes of dorsal palatal displacement may include palatal hypoplasia, palatal myositis, 9th and 10th cranial nerve deficits, pharyngitis, and secondary causes to include disorders of the guttural pouches and parapharyngeal structures.

The Guttural Pouches. The guttural pouches—large, thin-walled, air-filled extensions of the pharynx—are radiographically out-

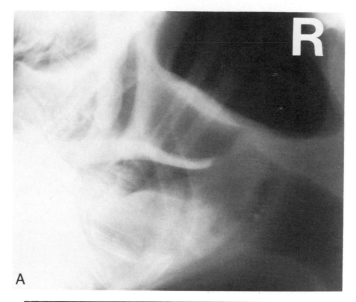

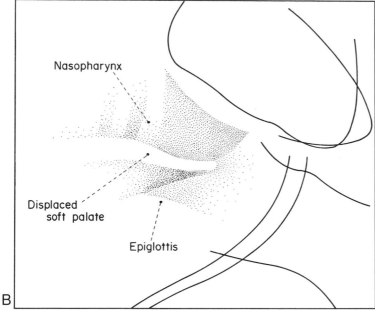

Figure 29–10. *A,* dorsal displacement of the soft palate secondary to palatal hypoplasia, lateral view. *B,* companion line drawing.

standing. Unfortunately, their superimposition and close relative proximity afford minimal opportunity for radiographic separation in all but the ventrodorsal view. This view, optimally obtained with the head forcefully extended, requires the use of general anesthesia. Accordingly, assessment is usually based on a lateral projection only, a practical consideration reflected in the presentation of the following material.

The roentgen signs of guttural pouch disease include increased air content; decreased air content; fluid level; deformity; intraluminal mass; extraluminal gas or fluid level, and pharyngeal compression and laryngo-tracheal displacement.

One or both guttural pouches may be distended with gas, fluid, or a combination. Severe gaseous distension, also known as tympany, is most frequently seen in foals and young horses; its cause is speculative. The degree of swelling is often so great that it compresses the pharynx and displaces the larynx and proximal trachea ventrally. This relocation may severely retard breathing (Fig. 29–11). Subtotal fluid accumulation in the guttural pouch is usually associated with a fluid level that is often quite striking radiographically (Fig. 29–12). It is not possible, however, to distinguish the nature of the fluid. Fortunately, the possibilities are few in number, with the two primary considerations being exudate (empyema) and hemorrhage. Hemor-

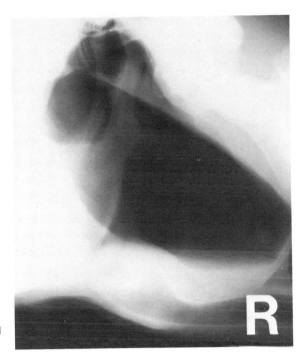

Figure 29–11. Congenital gas distension of the guttural pouches, lateral view.

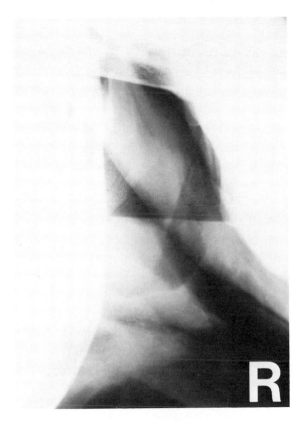

Figure 29–12. Fluid level resulting from guttural pouch infection, lateral view.

rhage is often associated with erosion of the internal carotid artery secondary to guttural pouch mycosis, although it may occur in conjunction with a bacterial infection, regional trauma, or a penetrating foreign body.

Occasionally, gas or fluid levels are identified in proximity, but external to the guttural pouches (Fig. 29–13). Inferentially, a guttural pouch origin should be considered, although other gas-containing structures, such as the pharynx, larynx, and trachea, may also leak air after perforation. In the case of the guttural pouches, it is usually an infection that results in necrosis of the guttural pouch wall and subsequent escape of its gas and infectious content. Fistulas and sinuses sometimes form and often are amenable to sinography. Bacterial gas formation occurs rarely.

Intraluminal masses are identified occasionally if they are of sufficient size and are surrounded by air (Fig. 29–14). Possible causes of such masses include chondroids, inflammatory tissue masses, and blood clots. Theoretically, tumors may appear similarly; however, I have no personal knowledge of such occurring.

Large volumes of luminal fluid may somewhat or entirely obscure one or both guttural pouches. It may be especially difficult to establish the laterality of such lesions, because they frequently compress the uninvolved pouch as well as the pharynx, larynx, and proximal trachea (Fig. 29–15).

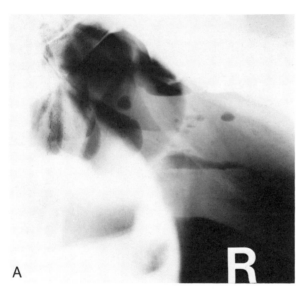

A

Figure 29–13. *A,* extraluminal gas accumulations and fluid levels developed secondary to chronic guttural pouch infection, fistulation, and extension of the infection into the proximal cervical region, lateral view. *B,* companion line drawing.

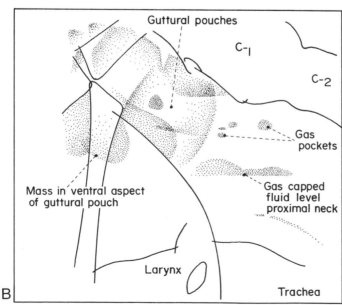

B

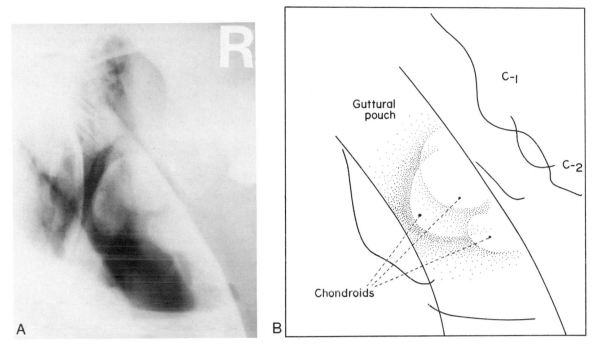

Figure 29–14. *A*, multiple luminal masses (chondroids), lateral view. *B*, companion line drawing.

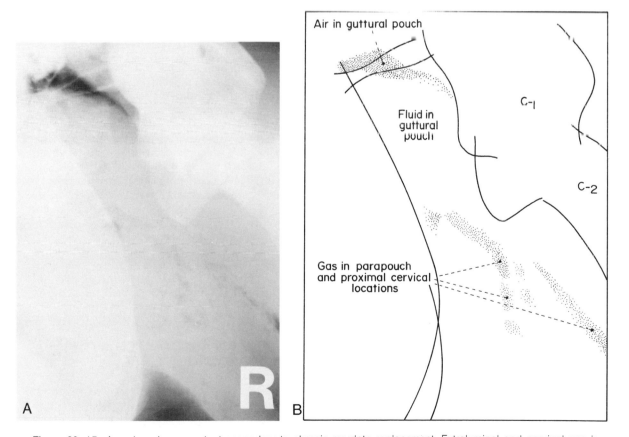

Figure 29–15. *A*, reduced gas content secondary to chronic exudate replacement. Extraluminal and cervical gas is secondary to associated necrosis and gas escape, lateral view. *B*, companion line drawing.

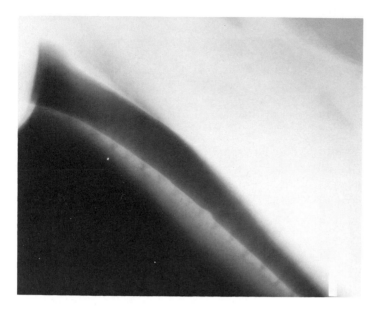

Figure 29–16. Lateral view. Normal equine cervical trachea.

ROENTGEN SIGNS OF TRACHEAL DISEASE

The radiologic appearance of tracheal disease in the horse is not well-described; consequently, its description is based in large part on personal experience. The normal equine cervical trachea may be imaged sufficiently to detect the following structures: the caudal aspect of the larynx, the tracheal lumen, the inner tracheal surface (mucosa), the tracheal rings, and the annular ligaments (by inference the space between tracheal rings) (Fig. 29–16). The absence or alterations of these normally visible shadows form the radiologic basis for a diagnosis of tracheal disease.

Roentgen signs of tracheal disease include extraluminal gas (usually linear but sometimes focal); mediastinal gas (secondary to tracheal leakage); decreased definition or absence of normally visible tracheal soft tissues; luminal alteration; and deformity, deviation, or displacement. The cervical trachea is an uncommon site of primary radiographically discernible pathologic processes. Far more frequent are the mass-related secondary effects generated by contiguous structures, such as the guttural pouch and esophagus; these effects are primarily dislocating (Figs. 29–11 and 29–15).

The most common roentgen sign of primary tracheal disease, in our experience, is extraluminal gas. Some causes of this finding include tracheal air that escapes after transtracheal aspiration, tracheal fracture after blunt trauma, tracheal perforation after penetrating trauma, and tracheal necrosis/perforation associated with tracheal or paratracheal infection or abscess formation (Figs. 29–17 and 29–18); the latter may result in fistula formation. Gas may

also be seen along the outer margin of the trachea after laryngeal or tracheal surgery, and as a complication of wound dehiscence. It is highly unusual for air to reach the tracheal perimeter as a result of atmospheric dissection after a lacerative injury. In the event such a finding is made under these circumstances, it is strongly recommended that upper airway leakage be sought.

Mediastinal gas (pneumomediastinum) is usually the result of tracheal fracture or perforation, the escaping gas dissecting caudally into the mediastinum along the deep fascial planes of the neck (see Fig. 31–21). The origin may, however, be the thoracic trachea or bronchi. Occasionally, air may arise from ruptured alveoli, dissecting in a retrograde fashion along the vascular adventitia into the mediastinum.

Decreased definition of the normally visible tracheal soft tissues may be seen with infection or trauma. Paratracheal disease may result in the formation of a positive silhouette sign, effectively mimicking tracheal disease. The usual absence of a right angle view often makes it impossible to make the necessary distinction. Luminal alterations in the form of tracheal stenosis, collapse, or masses rarely occur.

DISORDERS ASSOCIATED WITH NORMAL RADIOGRAPHIC FINDINGS

Larynx. In the horse, there frequently are no radiographic abnormalities associated with epiglottic entrapment (Fig. 29–19). Subsequent endoscopic examinations of the same horses have shown varying degrees of entrapment or, more usually, restricted or limited epiglottic

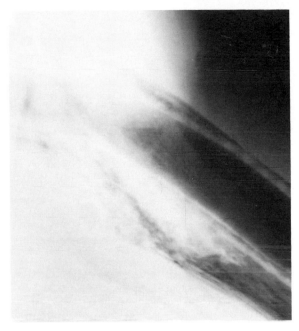

Figure 29–17. Extraluminal gas escaping the cranial cervical trachea 3 hours after transtracheal aspiration, lateral view.

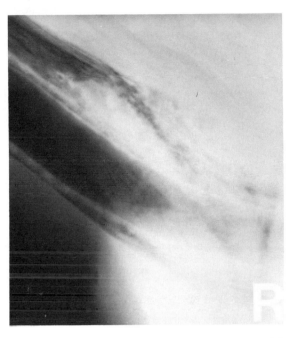

Figure 29–18. Extraluminal gas escaping the caudal cervical trachea after a penetrating wound, lateral view.

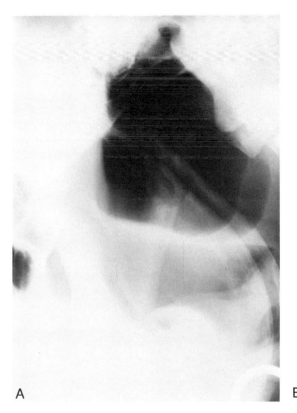

A

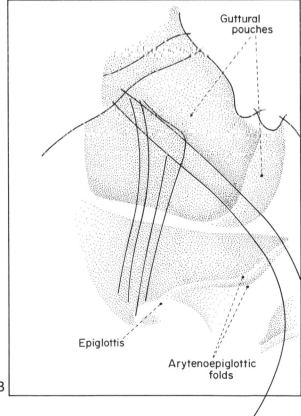

Guttural pouches

Epiglottis

Arytenoepiglottic folds

B

Figure 29–19. A, lateral view. Normal appearing larynx, which on subsequent endoscopy showed restricted epiglottic motion. B, companion line drawing.

movement. These findings have usually been attributed to a slight inward folding of the arytenoepiglottic folds. The point is that as with any radiographic examination designed to evaluate altered anatomy, the alteration must be of sufficient magnitude to be recognizable; subtle changes or slight variations from normal are likely to go undetected. For this reason, not only should endoscopy be performed in all cases of suspected epiglottic entrapment, but also it should precede the radiographic examination; the chances of finding a radiographic abnormality are therefore greatly enhanced.

Laryngeal hemiplegia cannot be diagnosed radiographically, nor can all but the most extreme epiglottic inflammations. Even this type of inflammation may not result in detectable change.

Pharynx. Pharyngeal lymphoid hyperplasia has not been recognized radiographically, irrespective of extent. Pharyngeal cysts are undetectable, unless they are sufficiently large and are projected in profile. The same may be said for other pharyngeal masses, such as abscesses or granulomas. Fluid in the pharyngeal cavity usually goes unrecognized, irrespective of its nature.

Trachea. Tracheitis has not been described radiographically, with or without the use of contrast medium. Tracheal fluid, even in large volumes, is not detectable radiographically in my experience. Small luminal masses (less than 1 cm) typically remain unidentified. Tracheograms show only major lesions and rarely identify perforations, including those that produce substantial air leakage.

Suggested Reading

Larynx

Farrow CS, and Barber SM: Paralaryngeal abscess with laryngeal fistulation in a horse (What is your diagnosis?). J Am Vet Med Assoc 179:830, 1981.

Haynes PF, Snider TG, McClure JR, et al: Chronic chondritis of the equine arytenoid cartilage. J Am Vet Med Assoc 177:1135, 1980.

Linford RL, et al: Radiographic assessment of epiglottic length and pharyngeal and laryngeal diameter in the Thoroughbred. Am J Vet Res 44:1660, 1983.

Pharynx

Blythe LL, et al: Palatal myositis in horses with dorsal displacement of the soft palate. J Am Vet Med Assoc 183:781, 1983.

Haynes PF: Persistent dorsal displacement of the soft palate associated with epiglottic shortening in two horses. J Am Vet Med Assoc 179:677, 1981.

Koch C: Disease of the larynx and pharynx of the horse. Comp Contin Ed Pract Vet 2:573, 1980.

Guttural Pouch

Bayly WM, and Robertson JT: Epistaxis caused by foreign body penetration of a guttural pouch. J Am Vet Med Assoc 180:1232, 1982.

Cook WR: The auditory tube diverticulum (guttural pouch) in the horse: its radiographic examination. J Am Vet Radiol Soc 14(2):51, 1973.

Freeman DE: Diagnosis and treatment of diseases of the guttural pouch (Part 1). Comp Contin Ed Pract Vet 2:53, 1980.

Freeman DE: Diagnosis and treatment of diseases of the guttural pouches (Part 2). Comp Contin Ed Pract Vet 2:525, 1980.

Lingard DR, Gosser HS, and Monfart TN: Acute epistaxis associated with guttural pouch mycosis in two horses. J Am Vet Med Assoc 164:1038, 1974.

Trachea

Farrow CS: Pneumomediastinum in the horse: A complication of transtracheal aspiration. J Am Vet Radiol Soc 17:192, 1976.

CHAPTER 30

THE PLEURAL SPACE

RON D. SANDE

Radiographic examination of the equine thorax has received minimal attention because of the limited availability of adequate diagnostic facilities. The pleural space of the equine is as complex as that of any species, and its examination is complicated by the large size of the patient. Parallax and magnification are serious problems given the magnitude of pathologic change that is necessary to be considered radiographically significant.

ANATOMY

The pleural cavity is a potential space on each side of the thorax. The pleurae are serous membranes that line the walls of the thorax and the diaphragm, form the laminae of the mediastinum, and are reflected onto the surface of the lungs.

The laminae of the mediastinal pleurae cover the organs in the mediastinal space. In some areas, the laminae may be apposed. The visceral pleurae are those that are reflected onto the surface of the lungs and cover all but a small portion of the mediastinal surface at the hilus of each lung. Behind the hilum of the lung there is an area where the apposing lungs are attached and thus interrupt the mediastinum. The visceral pleurae form folds that reflect from the mediastinum and the diaphragm to the lung and constitute the pulmonary ligament. The right visceral pleura and lung form the fold of the vena cava (plica vena cava), and a small fold for the right phrenic nerve.[2]

The remaining pleural components are called parietal pleural; that which covers the diaphragm may be called diaphragmatic, and that which is attached to the thoracic wall may be called costal pleura. Regardless of the nomenclature used to describe anatomic locations, the pleural sac is continuous tissue.

The lines of pleural reflection are important landmarks in diagnostic imaging. The parietal pleura is reflected along three major boundaries. The sternal line of reflection is where the costal pleura reflects dorsally to become the visceral pleura of the mediastinum. The vertebral line of reflection is where the costal pleura turns ventrally to form the mediastinal pleura.

Perhaps the most important pleural reflection in diagnostic imaging is the diaphragmatic reflection, where the parietal pleura of the costal surface extends to the surface of the diaphragm and forms the costodiaphragmatic recess or phrenicocostal sinus. This line is the demarcation between the thorax and the abdomen. Externally, the anatomic limits can be determined by a line connecting the following points: the 17th intercostal space at the level of the tuber coxae; the 15th intercostal space at the level of the tuber ischii; the 13th intercostal space at the dorsoventral midpoint; the 11th intercostal space at the level of the point of the shoulder; and a gradually descending line to the point of the elbow. Although it may be difficult to visualize radiographically, this line should be found ventrally at the level of the costochondral junctions caudal to the ninth rib, where it courses caudal and dorsal at a gradually increasing distance from the sternal ends of the ribs to the level of the midshaft of the last rib. It then reflects slightly cranial and dorsal to terminate at the vertebral end of the last intercostal space.

The normal pleural space contains clear serous fluid of sufficient quantity to moisten the surface of the sacs. The pleural space is a capillary space between the visceral and parietal pleura that is a lubricating surface. The minimal quantity of liquor pleurae normally present is not detectable by radiographic imaging or by using diagnostic ultrasound.

RADIOGRAPHY

Radiographic examination of the equine thorax has become a routine procedure. In the past, this procedure was usually limited to teaching hospitals. Advances in technology associated with intensifying screens have effectively increased the capability of mobile x-ray equipment. Despite the sophistication of equipment, it is still difficult to image the cranioventral thorax.

Radiographic examination of the thorax for the purpose of evaluating the pleural space is performed with the same technique as that used to evaluate other thoracic structures. Horizontal beam projections are made with the patient standing. Right and left lateral projections should be obtained. The average horse (450 kg) requires at least three and perhaps four cassette (35 by 43 cm) positions on each side for complete examination.[1] The radiographic technique is the operator's choice; however, a grid or an air gap is advised. Ventrodorsal projections may be attempted if the patient is recumbent, although the procedure may be difficult, unrewarding, and dangerous for the patient.

Survey examination for diseases of the pleural space should at least include one right and one left lateral projection of the caudal ventral portion of the thorax. The need for additional projections may be determined based on the preliminary findings and the severity of the disease.

Radiographic Interpretation

Magnification inherent to radiographic examination of the equine thorax results in progressive loss of detail of structures closer to the x-ray tube. Right and left lateral projections permit evaluation of each side of the thorax. Because radiographic detail is better when structures are closer to the film, one may be able to localize lesions in their approximate sagittal plane. A lesion that is near the thoracic wall may be clear and crisp in one lateral projection (see Fig. 30–4A) and on the opposite projection it is blurred beyond recognition (see Fig. 30–4B). A lesion located at the midline appears similar or identical, regardless of the projection. Details of lesions within the pulmonary parenchyma vary according to the sagittal plane in which they exist.

Accumulation of fluid within the pleural space or mediastinum is often a generic finding. Differentiation of transudate, exudate, or blood is impossible without performing thoracentesis. Many folds and pockets exist within the mediastinum and pleural sacs. Fluid may accumulate in preferred areas and thus become visible earlier in the course of the disease. The horse is seldom found in other than a standing position, and as expected, accumulation of fluid is most often dependent. The earliest sign of fluid in the pleural space is loss of detail in the ventral thorax caudal to the heart. The area cranial to the heart is more difficult to evaluate. Loss of vascular detail within the lung lobes nearest the ventral margins may be the earliest indication of pleural effusion. The volume of fluid required for radiographic detection varies with the size of the patient and the quality of the study. Perhaps no less than 1 to 2 liters of fluid in any compartment will be detected in a 450-kg patient. Greater volumes of fluid result in loss of detail progressing dorsally in the thorax, causing a silhouette sign of the respective borders of the diaphragm and heart. Despite the opinion that fluid moves freely through the mediastinum, it is common to find compartmentalization of the fluid or unilateral hydrothorax; the latter is most often associated with inflammatory conditions and is best studied by using diagnostic ultrasound. Subcardiac fat in the mediastinum causes accentuation of the costal border of the lungs in the caudal thorax. This normal finding is often misinterpreted as the accumulation of fluid.

A common error in radiographic interpretation is made when one expects to find a "fluid line" with hydrothorax. Because of the capillarity and surface tension, a horizontal fluid-line is not present unless there is also free air in the pleural space.

Pneumothorax has multiple etiologies, although the sources of air are limited to the lung, esophagus, or external body surface. The presence of gas-forming bacteria provides a forum for academic discussion, but radiographic diagnosis is not likely to be made before the death of the patient. It is quite common to find entrapped gas within an abscess.

Air in the pleural sacs or mediastinum compartmentalizes rapidly according to the preferred space available. The mass of pulmonary and cardiac tissue in the horse results in dependent displacement of tissue in relation to air. Free air quickly locates in the dorsal thoracic gutter. Crisp visualization of the dorsal lung margins indicates air in the pleural spaces. Right and left lateral projections may be necessary to identify the pulmonary margins accurately and to determine the location of the pneumothorax.

Pleurography may be performed by injection of water-soluble contrast medium into the pleural space. Approximately 300 ml of solution with an iodine concentration of 300 to 400 mg/ml provides adequate visualization. Indications for the use of this technique include diaphragmatic hernia and noneffusive mass lesions. The occasions for selecting this technique are rare and the interpretation of findings are dependent on the type of the suspected lesion.

DIAGNOSTIC ULTRASOUND

Diagnostic ultrasound may be used for primary examination of the thorax or to augment radiographic findings. Although air in the lung prohibits penetration of the ultrasound beam, one may successfully study the parietal and pulmonary visceral pleurae. The cardiac notch on both sides of the thorax provides a window through which one can study a segment of the mediastinum, the pericardium, and the heart.

The radiographic detection of fluid in the thorax is usually a generic finding. Diagnostic ultrasound can be used to locate and determine the boundaries of the fluid-filled spaces. Ultrasound examination is used to study tissue texture or fluid composition and may be used to guide catheter placement for thoracentesis.

Hair must be removed over the area to be examined, and a suitable conducting medium is applied to the skin to ensure coupling of the transducer with the underlying tissue. It is necessary to scan at intercostal spaces because conduction of sound through bone is significantly different than soft tissue, and results in no image formation deep to the bone surface.

Two-dimensional real-time imaging with linear array or mechanical sector transducer technology is more popular than static B-mode scans. Phased array transducers have the additional advantage of variable focus and the sound beam is steerable. The appropriate literature should be consulted for a more complete un-

derstanding of this valuable imaging modality.[3, 5-7] (See Chapter 46.)

DISEASES OF THE PLEURA AND PLEURAL SPACE

Pleural Effusion. The pathogenesis of this condition is complex and the etiologies are manifold.[4] Radiographic signs vary according to the volume of fluid present. Small volumes of fluid result in increased opacity and loss of detail in the ventral caudal thorax. The ventral margins of the lung may be outlined and the vascular detail within the lung may be decreased (Fig. 30–1). Increased volume of fluid results in progressive silhouette sign of the border of the diaphragm, the heart, and the vena cava. Concomitant collapse of the lungs results in a greater increase in pulmonary opacity and loss of detail due to excursion of air from the pulmonary parenchyma.

Radiographic evidence of fluid in the pleural spaces or mediastinum does not provide definitive information that may be of use when differentiating the disease processes. Despite the radiographic findings, thoracentesis is necessary.

Diagnostic ultrasound may be used for additional examination of the thorax, and proves most valuable in guiding thoracentesis. Pleural fluid results in separation of the visceral surface

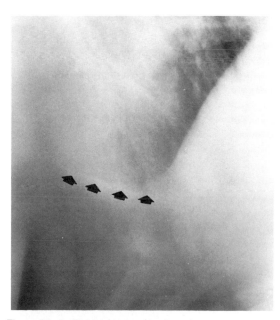

Figure 30–1. Right lateral projection of an equine thorax with early pleural effusion. The ventral margin of the lung is visible *(arrows)*. There is a silhouette sign of the ventral heart and diaphragm and loss of detail of the distal right middle pulmonary vasculature.

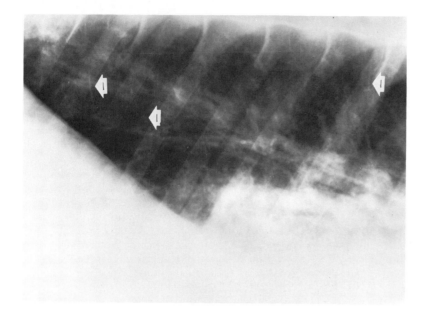

Figure 30–2. Left lateral projection of an equine thorax with chronic pleuritis. There is a silhouette sign of the heart, ventral diaphragm, and caudal vena cava. Fibrin can be identified as opaque white lines with vertical orientation *(arrows).*

of the lung from the costal pleura. Transudate is relatively anechoic when compared to the composite, echoic appearance of exudate. Ultrasound examination permits visualization of the thoracic and abdominal surfaces of the diaphragm simultaneously, which allows ascites to be detected if it is present.

Pleuritis. Radiographic signs of acute or subacute pleuritis are often not differentiated from those of effusion. The presence of fibrin remains undetected unless it causes restriction of the lung margins. Because the equine lung is not divided by deep fissures, it is difficult to demonstrate the scalloped borders characteristic of restrictive pleuritis. Accumulation of fibrin may be detected when pleural adhesions and fibrin sheets form and the pleural fluid regresses. The fibrin tags tend to orient vertically within the pleural space or are at least more easily identified when their axes are orthogonal to the vessels and airways within the lung (Fig. 30–2).

Diagnostic ultrasound examination demonstrates the presence of fluid-containing echogenic material. Fibrin tags attached to the lung extend into the pleural fluid. The visceral pleurae appear brightly echogenic and strands or sheets of fibrin are suspended in the fluid compartment. Two-dimensional real-time imaging provides a vivid demonstration of the dynamics that occur. Static images of these events are less exciting (Fig. 30–3).

Pleural and Extrapleural Masses. Differentiation of the etiologies of pleural and mediastinal masses should be made on the basis of clinical signs, thoracentesis, and biopsy. In the absence of excessive free fluid, a pleural mass may be visualized, radiographically. The loca-

tion of the mass can be determined by using opposing projections are previously described (Fig. 30–4). Tissue masses extending from the pleural surface or in contact with the costal pleura may be examined by using diagnostic ultrasound. Tissue texture may provide an indication of the nature of the mass (Fig. 30–5).

Pneumothorax. The diagnosis of pneumothorax does not identify the actual location of air within the thorax nor does it define the etiology. The etiologies are numerous, and among the most common is jugular venipuncture with subsequent tension pneumomediastinum. Free gas in the thorax quickly seeks the dorsal free spaces. The standing lateral, hori-

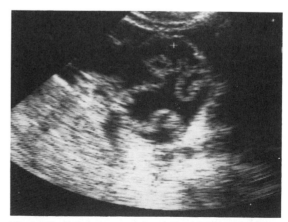

Figure 30–3. Sonogram of the right pleural space at the sixth intercostal space. The near field contains composite fluid with a large sheet of fibrin that has a serpentine appearance. No normal structures can be visualized.

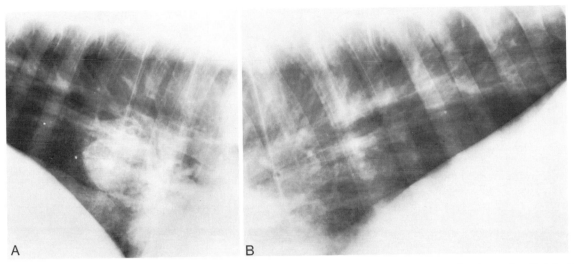

Figure 30–4. *A,* Left lateral projection of an equine thorax. There is a mass lesion with well-defined margins. Detail of the caudal vena cava and diaphragm are preserved. There is loss of detail in the pulmonary parenchyma cranial and ventral to the mass. *B,* Right lateral projection. There is slight loss of detail in the lower left corner of the image. The mass lesion is magnified and superimposed in that area.

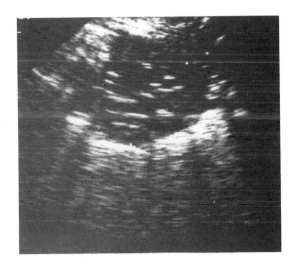

Figure 30–5. Sonogram at the left sixth intercostal space of the equine thorax shown in Figure 30–4. A circumscribed area of composite fluid is present in the lung adjacent to the pleural surface. An ultrasound-guided biopsy yielded purulent material containing *Streptococcus zooepidemicus.*

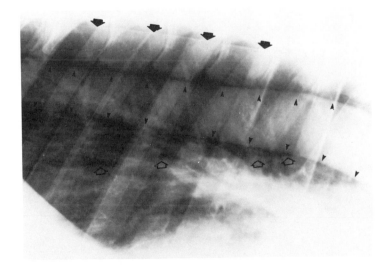

Figure 30–6. Left lateral view of the thorax of a horse with pneumothorax. Radiographic signs include visible lung border *(solid arrows),* dorsal margin of the esophagus *(open arrows),* and increased detail of the margins of the aorta *(arrowheads).*

zontal beam projection demonstrates air in the dorsal gutters of the thorax. Therefore, the first sign of pneumothorax is an increase in detail of the margins of the lungs. Increased volume of air results in dependent retraction of the lung and decreased opacity in the dorsal thorax (Fig. 30–6). Air within the mediastinum outlines the aorta and does not displace the lung margins. Large volumes of air result in confusing patterns, but with careful examination it is possible to discriminate the esophagus from the area of mediastinal pulmonary adhesion. Entrapment of air in the more dependent areas of the pleura or mediastinum is a sign of inflammatory disease and is usually associated with a cavitated abscess.

References

1. Farrow CS: Radiography of the equine thorax: Anatomy and technic. J Am Vet Radiol Soc 22:62, 1981.
2. Getty R: Sisson and Grossman's The Anatomy of the Domestic Animals. Philadelphia, WB Saunders, 1975, pp. 514–518.
3. Powis RL: Ultrasound physics for the fun of it. Cleveland, OH, Technicare Corp., 1980.
4. Smith BP: Pleuritis and pleural effusion in the horse: A study of 37 cases. J Am Vet Med Assoc 170:208, 1977.
5. Rantanen NW: Ultrasound appearance of normal lung borders and adjacent viscera in the horse. Vet Radiol 22:217, 1981.
6. Rantanen NW, and Ewing RL: Principles of ultrasound application in animals. Vet Radiol 22:196, 1981.
7. Rantanen NW, Gage L, and Paradis MR: Ultrasonography as a diagnostic aid in pleural effusion of horses. Vet Radiol 22:211, 1981.

CHAPTER 31

THE LUNG

CHARLES S. FARROW

RADIOGRAPHY AND RELATED ANATOMY

The thorax of a young foal may be completely imaged by using a single 14 by 17 in x-ray film (Fig. 31–1). By comparison, four films of this size are needed to image the thorax of an adult horse completely (Figs. 31–2 to 31–5). All films are exposed on full inspiration, with the animal standing and its right side against the receiver system.

DIAGNOSTIC STRATEGY

Although radiographs of the equine thorax are obtained with increasing frequency, they are still considered by most students and clinicians as one of the most difficult survey radiographic examinations to interpret. The trained radiologist often looks over a radiograph of the thorax in an apparently random fashion. When an abnormality is found, the subsequent analysis is dictated by the possibilities that come to mind for that particular shadow. For example, if a nodule in the lung is seen, the shape of the nodule is assessed, and evidence of other lung lesions and spread of disease to other parts of the thorax is sought. This problem-oriented approach—the observer constantly asking himself questions, not only about the shadows seen but also about the patient's clinical findings—is the quickest and most accurate way of achieving a diagnosis. This approach takes time to learn, however, and in the early stages, a routine is necessary to avoid missing valuable radiologic signs. The order in which the structures are evaluated is unimportant; what matters is that a routine is followed. Otherwise important abnormalities may be overlooked. One way of examining radiographs of the equine thorax is presented below.

Assessment of Technical Quality. This is necessary because incorrect exposure or faulty centering or projection may either hide or mimic disease. This fact is especially true of underexposed radiographs, in which normal lung opacity tends to be accentuated, thereby creating the impression of interstitial disease. Conversely, the overexposed radiograph appears hyperlucent, closely resembling an emphysematous lung or other forms of chronic obstructive lung disease.

Radiographs of the thorax must be made on inspiration; those made on expiration may be difficult to interpret because of a relative increase in lung opacity produced by a relative reduction in lung volume. Additionally, the heart appears larger and the pulmonary vasculature becomes less distinct. Loss of clarity or blurring produced by patient or physiologic

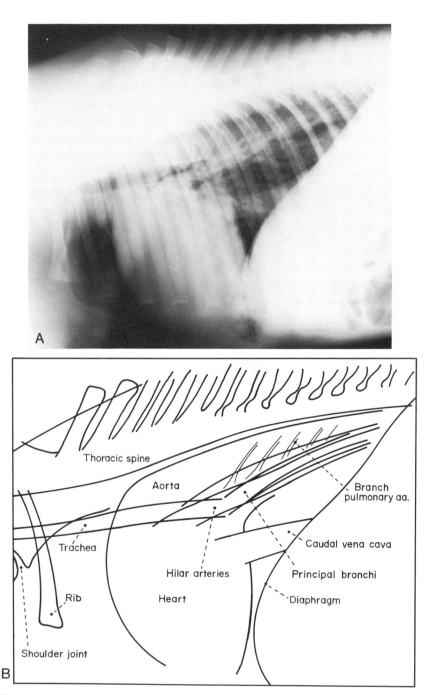

Figures 31–1. *A*, normal foal thorax, right lateral projection. *B*, companion line drawing,

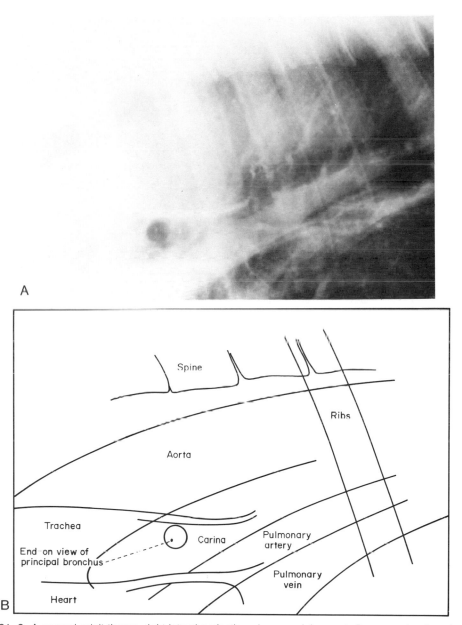

Figure 31–2. *A*, normal adult thorax, right lateral projection, dorsocranial aspect. *B*, companion line drawing.

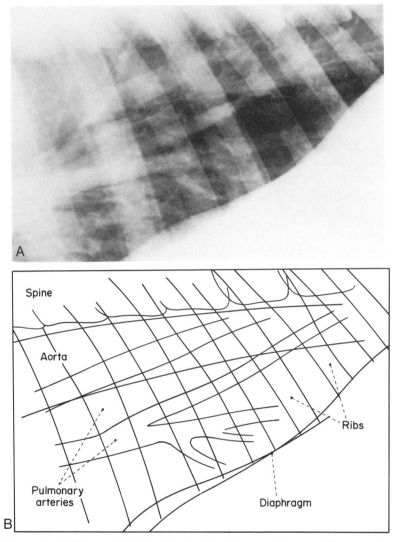

Figure 31–3. *A*, normal adult thorax, right lateral projection, dorsocaudal aspect. *B*, companion line drawing.

movement must be avoided because it results in severe image degradation.

Examination of Radiographs, Individually and Collectively

Dorsocranial View. The dorsal aspect of the heart, the ascending aorta, and the major pulmonary arteries and veins are evident in this view. Also seen are the trachea, the trachial bifurcation (the carina), and the principal bronchi. The lung may be seen, but it is difficult to evaluate because of the extensive superimposition of cardiovascular tissue. Caution is advised regarding the evaluation of cardiac size in this view.

Dorsocaudal View. This view includes a large part of the lung. It is important to recognize that normal interstitial lung opacities in the horse are particularly outstanding, especially when compared to the dog. The vascular course and caliber are relatively constant, with the branch pulmonary arteries and veins most subject to perceptible change associated with circulatory derangement from whatever cause. The diaphragm usually appears flattened or slightly convex cranially, with some variation depending on the degree of inspiration at the time of the exposure.

Ventrocranial View. The bulk of the heart, aortic root, cranial mediastinum, and thoracic trachea are included in this view. The scapulae and one or both humeri usually are seen cranially. Background shadows are those of the lung and associated vasculature. Lung structures may be overexposed and difficult to see clearly because of the high kilovoltage required to penetrate the thick cardiovascular tissues and the musculature of the partially superimposed proximal forelimbs.

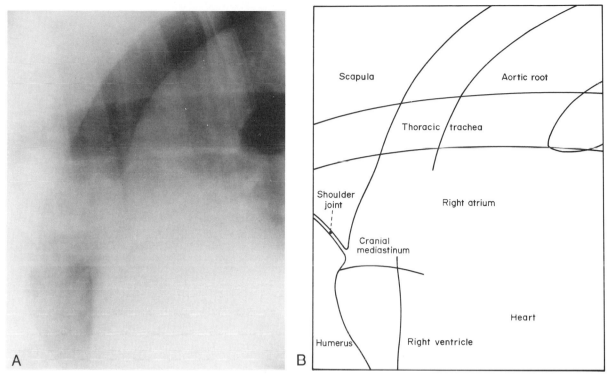

Figure 31–4. *A*, normal adult thorax, right lateral projection, ventrocranial aspect. *B*, companion line drawing.

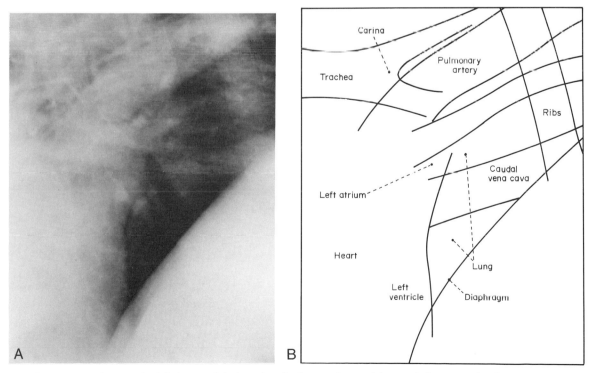

Figure 31–5. *A*, normal adult thorax, right lateral projection, ventrocaudal aspect. *B*, companion line drawing.

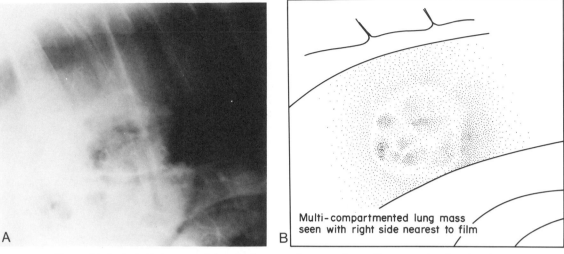

Figure 31–6. *A*, right dorsocranial projection reveals a mycetoma. *B*, companion line drawing.

Ventrocaudal View. This view outlines the caudal part of the heart, the left atrium, and the larger pulmonary veins. The caudal vena cava and ventral part of the diaphragm are also visible. The latter structures join the caudal border of the cardiac silhouette to form a triangle through which the lung can be evaluated.

Of the four described views, the dorsocaudal and ventrocaudal views are most apt to reveal any pathologic processes in the lung. Cardiovascular assessment is optimized by centering the heart on a single 14 by 17 in film.

Extra Views

Spot Films and Alternate Side Radiography. Optimal imaging is obtained when a lesion or region of interest is centered radiographically.

Thus, once such a lesion has been located in a standard radiographic series, it is often advisable to obtain a spot radiograph in an effort to improve image clarity. Clarity may be further enhanced by reducing the distance between the lesion and the film, thereby reducing magnification and improving the sharpness and detail of the image. Because it is often difficult to establish whether a lesion is in the right or left hemithorax on the initial right lateral projection, a left lateral spot radiograph is often instrumental in making such a distinction (Figs. 31–6 and 31–7).

Penetrated Radiographs. By using a more penetrating x-ray beam, it is possible to see more details of certain types of lesions, such as

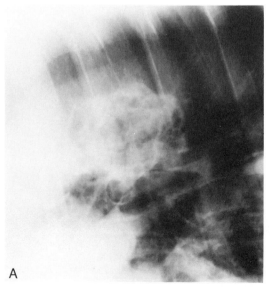

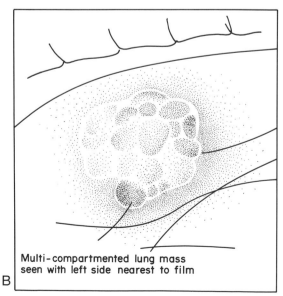

Figure 31–7. *A*, left dorsocranial projection shows a mycetoma. *B*, companion line drawing.

a cavitated lung abscess. Additional benefit from a penetrated radiograph is greatest when relatively low kilovoltage techniques are used routinely.

Inspiration-Expiration Sequence. In cases of suspected chronic obstructive lung disease, air trapping may be inferred radiographically on the basis of minimal or no difference in lung volume in two sequential films, one on maximal inspiration and then one on maximal expiration. This maneuver is especially useful in animals that have otherwise normal radiographic findings. Obviously, care must be taken to be certain that each radiograph was exposed on opposite phases of the respiratory cycle when these sequential examinations are compared.

SPECIAL PROCEDURES

Esophageal Marking Study. A barium swallow is useful in the indirect detection of mediastinal and some pulmonary lesions. On the basis of the altered course or configuration of the thoracic esophagus, provoking lesions, especially masses, may be inferred. Dorsal elevation of the contrast medium-filled esophagus is also reliable evidence of cardiac enlargement, especially of the left atrium. The procedure is inexpensive and has minimal risk.

Bronchography. Bronchography involves the introduction of sterile barium sulfate into the bronchial tree. There are various ways of instilling the contrast medium—via a catheter introduced into the trachea through the nose or mouth, or alternatively, after puncture of the proximal part of the upper airway.

The major indication for bronchography is assessment of bronchiectasis. Bronchograms may also be used to demonstrate obstruction of the major conducting bronchi, although this assessment may be better accomplished by bronchoscopy. Bronchography is of questionable use in bronchitis, even in its chronic form. Bronchography is of minimal use in establishing the nature of pulmonary mass lesions, because regardless of etiology, they all tend to obstruct the surrounding airways to some extent. The procedure is moderately expensive and has some risk, as regards the required use of general anesthesia. The contrast material that may remain in the lung has minimal significant consequence.

Pulmonary Angiography. Pulmonary vasculature may be evaluated by making serial radiographs after the rapid injection of angiographic contrast medium into the pulmonary artery through a catheter. Catheterization is carried out under fluoroscopic control with continuous electrocardiographic monitoring. The principal use of angiography is in demonstration of congenital vascular anomalies; occasionally, it is used to demonstrate obstruction of the pulmonary vasculature. The procedure is expensive and carries a small, but definite risk.

Radionuclide Lung Scanning. There are two different kinds of lung scans that can be obtained by using the gamma camera, perfusion and ventilation scans. For perfusion scans, macroaggregates of albumin labeled with an isotope, such as technetium 99m, are injected intravenously. These particles become trapped in the pulmonary capillaries, their pattern reflecting blood flow. A ventilation scan images the flow and distribution of air in the lungs. For this study, the patient must inhale a radioactive gas, such as xenon 133.

The major indication for perfusion scans is the assessment of the blood flow to the lungs, particularly so to diagnose pulmonary embolism. In pulmonary embolism, one or more filling defects are seen on the perfusion scan. Because many other lung abnormalities, e.g., pneumonia, emphysema, and pleural effusion, also give rise to perfusion defects, the perfusion scan may be combined with a ventilation scan. By comparing the two scans, it is possible to diagnose pulmonary embolism by demonstrating parts of the lung that are ventilated but not perfused.

ROENTGEN SIGNS OF PULMONARY DISEASE

Pulmonary lesions may be classified according to distribution within the lungs as local, re-

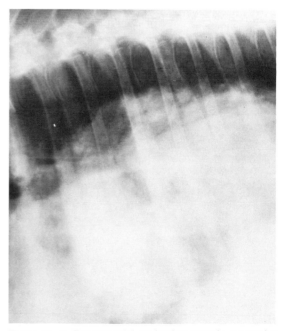

Figure 31–8. Dorsocaudal projection reveals a massive pulmonary abscess.

gional, or diffuse. Examples of such diseases may be further categorized according to the part of the lung involved, e.g., interstitium, terminal air spaces, conducting airways, and pulmonary vasculature. Relegation of a given examination to one of the above anatomic categories is dependent on the associated radiographic signs—abnormal shadow configurations that may be directly or indirectly related to one or more pulmonary diseases or disease mechanisms. In diffuse lung disease, this analytic method is termed pattern recognition. Its primary purpose is to limit the number of differential diagnoses required for a given examination while freeing the radiograph interpreter from the restraints of memorization diagnosis.

Pulmonary Mass Lesions. Detectable pulmonary mass lesions in the horse are usually large, cavitated, or both (Fig. 31–8). Many mass lesions, such as abscesses, may go undetected radiographically because of the masking influence of the heart and associated great vessels (Fig. 31–9). Other lesions are obscured by associated lung or pleural disease, particularly when they occur in the ventral part of the thorax. Pulmonary atelectasis secondary to pleural effusion may resemble a mass lesion, as may patchy consolidation. The majority of lung masses in the horse are abscesses, many of which are cavitated. The latter feature usually renders the lesion more outstanding, particularly when a fluid line is present (Figs. 31–9 and 31–10). Mycetoma occur occasionally and are usually associated with internal compartmentalization without fluid lines (Figs. 31–6 and 31–7). Cavitary lesions have been described

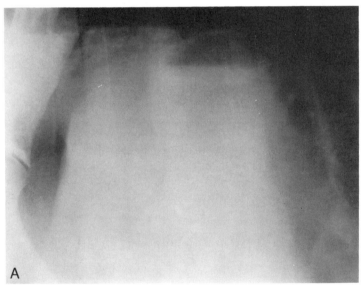

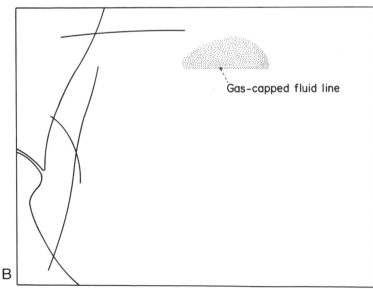

Figure 31–9. *A*, ventrocranial projection demonstrates a cavitated lung abscess. *B*, companion line drawing.

Gas-capped fluid line

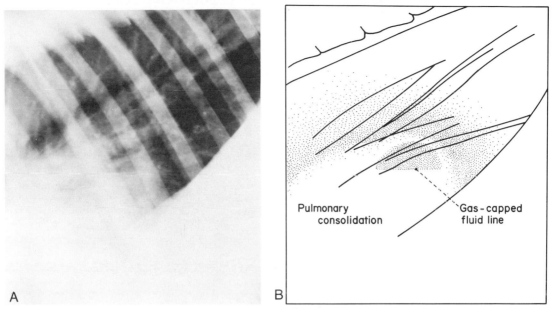

Figure 31–10. *A*, dorsocaudal projection reveals a cavitated lung abscess. *B*, companion line drawing.

Figure 31–11. *A*, typical radiographic pattern of pneumonia in a foal. *B*, companion line drawing.

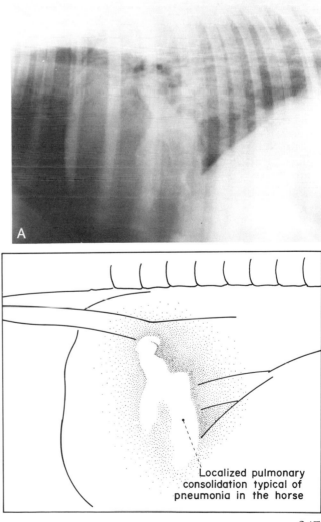

in association with exercise-induced pulmonary hemorrhage in race horses; the lesion typically occurs in the dorsocaudal aspect of the lung. Primary lung tumors are rare in the horse, and metastatic lesions occur only occasionally; the latter more often assume an interstitial pattern. Mediastinal masses may be difficult to distinguish from pulmonary lesions when they displace an adjacent mediastinal structure, such as the trachea. Most lung masses are associated with additional lung disease.

Regional Lung Disease. Regional lung disease is commonly encountered in the horse. It is usually of bacterial nature and results in pulmonary consolidation. The ventrocaudal lung is most often affected, frequently producing a positive silhouette sign with the heart (Fig. 13–11). In some instances, the silhouette effect creates an initial impression of cardiomegaly. Patchy consolidation may be difficult to differentiate from abscess formation. Followup examinations often serve to resolve this question, in that consolidation is usually progressive whereas abscesses are often static.

Interstitial Disease. The pattern of interstitial disease may be defined as the constellation of radiographic findings indicating disease in the connective tissue compartment of the lung, the pulmonary interstitium. The pulmonary interstitium is that portion of the lung that acts as a scaffold on which the pulmonary vasculature and airways are supported. The roentgen signs of interstitial disease include increased background lung opacity, usually discrete; indistinctness of pulmonary airways and vasculature; widespread small shadows (may range from reticular to granular, to nodular, or to various combinations of these findings); and capacity to change lung volume with varied respiration (maintenance of terminal air spaces).

Examples of interstitial diseases in the horse include viral, bacterial, mycotic, parasitic, and hypersensitivity pneumonias (Fig. 31–12). The extent of interstitial involvement and that of the other lung compartments is dependent on the stage of a given disease at the time the horse is examined, as well as the nature of the infecting organism or offending inhalant. Some diseases, such as bronchitis and bronchiolitis, that primarily affect the conducting airways may also have an interstitial pattern (Fig. 31–13). Pulmonary fibrosis resulting from both disease and aging is typically seen as an increase in background lung opacity. Pulmonary edema and bleeding disorders appear as interstitial diseases in their earlier stages, before progressing to more typical air space patterns. Neonatal and adult respiratory distress syndromes may appear as interstitial patterns during their initial development. Because almost all air-space dis-

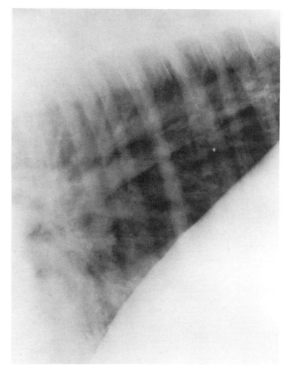

Figure 31–12. Dorsocaudal projection. Increased background lung opacity and indistinct pulmonary airways and vasculature are evident. Pathologic diagnosis: viral pneumonia.

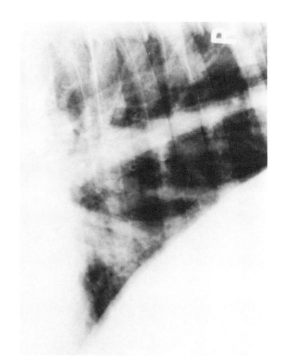

Figure 31–13. Dorsocaudal view. Increased background lung opacity and loss of normal vessel clarity are evident. Pathologic diagnosis: chronic bronchiolitis, allergic?

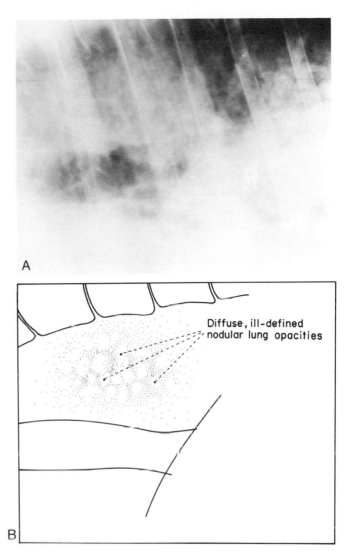

Figure 31–14. *A*, right lateral projection centered at the carina reveals a nodular interstitial pattern. Pathologic diagnosis: metastatic carcinoma. *B*, companion line drawing.

eases must first penetrate the pulmonary interstitium before infiltrating the alveoli, theoretically at least, all such diseases show an interstitial disease pattern at some time during their development. Most air-space diseases will not show sufficient clinical signs of illness, however, until the air space has become involved. Metastatic lung disease is often nodular during its early stages (Fig. 31–14), but may tend to assume an air-space pattern later.

Terminal Airspace (Alveolar) Disease. The alveolar pattern of disease may be defined as the collective radiographic findings that indicate disease affecting the terminal air space. The terminal air space in the horse is that portion of the lung distal to the terminal bronchiole, essentially the alveoli. Terminal air-space disease results from the filling of alveoli with exudate, transudate, blood, or tissue, which replaces the normal air content. The roentgen signs of terminal air space disease include in-

creased foreground lung opacity, often discrete; accentuation of pulmonary airways (air bronchograms); regional or widespread, often symmetric, medium-sized shadows that tend to coalesce; silhouette sign (consolidation); failure of the affected lung to show volume change with varied respiration (inability to ventilate terminal air spaces).

Bacterial pneumonia is the most common airspace disease seen in the horse. The condition is usually bilateral and is often associated with abscess formation, (Fig. 31–15). Air bronchograms are often present, but they tend to be less discrete than in other species, probably due to a combination of factors, including patient size, pulmonary anatomy, and the absence of a dorsoventral or ventrodorsal projection (Fig. 31–16). When the disease is unilateral, a negative silhouette sign may be found, indicated by the transparent appearance of the consolidated lung. This effect is enhanced when

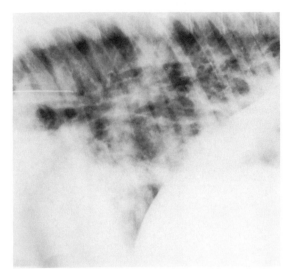

Figure 31–15. Dorsocaudal projection showing a large cavitary lesion, multiple patchy opacities, accentuated bronchial markings, and decreased vascular detail compatible with a mixed air space/interstitial pattern associated with abscess formation. Pathologic diagnosis: gangrenous pneumonia with cavitating abscess formation.

the affected lung is positioned on the side opposite the receiver system. As mentioned previously, many pulmonary diseases, including pneumonia, go through a pattern evolution, beginning with an interstitial display, progressing to a transitional appearance, and culminating in an air-space pattern.

Other lung disorders often represented by air-space patterns include mycotic pneumonia, inhalation pneumonia, bleeding disorders, smoke inhalation, respiratory distress syndrome, and pulmonary edema, both cardiogenic and noncardiogenic in origin.

Conducting Airway Disease. The airway pattern may be defined as the spectrum of radiographic findings indicative of diseases that affect the conducting airways. The conducting airways in the horse include the principal bronchi, subsidiary bronchi, and proximal and terminal bronchioles; respiratory bronchioles are rare and poorly developed. Conducting airway disease may involve the endobronchial, bronchial, or peribronchial tissues, as well as any combination of these tissues. The roentgen signs of conducting airway disease are accentuation of airway markings, which include line shadows (tram lines) and ring shadows (peribronchial cuffing, peribronchial thickening); increased airway diameter; increased number of airways; and abnormal airway configuration.

Many of the common diseases of the conducting airways, such as bronchitis and bronchiolitis, usually produce minimal or no radiographic change, irrespective of the infecting organism. Not until these diseases become prolonged and severe are they associated with radiographic signs. Even under these circumstances, the visible radiographic alterations may be nonspecific, often appearing as nondescript interstitial patterns.

When present, line and ring shadows are reliable radiographic signs of conducting airway disease, although they are usually nonspecific (Fig. 31–17). It is often difficult to access the airways accurately because of associated lung disease, sometimes to the extent that the airway

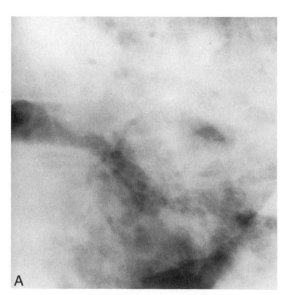

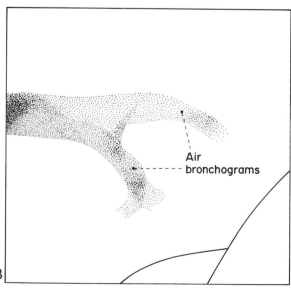

Figure 31–16. *A*, ventrocaudal view reveals massive pulmonary consolidation with air bronchogram formation centrally compatible with an air space pattern. Pathologic diagnosis: chronic suppurative bronchopneumonia. *B*, companion line drawing.

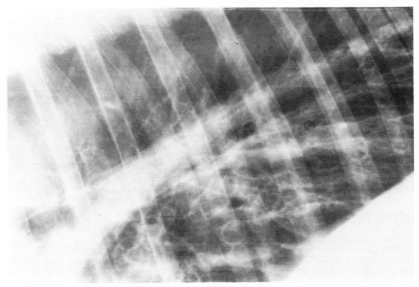

Figure 31–17. Dorsocaudal projection demonstrates widespread line and ring shadows and diminished pulmonary vasculature compatible with airway pattern. Pathologic diagnosis: chronic bronchiectasis and emphysema.

pattern may go undetected (Fig. 31–18). Bronchography is often useful in such situations (Fig. 31–19). Uncomplicated bronchiectasis is fairly specific and is typically seen as multiple, large dilated airways.

Some older horses have radiographically prominent airways, presumably due to age-associated bronchial peribronchial metaplasia (Fig. 31–20). Thin horses invariably show outstanding bronchial markings as a function of a reduced perithoracic tissue mass. It is imperative, but not always possible, to recognize the

difference between prominent and abnormal airways.

Pneumomediastinum is a common radiographic finding in horses after transtracheal aspiration (Fig. 31–21). Although potentially hazardous, pneumomediastinum rarely results in complications.

Vascular Disease. The vascular pattern may be defined as the roentgen findings typically associated with disorders of the pulmonary vasculature. Such disorders may be either primary or secondary, with the latter being more com-

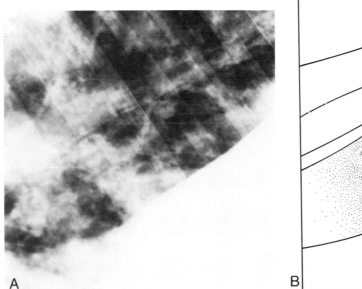

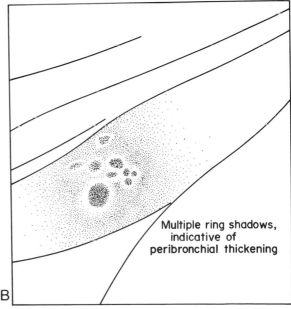

Multiple ring shadows, indicative of peribronchial thickening

Figure 31–18. *A*, dorsoventral projection shows mixed airway and air space pattern. *B*, companion line drawing.

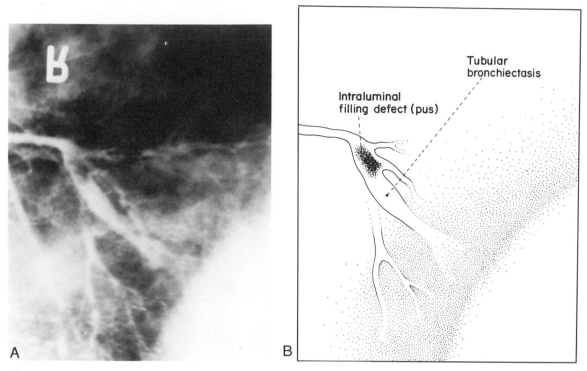

Figure 31–19. *A,* bronchogram (ventrocaudal projection) reveals severe bronchial disease. Pathologic diagnosis: bronchiectasis and bronchopneumonia. *B,* companion line drawing.

Figure 31–20. *A,* dorsoventral projection illustrates prominent bronchial markings in a normal, aged horse.

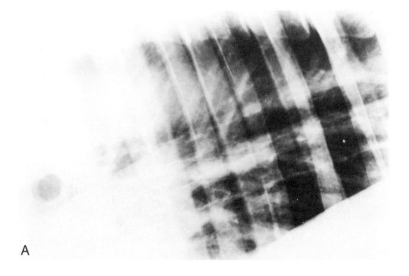

Illustration continued on opposite page

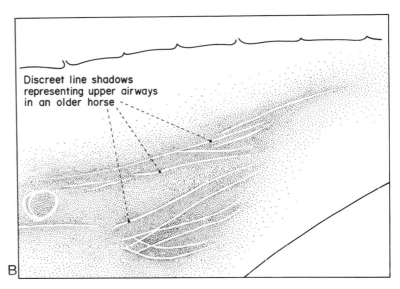

Figure 31–20 *Continued*. *B*, companion line drawing.

Discreet line shadows representing upper airways in an older horse

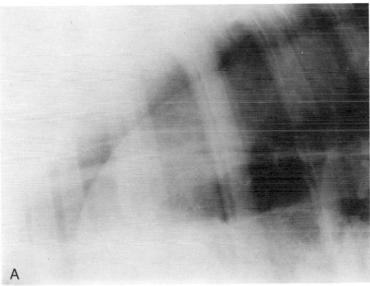

Figure 31–21. *A*, dorsocranial projection reveals pneumomediastinum after transtracheal aspiration. *B*, companion line drawing.

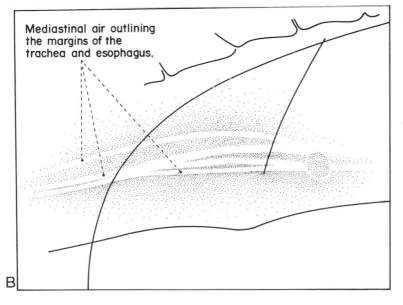

Mediastinal air outlining the margins of the trachea and esophagus.

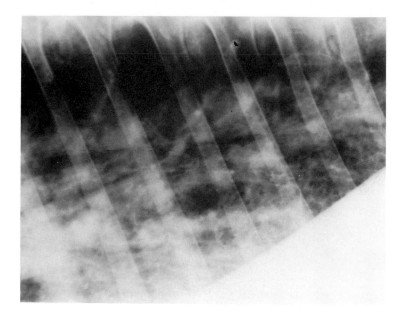

Figure 31–22. Dorsocaudal projection demonstrates increased vessel size and number compatible with pulmonary overcirculation secondary to a left to right intracardiac shunt. Pathologic diagnosis: ventricular septal defect.

mon, e.g., pulmonary congestion secondary to left heart failure. The roentgen signs of pulmonary vascular disease include increased number of pulmonary vessels, increased size of pulmonary vessels, abnormal vascular configuration, and pulmonary edema.

The majority of vascular patterns in the horse are secondary to congenital heart disease, particularly septal defects that produce left to right shunting (Fig. 31–22). Shunt vasculature may be of two types: failure and non-failure compatible. Failure-compatible shunt vasculature is poorly marginated and is generally indistinct as a result of perivascular leakage and concomitant reduction in perivascular contrast. Non-failure-compatible shunt vasculature is relatively well

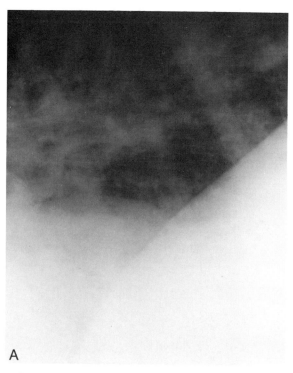

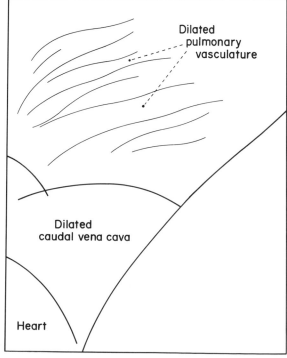

Figure 31–23. *A,* ventrocaudal projection shows a dilated and distorted caudal vena cava compatible with right heart failure. Pathologic diagnosis: congestive cardiomyopathy.

marginated, without any abnormal perivascular opacity. The branch pulmonary anteries best seen in the dorsocaudal projection are the most easily evaluated relative to their diagnostic criteria.

Alterations in the great vessels of the heart are difficult to appreciate in the adult horse. An exception is the caudal vena cava, which may reflect circulatory disturbance by virtue of changes in size and shape best seen in the ventrocaudal projection (Fig. 31–23).

Bleeding disorders of whatever cause alter the appearance of the pulmonary vasculature, often resembling pulmonary edema. Most inflammatory lung disease results in some degree of pulmonary hyperemia, which may be detected radiographically as an increase in both the size and number of the pulmonary vessels.

PULMONARY DISEASE ASSOCIATED WITH A NORMAL RADIOGRAPH

Respiratory disease, sometimes of life-threatening severity, may be present even when the findings from radiographs of the thorax are normal. In some instances, however, this diagnostic information is valuable in that it may exclude those diseases in which clinical signs of thoracic disease are usually associated with radiographic abnormalities. In some horses, a given radiographic examination is normal because a particular disease has simply not progressed to a point at which it is radiographically evident. In such instances, examination of previous radiographs or the making of subsequent comparison studies may resolve the problem.

The accuracy of pattern recognition techniques employed in the radiographic diagnosis of pulmonary parenchymal diseases currently constitutes a point of contention in radiographic circles. Nevertheless, it has been recognized that definite limitations exist with regard to the radiographic visibility of both interstitial and alveolar lesions. Even under ideal conditions, expert observers find that some lesions are below the threshold of visibility, or may be hidden behind or juxtaposed to bony or vascular shadows. A solitary uncalcified lesion less than 6 mm in diameter is rarely identified. When the lesion has enlarged, it may then be detected on a subsequent examination. Pathologically confirmed nodules as large as 2 cm in diameter may be overlooked, particularly if they are situated over the convexity of the lung or in the paramediastinal area, in which the rib cage, large vessels, and mediastinal contents obscure their images. In contrast, multiple micronodular opacities of no more than 1 or 2 cm in diameter are usually identifiable, possibly because they are superimposed on one another. Conditions frequently associated with normal radiographic findings are tracheitis, bronchitis, alveolitis, emphysema, chronic obstructive lung disease, hypersensitivity syndromes, and acquired heart disease in its less advanced stages.

Suggested Reading

Farrow CS: Equine thoracic radiology. J Am Vet Med Assoc 179:776, 1981.

Farrow CS: Radiography of the equine thorax: Anatomy and technic. Vet Radiol 22:62, 1981.

Farrow CS: Radiographic aspects of inflammatory lung disease in the horse. Vet Radiol 22:107, 1981.

Farrow CS: Pneumomediastinum in the horse: A complication of transtracheal aspiration. Vet Radiol 17:192, 1976.

Farrow CS: Inhalation pneumonia in a horse. Can Vet J 23:340, 1982.

Kangstrom LE: The radiological diagnosis of equine pneumonia. Vet Radiol 9:80, 1968.

Morris DD, and Beech J: Disseminated intravascular coagulation in six horses. J Am Vet Med Assoc 183:1067, 1983.

Pascoe JR, O'Brien TR, Wheat JD, Meagher DM: Radiographic aspects of exercise-induced pulmonary hemorrhage in racing horses. Vet Radiol 24:85, 1983.

Silverman S, Poulos PW, Suter PF: Cavitary pulmonary lesions in animals. J Am Vet Radiol Soc 17:134, 1976.

Walker M, and Goble D: Barium sulfate bronchography in horses. Vet Radiol 21:85, 1980.

SECTION 8

ABDOMEN– COMPANION ANIMALS

CHAPTER 32

ABDOMINAL MASSES

CHARLES R. ROOT

INTRODUCTION

Normal abdominal radiographic anatomy is well covered elsewhere.[2, 4, 5, 7, 8, 10, 13, 14] Successful radiographic differentiation of abdominal masses depends upon a good working knowledge of normal radiographic anatomy as well as an appreciation for the normal anatomic variations of major abdominal visceral structures. It must be borne in mind that some organs are nearly always seen, some organs are almost never seen, some are typically only partially seen, and some are seen only if abnormal. In instances in which no lesions are appreciated in the visualized portion of an organ, the remainder of the organ should be assumed to be normal *in the context of radiographic differentiation of abdominal masses*. In other words, one must assume normalcy unless there is direct radiographic evidence to the contrary.

Routine radiography of the abdomen should include ventrodorsal and lateral projections. Right-side dependency allows the tail of the spleen to gravitate across the midline and thereby be more frequently visualized than with the left side down; likewise, in left lateral recumbency, the gas-filled pyloric part of the stomach, which can serve as an important landmark is usually seen. Normally visible structures may not be obvious for a variety of reasons, and there is a great temptation to perform contrast radiography in such instances. Before resorting to contrast radiography to enhance visualization of poorly delineated abdominal visceral structures, however, one should consider positional radiography. This alternative often obtains definitive results quicker and with less manipulation or expense than most contrast radiographic procedures. It may consist simply of radiography in the opposite lateral, dorsoventral, or oblique view, but it also can include horizontal beam projections depending on the suspected nature and location of the lesion.

SPECIAL PROCEDURES

If better visualization of abdominal visceral structures is desired, and positional radiography is contraindicated or has been unsuccessful, various contrast radiographic procedures may be performed. Special radiographic procedures that have proved helpful in radiographic differential diagnosis of certain abdominal masses include pneumoperitoneography,[3, 7, 9, 14] excretory urography,[11] upper GI series,[12] urethrography,[14] cystography,[11] and celiography.[6]

Celiography deserves further attention here, since its use may not be familiar to most veterinarians; it involves the injection of water-soluble contrast medium into the peritoneal cavity. Indications for celiography include

(1) delineation of adjacent visceral organs in the presence of poor abdominal visceral detail, and (2) confirmation of suspected hernias (diaphragmatic, inguinal, ventral, umbilical, and so forth). Although contraindications are few, if peritonitis is suspected, contrast medium should not be injected. The procedure requires very little special equipment; organic iodide contrast medium, sterile syringes and needles, and local anesthetic are all that is needed. Also, the mechanics of the procedure are simple, requiring injection of 350 to 400 mg organic iodide solution per kg of body weight into the peritoneal cavity.

The injection site (at the right lateral aspect of the umbilicus) is clipped and scrubbed with antiseptic solution. The animal is held in left lateral recumbency (to allow the spleen to shift away from the ventral body wall), and contrast medium is injected into the peritoneal cavity. After injection, multiple projections of the abdomen are obtained, including left lateral, right lateral, dorsoventral, and ventrodorsal views. Oblique projections, passing tangentially to suspected lesions in the body wall, are valuable. Horizontal-beam projections, although generally not necessary, can be done after conventional projections have been viewed. The radiographs are then carefully evaluated and compared with the survey radiographs, carefully tracing the many contrast interfaces and relating them to visceral structures and peritoneal boundaries. One should be aware that the contrast medium is absorbed rather rapidly from the peritoneal cavity and excreted by the kidneys. If one waits too long to make supplemental projections, therefore, an excretory urogram may be all that remains of the contrast medium.

RADIOGRAPHIC SIGNS

Several abdominal visceral structures undergo tremendous variation in size under normal circumstances. These are the stomach (after ingestion), the urinary bladder (especially in a house-trained pet), and the uterus (in the pregnant female). Each of these structures, of course, may be pathologically enlarged, and it may be difficult to radiographically differentiate between normal and abnormal enlargement. Most of the rest of the normally visible abdominal visceral structures are enlarged only if abnormal. Further, pathologic enlargement of certain structures (such as the pancreas, the ovaries, the mesenteric lymph nodes, and the adrenal glands) is the only reason they are ever identified radiographically.

The edges of enlarged visceral structures may not be directly visible radiographically. In such instances, enlargement must be inferred by the direction and degree of displacement of adjacent structures. Such displacement may be appreciable even in the presence of diminished abdominal visceral detail due to ascites, emaciation, mesenteric contusion, or other conditions in which visceral contrast is destroyed.

The following is a discussion of the typical radiographic signs associated with specific abdominal viscera. There will be exceptions to the general pattern of visceral displacement, but they are rare. The most common exceptions to typical radiographic signs of abdominal masses are due to extreme enlargement of the organ or structure in question.

Stomach

Enlargement of the stomach (Fig. 32–1), whether postprandial or pathologic, causes caudal displacement of the small bowel, the transverse colon, and the spleen. Splenic displace-

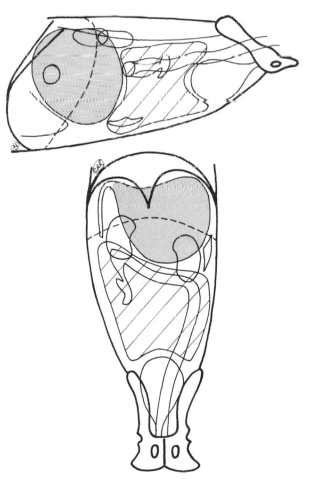

Figure 32–1. The radiographic signs of gastric enlargement and the effect of the enlarged stomach on adjacent viscera.

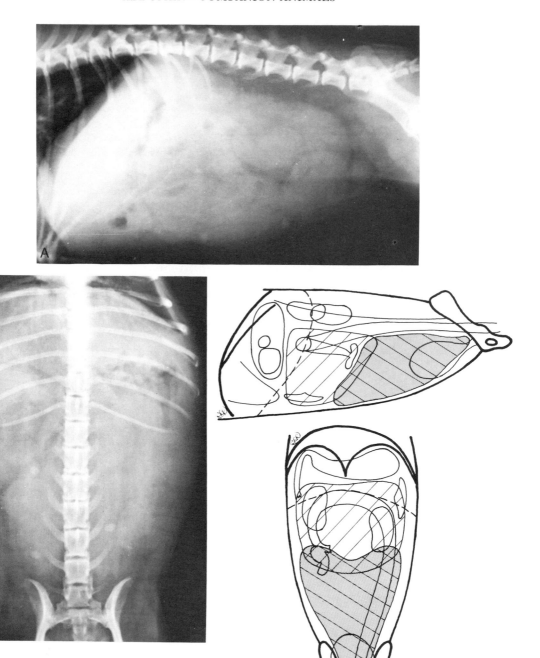

Figure 32–2. Lateral *(A)* and ventrodorsal *(B)* abdominal radiographs of a female dog with typical signs of pyometra. Notice the convoluted loops of tubular fluid opacity in the caudoventral abdomen. The small bowel is craniodorsally and centrally displaced. The descending colon is often displaced dorsally as depicted in the associated diagram *(C)*. *(A* and *B* from Root CR: J Am Vet Radiol Soc *15:*26, 1974, with permission.)

ment in the presence of gastric torsion is variable and may be accompanied by considerable splenomegaly.

Uterus

Uterine enlargement is generally not appreciated radiographically until it exceeds the di-

ameter of the adjacent small bowel. Further enlargement of the uterine body and horns causes craniodorsal displacement of the small bowel in the lateral projection and mesocranial gathering of the small bowel in the ventrodorsal view (Fig. 32–2). Tortuous or convoluted homogeneous tubular opacities in the caudoventral abdomen are often seen to be responsible for this specific pattern of enteric displacement. Further, there may be separation of the ventral aspect of the colon and the dorsal aspect of the urinary bladder by distension of the body of the uterus in the vesicocolonic space. Late pregnancy should be easily determined by the presence of fetal skeletal mineralization, a finding that is generally first present at 40 to 45 days of gestation in dogs and cats.[2, 4, 5]

Urinary Bladder

Distension of the urinary bladder (Fig. 32–3) usually produces a homogeneous space-occupying opacity in the caudoventral abdomen. In the lateral projection, a full urinary bladder usually causes cranial displacement of the small bowel and dorsal displacement of the descending colon. In the ventrodorsal projection, the descending colon may be displaced either to

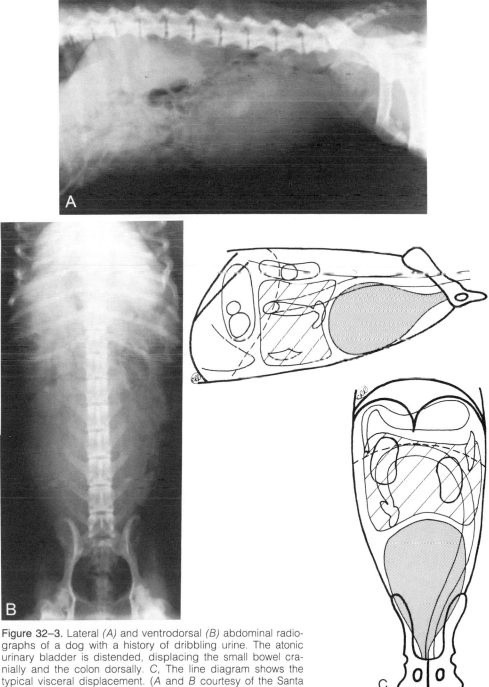

Figure 32–3. Lateral *(A)* and ventrodorsal *(B)* abdominal radiographs of a dog with a history of dribbling urine. The atonic urinary bladder is distended, displacing the small bowel cranially and the colon dorsally. *C,* The line diagram shows the typical visceral displacement. *(A and B courtesy of the Santa Cruz Veterinary Hospital.)*

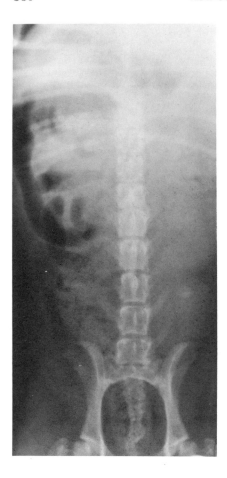

Figure 32–4. Ventrodorsal lumbar vertebral radiograph of a dog. Notice that the caudal part of the descending colon is on the right side. This is not uncommon, especially when the urinary bladder is full, when the colon is redundant, and when the animal was in right lateral recumbency immediately before being placed on its back for the ventrodorsal radiographic projection. (Courtesy of the Seattle Veterinary Hospital for Surgery.)

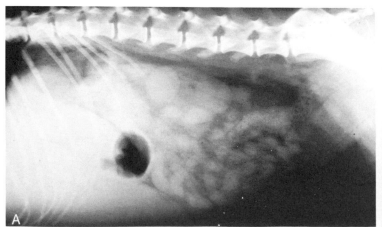

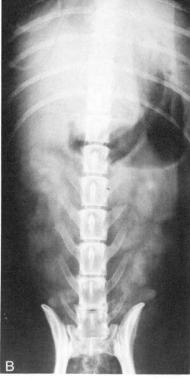

Figure 32–5. Lateral *(A)* and ventrodorsal *(B)* abdominal radiographs of a dog with generalized hepatic enlargement due to diabetes mellitus.

Illustration continued on opposite page

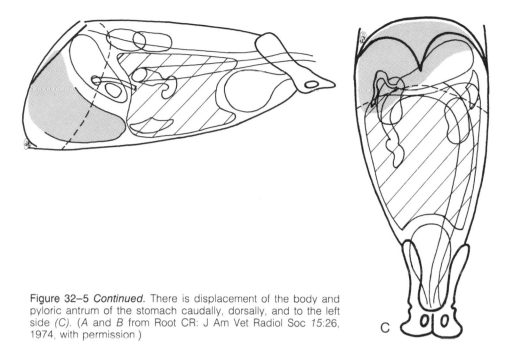

Figure 32–5 *Continued.* There is displacement of the body and pyloric antrum of the stomach caudally, dorsally, and to the left side *(C)*. *(A* and *B* from Root CR: J Am Vet Radiol Soc *15*:26, 1974, with permission.)

the right or to the left of the urinary bladder, depending upon which side of the body was dependent immediately before the patient was placed in dorsal recumbency, and whether or not the colon is redundant. A full urinary bladder can entrap a redundant descending colon to the right of the midline if the animal was in left lateral recumbency immediately before being placed upon its back for the ventrodorsal projection (Fig. 32–4).

Diffuse Hepatomegaly

Generalized enlargement of the liver produces characteristic displacement of the pylorus and pyloric antrum caudally, dorsally, and to the left (Fig. 32–5). In the lateral projection, the gastric axis (an imaginary line connecting the fundus, body, and pylorus of the stomach) should be parallel to the ribs and perpendicular to the spine, or somewhere between those two extremes. In the ventrodorsal projection, the

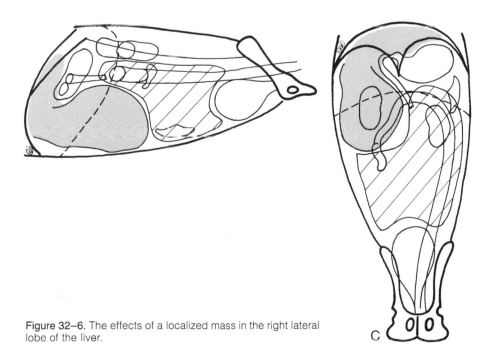

Figure 32–6. The effects of a localized mass in the right lateral lobe of the liver.

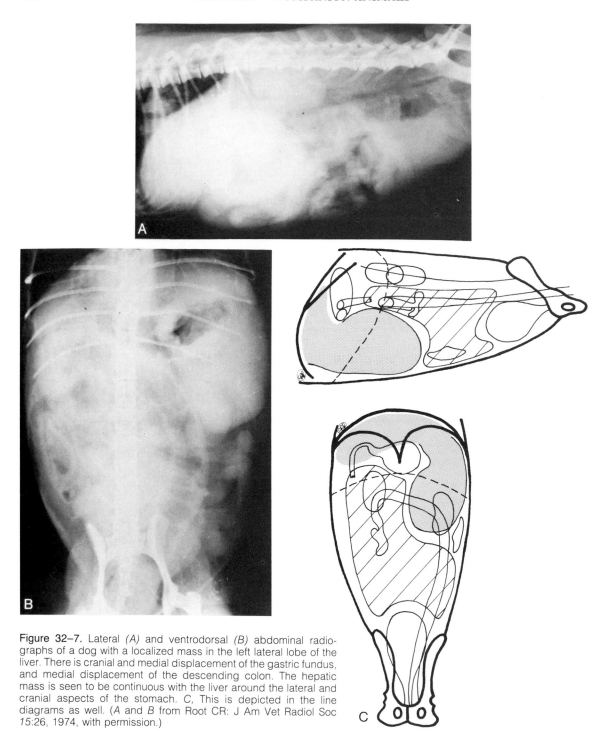

Figure 32–7. Lateral *(A)* and ventrodorsal *(B)* abdominal radiographs of a dog with a localized mass in the left lateral lobe of the liver. There is cranial and medial displacement of the gastric fundus, and medial displacement of the descending colon. The hepatic mass is seen to be continuous with the liver around the lateral and cranial aspects of the stomach. *C,* This is depicted in the line diagrams as well. *(A* and *B* from Root CR: J Am Vet Radiol Soc *15*:26, 1974, with permission.)

gastric axis should be perpendicular to the spine of the dog. Since the pylorus may normally be more caudal in the cat, it can be approximately 30 degrees from perpendicular to the spine in that species, especially in the ventrodorsal projection. In many instances, the enlarged cau-

doventral edge of the abnormal liver can be directly visualized as it projects beyond the costal margin. However, in instances in which poor abdominal visceral detail prevents direct visualization of the edge of the liver, disturbances in the gastric axis are readily apparent if the gastric contents can be seen. Occasionally, contrast gastrography may be necessary to fully appreciate generalized hepatomegaly.

Focal Lobar Hepatic Masses

Masses developing in the right lateral or right middle lobe of the liver, in the absence of diffuse hepatomegaly, often produce rather specific visceral displacements (Fig. 32–6). There is dorsomedial displacement of the pyloric antrum, pylorus, proximal descending duodenum, and ascending colon. Further, there is caudodorsal displacement of the adjacent small bowel loops and, if the hepatic mass is pedunculated and sufficiently large, craniodorsal displacement of the body of the stomach.

Left lateral or left middle lobar hepatic masses are also quite specific in displacement of adjacent viscera (Fig. 32–7). The head of the spleen, the adjacent small intestine, and the gastric fundus are displaced dorsomedially. The tail of the spleen is variably displaced, but the fundus of the stomach may be strikingly displaced craniodorsally if entrapped by a pedunculated hepatic mass of sufficient size lying to the left.

Central lobar liver masses are rare but usually cause the body of the stomach to be displaced caudodorsally, creating extrinsic indentation of its lesser curvature (Fig. 32–8). Contrast radiography of the stomach may be necessary to fully appreciate this radiographic sign.

Diffuse Splenomegaly

Generalized enlargement of the spleen, if mild, is difficult to verify radiographically. The spleen undergoes considerable nonpathologic variation in size, and there appears to be some overlap of maximum normal and minimal pathologic size. Radiographic assessment of splenic size is subjective, at best. The most acceptable criterion appears to be that a spleen should be considered enlarged if its edges are rounded and if it obviously displaces adjacent viscera (Fig. 32–9).

Splenic Masses

Masses originating in the head of the spleen cause caudodorsal displacement of the adjacent small intestine in the lateral projection. In the ventrodorsal projection, splenic head masses cause the small bowel to be displaced caudally and to the right. Also, since the gastrosplenic ligament renders the head of the spleen relatively immobile, masses of the head of the spleen are often associated with extrinsic cranial displacement of the greater curvature of the stomach, especially in the ventrodorsal view (Fig. 32–10).

Masses that originate in the body or tail of the spleen are much less consistent in their displacement of the small bowel than are those of the head of the spleen. This is due to the fact that the tail and body of the spleen are much more mobile than the head. The small bowel may be displaced in any number of

Text continued on page 368

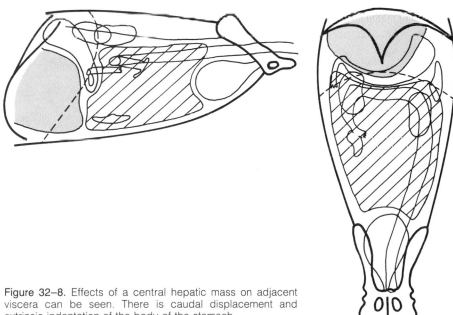

Figure 32–8. Effects of a central hepatic mass on adjacent viscera can be seen. There is caudal displacement and extrinsic indentation of the body of the stomach.

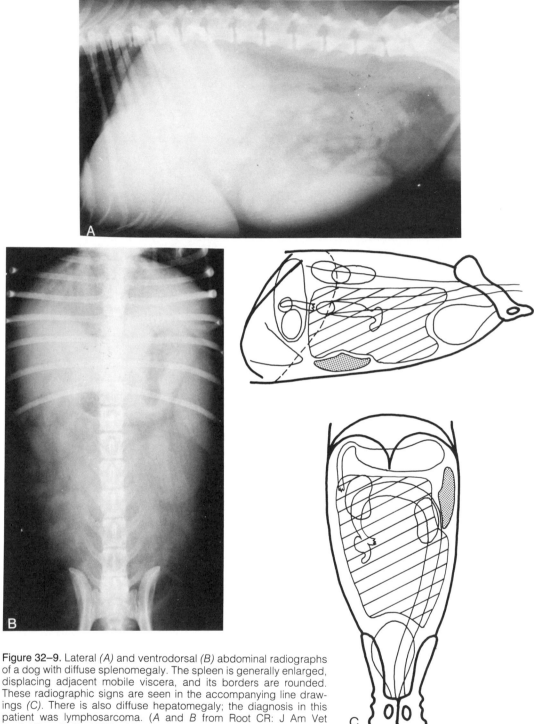

Figure 32–9. Lateral *(A)* and ventrodorsal *(B)* abdominal radiographs of a dog with diffuse splenomegaly. The spleen is generally enlarged, displacing adjacent mobile viscera, and its borders are rounded. These radiographic signs are seen in the accompanying line drawings *(C)*. There is also diffuse hepatomegaly; the diagnosis in this patient was lymphosarcoma. (*A* and *B* from Root CR: J Am Vet Radiol Soc *15:*26, 1974, with permission.)

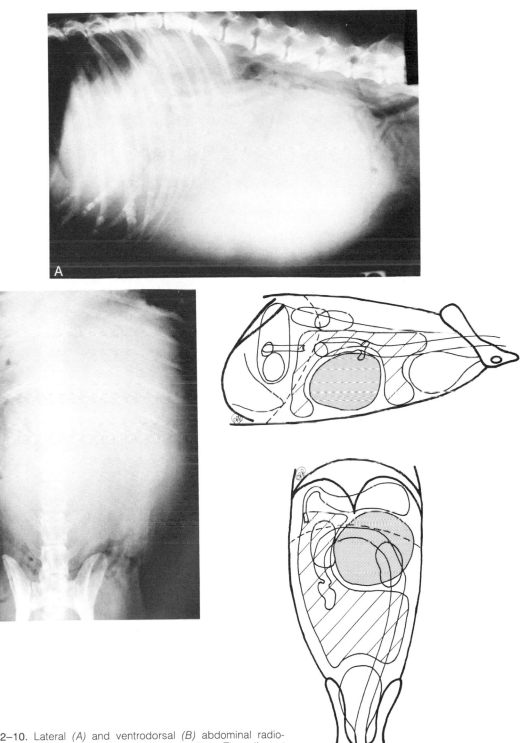

Figure 32–10. Lateral *(A)* and ventrodorsal *(B)* abdominal radiographs of a dog with a mass in the head of the spleen. The adjacent small bowel loops are for the most part displaced caudally by the mass *(C).* (*A* and *B* from Root CR: J Am Vet Radiol Soc *15*:26, 1974, with permission.)

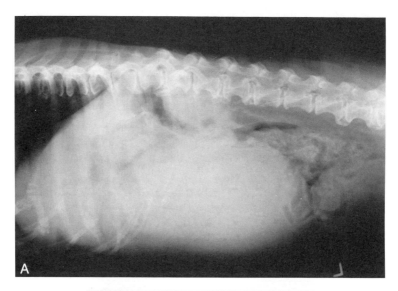

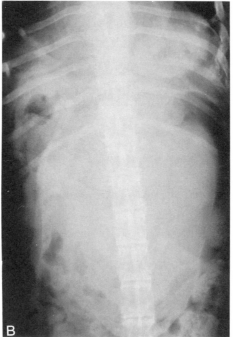

Figure 32–11. Lateral *(A)* and ventrodorsal *(B)* abdominal radiographs of a dog with a splenic hematoma. The small bowel is displaced primarily caudally. Histopathology is necessary to differentiate benign from malignant splenic masses.

Illustration continued on opposite page

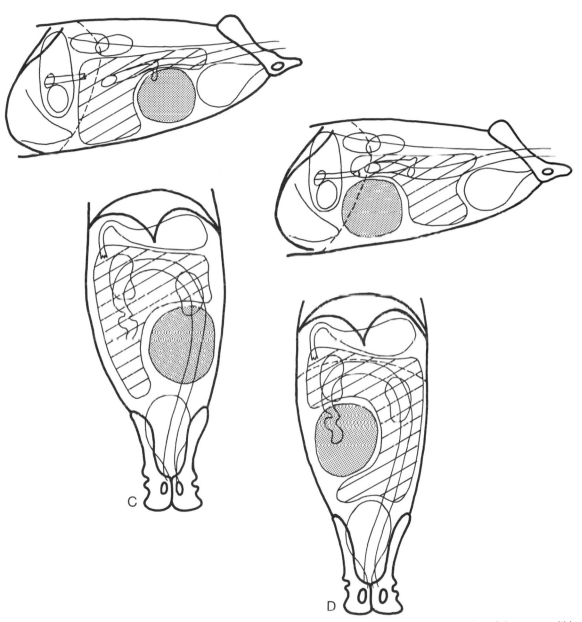

Figure 32–11 *Continued.* *C* and *D*, Visceral displacement is variable, depending upon the location of the mass within the spleen.

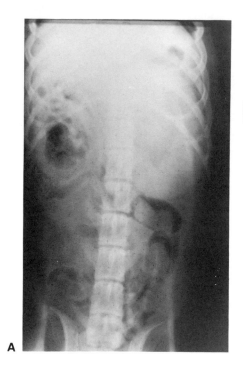

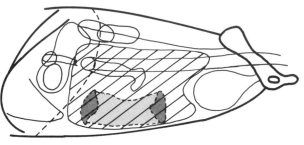

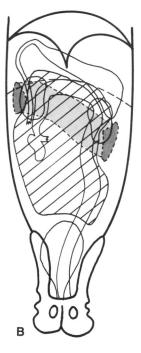

Figure 32–12. Ventrodorsal (A) abdominal radiograph of a dog with torsion of the spleen. Contrary to its occurrence in some animals, the descending duodenum is not displaced medially. However, both ends of the spleen are seen end-on, the organ having assumed a C-shape owing to rotation about its own vascular pedicle. This is diagrammed in B along with medial displacement of the descending duodenum, which is sometimes seen in torsion of the spleen. This patient was in a relatively acute phase of the syndrome; later, the radiographic signs may become much more vague, especially after body fluids have begun to effuse through the splenic capsule. (A courtesy of the Santa Cruz Venterinary Hospital.)

directions or combinations of direction (Fig. 32–10). There is generally dorsal displacement of some portion of the small bowel in the lateral projection. However, there may also be predominantly caudal or predominantly cranial displacement as well as combinations of cranial and caudal enteric displacement. In the ventrodorsal projection, depending on the exact location of the splenic mass, the small intestine may be displaced to the left, to the right, caudally, cranially, or peripherally. In fact, subsequent radiographs of positional radiography may show considerable change in enteric visceral displacement. Furthermore, the amount of time a patient is kept in a certain position before radiographs are made may greatly influence the position of the splenic mass.

Splenic Torsion
The radiographic signs (Fig. 32–12) of torsion of the spleen have only recently been described.[1, 7] Although the syndrome has yet to be fully appreciated from a pathogenic and morphologic point of view, it may be either secondary to gastric volvulus or independent of other abdominal lesions. In animals in which splenic torsion has existed for several days, only a poorly marginated, generalized, pronounced splenomegaly may be appreciated.[7] In patients with more recent splenic torsion, it is possible to appreciate caudal displacement of the gastric fundus; the spleen is often dramatically and diffusely enlarged and may be drawn into a C shape as a result of rotation about its own pedicle. There is often medial displacement of the descending duodenum and ascending colon, if the tail of the spleen is located between the body wall and the right lateral aspect of the enteric viscera. These radiographic signs are difficult to appreciate if the duration of the condition has resulted in ascites due to effusion from the splenic capsule.

Mesenteric or Enteric Masses
Circumscribed masses originating in the mesentery and those originating from the gut wall often produce similar radiographic signs of vis-

ceral displacement. Location of such masses is variable and often unstable in serial or positional radiographs. Therefore, visceral displacement is rarely predictable. Masses originating from the root of the mesentery, however, generally produce characteristic peripheral enteric displacement in the ventrodorsal projection and dorsal, cranial, and caudal displacement of the intestine in the lateral projection (Fig. 32–13). They are easily confused with certain splenic masses, especially those originating from the tail or body of the spleen, and may require

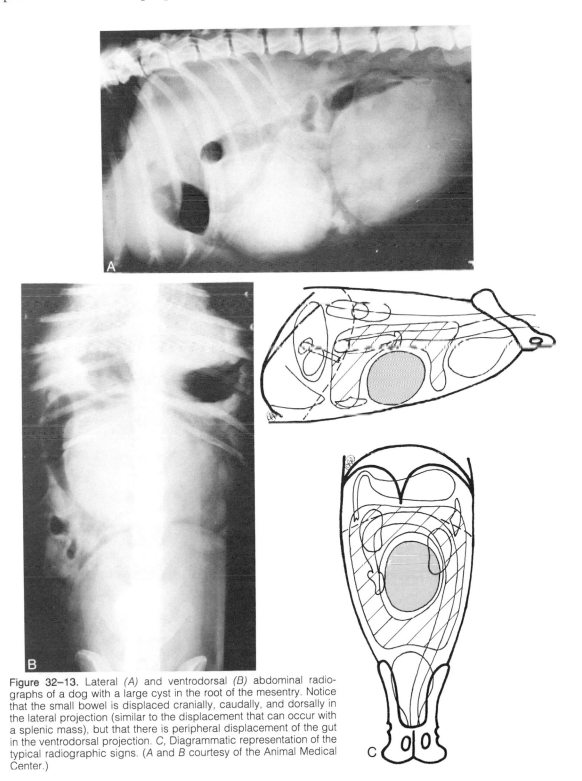

Figure 32–13. Lateral *(A)* and ventrodorsal *(B)* abdominal radiographs of a dog with a large cyst in the root of the mesentry. Notice that the small bowel is displaced cranially, caudally, and dorsally in the lateral projection (similar to the displacement that can occur with a splenic mass), but that there is peripheral displacement of the gut in the ventrodorsal projection. *C,* Diagrammatic representation of the typical radiographic signs. *(A and B courtesy of the Animal Medical Center.)*

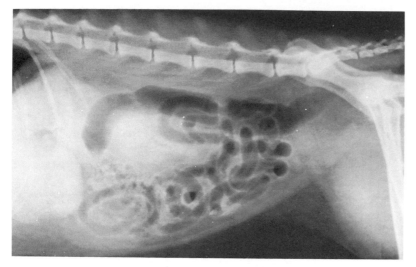

Figure 32–14. Lateral abdominal radiograph of a cat with colic lymphadenopathy due to lymphosarcoma. Notice the ventral displacement of the ascending portion of the colon (feces-filled) and the caudal and ventral displacement of the adjacent small bowel. These radiographic signs are quite specific for enlargement of the colic lymph node in the cat. As the mass enlarges, enteric displacement may change to become cranial and dorsal. (Courtesy of the Santa Cruz Veterinary Hospital.)

positional films for differentiation. Masses derived from enlargement of the colic lymph node cause ventral and dextrolateral displacement of the ascending colon. Such ventral colonic displacement is best seen with the patient in left lateral recumbency (Fig. 32–14).

Pancreatic Masses

Masses evolving from pancreatic tissue are special cases of enteric masses, but they may produce rather specific radiographic signs depending upon the location of the mass within the pancreas. If the mass originates in the head of the pancreas (Fig. 32–15), there is almost always lateral displacement of the descending duodenum and extrinsic displacement of the caudodextral wall of the pyloric antrum of the stomach in the ventrodorsal projection. In the lateral projection, the duodenum is displaced ventrally. If the mass originates from the tail of the pancreas, there is usually no extrinsic distortion of the gastric wall, but the adjacent portion of the descending duodenum is displaced ventrally and to the right. Appreciation of these radiographic signs depends upon visualization of the duodenum, sometimes requiring the administration of barium sulfate suspension.

Kidney Masses

Visualization of the entire contour of the right kidney is rarely possible in survey radiographs. However, if its caudal pole is not visible, and

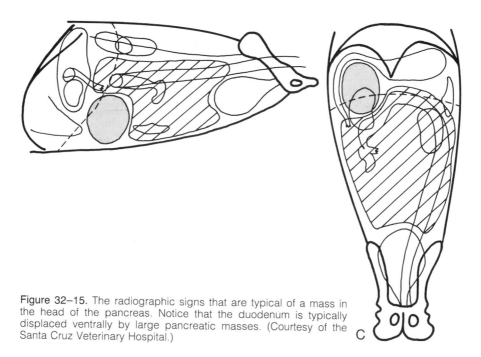

Figure 32–15. The radiographic signs that are typical of a mass in the head of the pancreas. Notice that the duodenum is typically displaced ventrally by large pancreatic masses. (Courtesy of the Santa Cruz Veterinary Hospital.)

if there is a homogeneous fluid opacity on the right side of the craniodorsal portion of the abdomen, enlargement of the right kidney should be suspected, and adjacent visceral displacement should be assessed. Enlargement of the right kidney produces medial and ventral displacement of the descending duodenum and ascending colon. There is also levoventral displacement of the adjacent portion of the small intestine (Fig. 32–16).

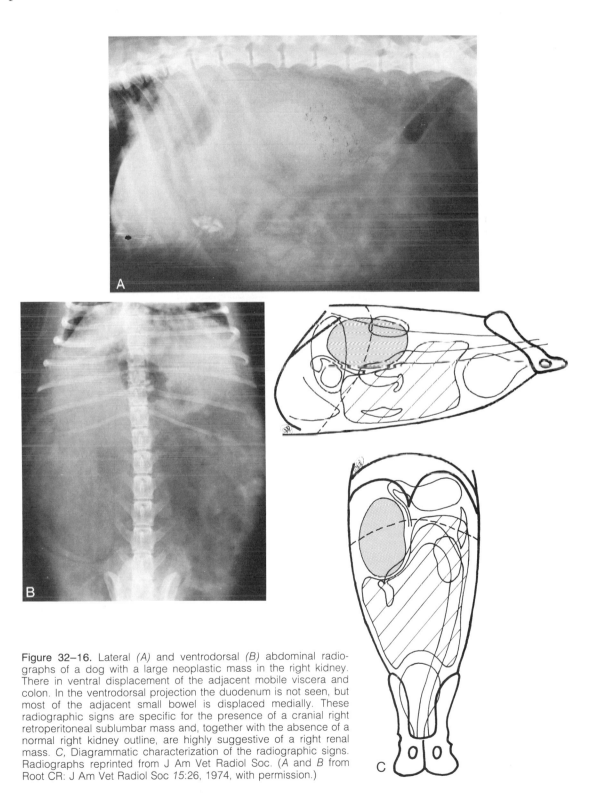

Figure 32–16. Lateral *(A)* and ventrodorsal *(B)* abdominal radiographs of a dog with a large neoplastic mass in the right kidney. There in ventral displacement of the adjacent mobile viscera and colon. In the ventrodorsal projection the duodenum is not seen, but most of the adjacent small bowel is displaced medially. These radiographic signs are specific for the presence of a cranial right retroperitoneal sublumbar mass and, together with the absence of a normal right kidney outline, are highly suggestive of a right renal mass. *C,* Diagrammatic characterization of the radiographic signs. Radiographs reprinted from J Am Vet Radiol Soc. (*A* and *B* from Root CR: J Am Vet Radiol Soc *15:*26, 1974, with permission.)

Direct visualization of the contour of the left kidney is much more reliable than that of the right kidney. Inability to visualize the normal left kidney in either projection may be the first radiographic sign associated with a left renal mass. Moreover, there is ventral and medial displacement of the descending colon and adjacent small bowel (Fig. 32–17).

Renal masses, even those of considerable size, remain dorsal in the abdomen. The kidneys are truly retroperitoneal structures and, like all retroperitoneal structures, are prevented from migrating ventrally by the tough retroperitoneal fascia. Fortunately, neoplastic or inflammatory enlargement of the other retroperitoneal structures is very rare. In instances of retroperitoneal masses of other than renal origin, visualization of the ipsilateral kidney should not be impaired. Renal displacement in such instances depends upon the location of the mass. Adrenal masses and masses originating from the epaxial spinal musculature are exam-

ples of extrarenal retroperitoneal space-occupying lesions. One note of caution is appropriate at this point: Adrenal pheochromocytoma may invade and replace ipsilateral kidney tissue (Fig. 32–18).[10] Inasmuch as renal masses tend to remain dorsal, progressive enlargement causes ventral displacement of the adjacent mobile visceral structures. The alimentary tract is suspended centrally by various forms of the mesentery (mesoduodenum, mesojejunum, mesoileum, and mesocolon). Since the kidneys are lateral to the root of the mesentery, visceral displacement mesad is produced as the kidneys enlarge.

Ovarian Masses

Right ovarian masses are associated with a well-circumscribed homogeneous opacity cranial to the right kidney, separate and distinct from the caudate lobe of the liver. They produce medial, but not ventral, displacement of the descending duodenum and ascending colon. Furthermore,

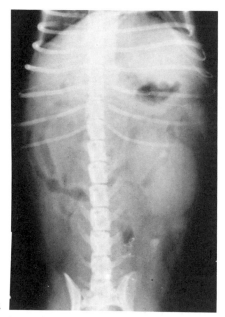

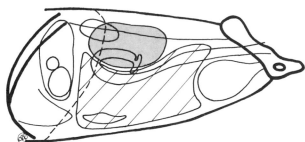

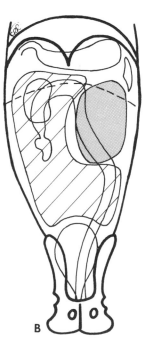

Figure 32–17. Ventrodorsal *(A)* abdominal radiograph of a dog with hydronephrosis of the left kidney. With left renal enlargement *(B)*, small bowel is often displaced medially and ventrally. *(A courtesy of Louisiana State University.)*

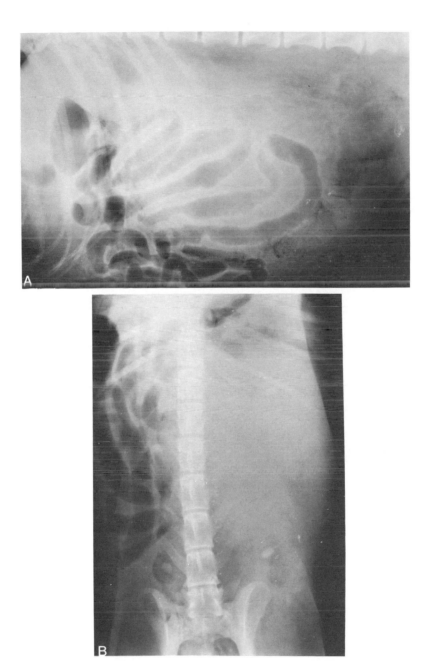

Figure 32–18. Lateral *(A)* and ventrodorsal *(B)* abdominal radiographs of a dog with a large mass in the left sublumbar region; notice the typical visceral displacement. The left kidney is not seen, and there is ventral and caudal displacement of the metallic sutures placed during ovariohysterectomy. This lesion proved to be an adrenal pheochromocytoma that had invaded and replaced the left kidney by vascular extension. (From Root CR: J Am Vet Radiol Soc *15*:26, 1974, with permission.)

there will be ventral deviation of the caudal pole of the right kidney if the ovarian mass is large enough.

Left ovarian masses, in addition to producing a space-occupying soft tissue opacity cranial to the left kidney, usually produce medial (but not ventral) displacement of the descending colon and adjacent small bowel (Fig. 32–19). The caudal pole of the left kidney may be tipped ventrally, depending upon the size and location of the mass.

At first consideration, masses originating in the ovaries would seem to be capable of producing visceral displacement identical to that produced by kidneys. *They do not*, and a note of explanation is in order. The ovaries are not retroperitoneal structures. Therefore, as they enlarge, they are free to gravitate ventrally between the body wall and the mobile enteric viscera. The ovarian ligament stretches, permitting the mass to gain access ventral to the adjacent enteric structures (the descending colon on the left, and the ascending colon and descending duodenum on the right). As a result, those structures appear radiographically to be in their respectively normal locations in the lateral projection, but they are displaced medially in the ventrodorsal view. Since the ovarian ligament is attached to the caudal pole of the kidney, a sufficiently pendulous ovary will produce ventral deviation of the caudal pole of the ipsilateral kidney.

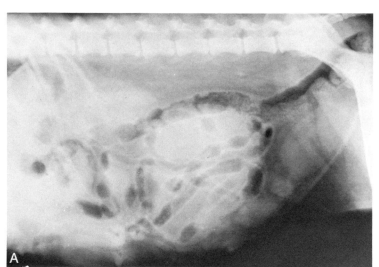

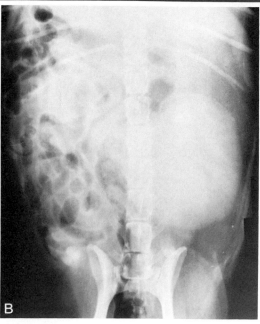

Figure 32–19. Lateral *(A)* and ventrodorsal *(B)* abdominal radiographs of a dog with a neoplasm of the left ovary. There is medial, *but not ventral,* displacement of the descending colon. The caudal pole of the left kidney is tipped ventrally.

Illustration continued on opposite page

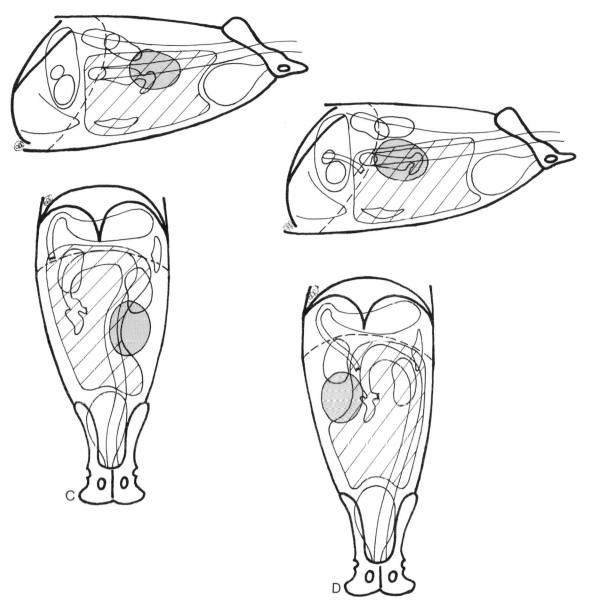

Figure 32–19 *Continued.* The line drawings show the typical radiographic signs of left *(C)* and right *(D)* ovarian masses. (*A* and *B* from Root CR: J Am Vet Radiol Soc *15*:26, 1974, with permission.)

Prostate Gland

The prostate gland is normally intrapelvic and is, therefore, usually not seen radiographically. However, house-trained pets may be able to distend the urinary bladder enough to pull the prostate gland cranial to the brim of the pubis; emptying the urinary bladder should allow the prostate gland to regain its normal position in the pelvic canal in such instances. Generalized or symmetric enlargement of the prostate gland produces cranial displacement of the urinary bladder and, possibly, dorsal displacement of the rectum (Fig. 32–20). The ventrodorsal projection is often of little value in assessment of

diseases of the prostate gland, but it should be noted that prostatomegaly (in the absence of distension of the urinary bladder) can displace the colon to either side of the midline. If the prostate is painful, the colon may be full of fecal material, since the animal may be obstipated.

Eccentric enlargement of the prostate gland, as produced by prostatic cysts or some neoplastic infiltrates, has a variable effect on the adjacent caudal abdominal visceral structures (Fig. 32–21). Depending upon the location or site of origin of the prostatic cyst, the urinary bladder may be displaced either cranioventrally or craniodorsally. Contrast radiography is usually nec-

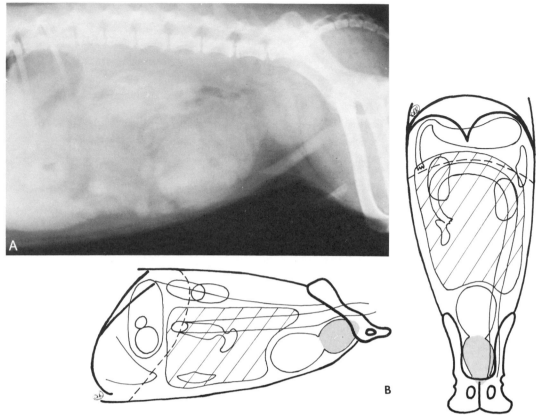

Figure 32–20. Lateral abdominal radiograph *(A)* of a dog with symmetric prostatomegaly. The ventrodorsal projection is generally noncontributory in this condition. The urinary bladder is displaced cranially, and the prostate gland can be seen at the brim of the pelvis. Often, there is mild dorsal displacement of the pelvic portion of the descending colon, as seen in *B*. *(A* from Root CR: J Am Vet Radiol Soc *15:*26, 1974, with permission.)

Figure 32–21. Lateral abdominal radiograph *(A)* and cystogram *(B)* of a dog with a prostatic cyst.

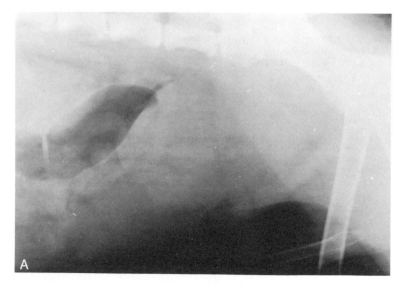

Figure 32–21 *Continued.* In this animal the prostatic cyst is between the colon and the urinary bladder, whereas in other dogs the prostatic cyst may be between the urinary bladder and the ventral body wall (*C* and *D*). Cystography usually must be done to differentiate prostatic cysts from the urinary bladder. The descending colon is usually displaced dorsally. The ventrodorsal projections (*C* and *D*) generally do not contribute significantly to evaluation of this lesion. (*A* and *B* from Root CR: J Am Vet Radiol Soc *15*:26, 1974, with permission.)

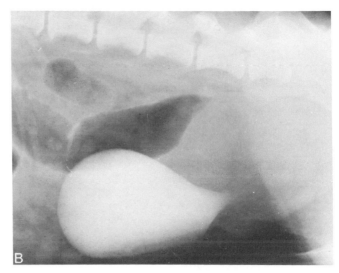

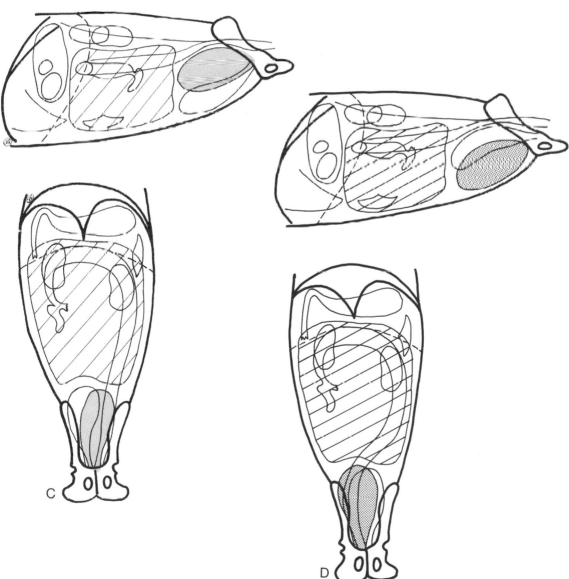

essary to differentiate between the urinary bladder and the lesion in such instances.

Caudal Sublumbar Masses

Masses originating in the caudal sublumbar region are treated separately, as their radiographic signs are quite specific (Fig. 32–22). In general, there are few lesions that produce the radiographic signs associated with caudal sublumbar masses. Most such lesions are caused by iliac lymphadenopathy, caudal sublumbar muscular masses, or inflammatory granuloma/abscess formation. The descending colon is displaced ventrally in the lateral projection. There is usually a broadly based homogeneous mass in the sublumbar space, but its opacity may be interrupted by gas pockets if the lesion is a granulomatous response to a foreign body, such as a migrating grass awn or a porcupine quill. The ventrodorsal projection is usually noncontributory, but the rectum may be displaced either to the left or to the right.

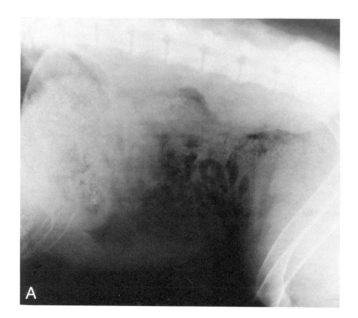

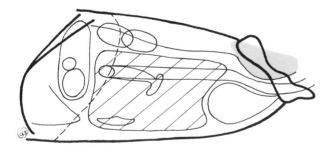

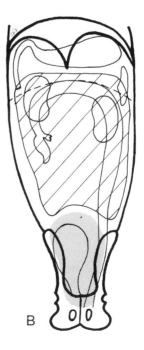

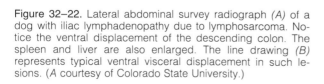

Figure 32–22. Lateral abdominal survey radiograph *(A)* of a dog with iliac lymphadenopathy due to lymphosarcoma. Notice the ventral displacement of the descending colon. The spleen and liver are also enlarged. The line drawing *(B)* represents typical ventral visceral displacement in such lesions. *(A* courtesy of Colorado State University.)

References

1. Blevins WE: Personal communication, 1985.
2. Douglas SW, and Williamson HD: Veterinary Radiological Interpretation. Philadelphia, Lea & Febiger, 1970.
3. Ferron RR: Low-cost, pocket-sized CO_2 dispenser for medical use. J Am Vet Radiol Soc 17:18, 1976.
4. Gillette EL, Thrall DE, and Lebel JL: Carlson's Veterinary Radiology, 3rd ed. Philadelphia, Lea & Febiger, 1977.
5. Kealy JK: Diagnostic Radiology of the Dog and Cat. Philadelphia, WB Saunders, 1979.
6. Morgan JP: Celiography with iothalamic acid. J Am Vet Med Assoc 145:1095, 1964.
7. O'Brien TR: Radiographic Diagnosis of Abdominal Disorders in the Dog and Cat. Philadelphia, WB Saunders, 1978.
8. Owens JM: Radiographic Interpretation for the Small Animal Clinician. St Louis, Ralston Purina Co, 1982.
9. Root CR: Abdominal masses: the radiographic differential diagnosis. J Am Vet Radiol Soc 15:26, 1974.
10. Root CR: Interpretation of abdominal survey radiographs. Vet Clin North Am 4:763, 1974.
11. Root CR: The urinary system. In Ticer JW (Ed): Radiographic Technique in Veterinary Practice, 2nd ed. Philadelphia, WB Saunders, 1984.
12. Root CR: The gastrointestinal tract. In Ticer JW (Ed) Radiographic Technique in Veterinary Practice, 2nd ed. Philadelphia, WB Saunders, 1984.
13. Schebitz H, and Wilkens H: Atlas of Radiographic Anatomy of Dog and Cat, 3rd ed. Berlin, Paul Parey, 1977.
14. Ticer JW (Ed): Radiographic Technique in Veterinary Practice, 2nd ed. Philadelphia, WB Saunders, 1984.

CHAPTER 33

THE PERITONEAL SPACE

DON L. BARBER
MARY B. MAHAFFEY

ANATOMY

Limits of the abdominal cavity include the diaphragm cranially; the pelvic inlet caudally; the sublumbar muscles, spine, and crura of the diaphragm dorsally; and the muscles of the abdominal wall and diaphragm laterally and ventrally. The cranial abdominal cavity extends into the caudal rib cage. The peritoneum is a thin, serous membrane that lines the abdomen, covers the viscera, and forms the peritoneal space or cavity. The peritoneum can be divided into parietal, visceral, and connecting peritoneum, which are all continuous.[3] The parietal peritoneum covers the inner surface of the abdomen and generally is closely adhered to abdominal musculature. The parietal peritoneum separates extra- and intraperitoneal spaces. The visceral peritoneum covers the organs of the abdominal cavity either in whole or in part. The connecting peritoneum includes mesenteries, omenta, and ligaments within the abdomen. The peritoneal space is more of a potential cavity that normally contains only a small amount of fluid for lubrication to facilitate motion of viscera. The retroperitoneal space occupies the dorsal portion of the abdomen and is extraperitoneal. Kidneys, ureters, major blood vessels, and lymph nodes are located in the retroperitoneal space. Fat is usually deposited throughout the abdominal cavity and is particularly localized in the falciform ligament, greater omentum, mesentery, and retroperitoneal space.

RADIOGRAPHIC TECHNIQUE

Good quality radiographs are important for radiographic visualization of some peritoneal diseases, especially for recognition of subtle abnormalities. Abdominal preparation is important and is discussed elsewhere.[15] Exposure factors are also important. Both overexposure and underexposure can create false results by obscuring or simulating peritoneal diseases. Intra-abdominal contrast and organ visualization are dependent on the difference in opacity between soft-tissue viscera and intra-abdominal fat. This difference in opacity is less than that between bone and soft tissue and between soft tissue and air as would be seen in radiography of the musculoskeletal system and thorax, respectively. Thus, the abdomen is relatively low in inherent contrast, and radiographic exposure techniques or recording systems that enhance this contrast should be used.

Respiratory motion can cause unsharpness of images that may simulate peritoneal disease. Respiratory motion can be minimized by making the exposure during the respiratory pause after expiration and by using a relatively short

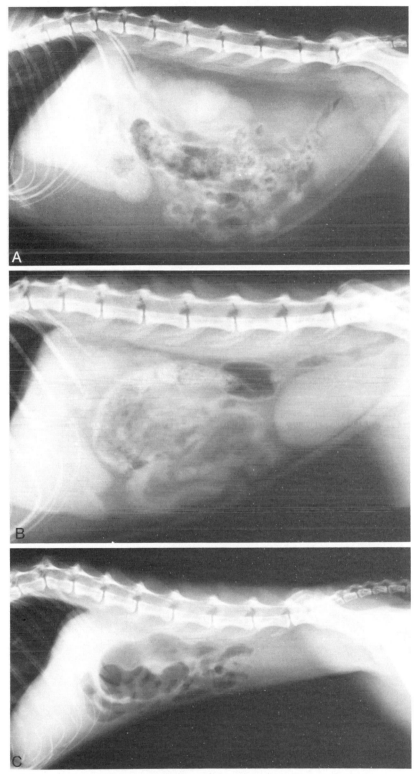

Figure 33–1. Lateral views of the abdomen. *A,* obese cat. Extensive fat deposition in the falciform, omental, mesenteric, and retroperitoneal areas provides interposed opacity between viscera of soft-tissue opacity. *B,* normal cat. Fat deposition is less than in *A,* but is adequate to separate and allow visualization of viscera. *C,* emaciated cat. Without interposed fat, viscera silhouette, producing a uniform, homogeneous, soft-tissue opacity throughout the abdomen, except for gas in the bowel loops.

exposure time. Proper patient positioning can also enhance visualization of intra-abdominal structures. If possible, hind limbs should be positioned so that the femora are perpendicular to the spine for both lateral and ventrodorsal views. Flexion at the hips can cause superimposition of femoral muscle mass over the caudal abdomen. Pronounced extension at the hips can produce a taut abdominal wall, crowding of abdominal viscera, and difficulty in visualizing specific organs.

NORMAL RADIOGRAPHIC APPEARANCE

Excluding air within the gastrointestinal tract, abdominal viscera are of soft-tissue opacity. Thus, on conventional survey radiographs, abdominal viscera appear as the same tissue opacity, and variations are the result of variations in thickness of individual organs and of various summation shadows. The presence of intra-abdominal fat is important for visceral organ visualization because the fat provides an interposed opacity between viscera, creates a differential opacity interface, and thus allows soft-tissue viscera to be visualized on survey radiographs. Fat in the falciform ligament, greater omentum, mesentery, and retroperitoneal space usually provides adequate interposed opacity between viscera. Without interposed fat, intra-abdominal viscera silhouette to produce a uniform, homogeneous, soft-tissue opacity throughout the abdomen. In mature animals, the amount of fat deposition varies from lean to obese animals (Fig. 33–1). Although thin animals have a small amount of fat that separates viscera, there is usually enough fat present to allow organ visualization. Obese animals may have tremendous fat accumulation separating abdominal viscera; however, organ visualization may also depend on conformation of the patient. For example, in narrow, deep-chested breeds of dogs, it may be difficult to visualize intra-abdominal organs on the ventrodorsal radiograph. This difficulty may be due in part to problems with exposure, such as overexposure of the small caudal abdomen or underexposure of the deep cranial abdomen. The narrow conformation, however, may also contribute to poor separation of viscera. Young dogs and kittens less than a few months of age have minimal intra-abdominal fat, poor organ separation, and uniform homogeneous soft-tissue opacity throughout the abdomen.

The diaphragm is the cranial limit of the abdominal cavity. The cranial surface of the diaphragm is visible because of the differential opacity interface provided by air in the lungs. The caudal surface of the diaphragm silhouettes with the cranial surface of the liver and is thus not usually visualized. The dorsal limit of the abdominal cavity is defined by the sublumbar

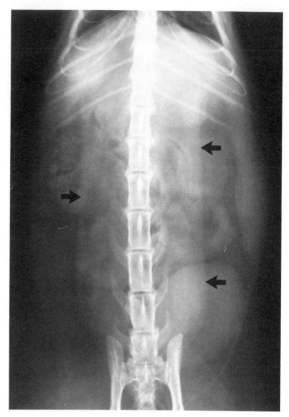

Figure 33–2. Ventrodorsal view of the abdomen of a normal cat. Note the margins of the large lumbar muscle mass *(arrows).*

musculature and spine. The sublumbar musculature is usually well defined in normal animals, contrasts well with retroperitoneal fat, and is usually visualized on lateral radiographs. Cats have a relatively large lumbar muscle mass, which can usually be visualized on ventrodorsal radiographs (Fig. 33–2). The abdominal wall may be seen because of the contrasting opacity of intraperitoneal fat internally and subcutaneous fat externally. Increasing fat deposition can produce separation and visualization of specific muscle bundles. The entire abdominal wall is not routinely visualized because the wall is only visualized when muscle layers are projected tangentially.

ABNORMAL RADIOGRAPHIC FINDINGS

Increased Fluid Opacity. Increased amounts of fluid within the peritoneal cavity cause increased soft-tissue opacity within the abdomen, which in turn causes a loss of the differential opacity interface between viscera that is normally provided by fat. Loss of this differential interface may actually be due to lack of fat, to increased fluid, or to both. Phrases commonly used to describe the radiographic appearance of this phenomenon include loss of intra-abdominal contrast, increased intra-abdominal soft-tissue opacity, increased intra-abdominal fluid opacity, and decreased visualization of serosal surfaces. Causes of this loss of intra-abdominal contrast include lack of fat, abdominal effusion, peritonitis, peritoneal neoplasia, and wet hair. A wet hair coat superimposed over the abdomen can create irregular opacities that appear to be within the abdomen. This possibility should be readily excluded by physical examination.

Lack of intra-abdominal fat may be due to the age of the animal or to emaciation. Immature dogs and kittens less than a few months of age lack sufficient fat to provide intra-abdominal contrast, and thus the abdomen appears as relatively uniform, homogeneous, soft-tissue opacity. The abdomen may also be somewhat pendulous in such normal, immature patients. Emaciation causes a similar homogeneous, soft-tissue opacity throughout the abdomen due to lack of fat (Fig. 33–1C). In emaciated patients, the abdomen is often tucked up, which can be visualized on the radiographs; however, the possibility of coexistent peritonitis can not be excluded.

Abdominal effusion refers to increased fluid accumulation within the abdomen. Fluid opacity between abdominal viscera silhouettes with the viscera and thus causes a loss of intra-abdominal contrast. Classification of abdominal effusion is broad and includes various types of transudates, exudates, blood, urine, bile, and chyle.[2] Differences do exist in some fluid opacities based on their attenuation coefficients.[13] Differences in attenuation coefficients as small as 0.5 per cent can be detected with computed tomography.[8] Conventional radiography is limited to the perception of differences of 2 to 4 per cent in object contrast.[22] Differences in contrast between ascitic fluid and visceral organs may be as much as 5 per cent, and thus structures such as the liver margin may occasionally be visualized on conventional survey radiographs, even when surrounded by fluid.[14] In practice, however, these differences are rarely recognized, and all abdominal fluids are thought to be of water or soft-tissue opacity, comparable to the visceral organs. Recognized differences in opacity are more likely due to differences in volume. Peritonitis can also cause loss of intra-abdominal contrast with its associated edema and inflammation of serosal surfaces and adjacent fat. In addition, abdominal effusion is usually present with peritonitis. Peritoneal seeding of neoplastic foci can also cause a loss of intra-abdominal contrast because of the soft-tissue opacity of the nodules as well as possible coexistent effusion.

The radiographic appearance of the aforementioned conditions depends on the cause, severity of the disease, and amount of fluid present. A large volume of abdominal fluid appears as a homogeneous fluid opacity uniformly distributed throughout the abdominal cavity (Fig. 33–3). The homogeneous appearance is due to the total silhouette with all soft-tissue structures within the abdomen. A large volume of fluid often causes abdominal distension, with outward protrusion of the contour of the abdominal wall. Care must be taken because radiographs of normal immature animals may exhibit similar findings. A large volume of fluid may also displace the diaphragm cranially. If relatively mobile segments of bowel contain gas, they often float to the highest or uppermost area within the abdominal cavity. If the abdomen is pendulous and distended, these segments are often near the center of the abdomen on both lateral and ventrodorsal views. The radiographic appearance is that of effusion, and the presence or absence of coexistent peritonitis

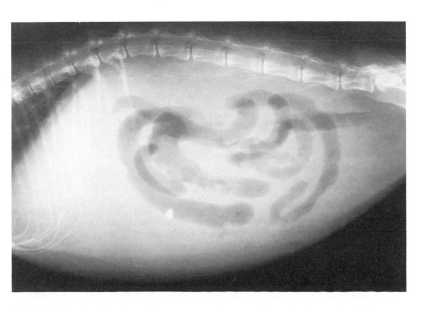

Figure 33–3. Lateral view of the abdomen of a cat with a large volume of abdominal fluid. Homogeneous fluid opacity is uniformly distributed throughout a distended abdomen. Diagnosis: feline infectious peritonitis.

cannot be ascertained radiographically. Peritoneal irritation may cause dilatation of the bowel; however, this dilatation may be due to many other causes, some of which are also associated with abdominal effusion.[17] Thus, bowel distention in the presence of abdominal effusion is not a specific indication of peritonitis. Large amounts of abdominal fluid are often the result of transudates of cardiac or hepatic disease or of rupture of the urinary bladder.

Smaller amounts of abdominal fluid or peritonitis may produce a mottled, hazy, or irregular fluid opacity on survey radiographs (Fig. 33–4). Individual viscera may be visualized, but there is indistinctness or blurring of the margins of soft-tissue structures. With small amounts of fluid, this appearance may be due to interdigitation of fluid with folds in the greater omentum and small bowel but without a total silhouette effect.[12] Inflammation of the peritoneum or fat may produce a similar effect. Smaller amounts of effusion may be due to early fluid accumulation of a generalized process or to more localized diseases. Examples include rupture of the urinary bladder with a small amount of urine in the caudal to midventral abdomen, pancreatitis, and laparotomy. Manipulation of viscera during laparotomy produces physiologic changes within the abdomen that may appear comparable to peritonitis on radiographs, and these changes may be modified by the amount of induced tissue trauma.[12] Solutions containing water, electrolytes, and relatively low molecular weight components are absorbed by the peritoneal membrane within 24 hours.[1] Proteinaceous fluids such as serum, blood, and lymph are absorbed more slowly and may be identified sonographically until 12 days after laparotomy.[11]

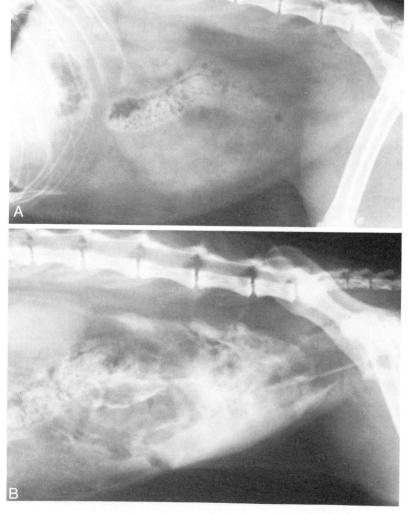

Figure 33–4. A, lateral survey radiograph of the abdomen of a cat that had been hit by a car. Mottled, hazy, or irregular fluid opacity within the ventral half of the abdomen produces indistinctness or blurring of the margins of soft-tissue structures. Note that the retroperitoneal space is normal and that a hip is luxated dorsally. B, lateral cystogram of the same cat documents rupture of the urinary bladder and demonstrates how the fluid may interdigitate with bowel loops and mesentery.

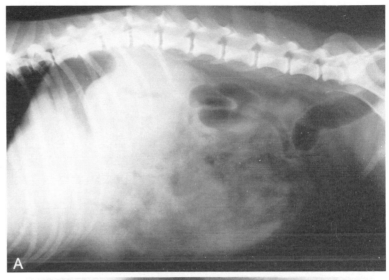

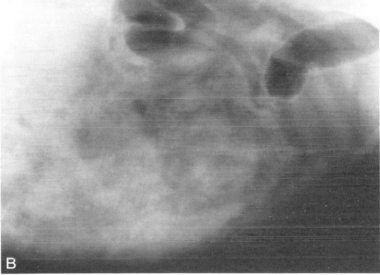

Figure 33–5. *A*, lateral radiograph of a dog with mottled or irregular fluid opacity within the midventral abdomen that appears as an ill defined nodular pattern. *B*, close-up view. Diagnosis: splenic leiomyosarcoma with peritoneal seeding.

It is important to recognize that these changes can be visualized after laparotomy and that they not be mistaken for more significant complications. Static or progressive fluid accumulation during this period would be abnormal.

Mottled or irregular fluid opacity within the abdominal cavity may also appear as an ill-defined nodular or granular pattern (Fig. 33–5). This pattern may be caused by seeding of the peritoneum with multiple, metastatic neoplastic foci. Examples of tumors associated with such spread include hemangiosarcoma of the spleen and carcinomas of various abdominal organs. The terms abdominal or peritoneal carcinomatosis may be used to describe any cancer disseminated throughout the abdomen,[9] or may be limited only to carcinomas with this distribution.[16]

The distribution of radiographic changes of peritoneal disease may be either generalized or localized. Localized changes can be due to a variety of causes, but are most often due to a small amount of fluid or to localized peritonitis (Fig. 33–6). One of the more common causes of localized peritoneal disease is acute pancreatitis. The frequency and appearance of radiographic changes caused by acute pancreatitis are variable.[4, 7, 20] Changes can usually be localized to the right cranial abdomen, where the right lobe of the pancreas is closely associated with the proximal duodenum and pyloric antrum, or to midline just caudal to the stomach where the left lobe of the pancreas is located. The major radiographic abnormality is usually an increased, irregular, soft-tissue opacity in the right mid to cranial abdomen, indicating localized peritonitis (Fig. 33–7A). The proximal descending duodenum may be displaced ventrally or toward the right to produce a broad curvature; the pylorus of the stomach may be displaced toward the left (Fig. 33–7B). Less frequently, the transverse colon may be dis-

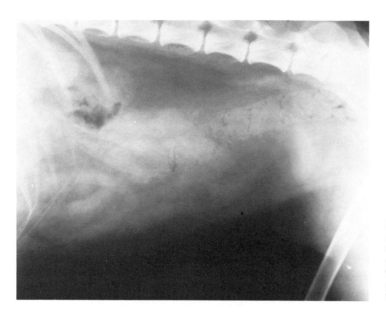

Figure 33–6. Lateral view of a dog with subtle changes due to peritonitis or to a small amount of fluid. Also note the greater detail in the retroperitoneal in comparison with the intraperitoneal space. Diagnosis: pyometra with small perforation and peritonitis.

placed caudally. Bowel loops adjacent to the pancreas, such as the proximal descending duodenum, may contain gas, have loss of tone, and be dilated; spasticity of the duodenum has also been described. Foci of mineralization may occur in areas of fat necrosis with repeated bouts of acute pancreatitis.[7]

The shape or contour of the abdomen should also be evaluated. Large amounts of abdominal effusion result in a pendulous abdomen. The abdomen may also be pendulous due to other causes, such as obesity or the muscle weakness of Cushing's syndrome. Emaciation usually causes the abdomen to appear tucked up. Trauma of the abdominal wall or localized abdominal pain may produce asymmetric contraction of abdominal muscles.[12]

Large volumes of intra-abdominal fluid obscure the retroperitoneal space, even if the fluid is confined to the intraperitoneal space. This occurrence may be due to superimposition by the large fluid volume. The retroperitoneal space can be visualized normally with smaller amounts of intraperitoneal fluid (Fig. 33–4). Fluid accumulation can also be confined to the retroperitoneal space, with a normal appearance

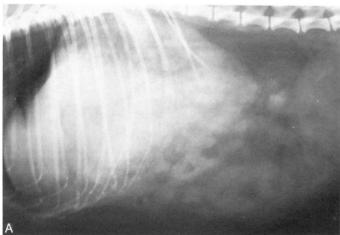

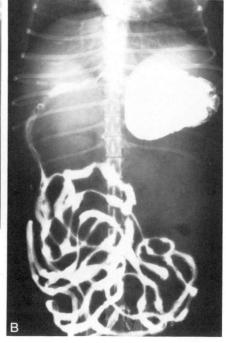

Figure 33–7. A, lateral survey radiograph of a dog with increased, irregular soft-tissue opacity in the mid to cranial abdomen due to localized peritonitis. B, ventrodorsal view, upper gastrointestinal tract series. The pylorus is displaced to the left and the proximal duodenum is broadly curved. Diagnosis: pancreatitis with peripancreatic abscess.

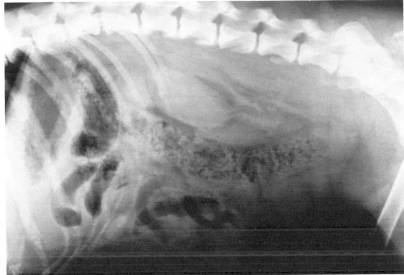

Figure 33–8. Lateral view of the abdomen of a dog that had been hit by a car. There is fluid opacity in the retroperitoneal space with blurring of the margin of the lumbar musculature. Note the greater intraperitoneal detail. There is also a sacral fracture with dorsal displacement. Diagnosis: retroperitoneal hemorrhage.

of the remainder of the abdomen (Fig. 33–8). The most common causes of isolated retroperitoneal effusion are hemorrhage and urine leakage from renal, ureteral, or urethral trauma.

Mineral Opacity. Mineralization of individual organs is discussed elsewhere in this text. Mineral opacities of the peritoneum are uncommon and changes are rarely specific. Bone fragments may perforate the bowel and be located outside of the bowel lumen.

Metal Opacity. The radiographic recognition of surgical equipment or supplies retained within the abdomen after surgery is dependent on their radiopacity. In most cases, their identification does not pose a diagnostic problem, with the exception of retention of surgical sponges and laparotomy pads.[18] Unless these supplies are individually labeled with radiopaque markers, their radiographic identification is difficult.

Free Abdominal Gas. Free abdominal gas refers to gas within the abdominal cavity that is not contained within a specific organ or structure but is free and thus movable. Although there may be many causes of free abdominal gas, the two most common categories are penetration of the abdominal wall, either by laparotomy or penetrating wounds, and perforation of a hollow organ, such as the bowel. Laparotomy is the most common cause of free abdominal gas, and the history is usually known in such cases. A moderate amount of gas comparable to that introduced during laparotomy may persist within the abdomen for as many as 19 days in normal dogs.[19] Penetrating abdominal wounds are usually diagnosed by findings at physical examination or the radiographic finding of lead fragments from a gunshot. Differentiating whether any associated free abdominal gas

is due solely to penetration of the abdomen or concurrent hollow organ rupture is difficult. Rupture of the gastrointestinal tract is the most common cause of free abdominal gas due to rupture of a hollow organ; however, not all bowel perforations produce free abdominal gas.[21]

A small volume of free abdominal gas is difficult to recognize on conventional radiographs made with a vertically directed x-ray beam. The gas may be localized around the intestine, the mesentery, or the omentum. Gas bubbles may be small and irregular in shape because of interdigitation between bowel loops and mesentery.[12] If the volume is of sufficient size, the gas may coalesce into a larger gas bubble. This larger bubble may still be difficult to recognize on a radiograph made with a vertical x-ray beam, because it is superimposed over other abdominal viscera. In addition, this larger bubble may simulate a gas-containing organ, such as the stomach. Such free abdominal gas usually floats to the highest point within the abdominal cavity, which varies with conformation of the patient. In lateral recumbency, this point is usually under the caudal ribs or in the midabdomen. The concurrent presence of abdominal effusion may make recognition of this bubble easier, because the fluid provides a more uniform, homogeneous soft-tissue background opacity (Fig. 33–9A). A large volume of free abdominal gas is readily visualized on survey radiographs, because the gas provides contrast to outline serosal surfaces of viscera, such as bowel loops, the stomach, and the diaphragm (Fig. 33–9B).

Because free gas rises to the highest portion within the abdominal cavity, free gas may be isolated from superimposed structures by using

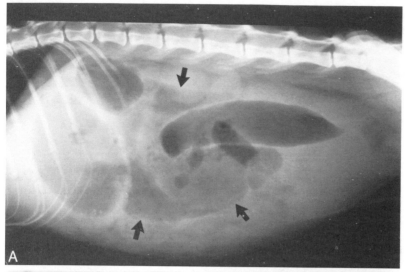

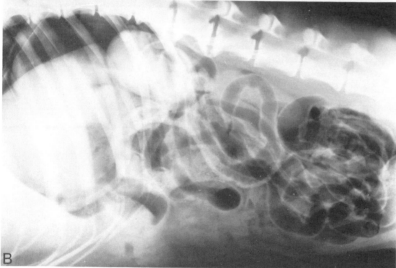

Figure 33–9. *A,* lateral survey radiograph of a cat with abdominal effusion and a moderate amount of free intra-abdominal gas. *Arrows,* margins of the gas pocket. *B,* lateral survey radiograph of the abdomen of a dog immediately after laparotomy. There is a large volume of free abdominal gas that outlines the caudal surface of the right crus of the diaphragm, the cranial pole of the right kidney, the caudal surface of part of the liver, and serosal surfaces of some bowel loops.

a horizontally directed x-ray beam. With a small volume of gas, it may be preferable to position the patient for 10 minutes before exposure to allow most of the gas to migrate and coalesce at the uppermost portion. The most commonly used projection to document a small volume of free abdominal gas is the ventrodorsal view, obtained with the patient in left recumbency with the use of a horizontally directed x-ray beam. The gas bubble is usually localized under

the highest portion of the right abdominal wall (Fig. 33–10), which is usually under the caudal ribs. With larger volumes of gas, the bubble may extend well under the diaphragm or along the abdominal wall caudally. Raising or lowering either end of the animal shifts the point of gas accumulation. Exposure factors should be lowered to underexpose the abdomen, and the right abdominal wall should be centered in the x-ray beam to avoid superimposition of abdom-

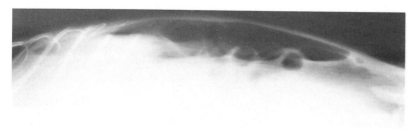

Figure 33–10. Ventrodorsal view of the abdomen with the patient in left recumbency and the use of a horizontally directed x-ray beam (same cat as in Fig. 33–9A). The free abdominal gas pocket is located under the right abdominal wall and is projected separately from rather than superimposed over the abdominal fluid. Diagnosis: ruptured stomach.

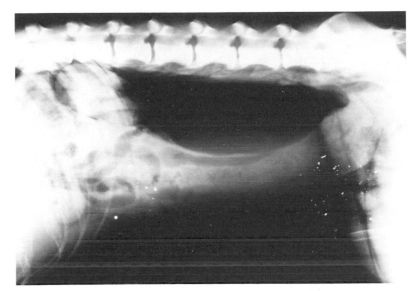

Figure 33–11. Lateral view of a dog that had been shot in the caudal abdomen. There is a large volume of gas confined to the retroperitoneal space. There is also gas dissecting along the aorta (ventral to T12) and along the fascial planes of the hind limb.

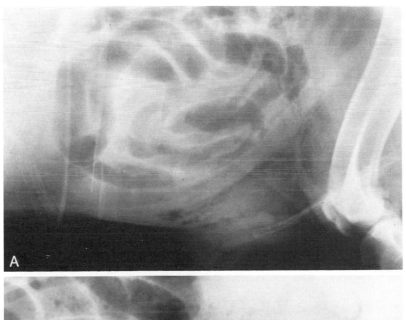

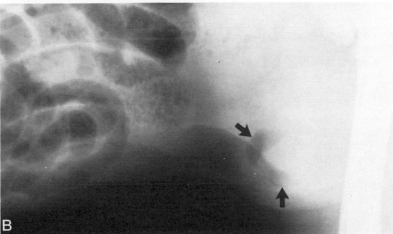

Figure 33–12. A, lateral view of the abdomen of a dog that had been hit by a car. Mottled; irregular gas pattern of the soft tissues ventral to the abdominal wall was due to abrasions and lacerations. B, lateral view of the abdomen of a dog with a sharply marginated, tubular gas pocket (arrows) ventral to the abdominal wall due to an inguinal hernia.

inal organs created by divergence of the beam at its periphery. The ventrodorsal view with the animal in right recumbency is not recommended because the gas bubble rises to the left side and could be confused with gas within the fundus of the stomach. An upright view with the animal standing on its hind legs may demonstrate the gas between the diaphragm and liver. The use of such a view initially, however, may cause the gas to be trapped caudal to the liver and thus prevent its rise beneath the diaphragm. It was recently noted that the lateral view with the patient in dorsal recumbency and the cranial abdomen elevated may be the most sensitive technique to document free abdominal gas in dogs and cats.[5] Other views and sequences of patient manipulation have been described and may allow the radiographic demonstration of as small an amount as 1 to 2 ml of free abdominal gas.[10]

Gas may also accumulate in the retroperitoneal space. Retroperitoneal gas is most often due to extension of a pneumomediastinum or to penetration of the abdominal wall, either by penetrating wounds or surgical procedures. Retroperitoneal gas is confined to the retroperitoneal space in the dorsal abdomen and is best visualized on a lateral radiograph (Fig. 33–11).

Abdominal Wall Abnormalities. It is often difficult to visualize abnormalities of the abdominal wall radiographically. The abdominal wall is seen only in those limited areas in which the wall is projected tangentially. Trauma may cause hemorrhage and edema of the abdominal wall, which may be visible radiographically as soft-tissue opacity causing localized loss of muscle definition.[12] Muscle rigidity due to pain may also cause distortion and loss of separation of muscles. If unilateral, pain may cause unilateral muscle wall contraction with curvature of the trunk. Mineralization may occasionally be visualized in the soft tissues surrounding the abdomen. As an example, calcinosis associated with Cushing's syndrome may produce nodular or linear calcification of soft tissues that may be visualized radiographically, most often dorsally and in the ventral abdominal wall.[6] Gas may be seen in the soft tissues surrounding the abdomen from a variety of causes. Abrasions with lacerations often produce a mottled, irregular gas pattern (Fig. 33–12A). Tubular or round gas pockets may be contained within herniated bowel loops (Fig. 33–12B). Gas that dissects along fascial planes is most often due to large open wounds or to upper airway perforation or pneumomediastinum. These patterns, however, are not pathognomonic for the cause of the gas accumulation.

References

1. Boen ST: Peritoneal Dialysis in Clinical Practice. Springfield, Charles C Thomas, 1964.
2. Ettinger SJ: Peritoneal diseases. *In* Ettinger SJ (Ed): Textbook of Veterinary Internal Medicine. Philadelphia, WB Saunders, 1975.
3. Evans HE, and Christensen GC: Miller's Anatomy of the Dog, 2nd Ed. Philadelphia, WB Saunders, 1979.
4. Gibbs C, Denny HR, Minter HM, et al: Radiological features of inflammatory conditions of the canine pancreas. J Small Anim Pract 13:531, 1972.
5. Guffy, MM: Personal communication, 1984.
6. Huntley K, Fraser J, Gibbs C, et al: The radiological features of canine Cushing's syndrome: A review of forty-eight cases. J Small Anim Pract 23:369, 1982.
7. Kleine LJ, and Hornbuckle WE: Acute pancreatitis: The radiographic findings in 182 dogs. J Am Vet Radiol Soc 19:102, 1978.
8. McCullough EC, Baker Jr HL, Houser OW, et al: An evaluation of the quantitative and radiation features of a scanning x-ray transverse axial tomograph: The EMI scanner. Radiology 111:709, 1974.
9. McDermott W: Diseases of the peritoneum. *In* Beeson P, and McDermott W (Eds.): Textbook of Medicine, 13th Ed. Philadelphia, WB Saunders, 1971.
10. Miller RE, and Nelson SW: The roentgenologic demonstration of tiny amounts of free intraperitoneal gas: Experimental and clinical studies. AJR 112:574, 1971.
11. Neff CC, Simeone JF, Ferrucci Jr JT, et al: The occurrence of fluid collections following routine abdominal surgical procedures: Sonographic survey in asymptomatic postoperative patients. Radiology 146:463, 1983.
12. O'Brien TR: The Radiographic Diagnosis of Abdominal Disorders of the Dog and Cat. Philadelphia, WB Saunders, 1978.
13. Phelps ME, Hoffman EJ, Ter-Pogossian MM: Attenuation coefficients of various body tissues, fluids, and lesions at photon energies of 18 to 136 KeV. Radiology 117:573, 1975.
14. Proto AV, and Lane EJ: Visualization of differences in soft tissue densities: The liver in ascites. Radiology 121:19, 1976.
15. Root CR: Interpretation of abdominal survey radiographs. Vet Clin North Am 4:763, 1974.
16. Root CR, and Lord PF: Peritoneal carcinomatosis in the dog and cat: Its radiographic appearance. J Am Vet Radiol Soc 12:54, 1971.
17. Silen W, and Skillman JJ: Gastrointestinal responses to injury and infection. Surg Clin North Am 56:945, 1976.
18. Spiegel SM, and Palayew MJ: Retained surgical sponges: Diagnostic dilemma and an aid to their recognition. Radiographics 2:53, 1982.
19. Stickle, R.: Peritoneal air in the dog. Scientific Program of the American College of Veterinary Radiology, Chicago, 1983.
20. Suter, PF, and Lowe R: Acute pancreatitis in the dog. A clinical study with emphasis on radiographic diagnosis. Acta Radiol [Suppl] (Stockh) 319:195, 1970.
21. Suter, PF, and Olsson SE: The diagnosis of injuries to the intestines, gall bladder and bile ducts in the dog. J Small Anim Pract 11:575, 1970.
22. Ter-Pogossian MM, Phelps ME, Hoffman EJ, et al: The extraction of the yet unused wealth of information in diagnostic radiology. Radiology 113:515, 1974.

CHAPTER 34

THE LIVER AND SPLEEN

ROBERT D. PECHMAN, JR.

Radiographic diagnosis of diseases of the liver or spleen depends on recognizing abnormalities in size, shape, position, margination, and radiopacity of these organs. Alterations in size, shape, and margination are common survey radiographic signs of hepatic or splenic disease. Positional changes of these organs are not common, and alterations in radiopacity of the liver and spleen are rare.[1] Abnormalities detected on survey radiographs most often are not specific for any particular disease process; the liver or spleen may appear radiographically normal even in the face of severe disease.

Several radiographic procedures have been devised in an attempt to improve the radiographic diagnosis of hepatic or splenic diseases. Pneumoperitonography enhances abdominal contrast for more precise evaluation of hepatic and splenic size and margination changes.[2] Portography allows evaluation of the portal venous circulation and detection of portosystemic shunting of blood.[3] Cholangiography and cholecystography are useful in evaluating the biliary system.[4, 5] Angiography may be used to assess the blood supply and structure of these two highly vascular organs.[6]

In recent years, alternative imaging techniques have become available that greatly enhance the assessment of hepatic and splenic diseases. Radioisotope scanning of the liver and spleen can be used to evaluate the internal structure of both of these organs or the hepatobiliary system;[2] ultrasonic imaging is particularly effective.[7] These alternative imaging techniques are often less invasive than radiographic contrast medium examinations, but sophisticated, expensive imaging equipment is required, and thus use of these techniques is currently limited to large institutional veterinary practices.

THE LIVER

The liver is the largest solid organ in the abdomen and occupies the most cranial aspect of the abdomen. The depth of the abdomen is greatest in the region of the liver. Radiographic exposures must be adequate to penetrate the liver, yet not so great as to eliminate the slight natural contrast between the liver and the other organs in the cranial abdomen. Evaluation of liver size and shape requires evaluation of the liver borders that can be visualized as well as borders that are not seen directly but are indicated by the position of adjacent organs (Fig. 34–1).[1]

The convex cranial margin of the liver is in close contact with the diaphragm, which is delineated cranially by adjacent air-filled lung. The right and left lateral margins of the liver

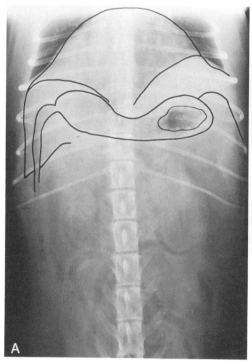
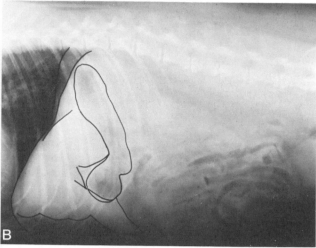

Figure 34–1. Ventrodorsal *(A)* and lateral *(B)* radiographs of the abdomen of a normal dog. The liver borders are outlined. The margins of the liver are smooth and the caudal ventral edge is sharp. The stomach and descending duodenum *(outlined)* are in their normal locations and define the caudal surface of the liver. The stomach is perpendicular to the spine in the ventrodorsal projection and follows the arch of the ribs in the lateral projection.

are near the abdominal wall, but may be detected if there is adequate intra-abdominal fat. The ventral border of the liver is usually well defined by the fat in the falciform ligament. The dorsal border of the liver is usually not visualized. The concave caudal border of the liver is not directly visualized on survey radiographs, but its position can be estimated by its relationship to the right kidney, stomach, and cranial flexure of the duodenum. In lateral radiographs, the dorsocaudal border of the liver is adjacent to the cranial pole of the right kidney; the cranial wall of the stomach defines the caudal margin of the liver in the midabdominal region; the caudal ventral border of the liver is formed by the left lateral liver lobe. The triangular liver shadow ventral to the pyloric antrum is formed by the right medial liver lobe cranially and the left lateral liver lobe caudally (see Reference 9).[1]

In ventrodorsal radiographs, the caudal border of the right lateral liver lobe is indicated by the cranial duodenal flexure. The cranial pole of the right kidney defines the caudal border of the caudate liver lobe and the gastric fundus indicates the caudal border of the left lateral liver lobe. The caudal borders of the right medial, quadrate, and left medial liver lobes are adjacent to the lesser curvature of the stomach.[1, 2, 8, 9]

The apparent shape and position of the liver can be affected by the phase of respiration during which the radiograph is made; the age,

breed, and thoracic conformation of the patient, and the position of the patient during radiography.[1, 2] The left liver lobes move caudally during radiography in right lateral recumbency, and the entire liver may move caudally if radiographs are made at peak inspiration. In animals with a deep, narrow chest conformation, the liver may be entirely within the portion of the abdomen lying under the caudal rib cage, whereas the liver may extend slightly beyond the costal arch in animals with a shallow, wide thoracic conformation. The liver is usually larger in young animals than in adults.[2] The liver may be separated from the ventral abdominal wall by a substantial distance due to fat in the falciform ligament, particularly in obese cats. Ligaments that attach the liver to the diaphragm may weaken and stretch in aged or obese dogs, allowing the liver to slide caudoventrally and extend beyond the costal arch.[9] All of these normal variants must be recalled when survey radiographs of the liver are assessed.

Alterations in Liver Size

Alterations in liver size may be found in primary liver diseases or secondary to diseases of other organ systems. Survey radiographs may depict increases or decreases in liver size, but rarely delineate the cause of the size alteration. Radiographic assessment of liver size is fraught with error and, at best, is inexact and subjective.

Hepatomegaly is usually easier to identify than is microhepatica.

Hepatomegaly is a reliable radiographic sign of liver disease (Fig. 34–2).[1] Hepatomegaly may be diffuse, with fairly uniform enlargement of all lobes, or it may be focal, with enlargement of only a single lobe. Severe diffuse hepatomegaly causes a substantial portion of the caudal liver margin to project beyond the costal arch, an obvious increase in size, and, most importantly, rounding of the caudal liver edges in the lateral radiograph. The stomach is displaced caudodorsally in the lateral projection and caudally and toward the left in the ventrodorsal projection. The right kidney, cranial duodenal flexure, and transverse colon are displaced caudally in the ventrodorsal view.[1, 8] Diffuse hepatomegaly may be due to inflammatory or neoplastic diseases, hepatic venous congestion, fat infiltration, cholestasis, cirrhosis, amyloidosis, or storage diseases.[1, 2]

Focal hepatomegaly is depicted on survey radiographs by displacement of organs adjacent to the affected lobe, and the involved lobe is identified by recognizing which organ or part of an organ is displaced.[10] Right liver lobe enlargement displaces the body and pyloric regions of the stomach dorsally and toward the left while the gastric fundus remains in normal position; caudal and leftward displacement of the gastric fundus with indentation of the lesser curvature of the stomach may be seen with enlargement of the left liver lobes.[8, 10] Focal hepatomegaly, affecting only one or two lobes, may be caused by neoplastic diseases, regenerative nodules of cirrhosis, or localized masses, such as large hepatic abscesses or cysts.[1, 9, 10]

Microhepatica is more difficult to recognize radiographically than is hepatomegaly (Fig. 34–3).[1] Microhepatica may be indicated by cranial displacement of the stomach and decreased distance between the diaphragm and the stomach on the lateral and the ventrodorsal projections. Cranioventral slanting of the gastric shadow in the lateral projection and cranial displacement of the right kidney, cranial duodenal flexure, and transverse colon in the ventrodorsal view are additional radiographic signs of microhepatica. Reduced liver size is usually diffuse and may be due to chronic hepatic disease, fibrosis, hepatic cirrhosis, or congenital anomalies such as congenital portosystemic venous shunts. Importantly, reduced liver size may be seen in normal dogs and cats.[1]

Alterations in Liver Position

The liver is closely applied to the diaphragm and is held tightly by several ligaments. Changes in liver position are usually secondary to thoracic diseases or disruption of the diaphragm.[1] The liver may be located more cranially than normal when there is traumatic disruption of the diaphragm and herniation of liver lobes into the thoracic cavity. Congenital peritoneopericardial diaphragmatic hernias, in which a portion of the liver is within the pericardial sac, also result in cranial displacement

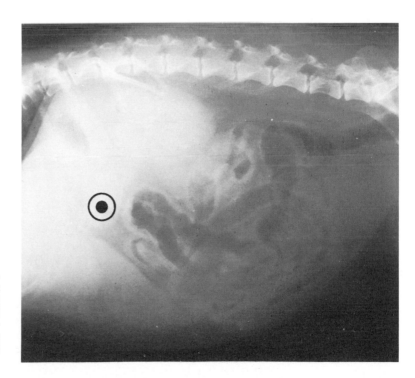

Figure 34–2. Generalized hepatomegaly in a dog with Cushing's disease. The liver extends caudal to the costal arch. There is dorsal and caudal displacement of the pyloric region of the stomach (●). The liver margins remain smooth and sharp.

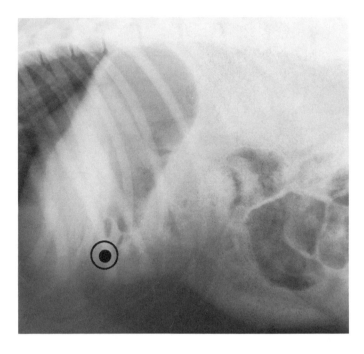

Figure 34–3. Microhepatica in a dog with chronic liver disease and hepatic fibrosis. The liver is slightly smaller than normal. The stomach (gas-filled) courses cranioventrally and there is slight cranial displacement of the pyloric region of the stomach (●). Microhepatica is ususally not dramatic, as in this dog, and caution should be exercised in making the diagnosis.

of the liver (Fig. 34–4).[2] In both diseases, the normal diaphragm shadow is incomplete on survey radiographs. Cranial displacement of the liver is indicated by the criteria used to define microhepatica.

Caudal displacement of the liver is usually due to intrathoracic diseases that displace the diaphragm, and consequently the liver, caudally. Abdominal radiographs made on full inspiration and of large pleural effusion demonstrate caudal displacement of the liver.[1, 2] Severe overinflation of the lungs, as may occur in chronic obstructive lung disease, also results in caudal displacement of the liver. The radiographic signs of caudal displacement of the liver are those associated with diffuse hepatomegaly—caudal displacement of adjacent organs.

Alterations in Liver Margins

Changes in the normally smooth and fairly pointed liver margins are usually associated with hepatomegaly,[1, 2] but they may be seen in some patients with reduced liver size. The caudal liver margins are often round and blunt in diseases that result in diffuse hepatomegaly: right heart failure, hepatic lipidosis, diffuse hepatic neoplasia or inflammation, and amyloidosis.[1, 2, 9]

Liver margins may be round, irregular, and "lumpy" in patients with hepatic neoplasia, particularly in patients with widespread hepatic metastases, and in cirrhosis with fibrosis and prominent regenerative nodules (Fig. 34–5).[1, 9] Solitary liver masses, such as neoplasms or abscesses near the organ surface, may produce

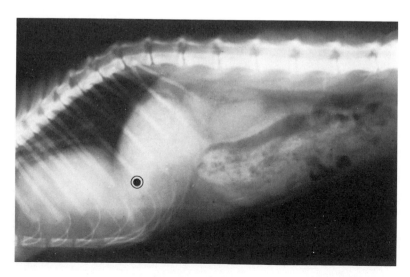

Figure 34–4. Lateral radiograph of the abdomen of a cat with a peritoneopericardial diaphragmatic hernia. The cardiac shadow is greatly enlarged and the ventral diaphragm shadow is not visible. The stomach is close to the diaphragm and there is cranial displacement of the pyloric region of the stomach (●). The caudoventral margin of the liver, normally ventral to the stomach, is not visualized. Radiographic signs of microhepatica are present. At surgery, approximately 80 percent of the liver was found in the pericardial sac.

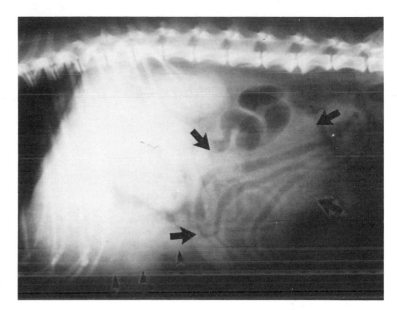

Figure 34–5. Nodular liver margins in a dog with splenic hemangiosarcoma and hepatic metastases. The neoplastic mass on the spleen is visible in the midabdomen *(arrows)*. The liver is enlarged and there is a "lumpy" appearance of the ventral border *(arrowheads)*. At surgery, the liver was found to contain numerous metastatic masses that were the cause of the nodular liver margins.

a single lump or hump on the normally smooth liver margin.[1] Liver masses resulting in significant displacement of adjacent organs are discussed in detail in another section of this text.

Alterations in Liver Radiopacity

The liver is normally of homogeneous soft-tissue opacity; increases or decreases in radiopacity are rare. Increased hepatic radiopacity is only caused by mineralization (Fig. 34–6). Hepatic mineralization, seen as miliary or discrete nodular radiopacities, may occur diffusely or may affect focal areas of one or more lobes.[1] Mineral opacities may be confined to the gallbladder or the biliary or cystic ducts in patients with cholelithiasis.[2, 11, 12] Nodular or miliary parenchymal mineralization may be associated with neoplasia, granulomatous diseases, or mineralized parasitic cysts.[1, 9]

Decreased liver opacity, which occurs rarely, is due to gas accumulation within the liver. Gas may accumulate in the gallbladder or biliary ducts or within the intrahepatic veins (Fig. 34–6).[1] Gas within the gallbladder, in the gall-

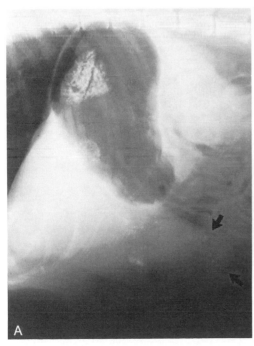

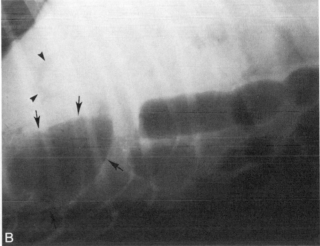

Figure 34–6. Alterations in liver opacity. Increased liver opacity *(A)* due to mineralization of granulomatous lesions of histoplasmosis. The liver is enlarged and the caudal edge is noticeably rounded *(arrowheads)*. Decreased hepatic opacity *(B)* due to gas accumulation within the gallbladder *(arrows)*, gallbladder wall, pericholecystic liver parenchyma, and dilated hepatic biliary duct *(arrowheads)*. This patient had emphysematous cholecystitis caused by *Clostridium* sp.

bladder wall, or in the pericholecystic liver parenchyma is usually secondary to cholecystitis caused by gas-forming organisms, but it can be due to an open communication with the lumen of the bowel.[1, 9, 13, 14] Gas in the hepatic veins appears as a linear branching pattern of gas opacities.[1] Gas within the vascular structures of the liver may occur secondary to gas embolization during pneumocystography or pneumourethrography, and may be seen when room air is used for diagnostic pneumoperitonography.[15] Detection of gas in hepatic vascular structures on survey radiographs is a grave sign.[1]

Contrast Medium Studies for Evaluation of the Liver

Numerous radiographic contrast medium techniques have been used in dogs and cats in attempts to improve the radiographic diagnosis of liver disease. Most of these techniques have fallen into disfavor, however, and are not often used. Newer imaging techniques, although generally restricted to usage in large institutions, have greatly improved the ability to detect and diagnose liver disease, and have replaced most contrast medium procedures.

Pneumoperitonography. This procedure is performed by injecting negative contrast medium, air, CO_2, or O_2 into the abdominal cavity. Multiple radiographs are made of the patient in a variety of positions with the use of vertical and horizontal x-ray beam projections to outline the liver lobes with the negative contrast medium. Pneumoperitonography is particularly useful in the evaluation of liver edges and margins and in the identification of liver masses.[2, 9]

Cholecystography and Cholangiography. These are positive-contrast medium techniques used to opacify the gallbladder and extrahepatic biliary ducts. The primary indication for cholecystography is icterus due to suspected extrahepatic biliary obstruction.[1] Oral or intravenous contrast media may be employed, but intravenous contrast media, such as iodipamide meglumine,* are preferred.[5, 9] A dosage of 0.5 to 0.6 ml per kilogram body weight of iodipamide meglumine administered by slow intravenous infusion over 30 minutes or longer has been recommended for use in dogs. Radiographs are made 1 and 2 hours after the start of the infusion.[1] For cats, a dosage of 0.3 to 1 ml per kilogram body weight has been recommended with radiographs made 2½ to 5 hours after the start of the infusion.[4]

Cholecystography is not often performed in dogs and cats because extrahepatic biliary obstruction as a cause of icterus is less common than is intrahepatic biliary obstruction. High serum bilirubin levels, icterus of hepatocellular origin, and known adverse reactions to iodinated contrast media are contraindications for cholecystography.[1]

Angiography. Hepatic arteriography is generally restricted in usage to large institutional veterinary practices. Image-intensified fluoroscopy and capabilities for making rapid serial radiographs are required for this procedure. Hepatic arteriography can be used to identify and localize intrahepatic masses, such as neoplasms, cysts, and abscesses. Hepatic venography can be used to opacify the hepatic sinusoids and may be combined with wedge hepatic vein pressure recordings to evaluate causes of ascites.[1, 6]

Hepatic venography is accomplished by selectively positioning a catheter in a hepatic vein. When the catheter is advanced as far as possible and is wedged in a hepatic vein, wedge hepatic vein pressures are recorded. Injection of contrast medium opacifies the hepatic sinusoidal system drained by the catheterized vein.[6]

Portography. Radiographic examination of the portal venous system can be accomplished by several techniques, many of which require equipment not often available in general veterinary practice.[3] A relatively simple technique—operative portography—is available, however, and can be easily performed without the need for sophisticated imaging equipment or arterial catheterization. Operative portography can be used to visualize the portal venous circulation for the diagnosis of congenital or acquired portosystemic shunts.[1, 3]

Operative portography is performed by surgically placing a catheter in a jejunal vein, in a splenic vein, or in the splenic pulp. Aqueous iodinated contrast medium is injected into the vein and a radiograph is made.[3] A lateral projection is usually adequate for diagnosis, but a ventrodorsal view may be helpful if surgical intervention is contemplated. The portal venous system is usually well defined with operative portography, and portosystemic shunts may be readily identified.

Several congenital and acquired portosystemic shunts have been described.[3] A portopostcaval shunt via the ductus venosus seems to be the most common congenital shunt; acquired portosystemic shunts may involve any of a large number of collateral venous channels (Fig. 34–7).[3]

Alternative Imaging of the Liver and Spleen

In recent years, radionuclide liver and spleen scans and ultrasonic examination of the liver

---

*Cholografin, E.R. Squibb & Sons, Princeton, NJ.

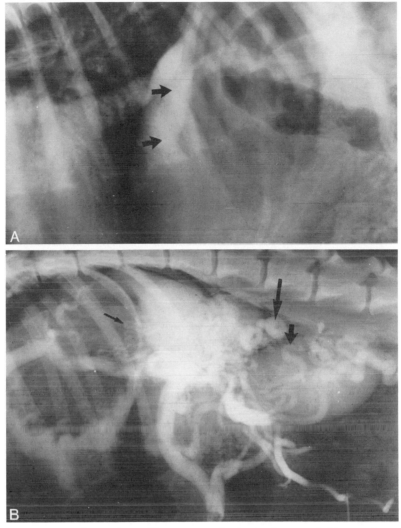

Figure 34–7. Contrast portograms in two dogs with portosystemic shunts. *A,* congenital patent ductus venosus *(arrows)* opacified after injection of contrast medium into the cranial mesenteric artery (cranial mesenteric arterial portography). *B,* numerous tortuous, collateral venous channels *(arrows)* in a dog with an acquired portosystemic shunt are opacified after injection of contrast medium into a jejunal vein (operative portography).

and spleen have been used in some teaching institutions.[2, 7, 9] Expensive, sophisticated imaging equipment is required; in the case of radioisotope studies, considerable expertise in the handling of radioactive substances, the patients, and their wastes after injection of the radionuclides is also necessary.

THE SPLEEN

The spleen is an elongated, flat, solid organ in the cranial left abdomen, lying just caudal to the stomach. The spleen consists of two main parts, the dorsal extremity (head) and the ventral extremity (tail). The dorsal extremity is less variable in position due to its short gastrosplenic ligament and its location between the gastric

fundus and the cranial pole of the left kidney. The ventral extremity is less tightly fixed in position and thus may vary greatly in location.[9, 16]

Radiographically, the spleen is an organ of solid, homogeneous soft-tissue opacity that is not uniformly visualized in lateral radiographs but can be seen regularly in ventrodorsal views of the abdomen (Fig. 34–8).[8, 10] The spleen is more likely to be seen in abdominal radiographs made with the animal in right lateral recumbency than in those made with the patient in left lateral recumbency.[8] When seen in the lateral projection, the spleen is near the ventral abdominal wall and just caudal to the liver shadow. In ventrodorsal radiographs, the spleen is a triangular structure of soft-tissue opacity

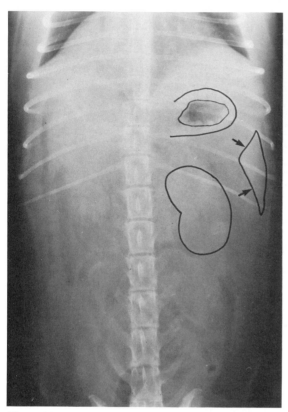

Figure 34–8. Ventrodorsal radiograph of the abdomen of a normal dog. The triangular opacity of the normal spleen *(outline* and *arrows)* is found midway between and slightly lateral to the gastric fundus and the left kidney. The spleen is reliably seen in this location in ventrodorsal radiographs of the abdomen.

that is slightly caudal and lateral to the gastric fundus.[8, 10] In some animals, particularly cats, the dorsal extremity of the spleen may be visualized in the lateral view as a small triangular soft-tissue opacity in the dorsal abdomen just caudal to the gastric fundus.

There are no reliable criteria for the radiographic determination of normal splenic size. Evaluation of splenic size is purely subjective.[10] Radiographically, the edges and margins of the normal spleen are smooth and sharp.

Alterations in Spleen Size

Because determination of normal splenic size is subjective, alterations in the size of this organ must be substantial to be recognized. The spleen may increase or decrease in size uniformly and diffusely, or the spleen may enlarge locally, as with a splenic mass (Fig. 34–9).

Diffuse splenic enlargement is often a physiologic response, which frequently occurs after the administration of medications. Phenothiazine tranquilizers and barbiturate anesthetics cause diffuse and often substantial splenic enlargement.[10] Diseases affecting the reticuloendothelial system, e.g., mastocytosis, lymphosarcoma, or histoplasmosis, also may produce diffuse splenic enlargement.[10, 17, 18] Diffuse splenic enlargement, by itself, is not a reliable sign of disease, because the possible causes are numerous and in many instances enlargement is a normal physiologic reaction. Diffuse splenic enlargement is often seen in patients with splenic torsion or gastric volvulus;[17] splenomegaly is not diagnostic for these conditions but is a supportive radiographic finding.

Primary and metastatic neoplasms are frequent causes of focal splenic enlargement.[10] Subcapsular hematomas also cause focal enlargement of this organ.[17] Splenic masses are recognized by their close association with the spleen in one or both views of the abdomen as well as by the displacement of adjacent organs that they cause.[8, 10] Radiographic diagnosis of splenic masses is discussed in Chapter 32.

Alterations in Spleen Position

Because the spleen is not rigidly fixed in position, the location of the spleen can vary greatly, even in normal dogs and cats.[8, 10] Pathologic alterations in spleen position may be seen in patients with traumatic hernias through which the spleen may pass. The dorsal extremity of the spleen is closely attached to the greater curvature of the stomach, so the spleen may be identified in the thorax of some animals with diaphragmatic hernias involving the stomach. Displacement of the stomach, as in gastric volvulus, may also displace the spleen. In patients with splenic torsion, the spleen may be found in an abnormal location, although identification of the spleen can be difficult due to abdominal effusion.[9]

Alterations in Splenic Shape or Margination

Changes in the margins or shape of the spleen are usually due to splenic masses. The masses distort the normally smooth, tongue-shaped spleen and produce irregularly lobulated margins. Masses may be neoplastic or may represent large hematomas.[17] Neoplastic masses tend to have lumpy margins with multiple lobulations; hematomas are usually smooth in outline and are spherical.[17] Margins of the spleen may become obscured or obliterated by fluid accumulation in the abdomen or around the spleen. This loss of visualization is particularly true in traumatic splenic rupture, with hemorrhage initially accumulating around the spleen; streaky,

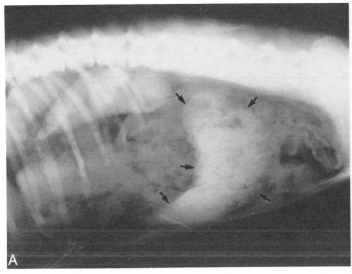

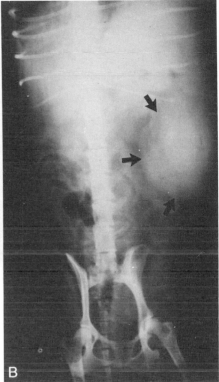

Figure 34–9. *A*, spleen is greatly enlarged in this dog and is clearly visualized due to intra-abdominal gas. The margins of the spleen are smooth *(arrows)* and no abdominal splenic mass is seen. Splenomegaly is due to the administration of a phenothiazine tranquilizer before this diagnostic pneumoperitoneum. *B*, normal splenic shadow is not visible in this dog. A large soft-tissue mass *(arrows)* is present where the normal spleen shadow is expected. Exploratory surgery revealed a large splenic neoplasm.

hazy areas of increased opacity obscure the normally sharp, clearly defined splenic margins.[9]

Alterations in Radiopacity of the Spleen

Changes in the radiopacity of the spleen are rare. Gas accumulation in the splenic pulp may be associated with splenic torsion and prolifer-

ation of gas forming organisms within the spleen (Fig. 34–10).

Contrast Medium Studies for Evaluation of the Spleen. Radiographic techniques involving the use of contrast medium are not often used to evaluate the spleen. Pneumoperitonography can be used to enhance abdominal contrast and to define the margins of the spleen more clearly. This procedure may be of value in patients with splenic masses, but it is not often performed.

Figure 34–10. Alteration in splenic opacity. The spleen contains mottled gas opacities *(small arrows),* and several veins also contain gas *(arrowheads)* in this dog with splenic torsion. Margins of the spleen are not visible because of intra-abdominal fluid. Free intra-abdominal gas is also present *(curved arrows). Clostridium* sp. were cultured from the spleen after it was surgically removed.

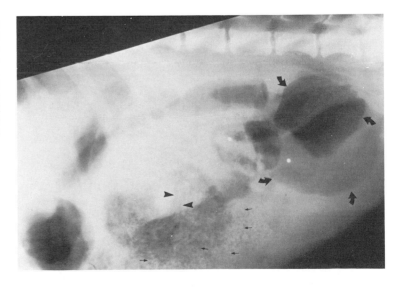

References

1. Suter PF: Radiographic diagnosis of liver disease in dogs and cats. Vet Clin North Am [Small Anim Pract] 12:153, 1982.
2. Hornbuckle WE, and Allan GS: Feline liver disease. *In* Kirk RW (Ed): Current Veterinary Therapy VII. Philadelphia, WB Saunders, 1980, pp. 891–895.
3. Suter PF: Portal vein anomalies in the dog: Their angiographic diagnosis. J Am Vet Radiol Soc 16:84, 1975.
4. Carlisle CH: A comparison of technics for cholecystography in the cat. J Am Vet Radiol Soc 18:173, 1977.
5. Allan GS, and Dixon RT: Cholecystography in the dog: The choice of contrast media and optimum dose rates. J Am Vet Radiol Soc 16:98, 1975.
6. Schmidt S, and Suter PF: Angiography of the hepatic and portal venous system of the dog and cat: An investigative method. Vet Radiol 21:57, 1980.
7. Nyland TG, and Park RD: Hepatic ultrasonography in the dog. Vet Radiol 24:74, 1983.
8. Root CR: Interpretation of abdominal survey radiographs. Vet Clin North Am 24:763, 1974.
9. O'Brien TR: Radiographic Diagnosis of Abdominal Disorders in the Dog and Cat. Chap. 10. Philadelphia, WB Saunders, 1978.
10. Root CR: Abdominal masses: The radiographic differential diagnosis. J Am Vet Radiol Soc 15:26, 1974.
11. Schall WD, Chapman Jr WL, Finco DR, et al: Cholelithiasis in dogs. J Am Vet Med Assoc 163:469, 1973.
12. Cantwell HD, Blevins WE, Hanika-Rebar C, et al: Radiopaque hepatic and lobar duct choleliths in a dog. J Am Anim Hosp Assoc 19:373, 1983.
13. Burk RL, and Johnson GF: Emphysematous cholecystitis in the nondiabetic dog: Three case histories. Vet Radiol 21:242, 1980.
14. Lord PF, Carb A, Halliwell WH, et al: Emphysematous hepatic abscess associated with trauma, necrotic hepatic nodular hyperplasia and adenoma in a dog: A case report. Vet Radiol 23:46, 1982.
15. Ackerman N, Wingfield WE, Corley EA: Fatal air embolism associated with pneumourethrography and pneumocystography in a dog. J Am Vet Med Assoc, 160:1616, 1972.
16. Evans HE, and Christensen GC: Miller's Anatomy of the Dog, 2nd Ed. Philadelphia, WB Saunders, 1979, pp. 835–838.
17. Brodey RS: The Spleen. *In* Archibald J (Ed): Canine Surgery, 2nd Ed. Santa Barbara, American Veterinary Publications, 1974, pp. 807–821.
18. Liska WD, MacEwen EG, Zaki FA, et al: Feline systemic mastocytosis: A review and results of splenectomy in seven cases. J Am Anim Hosp Assoc 15:589, 1979.

CHAPTER 35

ABDOMINAL LYMPH NODES

MARY B. MAHAFFEY
DON L. BARBER

NORMAL ANATOMY

Abdominal lymph nodes can be divided into two groups, parietal and visceral. Parietal (sublumbar) lymph nodes are those that lie along the dorsal wall of the abdomen in the retroperitoneal space. These lymph nodes receive afferent lymphatics from the spine, adrenal glands, kidneys, caudodorsal abdomen, pelvis, and pelvic limbs. Efferent vessels from these lymph nodes drain into the lumbar trunk, which in turn empties into the cisterna chyli. The more cranially located of these lymph nodes may bypass the lumbar trunk and drain directly into the cisterna chyli. Many of the lymph nodes are inconsistently developed and often are absent. The medial iliac lymph nodes, however, the largest lymph nodes of the sublumbar group, are constant. The medial iliac lymph nodes, previously known as the external iliac lymph nodes,[1] are located ventral to the vertebra and between the deep circumflex iliac and external iliac arteries. Although some authors state that the medial iliac lymph nodes lie ventral to the fifth and sixth lumbar vertebrae,[1] it is our experience and that of another author[3] that these lymph nodes are frequently located ventral to the sixth and seventh lumbar vertebral bodies. One lymph node is usually present on each side, but occasionally there are two lymph nodes on one or both sides. The medial iliac lymph nodes receive afferent lymphatics from the urogenital tract as well as other structures in the caudal abdomen, pelvis, and pelvic limbs.

The visceral group of abdominal lymph nodes drain the liver, spleen, pancreas, stomach, and intestine. The largest of this group are the cranial mesenteric lymph nodes, which receive afferent lymphatics from the jejunum, ileum, and pancreas. The efferent vessels of the visceral lymph nodes drain into the intestinal trunk, which then empties into the cisterna chyli.

Normal abdominal lymph nodes are not seen on survey radiographs because they are not of sufficient size or opacity to be seen as separate structures (Fig. 35–1).

ABNORMALITIES OF THE LYMPH NODES

Abdominal lymph nodes may be seen radiographically only if they are enlarged or mineralized. Abundant retroperitoneal fat present in most dogs also aids in providing adequate contrast between enlarged lymph nodes and surrounding soft-tissue structures. Of the parietal group of lymph nodes, the medial iliac nodes

401

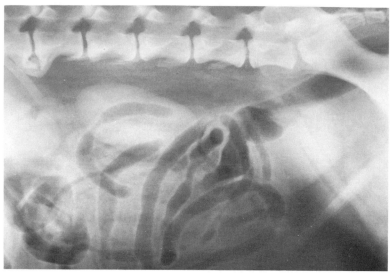

Figure 35–1. Lateral view of the abdomen of a normal dog. Note the fat opacity within the retroperitoneal space. The soft-tissue opacity along the ventral border of the spine is due to the sublumbar musculature, the aorta, and the caudal vena cava. The black dot overlying L_4 is a film artifact.

are usually the only nodes that enlarge to a degree that they can be seen radiographically. When enlarged, the lymph nodes appear as soft-tissue masses in the retroperitoneal space ventral to the sixth and seventh lumbar vertebrae (Fig. 35–2). If node enlargement is severe, the lymph nodes may extend more cranially

(Fig. 35–3). Frequently, enlarged lymph nodes displace the descending colon and rectum ventrally (Fig. 35–4). One should be cautioned, however, that a ventral course of the colon is not an indication of iliac lymph node enlargement, unless a soft-tissue mass is present where the lymph nodes are located; the colon may be

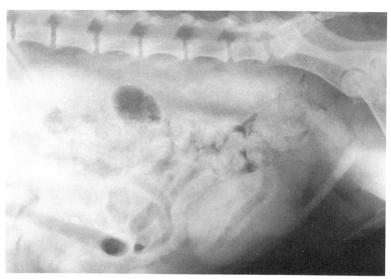

Figure 35–2. Lateral view of the abdomen of a dog with lymphosarcoma. The medial iliac lymph nodes are enlarged and appear as a soft-tissue mass with indistinct margins in the retroperitoneal space ventral to L_6 and L_7. The prostate gland is also enlarged.

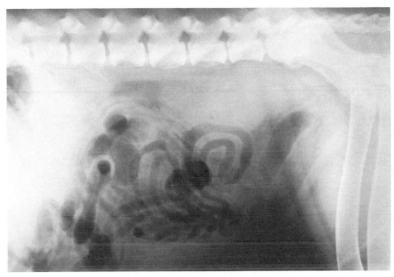

Figure 35–3. Lateral view of the abdomen of a dog with lymphosarcoma. Sublumbar lymph node enlargement is severe and appears as a soft-tissue mass in the retroperitoneal space extending caudally from L₄ into the pelvic canal.

normally positioned more ventral than usual without being displaced by a mass. Causes of lymph node enlargement include neoplasia, lymphadenitis, and hyperplasia.

Neoplastic lymph node involvement may be primary (lymphosarcoma) or metastatic (from caudal abdominal or pelvic neoplasms). Lymphosarcoma is the most common cause of medial iliac lymph node enlargement. Prostatic neoplasms frequently metastasize to the medial iliac lymph nodes.[2] In some animals, neoplastic lymph nodes may become mineralized. Prostatic infection could result in lymph node hyperplasia or lymphadenitis.

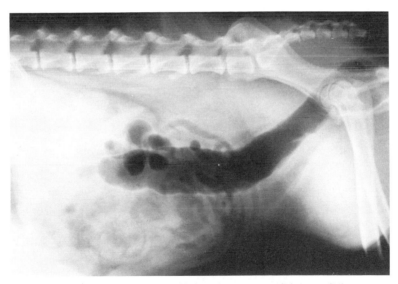

Figure 35–4. Lateral view of the abdomen of a dog with lymphosarcoma. A large soft-tissue mass (lymph nodes) in the retroperitoneal space extends from L₅ into the pelvic canal, displacing the air-filled colon ventrally.

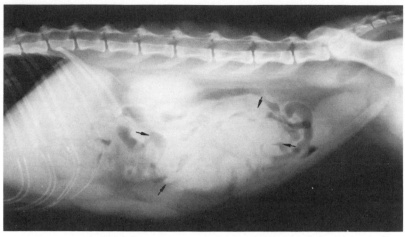

Figure 35–5. Lateral view of the abdomen of a cat with mesenteric lymph node enlargement. The enlarged lymph nodes appear as a single, ill-defined soft-tissue mass in the mid-abdomen *(arrows).*

Visceral abdominal lymph nodes are not usually seen on radiographs; they rarely enlarge to the degree that they can be seen radiographically, and also they silhouette with surrounding organs. The cranial mesenteric lymph nodes, however, may occasionally enlarge sufficiently so as to be seen as an ill-defined central abdominal mass displacing intestines peripherally (Fig. 35–5).

References

1. Evans HE, and Christensen GC: Miller's Anatomy of the Dog, 2nd Ed. Philadelphia, WB Saunders, 1979, p. 823.
2. Leav I, and Ling GV: Adenocarcinoma of the canine prostate. Cancer 22:1329, 1968.
3. O'Brien TR: Radiographic Diagnosis of Abdominal Disorders in the Dog and Cat: Radiographic Interpretation, Clinical Signs, Pathophysiology. Philadelphia, WB Saunders, 1978, p. 93.

CHAPTER 36

THE ADRENAL GLANDS

MARY B. MAHAFFEY
DON L. BARBER

NORMAL ANATOMY

The adrenal glands are located in the retroperitoneal space near the craniomedial border of the kidneys. The left adrenal gland is located more cranially with respect to its corresponding kidney than the right adrenal gland, which is located near the hilus of the right kidney. The right adrenal gland is bordered dorsally by the psoas minor muscle and the crus of the diaphragm, medially by the caudal vena cava, ventrolaterally by the right kidney, and cranioventrally by the right lateral liver lobe. The left adrenal gland is bordered dorsally by the psoas minor muscle, ventrally by the spleen, laterally by the left kidney, and medially by the aorta.[3] Because of their small size and soft-tissue opacity, the adrenal glands are not usually seen radiographically.

ABNORMALITIES OF THE ADRENAL GLANDS

Adrenal glands may be seen radiographically only when they are enlarged or mineralized. Reports of radiographically detectable adrenal tumors without metastases are scarce, and include descriptions of a nonmineralized pheochromocytoma[12] and of three mineralized carcinomas.[4, 15] Most adrenal tumors are not of sufficient size to be detected radiographically. An adrenal mass should be suspected, however, when a soft-tissue or partially mineralized mass is present craniomedial to a kidney; the kidney may be displaced caudolaterally by the mass. Masses of the right adrenal gland may be more difficult to detect than those of the left, because the right adrenal gland is in close proximity to the liver. Functional adrenal tumors (carcinomas and adenomas) have been reported to occur more commonly in the right (77 percent) than in the left adrenal gland.[14] This predilection for the right adrenal gland may be part of the reason that few adrenal tumors are seen radiographically. Left adrenal masses may displace the fundus of the stomach cranially, the transverse colon caudoventrally, and the left kidney caudally.

Adenomas are usually small, well circumscribed,[2] and not large enough to be seen on radiographs;[15] carcinomas tend to be larger.[2] Dystrophic calcification of adrenal tumors may occur and may be seen radiographically.[4, 15] Carcinomas may invade local tissues, including the caudal vena cava, and may metastasize to the liver, lymph nodes, and lungs.[5, 6, 13] When adrenal carcinomas are advanced, it may not be possible to determine the origin of the primary mass lesion radiographically. In such an instance, the metastases may be the major radio-

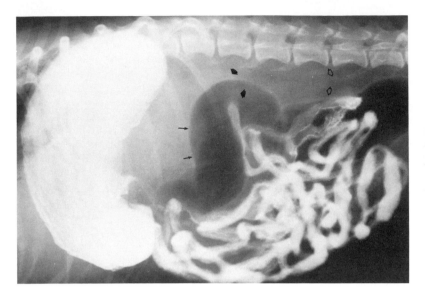

Figure 36–1. Lateral view during an upper gastrointestinal examination tract in a 9-year-old dog. The body of the stomach is displaced cranially, and the gas-filled transverse colon *(arrows)* and the left kidney are displaced caudally by a soft-tissue mass. The caudal poles of the left *(open arrowheads)* and right *(solid arrowheads)* kidneys are identified. The mass was due to metastasis from a pheochromocytoma.

graphic finding, although there may be an ill-defined soft-tissue mass in the craniodorsal abdomen (Fig. 36–1). Radiographic evidence of metastases to the liver, peritoneum, lungs, and other organs may also be seen.

Mineralization may occur in non-neoplastic adrenal glands (Fig. 36–2). Radiographically visible adrenal mineralization of unknown etiology was reported in a 1-year-old cat.[15] Histologic detection of adrenal calcification was reported in 3.5 percent of dogs, 30 percent of cats, and 50 percent of monkeys in one study,[11] and in 25 percent of cats[7] and 1 percent of dogs[9] in two other studies. Calcification occurred in the zona reticularis of the adrenal cortex in the dogs, monkeys, and cats; however, in some cats, calcification affected the entire adrenal cortex and extended into the medulla.[11] Adrenal

calcification was not correlated with clinical findings. The cause and pathogenesis of adrenal calcification are unknown. In man, adrenal calcification has been associated with intra-adrenal hemorrhage, tuberculosis, Addison's disease, tumors (benign and malignant), cysts, Niemann-Pick disease,[1] and Wolman's disease.[8]

It appears that calcification of the adrenal glands in cats is relatively common, but calcification in most animals is not sufficient to be seen radiographically. Mineralization of the adrenal glands of normal size is usually an incidental finding in cats and dogs.

Adrenal gland dysfunction usually causes secondary changes that are radiographically visible. Radiographic findings of Cushing's syndrome include hepatomegaly, bronchopulmonary mineralization, dystrophic mineralization of the

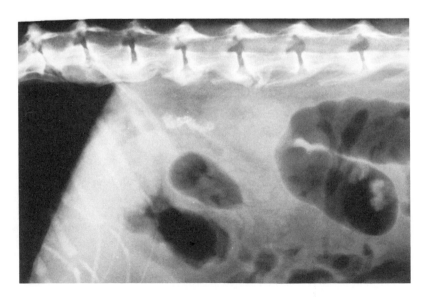

Figure 36–2. Lateral radiograph (close-up view) of the abdomen of a 13-year-old cat. Mineral opacities cranial to each kidney were adrenal glands with calcification of the zona reticularis. The cat was destroyed because of unrelated causes.

skin and other soft tissues, and rarely adrenal gland enlargement with mineralization, when functional tumors are present.[15] Esophageal dilation[15] and decreased heart size[10, 14] have been associated with Addison's disease. These findings are discussed elsewhere in this text.

References

1. Bergman SM, and Scouras GC: Incidental bilateral adrenal calcification. Urology 22:665, 1983.
2. Capen CC, Belshaw BE, and Martin SL: Endocrine disorders. In Ettinger SJ (Ed): Textbook of Veterinary Internal Medicine: Diseases of the Dog and Cat, Vol. 2. Philadelphia, WB Saunders, 1975, p. 1397.
3. Evans HE, and Christensen GC: Miller's Anatomy of the Dog, 2nd Ed. Philadelphia, WB Saunders, 1979, pp. 618–619.
4. Huntley K, Frazer J, Gibbs C, et al: The radiological features of canine Cushing's syndrome: A review of forty-eight cases. J Small Anim Pract 23:369, 1982.
5. Jubb KVF, and Kennedy PC: Pathology of Domestic Animals, 2nd Ed. New York, Academic Press, 1970, p. 427.
6. Kelly, DF, and Darke PGG: Cushing's syndrome in the dog. Vet Rec 98:28, 1976.
7. Marine D: Calcification of the suprarenal glands of cats. J Exp Med 43:495, 1926.
8. Raafat F, Hashemian MP, and Abrishami MA: Wolman's disease: Report of two new cases with a review of the literature. Am J Clin Pathol 59:490, 1973.
9. Rajan A, and Mohiyuddeen S: Pathology of the adrenal gland in canines (Canis familiaris). Indian J Anim Sci 44:123, 1974.
10. Rendano VT, and Alexander JE: Heart size changes in experimentally-induced adrenal insufficiency in the dog: A radiographic study. J Am Vet Radiol Soc 17:57, 1976.
11. Ross MA, Gainer JH, and Innes JRM: Dystrophic calcification in the adrenal glands of monkeys, cats, and dogs. Arch Pathol Lab Med 60:655, 1955.
12. Schaer M: Pheochromocytoma in a dog: A case report. J Am Anim Hosp Assoc 16:583, 1980.
13. Siegel ET: Endocrine Disorders of the Dog. Philadelphia, Lea & Febiger, 1977, p 166.
14. Scott DW: Hyperadrenocorticism (hyperadrenocorticoidism, hyperadrenocorticalism, Cushing's disease, Cushing's syndrome). Vet Clin North Am 9:3, 1979.
15. Ticer JW: Roentgen signs of endocrine disease. Vet Clin North Am 7:465, 1977.

CHAPTER 37

THE KIDNEYS AND URETERS

DANIEL A. FEENEY
GARY R. JOHNSTON

THE KIDNEYS

Survey radiographs as well as radiographic procedures with contrast medium can contribute much information toward the diagnosis of renal and ureteral diseases. The external boundaries of the kidneys can usually be identified on survey radiographs. This identification permits assessment of the size, shape, and radiographic opacity of the kidneys, which can aid in the diagnosis of disease processes. However, when the kidneys cannot be identified, when their boundaries cannot be defined, when their architecture cannot be assessed by survey radiographs, or when qualitative functional information is needed, excretory urography can provide the clinician with much information with minimal patient discomfort. To gain the maximal amount of information from any radiographic procedure, a rational approach to interpretation must be used. In general, the roentgen sign approach has stood the test of time and is quite easily understood. Roentgen signs are merely descriptions with the use of basic terms of radiopacity, geometry, or function of the affected organs. The roentgen sign method is employed throughout this chapter for interpretation of survey and contrast medium radiographs.

Roentgen signs applicable to organ radiopacity include the five basic radiopacities: air, fat, soft tissue (water), bone or mineral, and metal. Geometric roentgen signs include size, shape, position or location, number, and margination. The roentgen signs applicable to organ function include excretion, motility, patency, and integrity (particularly of tubular organs). The observer should scrutinize the radiograph for abnormalities of each specific organ and the cavity in which the organ lies. The abnormal roentgen findings identified should be compared with what is expected as the norm. These findings, in combination with information from the history, physical examination, and laboratory analyses should be combined, and a list of differential diagnoses (gamuts) should be formed in order of decreasing likelihood. Based on these ranked gamuts, the additional tests necessary (radiographic or other types) should be determined and performed as needed until a definitive diagnosis is achieved. Cost may be a limiting factor and the ideal approach may not necessarily be the most practical approach. The use of this suggested scheme for evaluation of survey radiographs, radiographic procedures involving contrast medium, or both enables the clinician to gain the maximal amount of information and to form the most applicable plan for subsequent work-up, if necessary.

The general goals of the chapter are to specify

the imaging procedures applicable to the kidneys and to place each of these procedures into perspective regarding indications, limitations, contraindications, and pitfalls when applicable. Subsequently, the normal radiographic findings based on roentgen signs are described. In addition, the abnormal radiographic findings are described and at least a partial list of gamuts, which should be considered as certain roentgen signs are encountered, are presented. Cited reference material should be consulted for more extensive review of the suggested disease processes.

Imaging Procedures

Survey radiographs are the simplest form of radiographic evaluation for small animals. The general indications for the use of survey radiographs to evaluate specific disease processes are outlined in textbooks of internal medicine.[1, 2] From a more general viewpoint, survey radiographs provide information on the external anatomy of the kidney when contrast (both abdominal and retroperitoneal) is adequate to permit their visualization. In addition, it is possible to assess any abnormal opacities near the kidneys, such as air or mineral, which may suggest a pathophysiologic mechanism for the clinical signs of renal disease encountered in that patient. Inadequate radiographic contrast, which is generally due to lack of retroperitoneal fat or presence of peritoneal or retroperitoneal fluid, limits visualization of the kidneys on survey radiographs.

The information available from survey radiographs can be maximized if the patient is properly prepared, i.e., withholding food for 24 hours and administering cleansing enemas at least 1 to 2 hours before radiography. To permit accurate localization within the three-dimensional patient, both lateral and ventrodorsal views should be used.[3] Because the right lateral view permits greater longitudinal separation of the radiographic images of the right and left kidneys, it is the projection most applicable to radiography of the upper urinary tract.[3] It must be emphasized that adequate technique and scrupulous attention to darkroom detail should be used to permit the best possible images to be obtained.

Because of the limitations of survey radiographs, especially when the patient is emaciated or has peritoneal or retroperitoneal fluid, excretory urography is the method of choice to define the anatomy and to assess qualitatively the function of the kidneys. It is a relatively simple means of verifying and localizing upper urinary tract disease and can be used to assess the reversibility of renal disease. Although excretory urography is not a quantitative measurement of renal function, it can be used to assess the relative function of the kidneys, and can be loosely interpreted to assess pathophysiologic mechanisms of renal failure.[4]

Excretory urography can be used in both azotemic and nonazotemic patients, provided hydration is adequate. As the degree of renal failure progresses, however, it may be necessary to increase the dose of contrast medium to provide adequate visualization of the kidneys. In any case, patient hydration should be assessed and determined to be at a normal level before the administration of any contrast medium.[4] It is possible that there may be a temporary decrease in the status of kidney function after excretory urography, and an indepth discussion of this is beyond this text. Clinical significance of this decreased function is considered minimal in the presence of adequate urinary output and patient hydration.

The technique of excretory urography is described in detail in Table 37–1. The patient should be prepared as for survey radiographs; food is withheld and cleansing enemas are administered.[4–6] Contrast medium is generally an iothalamate or diatrizoate contrast medium, which is given by bolus intravenous injection. The dose is 400 mg iodine per pound of body weight injected via preplaced cephalic venous or jugular venous catheter.[4–7] Catheter placement should be maintained for at least 15 to 20 minutes after administration of the contrast medium in that it provides a readily accessible route to the peripheral circulatory system in the event of a hypotensive reaction to the contrast medium. There are many suggested

TABLE 37–1. TECHNIQUE FOR INTRAVENOUS UROGRAPHY

Routine patient preparation
  24 hours without food; water ad libitum
  Cleansing enema at least 2 hours before radiography
Assess hydration status; proceed only if normal
Obtain survey radiographs
Infuse contrast medium intravenously via the cephalic or jugular vein as rapidly as possible (bolus injection)
  Dose: 400 mg iodine/lb body weight
  Contrast medium: sodium iothalamate or sodium diatrizoate
Obtain abdominal radiographs in the following sequence:
  Ventrodorsal views at 5 to 20 seconds, 5 minutes, 20 minutes, and 40 minutes post-injection for general assessment
  Lateral view at 5 minutes post-injection for general assessment
  Oblique views at 3 to 5 minutes post-injection for ureteral termination in urinary bladder
  Lateral and ventrodorsal views at 30 to 40 minutes post-injection to observe urinary bladder if retrograde cystography is contraindicated or impossible

(From Feeney DA, Barber DL, Johnston, GR, et al: The excretory urogram: Techniques, normal radiographic appearance and misinterpretation. Comp Contin Ed Pract Vet 4:233, 1982, with permission.)

filming sequences; in general, however, radiographs obtained immediately, 5, 20, and 40 minutes after injection of contrast medium yield the most information.[4, 5, 7]

The interpretative phases of the excretory urogram are the nephrographic and pyelographic phases. Opacification of the functional renal parenchyma is the nephrogram, and opacification of the renal pelves, pelvic diverticula, and ureters is the pyelogram. Each phase should be evaluated separately (based on subsequent information in this chapter). The sequence of these phases should then be compared in view of the normal findings yet to be described.

Although procedures in which radiographic contrast media are used provide considerable information relative to urinary tract disease, they may complicate some subsequent determinations for as many as 24 hours. For example, elevation of urine specific gravity by intravenously administered contrast medium may be erroneously interpreted as adequate renal concentrating ability.[8] In addition, although detailed in vivo studies are not available for all types of urinary pathogens, the influence of contrast media on growth of some urinary tract organisms cannot be ignored.[9] It is recommended, however, that the samples for culture and renal concentrating ability, as well as for urine sediment cytologic analysis, be performed before or at least 24 hours after (including several voidings) excretory urography.

Additional procedures that may provide information but require more sophisticated equipment or are more invasive include renal angiography,[10] ultrasonography,[11] and nephropyelostomy.[12] In renal angiography, contrast medium is placed into or near the renal artery to provide maximum opacification of the kidney and minimal superimposition of overlying vascular or parenchymal structures. This procedure does require catheterization of the aorta from an external vessel, and is most applicable to areas equipped with image intensification fluoroscopy and rapid film-changing equipment. Renal ultrasonography is a noninvasive technique in which sound is directed into the tissue and the reflected echoes are reconstructed into two-dimensional images. This procedure requires considerable expertise and sophisticated equipment, but information on renal architecture can be provided without the use of contrast medium. (A few renal ultrasonograms are shown throughout this chapter, and are paired with radiographs to aid reader understanding). Nephropyelostomy is a technique by which the renal pelvis is catheterized percutaneously.[12] This procedure can be used as a diagnostic and therapeutic tool, but the use of image intensification fluoroscopy, real-time ultrasonography, or both, is required.

TABLE 37–2. QUANTITATIVE APPEARANCE OF NORMAL CANINE AND FELINE EXCRETORY UROGRAMS[5]

Structure	Measurement*	Value†
Kidney	Length	Dog 3.00 ± 0.25 × L_2 2.50 to 3.50 × L_2 Cat 2.4 to 3.0 × L_2 4.0 to 4.5 cm
	Width	Dog 2.00 ± 0.20 × L_2 Cat 3.0 to 3.5 cm
Renal pelvis	Width	Dog 0.03 ± 0.017 × L_2 (generally ≤ 1.0 mm) Cat Not reported
Pelvic diverticula	Width	Dog 0.02 ± 0.005 × L_2 (generally ≤ 1.0 mm) Cat Not reported
Proximal ureter	Width	Dog 0.07 ± 0.018 × L_2 (generally ≤ 2.5 mm) Cat Not reported
Distal ureter	Width	Not reported in dogs or cats

*Measurements apply only to the ventrodorsal view.
†L_2, the length of the body of the second lumbar vertebral body as visualized on the ventrodorsal view.
(From Feeney DA, Barber DL, Johnston GR, et al: The excretory urogram: Techniques, normal radiographic appearance and misinterpretation. Comp Contn Ed Vet Prac 4:233, 1982. Modified and reprinted with permission.)

Normal Radiographic Findings

The normal radiographic findings for both the dog and cat that can be determined quantitatively are listed in Table 37–2. The normal number of kidneys is two.[6] The most widely used quantitation of normal kidney size in the dog and cat is that of renal length, which can usually be assessed on survey radiographs.[1, 3, 4, 5, 7, 13–15] In general, the dog kidney is approximately three times the length of the second lumbar vertebral body as visualized on the ventrodorsal view. Depending on which of the documented references are utilized, the normal range may extend from 2.75 to 3.25 times[7] or from 2.5 to 3.5 times[13] the length of the second lumbar vertebral body. In the cat, the most accepted renal length is that of 2.4 to 3.0 times the length of the second lumbar vertebral body,[14] but other values have been suggested.[15] Other quantitative measurements visible only on excretory urograms that may be used to assess the kidneys include measurement of the pyelographic variables, including width of the pelvic diverticula, renal pelvis, and proximal ureter. In general, the renal pelvis and pelvic diverticula in the dog do not exceed 1 to 2 mm in diameter, and the proximal ureter in the dog does not exceed 2 to 3 mm in diameter. More exact comparisons are given in Table 37–2, which are related to the length of the second lumbar vertebral body.

The shape of the dog kidney is somewhat elongated, resembling that of a bean, whereas that of the cat is somewhat more rounded, although still somewhat elongated.[1, 4–6] The normal radiographic appearance of the canine and feline kidneys are shown in Figures 37–1 and 37–2. The kidneys in both the dog and cat are located in the retroperitoneal space,[3] and are usually located along the longitudinal axis in association with the last thoracic and first three or four lumbar vertebrae.[1, 6] The right kidney is usually more cranial than the left and, as mentioned previously, this separation can be enhanced on the lateral view by using right lateral recumbent positioning during radiography.

Renal opacity on survey radiographs is that of homogeneous soft tissue.[1, 3] The visualization of the kidneys on survey radiographs relies upon the presence of retroperitoneal fat (perirenal fat) surrounding the kidneys, permitting a variation in radiation attenuation that when compared to the kidneys provides adequate inherent contrast. During excretory urography, the nephrogram is homogeneous, with the exception of the early combined vascular and tubular nephrograms, when the cortex is more radiopaque than the medulla.[4] The pyelogram in the normally functioning kidney is more radiopaque than the nephrogram (Figs. 37–1 and 37–2).

The dynamic aspects of excretory urography lie in the assessment of nephrographic opacification and fading sequences.[4, 16] The normal nephrogram should be most radiopaque within 10 to 30 seconds after bolus intravenous injection of the contrast medium. With increasing delay after injection, the nephrographic opacity should decrease progressively; less than 25 per cent of normal dogs have a detectable nephrogram 2 hours after injection. The pyelogram should be consistently opaque and the diameter of the ureter should vary with time due to peristalsis (Figs. 37–1 and 37–2). The degree of nephrographic and pyelographic opacification in combination with the opacification and fading patterns of the nephrogram can be used as a qualitative estimate of renal function.[6, 17] In general, the poorer the renal function, the less opacified are the nephrographic and pyelographic phases of the excretory urogram.

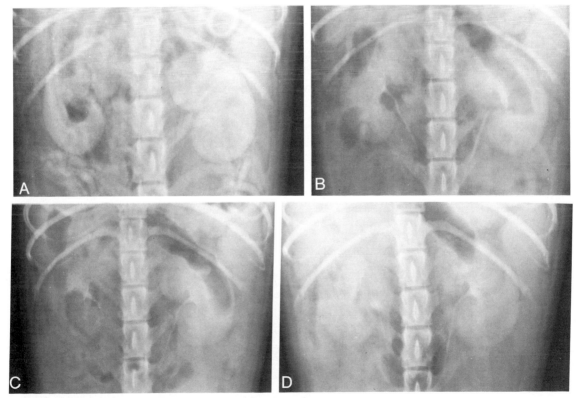

Figure 37–1. Ventrodorsal views of a normal dog after the administration of 400 mg iodine per pound body weight in the form of sodium iothalamate. A, 10 seconds; B, 5 minutes; C, 20 minutes; and D, 40 minutes after injection.

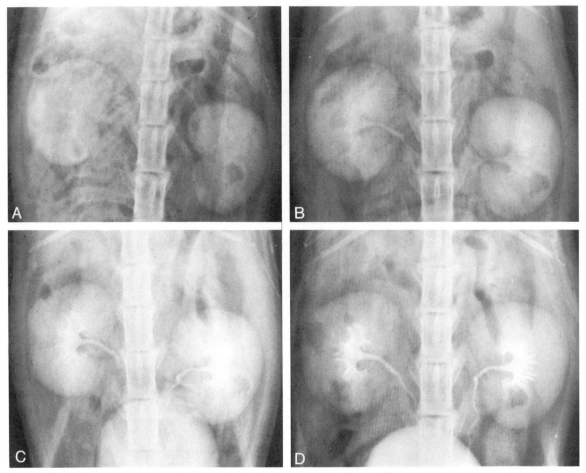

Figure 37–2. Ventrodorsal views of a normal cat after the administration of 400 mg iodine per pound body weight in the form of sodium iothalamate. A, 10 seconds; B, 5 minutes; C, 20 minutes; and D, 40 minutes after intravenous injection.

Abnormal Radiographic Findings

Number. Renal aplasia or agenesis may result in the inability to identify one of the kidneys, even on contrast radiographic procedures.[1, 2, 18] Unilateral renal agenesis may result in compensatory hypertrophy of the unaffected kidney (Fig. 37–3). There is also the possibility of more than the expected number of kidneys by the phenomenon of renal duplication.[19] It must also be considered that the inability to visualize a kidney radiographically may merely be the result of extreme hypoplasia, the consequences of chronic disease, or both.

Size, Shape, and Margination. The combination of these three factors, when applied to abnormal roentgen appearance of the kidneys, may aid the interpreter in identifying possible gamuts or limiting the possible considerations to a manageable number. These combinations and their differential considerations are discussed subsequently. In many of these differ-

ential diagnoses, surgical visualization or microscopic confirmation of the suspected diagnosis or both are mandatory.

Large, regularly shaped, and smoothly marginated kidneys can be encountered in conditions such as compensatory hypertrophy (Fig. 37–3).[2, 3] In addition, it may also be seen in infiltrative neoplasia, such as lymphosarcoma;[1–3] hydronephrosis, including that due to the renal parasite *Dioctophyma renale*;[1–3, 20] renal amyloidosis and glomerulonephritis;[1, 21] perirenal pseudocyst;[22] and possibly large solitary renal cyst.[23] Excretory urography aids in differentiating these possibilities by opacifying the functional renal parenchyma, thus permitting identification of abnormal areas. Characterization of the interface between the normal and abnormal areas is of value in differentiating solitary, well-defined abnormalities, such as a renal cyst, from infiltrative diseases, such as neoplasms.

Large, irregularly shaped kidneys with rough

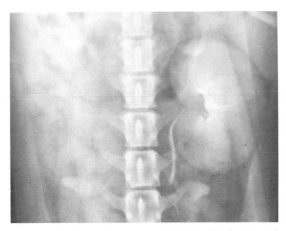

Figure 37–3. The left kidney is enlarged, but is anatomically and functionally normal. The right kidney is not visualized. The left kidney has undergone functional and anatomic compensatory hypertrophy.

margins must be subdivided into focal abnormalities or multifocal to diffuse renal involvement. If the above characteristics are focal, major consideration should be given to primary or metastatic renal neoplasms (Fig. 37–4),[1–3, 24] renal abscess,[3] renal hematoma,[3] and possibly perirenal pseudocyst.[2, 22] If the above combination of roentgen signs appear to be multifocal or diffuse throughout the kidney, diseases such as polycystic renal disease (Fig. 37–5),[1, 2, 25–28] feline infectious peritonitis,[2, 26] and renal lymphosarcoma[26, 29, 30] should be considered.

If the kidney size is normal, renal shape is regular, and margination is smooth, the presence of renal disease may not be excluded. Diseases such as amyloidosis,[1, 21] glomerulonephritis,[1, 2] and acute pyelonephritis[1] can still be encountered even in the presence of a radiographically normal kidney.

Figure 37–4. *A,* ventrodorsal view of a patient 5 minutes after contrast medium injection for excretory urography. In the midportion of the left kidney, there is a focal area of nephrographic nonopacification with compression and distortion of the renal pelvis and pelvic diverticula in the adjacent area. *B,* sagittal sonogram of the left kidney. The architectural abnormality of the kidney corresponds to the nonopacified area of the excretory urogram. The area is echogenic, suggesting that it is solid. Microscopic diagnosis: renal adenocarcinoma.

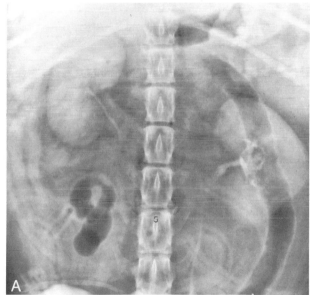

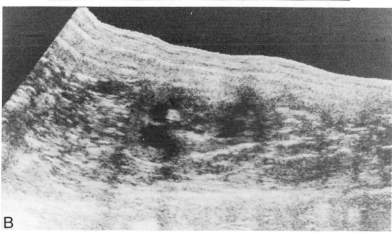

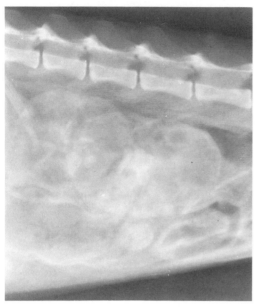

Figure 37–5. Lateral view of a cat 5 minutes after contrast medium injection for excretory urography. Kidneys are enlarged and nephrographic opacification is variable in a random patchy appearance. Microscopic diagnosis: feline polycystic kidney disease.

In the kidney that is of normal size but irregular shape with a rough outline, it must be determined whether the process is at one focus or is multifocal to diffuse. Focal variation in renal shape and margination in a normal-sized kidney merit consideration of renal infarct or focal inflammation and renal abscess.[31] Multifocal to diffuse irregularities in shape and margination in the normal-sized kidney are more likely due to chronic pyelonephritis,[1] polycystic renal disease,[32] or both.

The small kidney with regular shape and smooth margins may suggest renal hypoplasia but may also be the result of diseases such as glomerulonephritis,[1,2] amyloidosis,[1,2] and familial renal disease of specific dog breeds. Depending on the stage of familial renal disease, it has been suggested that this appearance of the kidney may be encountered in cocker spaniels,[1] Lhasa Apso and Shih Tzu dogs,[1] Doberman pinschers[33] and Samoyed dogs[34] and possibly in the Alaskan malamute[35] and the standard poodle.[36] An example of a small, regularly shaped kidney with smooth margins is shown in Figure 37–6, and represents one phase of the disease in the Shih Tzu breed.

A small kidney with an irregular shape and rough margins is most likely due to end-stage renal disease and may be from a myriad of causes. When the kidneys are small and renal function is poor, visualization by excretory urography is often limited, because it is a combination of glomerular filtration and tubular concentration that yields the increased contrast on the radiographic image. In addition, many of these patients have poor body stature due to their chronic disease, and retroperitoneal fat accumulations are less than optimal, which hinders critical evaluation of the kidneys on survey radiographs. Other diseases that must be considered include amyloidosis,[1,21] glomerulonephritis, and chronic pyelonephritis,[1] familial renal disease of the cocker spaniel,[37] Doberman pinscher,[38] Norwegian elkhound,[1,39] Lhasa Apso and Shih Tzu dogs,[40] German shepherd,[41] standard poodle,[36] and Alaskan malamute.[35] Nonspecific renal dysplasia[42] may manifest as a small, irregularly shaped kidney with rough margins, as may a large infarct or generalized renal ischemia.

Location. Kidneys may maintain relatively normal function while being abnormally located. Kidneys located at sites other than those expected in the retroperitoneal space near the thoracolumbar junction have been described and are referred to as ectopic.[3,43,44] In animals

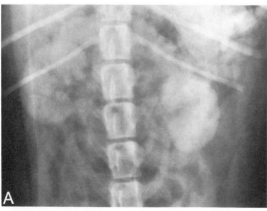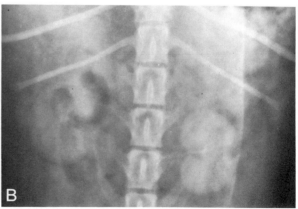

Figure 37–6. Ventrodorsal views 10 seconds (A) and 5 minutes (B) after contrast medium injection for excretory urography in a 1-year-old Shih Tzu. The kidneys are small, nephrographic opacity is poor, and pyelographic opacity is minimal at best. Microscopic diagnosis: Shih Tzu familial renal disease.

and man, kidneys have been identified in the thorax, intra-abdominal region (not the normal retroperitoneal space), and the pelvic canal. Excretory urography and possibly ultrasonography may be of assistance in confirming these unusually located masses as kidneys; excretory urography may aid in the assessment of the functional potential.

In addition to developmental displacement as an ectopic kidney, a kidney may be displaced by an adjacent mass.[3] In particular, adrenal masses may displace either kidney caudally, the right kidney may be displaced caudally by a liver mass, and the left kidney may be displaced caudally by a mass in the head of the spleen. This indirect method of assessing abdominal

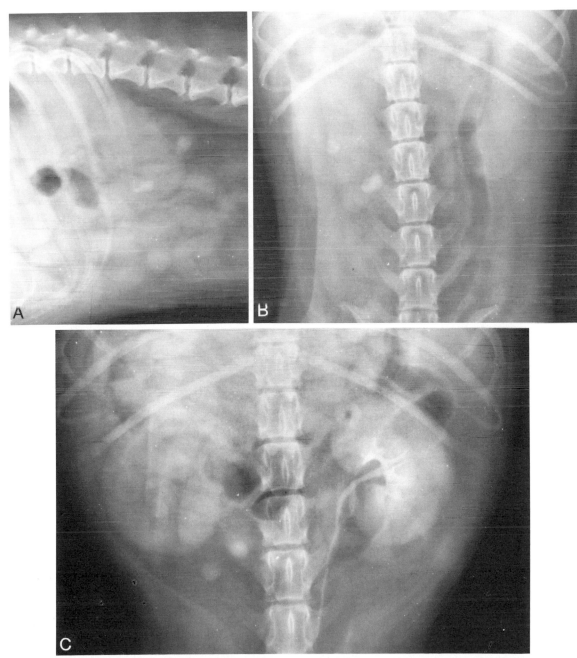

Figure 37–7. Lateral (A) and ventrodorsal (B) radiographs in which there are smoothly marginated, oval, white calcific opacities in the area of the right kidney and ureter. Ventrodorsal view (C) 5 minutes after injection of contrast medium for excretory urography. Peripheral opacification of the right nephrogram is identified without accompanying central or pyelographic opacification. Surgical diagnosis: right renal and ureteral calculi with ureteral obstruction and right renal hydronephrosis.

masses by adjacent organ displacement may be used as an aid in their differential diagnosis.

Radiopacity. On survey radiographs, variations in renal radiopacity (from the expected soft-tissue appearance) may be recognized. The most common opacities recognized include air or mineral. Air may result from vesicoureteral reflux from previous negative-contrast medium procedures involving the lower urinary tract, but may also be due to trauma to the perirenal area with leakage of air from intraperitoneal or extra-abdominal sources. Although highly unlikely, gas-forming bacteria may produce air within or around the kidney. Mineral radiopacity may be due to the presence of renal calculi (Fig. 37–7), which are usually magnesium am-

TABLE 37–3. POSSIBLE STRUCTURAL NEPHROGRAPHIC OPACIFICATION PATTERNS ASSOCIATED WITH CERTAIN RENAL DISEASES*

Opacification Pattern	Renal Disease
Uniform	Normal
	Compensatory hypertrophy
	Acute glomerular or tubulointerstitial disease
	Perirenal pseudocysts
	Hypoplasia
	Others(?)
Focal, nonuniform	Neoplasm
	Hematuria
	Cyst
	Single infarct
	Hydronephrosis
	Abscess
	Others(?)
Multifocal, nonuniform	Polycystic disease
	Multiple infarcts
	Acute pyelonephritis
	Chronic generalized glomerular or tubulointerstitial disease
	Feline infectious peritonitis
	Infiltrative neoplasia
	Others(?)
Nonopacification	Aplasia/agenesis†
	Renal artery obstruction†
	Nephrectomy or nonfunctional renal parenchyma†
	Insufficient or extravascular contrast medium injection
	Others(?)

*Best identified on radiographs exposed 5 to 20 seconds or 5 minutes after contrast medium injection. Do not overinterpret corticomedullary separation on early postinjection radiographs.

†Only unilateral conditions compatible with life.

TABLE 37–4. PYELOGRAPHIC APPEARANCE OF SOME COMMON DISEASES OF THE KIDNEY

Pyelonephritis
Acute:
Pelvic dilation
Proximal ureteral dilation
Absent or incomplete filling of diverticula
Chronic
± Pelvic dilation with irregular borders
Proximal ureteral dilation
Short-blunt diverticula
Hydronephrosis
Pelvic dilation
Dilation of pelvic diverticula (note: diverticula may not be distinguishable if pelvic dilation is severe)
Ureteral dilation
Neoplasia
Renal Parenchyma:
Distortion or deviation of renal pelvis, with ± dilation
Distortion or deviation of pelvic diverticula
Renal Pelvis:
Distortion or dilation of renal pelvis
Filling defects in renal pelvis
Uroliths
Filling defects in renal pelvis
Uroliths usually radiolucent compared to contrast medium
May be changes as seen in pyelonephritis
+ Pelvic dilation

(From Feeney DA, Barber DL, and Osborne CA: Advances in canine excretory urography. *In* 30th Gaines Veterinary Symposium, 1981. White Plains, Gaines Dog Research Center, with permission.)

monium phosphate in both dogs and cats.[3, 45] Other chemical types of calculi can be encountered with some frequency, however; the radiopacity may vary with the degree of mineralization and is not specific for chemical composition of the calculus. Other mineral opacities within the kidney that must be considered include mineralized cyst,[3] calcified tumors,[3] calcification of the renal parenchyma (nephrocalcinosis),[3, 46] and osseous metaplasia of the renal pelvis in the presence of renal disease.[47, 48] As previously mentioned, loss of retroperitoneal contrast due to emaciation, the presence of perirenal fluids (i.e., blood or urine), or both may impede or preclude visualization of the kidneys. The determination of the need for immediate excretory urographic analysis must be made on the basis of the assessment of the remainder of the body fat stores as well as the clinical history.

Excretory urography causes an increase in the radiographic opacity of the renal parenchyma by the accumulation of contrast medium within the renal tubules and vasculature. The opacity of the renal outflow tract is also increased because of urine that contains concentrated contrast medium. The identifiable structural alterations of both the nephrogram[4] and pyelogram[4] are described in Tables 37–3 and

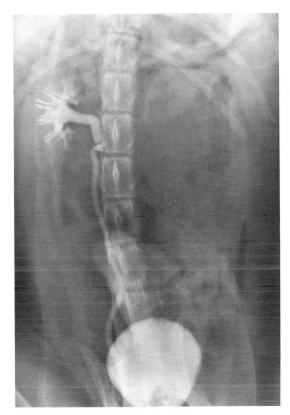

Figure 37–8. Ventrodorsal view 40 minutes after contrast medium injection for excretory urography. The right ureter, renal pelvis, and pelvic diverticula are symmetrically enlarged. The left kidney is dramatically enlarged, with only a rim of nephrographic opacification. The central portion of the left kidney is nonopacified, and there is no pyelogram. Necropsy confirmed moderate right and extreme left hydronephrosis secondary to ureteral obstruction by a transitional cell carcinoma of the bladder trigone and proximal urethra.

37–4, respectively; Figures 37–3 to 37–6 provide examples of structural nephrographic alteration. Figures 37–8 and 37–9 are examples of two common etiologies that result in structural alteration of the pyelogram. The use of Tables 37–3 and 37–4 in the separate evaluation of the nephrographic and pyelographic architecture is suggested as a beginning, and then common diagnoses (if any occur in both gamut lists) should then be pursued.

Function. The alterations in nephrographic opacification and fading sequences are described in detail in Table 37–5. In general, these changes are classified according to the degree of opacification encountered on the immediate postinjection radiograph as well as the relationship of the subsequently encountered nephrographic opacity in the patient in comparison to the initial opacification.[4, 16] Differential considerations for each of the nephrographic opacification sequences are listed, but those listed are not the only possibilities. It should be noted that early first (10 to 30 seconds) nephrographic opacification may be delayed in animals with acute and subacute pyelonephritis.[49, 50] Figure 37–10 is an example of an abnormal nephrographic opacity sequence, and should be compared to Figure 37–1.

Pyelographic alterations associated with changes in renal function generally manifest as poor or undetectable opacification of this phase of the excretory urogram. The opacity of the pyelogram is dependent on both the filtration of the contrast medium from the blood as well as the concentration of the contrast medium within the tubules. Loss of either of these capabilities within the kidneys (assuming adequate dosage and proper route of administration of contrast medium are performed) may result in a less than optimal pyelogram.

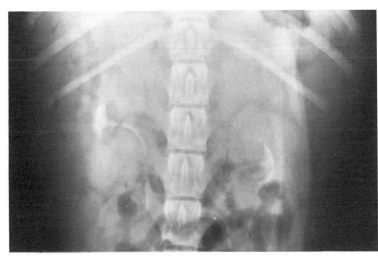

Figure 37–9. Ventrodorsal view 20 minutes after injection of contrast medium for excretory urography. The right and left renal pelves are dilated, but the pelvic diverticula cannot be identified. The ureters, particularly the right ureter, are mildly dilated. Radiologic diagnosis: bilateral chronic pyelonephritis.

TABLE 37–5. **POSSIBLE NEPHROGRAPHIC OPACIFICATION SEQUENCES ASSOCIATED WITH CERTAIN RENAL DISEASE PROCESSES**

Good initial opacification followed by progressively decreasing opacity:
  Normal
Fair to good initial opacification followed by progressively increasing opacity:
  Systemic hypotension due to contrast agents
  Acute renal obstruction (including precipitated Tamm-Horsfall mucoprotein in renal tubules)
  Contrast medium-induced renal failure
  Others
Fair to good initial opacification followed by persistent opacity:
  Acute renal tubular necrosis
  Contrast medium-induced renal failure
  Systemic hypotension due to contrast agents
  Others

Poor initial opacification followed by progressively decreasing opacity:
  Primary polyuric renal failure
  Inadequate contrast medium dose
  Others
Poor initial opacification followed by progressively increasing opacity:
  Acute extrarenal obstruction
  Systemic hypotension existing before to contrast medium administration
  Renal ischemia (arterial or venous)
  Others
Poor initial opacification followed by persistent opacity:
  Primary glomerular dysfunction (chronic)
  Severe generalized renal disease

(From Feeney DA, Barber DL, and Osborne CA: Functional aspects of the nephrogram in excretory urography: A review. Vet Radiol 23:42, 1982, with permission.)

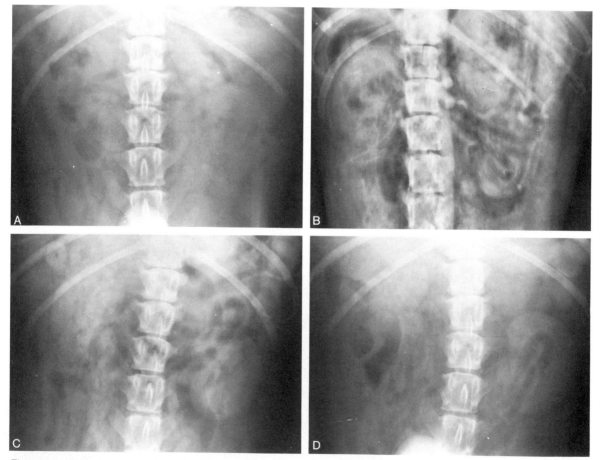

Figure 37–10. Ventrodorsal views immediately before (A), 10 seconds after (B), 5 minutes after (C), and 40 minutes after (D) injection of contrast medium for excretory urography. The size of the kidneys is normal but nephrographic opacification is poor and does not fade with time. Microscopic diagnosis: glomerulonephritis secondary to systemic lupus erythematosus.

Related Abnormal Radiographic Findings

Intra-abdominal Findings Related to Renal Disease. Other organs in the abdomen may be displaced secondary to renal masses.[51] In general, enlargement or a space-occupying mass originating within the left kidney displaces the colon ventrally and the small intestine downward and to the right.[4] Space-occupying masses or enlargement of the right kidney result in displacement of the small intestine (including the duodenum) downward, caudally, and toward the left. In patients with chronic renal disease, mineralization of the gastric rugae may occur.[46] Hypoproteinemia secondary to the nephrotic syndrome may result in ascites. Loss of retroperitoneal contrast due to effusion (urine or blood most often from renal trauma) may be noted on survey radiographs and confirmed at excretory urography (Fig. 37–11).

Extra-abdominal Findings Related to Renal Disease. Other tissues, including cutaneous and vascular structures, may undergo calcification secondary to chronic renal disease.[51] Hypertrophic osteopathy (previously referred to as hypertrophic pulmonary osteoarthropathy) may be encountered secondary to renal neoplasms in the absence of pulmonary metastases.[52, 53]

THE URETERS

Imaging Procedures

The general procedure for interpretation of the kidney should be used to evaluate the ureters. The gamut approach provides the most logical means of assessing radiographically identifiable abnormalities and their potential relationship to disease processes. In addition, the use of gamuts permits a rational approach to further

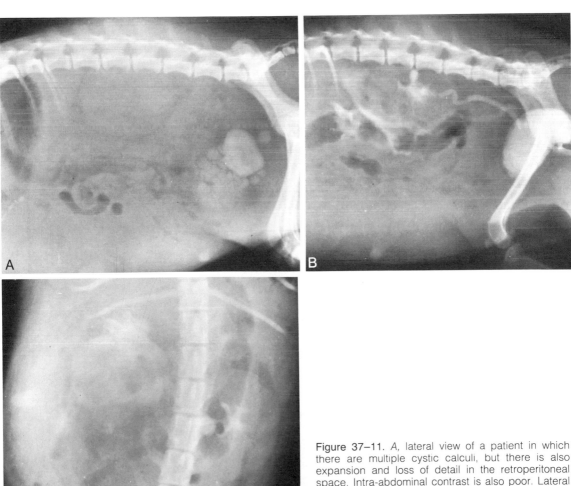

Figure 37–11. *A,* lateral view of a patient in which there are multiple cystic calculi, but there is also expansion and loss of detail in the retroperitoneal space. Intra-abdominal contrast is also poor. Lateral *(B)* and ventrodorsal *(C)* views 30 minutes after injection of contrast medium for excretory urography reveal prominent discontinuity of the right ureter with extravasation of contrast medium into the retroperitoneal space. Radiologic diagnosis: ruptured right ureter.

diagnostic procedures (radiographic or otherwise) that may be necessary to achieve a final diagnosis.

The imaging procedures described for the kidney are equally applicable to the ureter. These techniques are described in the preceding section.

Normal Radiographic Findings

The normal ureters are not visible on survey radiographs. As visualized at excretory urography, there are usually two ureters,[6, 7] and the size of each is usually less than 2 to 3 mm in diameter as these structures exit the kidney. The shape of the ureters is tubular, with segmentation secondary to ureteral peristalsis for propulsion of urine from the renal pelvis to the trigone region of the bladder.[4, 5] The ureters are primarily retroperitoneal,[54] but become intraperitoneal as they approach their termination at the bladder trigone.[55, 56] As mentioned previously, the normal ureters are not seen on survey radiographs, and care should be exercised in the interpretation of the end-on view of the deep circumflex iliac artery as a survey radiographic abnormality related to the ureter.[6] The normal findings for excretory urography relative to the ureter have been described (Figs. 37–1 and 37–2).[4-7] The function of the ureter is principally assessed relative to the segmentation peristalsis, which can be noted on serial radiographs or at fluoroscopy.[4, 5] In general, if the ureter can be visualized in its entirety from the pelvis of the kidney to the trigone of the bladder, the possibilities of poor ureteral peristalsis, ureteral dilatation, or both must be considered.

Abnormal Radiographic Findings

Number. As described previously, agenesis and aplasia of the kidneys and their associated ureters have been reported. Ureteral duplication in the presence of renal duplication in dogs has also been described.[19]

Size, Shape, and Margination. Information pertaining to the size of the ureter, its overall shape, and the mucosal margin characteristics can be combined to assist in the differential diagnosis of ureteral disease. In the following discussion, this triad of roentgen signs is used and, if possible, differential considerations of disease processes are listed.

A diffusely enlarged ureter with a regular shape and smooth mucosal margins is most likely due to ureterectasia as a result of obstruction[4, 6, 57, 58] or to ureteral atony induced by infection.[49, 57, 58] Ureteral atony secondary to periureteral inflammation or blunt abdominal trauma has also been described.[6, 54] Primary megaureter may result in these signs, but this condition has not been documented as a single entity in dogs or cats. Ureteral dilatation secondary to chronic vesicoureteral reflux is possible, but is considered unlikely.[59] A common finding in ectopic ureter is that of diffuse dilatation of the abnormal ureter.[6, 55] The cause of this dilatation has not been identified, but it is likely to be a combination of obstruction, inflammation, and a developmental anomaly.

A focally enlarged ureter with smooth margination is most consistent with a ureterocele or diverticulum (Fig. 37–12).[60-62] In most instances, the ureterocele is a dilation of the submucosal or intramuscular portion of the intravesical ureter as it approaches its point of emptying within the trigone of the urinary

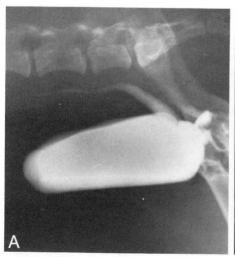
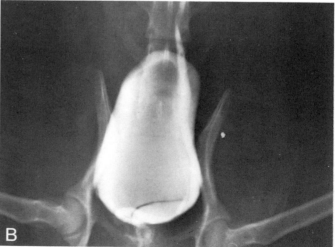

Figure 37–12. Lateral *(A)* and ventrodorsal *(B)* views of a patient 40 minutes after injection of contrast medium for excretory urography. The terminal portion of the left ureter is dilated in its intramural and submucosal path in the urinary bladder and terminates in the proximal urethra. Radiologic diagnosis: ectopic ureter with ureterocele.

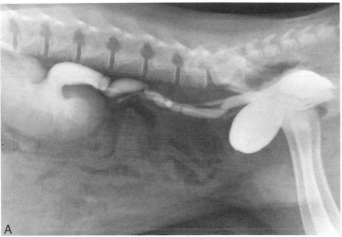
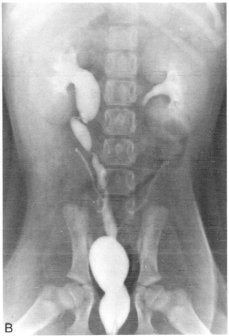

Figure 37–13. Lateral *(A)* and ventrodorsal *(B)* views of a patient 40 minutes after injection of contrast medium for excretory urography. The right ureter is extremely dilated as are the right renal pelvis and pelvic diverticula. The right ureter extends dorsal to the bladder trigone and ventral to the vestibule and terminates in the distal urethra. A previous retrograde vaginogram outlined the termination of this ureter as well as the urethral orifice, cervix, and uterine horns. Radiologic diagnosis: ectopic ureter.

bladder. The result is a space-occupying mass within the trigone region that must be differentiated from other bladder or trigonal abnormalities, including neoplasia.

Enlarged ureters of regular shape with roughened or irregular mucosal and mural margins along the entire ureter are suggestive of ureteral fibrosis secondary to chronic inflammation. If the process is focal, the major consideration is primary or metastatic neoplasia; ureteral neoplasia is uncommon.

A small ureter with regular and smooth margins is most likely due to inadequate contrast medium dose or primary renal oliguria, if the variation involves the entire ureter. If there is a focal decrease in size, compression from an extramural source must be considered. A small, irregularly shaped, rough-margined focal abnormality in a ureter is most likely suggestive of stricture. Stricture may be due to previous trauma, focal inflammation and secondary fibrosis, or neoplasia.

Location. The abnormal location of the ureter that is most often encountered is ectopic ureter, in which the distal portion of the ureter terminates at a point other than the bladder trigone.[55, 56] The most common site of abnormal ureteral termination is the vagina, followed in relative frequency by the urethra, bladder neck, and uterus. As mentioned in the preceding section, the affected ureter is usually abnormal throughout its length as well as at its sight of

termination; a representative example is shown in Figure 37–13. Another possible cause for abnormal location of the distal portion of the ureter is avulsion, usually due to trauma of the ureter from the bladder neck. In this instance, retroperitoneal effusion may also occur.

Radiopacity. On survey radiographs, the differential diagnostic considerations for air and mineral in the ureters are similar to those described for the kidney. Air in the ureters is most likely associated with vesicoureteral reflux during negative-contrast mediums studies of the urinary bladder. Mineralization of the ureter is rare; most mineral opacities in the area of the ureter represent calculi.[4, 6] Loss of retroperitoneal contrast may be an indirect indication of the accumulation of blood or urine or both, one cause of which may be ureteral rupture. This loss of retroperitoneal contrast must be interpreted in light of the body fat status in the remainder of the patient. An example of loss of retroperitoneal contrast due to ureteral rupture and retroperitoneal urine collection is shown in Figure 37–11.

During excretory urography, a reproducible filling defect in the contrast medium column in the ureter may be due to a calculus,[4, 6] a neoplasm, or a stricture secondary to disease or external compression. Assessment of the margination and opacity of these structures on survey radiographs in combination with the size, shape, and margination of the ureter at excretory urography can help to differentiate these considerations. Nonvisualization of a ureteral segment is usually normal, because it is due to peristalsis.[4, 5, 7] This segment of the ureter should, however, be visualized at some time in the sequence of radiographs. If the segment is not seen during the sequence, especially in the presence of contrast accumulation in the retroperitoneal space or loss of retroperitoneal contrast, ureteral rupture should be considered (Fig. 37–11).[54]

Function. Ureteral atony or hypotonia can be induced secondary to intraluminal infection, periureteral inflammation, trauma, or ureteral obstruction (Figs. 37–8 and 37–13).[4, 6, 50, 54, 57, 58] Differentiation among these possible etiologies requires complete assessment of the size, shape, and margination of the opacified ureter, as well as observation of the site and character of ureteral termination. Comparison with the results of urine cytology and culture is also of value.

Vesicoureteral reflux is the retroflow of urinary bladder contents into the ureter, either as a low pressure phenomenon in the presence of incompletely filled bladder or as a high pressure phenomenon in the presence of a filled bladder or during voiding.[59] Vesicoureteral reflux may be encountered in immature small animals and may be induced during retrograde radiographic procedures. Reflux may also be induced secondary to manual compression of the urinary bladder in an attempt to perform studies such as voiding urethrography. The major significance of vesicoureteral reflux lies in the potential of retroflow of urine contaminated with pathologic organisms from the urinary bladder toward the kidney.

On the basis of the information provided regarding techniques of evaluation, normal radiographic appearance in both survey and contrast radiography, and the differential diagnostic possibilities of the various abnormal findings, the examiner should now be equipped to formulate a differential diagnosis in a given case. Textbooks of internal medicine should be consulted for the specific nonradiographically oriented tests that may be of value when methods other than exploratory laporatomy or additional radiography are required to make a definitive diagnosis.

A final cautionary statement relative to contrast medium and its effect on renal function: Azotemia is not a contraindication to excretory urography, provided the patient is adequately hydrated. In other specific disease processes in humans, it has been suspected that excretory urography is contraindicated, but the major underlying factor contributing to the contrast medium-induced problem in these patients appeared to be poor urinary flow secondary to inadequate hydration. For information concerning the specific pathophysiology and management of patients with the unlikely occurrence of contrast medium-induced renal disease or failure, readers are directed to textbooks on renal disease.

References

1. Finco DR, Thrall DE, and Duncan JR: The urinary system. *In* Catcott EJ (Ed): Canine Medicine, 4th Ed. Santa Barbara, CA, American Veterinary Publications, 1979, pp. 419–500.
2. Finco DR, Barsanti JA, and Crowell WA: The urinary system. *In* Pratt PW (Ed): Feline Medicine. Santa Barbara, CA, American Veterinary Publications, 1983, pp. 363–410.
3. Allan G: Radiology in the diagnosis of kidney disease. Aust Vet Pract *12*:97, 1982.
4. Feeney DA, Barber DL, and Osborne CA: Advances in canine excretory urography. *In* Proceedings 30th Gaines Veterinary Symposium. Gaines Dog Research Center, White Plains, NY, 1981, pp. 8–22.
5. Feeney DA, Barber DL, Johnston GR, et al: The excretory urogram: Techniques, normal radiographic appearance and misinterpretation. Comp Contin Ed Vet Pract *4*:233, 1982.
6. Kneller SK: Role of excretory urography in the diagnosis of renal and ureteral disease. Vet Clin North Am *4*:843, 1974.
7. Feeney DA, Thrall DE, Barber DL, et al: Normal canine excretory urogram: Effects of dose, time and individual dog variation. Am J Vet Res *40*:1596, 1979.
8. Feeney DA, Osborne CA, and Jessen CR: Effects of radiographic contrast media on results of the urinalysis with emphasis on specific gravity. J Am Vet Med Assoc *176*:1378, 1980.
9. Ruby AL, Ling GV, and Ackerman N: Effects of sodium diatrizoate on the in vitro growth of three common canine urinary bacterial species. Vet Radiol *24*:222, 1983.
10. Barber DL: Renal angiography in veterinary medicine. J Am Vet Radiol Soc *16*:187, 1975.
11. Resnick MI, and Sanders RC: Ultrasound in Urology. Baltimore, Williams & Wilkins, 1979.
12. Ling GV, Ackerman N, Lowenstine LJ, et al: Percutaneous nephropyelocentesis and nephropyelostomy in the dog. Am J Vet Res *40*:1605, 1979.
13. Finco DR, Stiles NS, Kneller SK, et al: Radiologic estimation of kidney size in the dog. J Am Vet Med Assoc *159*:995, 1971.
14. Barrett RB, and Kneller SK: Feline kidney measurement. Acta Radiol [Suppl] (Stockh) *319*:279, 1972.
15. Bartels JE: Feline intravenous urography. J Am Anim Hosp Assoc *9*:349, 1973.
16. Feeney DA, Barber DL and Osborne CA: Functional aspects of the nephrogram in excretory urography: A review. Vet Radiol *23*:42, 1982.
17. Thrall DE, and Finco DR: Canine excretory urography: Is quantity a function of BUN. J Am Anim Hosp Assoc *12*:446, 1976.
18. Robinson GW: Uterus uncornius and unilateral renal agenesis. J Am Vet Med Assoc *147*:516, 1965.
19. O'Hardley P, Carrig PB, and Unshaw R: Renal and urethral duplication in a dog. J Am Vet Med Assoc *174*:484, 1979.
20. Senior DF: Parasites of the canine urinary tract. *In* Kirk RW (Ed): Current Veterinary Therapy VIII. Philadelphia, WB Saunders, 1980, pp 1141–1143.
21. Barsanti JA, and Crowell W: Renal amyloidosis. *In*

Kirk RW (Ed): Current Veterinary VII. Philadelphia, WB Saunders, 1980, pp. 1063–1066.

22. Brace JJ: Perirenal cysts (pseudocysts) in the cat. *In* Kirk RW (Ed): Current Veterinary Therapy VIII. Philadelphia, WB Saunders, 1983, pp. 980–981.

23. Stowater JL: Congenital solitary renal cyst in a dog. J Am Anim Hosp Assoc 11:199, 1975.

24. Caywood DD, Osborne CA, and Johnston GR: Neoplasms of the canine and feline urinary tracts. *In* Kirk RW (Ed): Current Veterinary Therapy. Philadelphia, WB Saunders, 1980, pp. 1203–1212.

25. McKenna SC, and Carpenter JL: Polycystic disease of the kidney and liver in the canine terrier. Vet Pathol 17:436, 1980.

26. Northington JW, and Juliana MM: Polycystic kidney disease in a cat. J Small Anim Pract 18:663, 1977.

27. Rendano VT, and Parker RB: Polycystic kidneys and peritoneal pericardial diaphragmatic hernia in a cat. J Small Anim Pract 17:479, 1976.

28. Crowell WA, Hubbell JJ, and Riley JC: Polycystic renal disease in related cats. J Am Vet Med Assoc 175:286, 1979.

29. Osborne CA, Johnson KH, Kurtz HJ, et al: Renal lymphoma in the dog & cat. J Am Vet Med Assoc 158:2058, 1971.

30. Batterschell D, and Garcia JP: Renal lymphosarcoma in a cat. Mod Vet Pract 50:51, 1969.

31. Barber DL: Radiographic evaluation of a focal inflammatory renal lesion. J Am Anim Hosp Assoc 12:451, 1976.

32. Chalifoux A, Phaneuf JB, Oliver N, et al: Glomerular polycystic kidney disease in a dog. Can Vet J 23:365, 1982.

33. Witcock BP, and Patterson JM: Familial glomerulonephritis in Doberman pinscher dogs. Can Vet J 20:211, 1070.

34. Bernard MA, and Valli VE: Familial renal disease in Samoyed dogs. Can Vet J 18:181, 1977.

35. Burk RL, and Barton CL: Renal failure and hyperparathyroidism in an Alaskan malamute pup. J Am Vet Med Assoc 172:64, 1978.

36. DiBartola SP, Chew J, and Boyce JT: Juvenile renal disease in related standard poodles. J Am Vet Med Assoc 183:693, 1983.

37. English PB, and Winter H: Renal cortical hypoplasia in a dog. Aust Vet J 55:181, 1979.

38. Chew DJ, DiBartola SP, Boyce JT, et al: Juvenile renal disease in Doberman pinscher dogs. J Am Vet Med Assoc 182:481, 1983.

39. Finco DR, Kurtz HJ, Low DG, et al: Familial renal disease in Norwegian elkhound dogs. J Am Vet Med Assoc 156:747, 1970.

40. O'Brien TD, Osborne CA, Yano BC, et al: Clinicopathologic manifestations of progressive renal disease in Lhasa Apso and Shih Tzu dogs. J Am Vet Med Assoc 180:658, 1982.

41. Finco DR: Congenital and inherited renal disease. J Am Anim Hosp Assoc 9:301, 1973.

42. Lucke VM, Kelly DF, Darke PG, et al: Chronic renal failure in young dogs—possible renal dysplasia. J Small Anim Pract 21:169, 1980.

43. Wells MJ, Coyne JA, and Prince JL: Ectopic kidney in a cat. Mod Vet Pract 61:693, 1980.

44. Johnson CA: Renal ectopia in a cat. J Am Anim Hosp Assoc 15:599, 1979.

45. Osborne CA, Klausner JJ, and Clinton CW: Analysis of canine and feline uroliths. *In* Kirk RW (Ed): Current Veterinary Therapy VIII. Philadelphia, WB Saunders, 1983, pp. 1061–1066.

46. Barber DL, and Rowland GN: Radiographically detectable soft tissue calcification in chronic renal failure. Vet Radiol 20:117, 1979.

47. Hall MA, Osborne CA, and Stevens JB: Hydronephrosis with hetero plastic bone formation in a cat. J Am Vet Med Assoc 160:857, 1972.

48. Miller JB, and Sande RD: Osseous metaplasia in the renal pelvis of a dog with hydronephrosis. Vet Radiol 21:146, 1980.

49. Fuller WJ: Subacute pyelonephritis with a unilaterally non-visualized pyelogram. J Am Anim Hosp Assoc 12:509, 1976.

50. Barber DL, and Finco DR: Radiographic findings in induced bacterial pyelonephritis in dogs. J Am Vet Med Assoc 175:1183, 1979.

51. Root CN: Interpretation of abdominal survey radiographs. Vet Clin North Am 4:763, 1974.

52. Caywood DD, Osborne CA, Stevens JB, et al: Hypertrophic osteoarthropathy associated with a typical nephroblastoma in a dog. J Am Anim Hosp Assoc 16:855, 1980.

53. Nafe LA, Herron AJ, and Burk RL: Hypertrophic osteopathy in a cat associated with renal papillary adenoma. J Am Anim Hosp Assoc 17:659, 1981.

54. Selcer BA: Urinary tract trauma associated with pelvic trauma. J Am Anim Hosp Assoc 18:785, 1982.

55. Faulkner RT, Osborne CA, and Feeney DA: Canine and feline urethral ectopia. *In* Kirk RW (Ed): Current Veterinary Therapy VIII. Philadelphia, WB Saunders, 1983, pp. 1043–1048.

56. Owen RR: Canine urethral ectopia. J Small Anim Pract 14:407, 1983.

57. Rose JG, and Gillenwater JY: Effects of obstruction on urethral function. Urology 12:139, 1978.

58. Rose JG, and Gillenwater JY: Effect of chronic ureteral obstruction and infection upon ureteral function. Invest Urol 11:471, 1974.

59. Klausner JS, and Feeney DA: Vesicoureteral reflux. *In* Kirk RW (Ed): Current Veterinary Therapy VIII. Philadelphia, WB Saunders, 1983, pp. 1041–1043.

60. Scott RC, Greene RW, and Patnaik AK: Unilateral ureterocele associated with hydronephrosis in a dog. J Am Anim Hosp Assoc 10:126, 1974.

61. Smith CW, and Park RD: Bilateral ectopic ureteroceles in a dog. Canine Pract 1:28, 1974.

62. Stowater JL, and Springer AL: Ureterocele in a dog. Vet Med/Small Anim Pract 74:1753, 1979.

CHAPTER 38

THE URINARY BLADDER

RICHARD D. PARK

SURVEY RADIOGRAPHIC EXAMINATION

The urinary bladder is a distensible, round to ovoid, hollow visceral organ in the caudal abdomen. It serves as a storage reservoir and voiding organ for urine.

Survey radiographic examination of the urinary bladder usually consists of lateral and ventrodorsal views. The lateral view provides the best radiographic visualization of the bladder. Good radiographic visualization is limited in the ventrodorsal view by superimposition of the spine and large bowel over the urinary bladder. Oblique views can be made to help compensate for poor radiographic visualization on the ventrodorsal view.

Normal Anatomy

The urinary bladder is divided grossly into three parts: the vertex (apex vesicae) cranially, the body (corpus vesicae) in the middle, and the neck (cervix vesicae) caudally (Fig. 38–1).[1-3] Three ligaments formed from peritoneal reflections hold the bladder loosely in position.[3] The middle bladder ligament (ligamenta vesicae medianum) extends along the ventral bladder surface and two lateral ligaments (ligamentae vesicae laterale) extend along the lateral bladder surfaces. These ligaments are often associated with large fat deposits facilitating radiographic visualization of the bladder neck and body. The cranial and dorsal surfaces of the bladder are radiographically visible because of adjacent fat within the omentum and mesentery (Fig. 38–2).

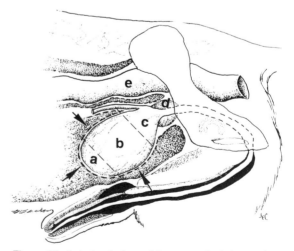

Figure 38–1. Lateral view of the normal abdomen in a male dog. a: vertex; b: body of the bladder; c: neck of the urinary bladder; d: prostate; e: large bowel. The broken line around the urinary bladder *(arrows)* represents the peritoneal reflection around and adherent to the serosal surface of the urinary bladder.

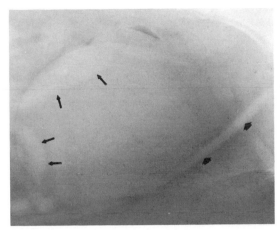

Figure 38–2. Lateral radiograph of a normal caudal abdomen in the dog. The bladder neck is well visualized because of fat within the bladder ligaments. The rectus abdominis muscle *(short arrows)* is ventral to the bladder. Superimposed bowel *(long arrows)* is over the cranial and dorsal borders of the bladder.

The urinary bladder wall is a musculomembranous structure consisting of mucosal, submucosal, and muscular layers, with the peritoneum closely adherent to the serosal surface providing a separate fourth layer. The muscle layers of the bladder wall and the mucosal surface of the bladder cannot be distinguished as separate structures on survey radiographs because the adjacent urine projects as the same radiographic opacity as the bladder wall.

Radiographic visualization of the urinary bladder is compromised by insufficient abdominal fat and superimposition opacities. Emaciated or young animals may not have sufficient abdominal fat deposits to provide good tissue contrast adjacent to the urinary bladder. Ingested material in the small bowel, fecal material in the large bowel, muscle tissue from the

hind legs, and bone from the spine and pelvis cause superimposition opacities that may obliterate all or part of the urinary bladder on a radiograph. These superimposition compromises can be eliminated or minimized by withholding food for 24 hours before the study, giving enemas to clear the large bowel, and pulling the hind limbs caudally while the radiograph is made.

The normal urinary bladder is a dynamic organ that varies in size, shape, and position. These normal variations within and between species should be known and taken into consideration when observing the urinary bladder radiographically.

Bladder size varies with the amount of urine in the bladder. After voiding, the bladder is small or not visible radiographically. With extreme distension, the cranial bladder border may extend to the umbilicus. Severe distension may occur in a normal bladder if the animal has not had an opportunity to void or will not void because of a strange or unfamiliar environment. The urinary bladder in the dog is usually oval, but with distension it becomes more ellipsoid (Fig. 38–3A). The feline urinary bladder is almost always ellipsoid (Fig. 38–3B).

The bladder is positioned within the abdomen, cranial to the pubis or pubis and prostate, dorsal to the rectus abdominus muscle, caudal to the small bowel and omentum, and ventral to the large bowel or large bowel and uterus. The urinary bladder in a dog may be displaced cranially from the pubis with extreme bladder distension. The long bladder neck in the cat cannot always be visualized radiographically. The urinary bladder in the cat therefore appears to be displaced cranially from the pubis approximately 2 to 3 cm.[1] A normal empty or small urinary bladder may be partially within the

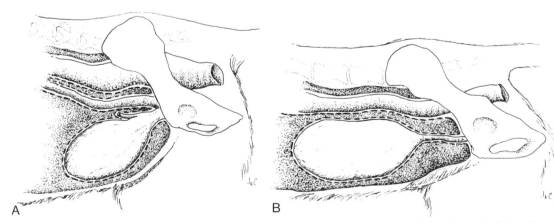

Figure 38–3. *A*, a normal bladder in a female dog. The bladder is adjacent to the pubis and is oval. *Broken line*, the peritoneal reflection around the bladder. *B*, normal bladder in a cat. The bladder is elliptic and has a long neck, which makes the bladder appear to be displaced cranially away from the pubis. *Broken line*, the peritoneal reflection around the bladder. (From Park RD: Radiology of the urinary bladder and urethra. Chap. 12. *In* O'Brien TR (Ed): Radiographic Diagnosis of Abdominal Disorders in the Dog and Cat. Davis, CA, Covell Park Vet. Co., 1981, with permission.)

pelvis; with moderate bladder filling, however, it usually moves to a position cranial to the pubis. Occasionally, a normal urinary bladder may remain partially within the pelvis even when distended.[5]

The urinary bladder projects as a structure of soft-tissue opacity radiographically. Any opacity greater or less than that of soft tissue detected within the bladder on survey radiographs is abnormal.

Radiographic Signs of Urinary Bladder Disease

Signs of urinary bladder disease on survey radiographs are somewhat limited. In many instances the signs indicate disease in adjacent structures. Signs that indicate disease of the urinary bladder or of adjacent structures are poor or nonexistent bladder visualization and abnormal bladder position, shape, size, and opacity (Table 38–1).

Inadequate or nonexistent radiographic visualization of the urinary bladder may occur with good or poor serosal detail in the caudal abdomen. The bladder is either empty or displaced from its normal position if it is not visualized, and the caudal abdominal serosal detail is good. Free peritoneal fluid is present or there is inadequate peritoneal fat if the bladder is indistinctly visualized, and serosal detail in the caudal abdomen is poor (Fig. 38–4).

The bladder can be abnormally displaced in all directions.[6] The cause of the displacement can often be determined radiographically by observing the surrounding structures (Fig.

TABLE 38–1. URINARY BLADDER: SURVEY RADIOGRAPHIC SIGNS

Radiographic Sign	Gamut of Condition(s) or Disease(s)	Radiographic Sign	Gamut of Condition(s) or Disease(s)
Visualization		*Abnormal Position*	Perineal hernia
Bladder not seen; abdominal serosal outlines are clear	Post-voiding	Caudal displacement	Large abdominal mass(es)
	Displaced bladder		Congenital anomalies
	Perineal hernia		"Short" urethra
	Inguinal hernia		Ectopic ureters
	Pelvic bladder		Congenital fistulas
	"Short" urethra		Normal pelvic bladder
	Ectopic ureter		
	Congenital fistulas	Dorsal displacement	Abdominal mass(es)
	Normal pelvic bladder	*Abnormal shape*	Mesenchymal neoplasia
Bladder not seen; abdominal serosal outlines are not clearly seen	Ruptured urinary bladder		Adjacent abdominal mass(es)
	Peritoneal fluid		Neoplasia
	Transudate		Abscess or granulomas
	Exudate	*Abnormal Size*	
	Hemorrhage	Increased size	Distal urinary obstruction
	Emaciated animal		Urethral obstruction
	Young animal less than 4 months of age		Bladder neck obstruction
Abnormal position			Neurologic deficiencies
Ventral displacement	Abdominal wall hernia	Decreased size	Congenital anomalies
	Inguinal hernia		Ectopic ureters
Cranial displacement	Prostatic disease		Fistulas
	Neoplasia		Diffuse bladder wall disease
	Prostatitis		Cystitis
	Prostatic cyst		Neoplasia
	Hypertrophy		Hemorrhage
	Enlarged uterus		
	Pyometra		
	Pregnancy	*Opacity Changes*	
	Sublumbar mass(es)	Increased	Calculi
	Large bowel distension		Bladder wall calcification
	Uterine "stump" granuloma or abscess		Neoplasia
	Persistent patent urachus or urachal ligament		Inflammation
		Decreased	Gas
			Iatrogenic
			Emphysematous cystitis

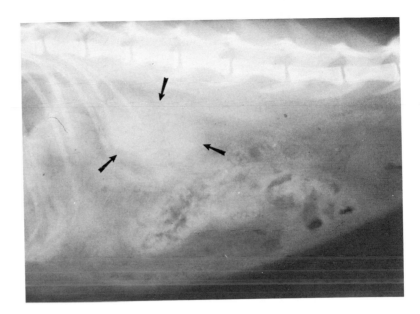

Figure 38–4. Lateral view of the abdomen of a cat. The kidneys are easily seen *(arrows)*. The serosal surfaces on the bowel and urinary bladder do not have distinct outlines because of free peritoneal fluid.

38–5). With severe bladder displacement, such as occurs with hernias, the bladder may not be seen on survey radiographs, but can be demonstrated with contrast cystography. A urinary bladder partially within the pelvic canal (Fig. 38–6) may be associated with congenital urinary tract anomalies[7] or may be a normal variation of position.[5]

Urinary bladder shape changes that can be observed on survey radiographs occur infrequently. Abdominal masses adjacent to the serosal surface of the bladder and occasionally leiomyomas or leiomyosarcomas originating from the bladder wall protrude from the serosal surface and produce discernible change in bladder shape (Fig. 38–7).[8] A pointed vertex with

the bladder appearing elongated may occur with a persistent urachal ligament in the cat.[9]

An abnormally small or large urinary bladder is difficult to diagnose from survey radiographs because of normal variation in bladder size. In most instances, a consistently small or large bladder with associated clinical signs is an indication that contrast studies should be performed. The cause for the small or large bladder can often be determined from the contrast examination(s).

Any change in radiographic opacity in the urinary bladder is abnormal and is usually easy to detect. Radiolucent opacity (gas) in the bladder may be iatrogenically introduced from catheterization. Small gas bubbles within the blad-

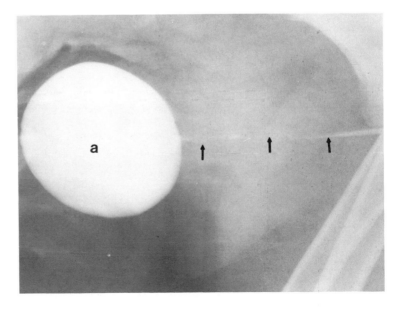

Figure 38–5. Positive-contrast cystogram, lateral caudal view, in a male dog. The urinary bladder (a) is displaced cranially from the pubis by a large prostatic mass. The urethra and bladder neck are filled with contrast medium *(arrows)*. Diagnosis: prostatic carcinoma.

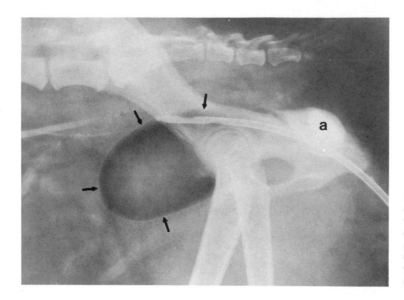

Figure 38–6. Lateral radiograph of the caudal abdomen and pelvis after intravenous urography and double contrast cystography. The urinary bladder is partially within the pelvis *(arrows)*. Contrast medium has accumulated in the vagina (a) because of an ectopic ureter.

Figure 38–7. Oblique view of the abdomen after double contrast cystography. A mass *(small arrows)* is present on the cranial aspect of the gas-filled bladder *(large arrows)*. The mass was a leiomyosarcoma originating from the bladder; it gave the bladder a bi-lobed appearance on the survey radiograph.

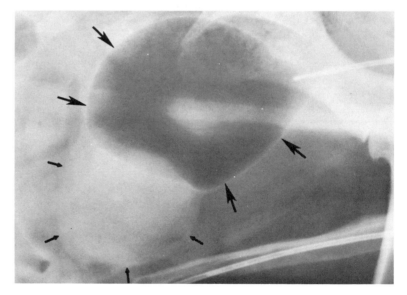

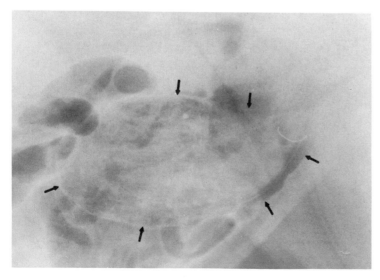

Figure 38–8. Lateral view of the abdomen of a dog with gas within the bladder wall, lumen, and bladder ligaments *(arrows)*. Gas in the surrounding bowel loops presents some difficulty in distinguishing gas within the bladder. The animal had cystitis caused by a gas-producing organism, but did not have diabetes mellitus.

TABLE 38–2. RADIOPACITY OF CYSTIC CALCULI ON SURVEY ABDOMINAL RADIOGRAPHS

Calculus Composition	Opacity
Calcium oxalate	Radiopaque
Calcium carbonate	Radiopaque
Triple phosphate	Radiopaque—small calculi may be nonradiopaque
Cystine	Nonradiopaque, but may have radiopaque stippling
Uric acid and urates	Nonradiopaque

der lumen are usually in the center of the bladder on the recumbent lateral view. Gas in the bladder lumen, wall, and occasionally within bladder ligaments occurs with emphysematous cystitis (Fig. 38–8). Emphysematous cystitis is produced by glucose-fermenting organisms and may be seen in association with diabetes mellitus.[10, 11] Occurrence of emphysematous cystitis without diabetes mellitus also has been reported.[12, 13] Most radiopacities associated with the bladder are calculi. Not all calculi are radiopaque (Table 38–2), however, and thus the absence of radiopacities within the bladder does not completely rule out the presence of cystic calculi

CONTRAST CYSTOGRAPHY

Retrograde contrast cystography is a fast, simple, and inexpensive technique that may provide valuable prognostic and diagnostic information about bladder disease. Indications for contrast cystography are obtained from clinical and radiographic signs. Clinical indications include frequent urination with small urine volumes, intermittent or chronic hematuria, and dysuria. Radiographic signs that indicate the need for contrast cystography include identification of increased or decreased opacity that may be associated with the urinary bladder, evaluation of caudal abdominal masses that may be associated with the urinary bladder, nonvisualization of the bladder after abdominal trauma, and evaluation of the urinary bladder that has an abnormal shape or location.

Voiding cystography is not discussed in detail; the reader is referred to other publications for additional information.[14-18] Voiding cystography, coupled with cystometry, is the technique of choice to investigate dynamic bladder diseases, such as urinary incontinence or other voiding abnormalities.

Technique

If possible, food should be withheld for 24 hours and a warm-water enema is administered before a cystogram is performed. Fecal material superimposed on the urinary bladder may obliterate valuable radiographic information.

All catheters and equipment should be sterilized and the genitalia should be cleansed before catheterizing the bladder. Equipment necessary for bladder catheterization is illustrated in Figure 38–9. To reduce bladder pain and spasm during cystography, 5 to 10 ml of 2 percent lidocaine (Xylocaine) without epinephrine may be injected before the procedure is performed.

Complications resulting from catheterization and cystographic procedures occur infrequently and are usually not detrimental to the animal. Iatrogenic trauma, bacterial contamination,[19] or kinked[20] and knotted urethral catheters may occur from improper catheterization techniques. Intramural accumulation of contrast medium in the bladder (Fig. 38–10) has been reported after maximal bladder distension with

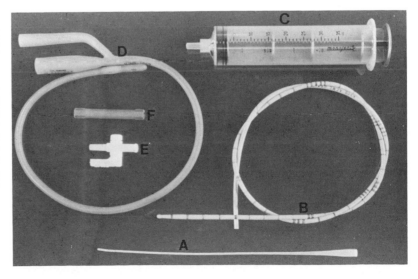

Figure 38–9. Equipment for bladder catheterization and cystographic procedures: A: Tom Cat catheter; B: male urethral catheter; C: a large volume syringe; D: a Foley (balloon-type) catheter; E: a three-way valve; and F: a catheter connector for use with the male urethral catheter. (From Park RD: Radiology of the urinary bladder and urethra. Chap. 12. *In* O'Brien TR (Ed): Radiographic Diagnosis of Abdominal Disorders in the Dog and Cat. Davis, CA, Covell Park Vet. Co., 1981, with permission.)

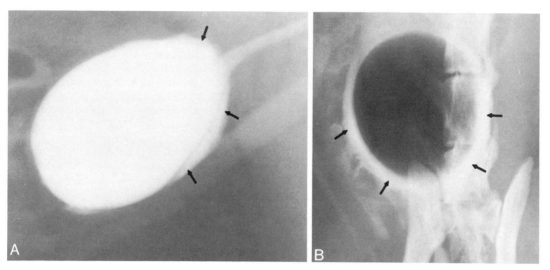

Figure 38–10. Positive- *(A)* and double-contrast *(B)* cystograms demonstrate subserosal accumulation of contrast medium *(arrows)*. This occurrence usually produces no severe or long-lasting complications, is produced by a high intraluminal bladder pressure, and is predisposed by bladder disease, particularly inflammation.

a Foley catheter.[21-24] Mucosal ulceration, inflammation, and granulomatous reactions may occur, but the changes are usually transitory and produce no serious clinical problems. The most serious complication from negative-contrast cystography is gas embolization into the circulatory system, which may result in death.[25, 26] Fortunately such complications occur only rarely and can be prevented by using nitrous oxide or carbon dioxide instead of room air.

Both negative- and positive-contrast media are used for contrast cystography. Negative-contrast media are room air, carbon dioxide, or nitrous oxide. Positive-contrast media are organic iodides in a 10 percent solution (Table 38–3) and barium sulfate. Complications from barium sulfate reflux make it less desirable as a contrast medium for cystography.[21, 27] Organic iodides are the recommended contrast media for cystography. The volume of contrast medium used for cystography varies with body weight, species, and pathologic process present. An approximation of 10 ml per kilogram body weight can be used. The injection should be terminated before the estimated volume has

TABLE 38–3. **ORGANIC IODIDES* AVAILABLE FOR CONTRAST CYSTOGRAPHY**

Brand Name	Generic Name	Manufacturer
Angio-Conray	80% Na iothalamate	Mallinckrodt†
Conray	60% Meglumine iothalamate	Mallinckrodt
Conray-30	30% Meglumine iothalamate	Mallinckrodt
Conray-400	66.8% Na iothalamate	Mallinckrodt
Hypaque Sodium 20%	20% Na diatrizoate	Winthrop‡
Hypaque Sodium 25%	25% Na diatrizoate	Winthrop
Hypaque Sodium 50%	50% Na diatrizoate	Winthrop
Hypaque-M 75%	25% Na diatrizoate and 50% meglumine diatrizoate	Winthrop
Hypaque-M 90%	30% Na diatrizoate and 60% meglumine diatrizoate	Winthrop
Hypaque Meglumine 60%	60% Meglumine diatrizoate	Winthrop
Renografin-60	52% Meglumine diatrizoate and 8% Na diatrizoate	Squibb & Sons§
Renografin-76‖	66% Meglumine diatrizoate and 10% Na diatrizoate	Squibb & Sons
Reno-M-60	60% Meglumine diatrizoate	Squibb & Sons
Renovist‖	35% Na diatrizoate and 34.3% meglumine diatrizoate	Squibb & Sons

*Should be diluted 0 to 10% solutions.
†Mallinckrodt Chemical Works, Diagnostic Products Division, P.O. Box 5439, St. Louis, MO 63160.
‡Winthrop Laboratories, 90 Park Avenue, New York, NY 10016.
§Squibb Laboratories, E. R. Squibb & Sons, Inc., Georges Road, New Brunswick, NJ 08903.
‖Approved for veterinary use by the U.S. Food and Drug Administration.

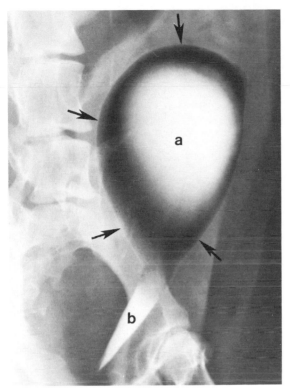

Figure 38-11. Oblique radiograph of a normal double-contrast cystogram. The urinary bladder wall *(arrows)* is clearly seen. The contrast "puddle" in the dependent portion of the bladder (a) and the contrast medium-filled urethra (b) are easily identified.

been administered if the bladder feels adequately distended by external palpation, if reflux occurs around the catheter, or if back pressure is felt on the syringe plunger. Four radiographic views of the caudal abdomen (one recumbent lateral, one ventrodorsal, and two recumbent obliques) should be made to examine the contrast medium–filled bladder adequately.

Cystographic Procedures

Retrograde positive- and double-contrast procedures are best for studying adynamic bladder conditions. Positive-contrast cystography is performed by injecting a 10 percent solution of an organic iodide compound into the bladder via a urethral catheter. The procedure is the method of choice for identifying the bladder location and demonstrating bladder tears or ruptures.

A double-contrast cystogram can be performed by injecting a small volume of positive-contrast medium into the bladder (10 to 15 ml) followed by bladder distension with negative-contrast medium (Fig. 38–11). Double-contrast cystography is superior for demonstrating pathologic conditions affecting the bladder wall and intraluminal filling defects. The selection of positive- or double-contrast cystography is based on clinical history, clinical signs, radiographic signs, and the character of aspirate obtained with bladder catheterization (Fig. 38–12).

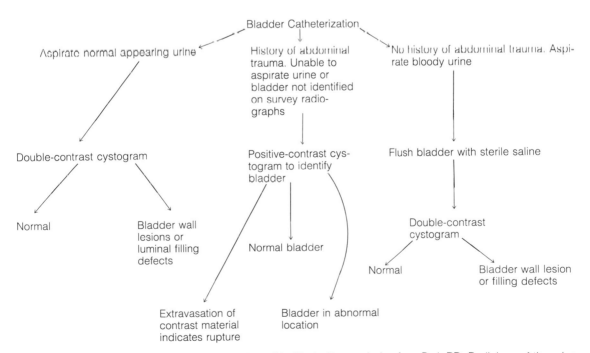

Figure 38–12. Selection of cystographic procedure. (Modified with permission from Park RD: Radiology of the urinary bladder and urethra. *In* O'Brien TR (Ed): Radiographic Diagnosis of Abdominal Disorders in the Dog and Cat. Davis, CA, Covell Park Veterinary Co., 1981, with permission.)

TABLE 38–4. RADIOGRAPHIC SIGNS OF PATHOLOGIC PROCESSES OF THE BLADDER

Disease	Mucosal Changes		Intramural Thickening		Filling Defect		Contrast Extravasation	
	Focal	Diffuse	Focal	Diffuse	Attached	Free	Smooth	Irregular
Chronic cystitis	Cranioventral	Occasional	Cranioventral	Occasional (cytoxan-induced cystitis)	Blood clots	Blood clots Calculi	—	—
Polypoid cystitis	Cranioventral	—	Cranioventral	—	Cranioventral	Blood clots	—	—
Acute cystitis	—	—	—	—	—	Occasional blood clots	—	—
Cystic calculi	Cranioventral from cystitis	—	Cranioventral from cystitis	—	—	Calculi and occasional blood clots	—	—
Neoplasia	Any location within bladder	Occasional	Any location within bladder	Occasional	Sessile, occasionally pedunculated	Blood clots	—	—
Bladder contusion	Any location	Large areas of bladder often involved	Any location	Large areas of bladder often involved	Bladder wall hematoma	Blood clots	—	—
Bladder rupture or perforation	—	—	—	—	—	Blood clots	—	Most extravasate is into peritoneal cavity
Traumatic diverticuli	—	—	—	—	—	Blood clots	Any location	—
Urachal diverticuli	Cranioventral associated with cystitis	—	Cranioventral associated with cystitis	—	—	—	Cranioventral	—

Radiographic Signs with Contrast Cystography

Radiographic signs observed with urinary bladder diseases are mucosal changes, intramural thickening, filling defects, and extravasation patterns (Table 38–4). These changes must be differentiated from air bubbles and inadequate bladder distension, which may produce misleading information. By noting the number, severity, and distribution of radiographic signs, a specific diagnosis can usually be postulated. If a specific diagnosis cannot be made, the bladder condition, as to normal or abnormal, can be demonstrated. If nonspecific radiographic signs are present or further confirmation is necessary, additional diagnostic tests can be made.

Mucosal Changes. The urinary bladder has a transitional epithelium, which appears smooth on a normal contrast cystogram. The transitional bladder epithelium is capable of metaplastic, neoplastic, and non-neoplastic proliferation.[28] Mucosal proliferation appears as an irregular outline along the inside bladder surface, and may be accentuated with inadequate bladder distension. The distribution of mucosal irregularity is usually focal, but it may be diffuse; it may vary in severity from a slight irregular "brush-type" surface to a severe "cobblestone" appearance (Fig. 38–13). Ulcers may be present with mucosal proliferation. On a double-contrast cystogram, ulcers can be identified if contrast medium adheres to the ulcerated surface.

Intramural Changes (Bladder Wall Thickening). A normal distended bladder has a wall approximately 1 mm thick. Intramural changes are best demonstrated with double-contrast cystography, and consist of increased bladder wall thickness that is usually focal but may be diffuse (Fig. 38–14). Bladder wall thickening may be caused by cellular infiltration or fibrous tissue proliferation. Cellular infiltration may result from inflammation, hemorrhage from trauma, or neoplasia. The bladder should be maximally distended to diagnose bladder wall thickening on cystography. Intramural bladder thickening causes decreased bladder distensibility, which may be symmetric with diffuse intramural bladder disease, or asymmetric with focal intramural bladder disease.

Filling Defects. A bladder filling defect is anything occupying space within the bladder lumen that alters normal filling; such a defect occupies space normally filled with contrast

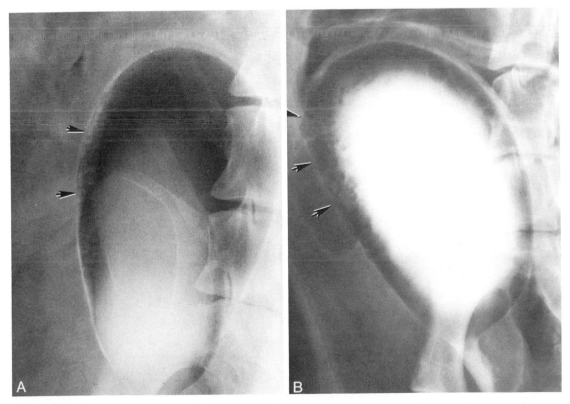

Figure 38–13. *A,* an oblique radiograph of the bladder during double-contrast cystography. There is mild mucosal irregularity along the right ventral bladder *(arrows)* caused by chronic bacterial cystitis. *B,* an oblique radiograph of the bladder during double contrast cystography. Severe mucosal irregularity and mild bladder wall thickening are present along the ventral right bladder *(arrows).*

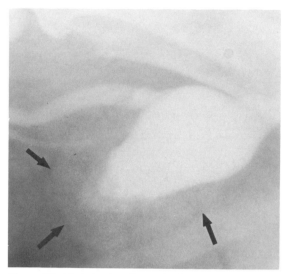

Figure 38–14. Lateral radiograph of the urinary bladder filled with positive contrast medium during intravenous urography. Diffuse bladder wall thickening is present as the result of cytoxan-induced cystitis. The serosal surface *(arrows)* is outlined by fat. Bladder distensibility is decreased by the severe intramural changes.

medium on a cystogram. All filling defects appear radiolucent when surrounded with positive-contrast medium. The size, shape, number, border contour, position within the bladder, and attachment to the bladder wall should be noted with all bladder filling defects. Observing these characteristics of filling defects helps to differentiate the nature of the filling defect and ultimately may prove helpful in arriving at a diagnosis (Table 38–5).

Filling defects can be categorized as free luminal filling defects and attached filling defects. Free luminal filling defects may be caused by air bubbles, calculi, or blood clots (Fig. 38–15). They are best demonstrated with double-contrast cystography and are seen within the dependent contrast puddle. Attached filling defects may be caused by neoplasia (Fig. 38–16), inflammatory polyps, blood clots, iatrogenic hematomas, and ureteroceles (Fig. 38–17).[29] Mucosal irregularity and ulcers are frequently present on the surface of large attached filling defects. Bladder wall infiltration may be diagnosed as a thickened bladder wall adjacent to the filling defect.[30] Although a specific diagnosis cannot always be made from the cystogram when attached filling defects are present, they can be identified by surgical removal, biopsy, or other diagnostic procedures.

Contrast Extravasation Patterns from the Urinary Bladder. Retrograde positive-contrast cystography best demonstrates extravasation patterns from the urinary bladder. Contrast medium extravasation may be within the urinary tract, communicating with other hollow visceral structures, or within the peritoneal cavity and surrounding soft tissues.

Contrast medium extravasation from the normal bladder confined within the urinary tract may be seen with vesicoureteral reflux, urachal anomalies, and traumatic bladder diverticuli (Fig. 38–18). Congenital urachal anomalies include diverticuli,[31] cysts, and persistent patent urachus.[32-35] The contrast medium borders produced by extravasation within the urinary tract are usually smooth and can be identified as extensions from the urinary bladder.

Contrast extravasation from the urinary bladder to adjacent hollow visceral structures may

TABLE 38–5. BLADDER FILLING DEFECTS

Lesion	Shape	Attachment	Border/Contour	Bladder Wall Infiltration (Thickening)
Calculi	Round to slightly irregular	Free in lumen	Indistinct	Variable. Usually cranioventral if associated with cystitis
Polyp	Pedunculated or convex	Stalk or sessile	Smooth or irregular, often with ulceration	Variable. Bladder wall may be thick at attachment site
Epithelial neoplasia	Irregular or convex	Sessile	Irregular, often with ulceration	Bladder wall often thick or infiltrated at base of attachment
Mesenchymal neoplasia	Convex	Sessile	Usually smooth	Originates within the bladder wall
Blood clots	Irregular	Variable. May be free luminal	Irregular and indistinct	Thickened bladder from primary disease process
Bladder wall hematoma	Convex	Sessile	Smooth to slightly irregular	Originates within the bladder wall
Ureterocele	Convex to round	Sessile	Smooth	Originates within the bladder wall of the trigone region

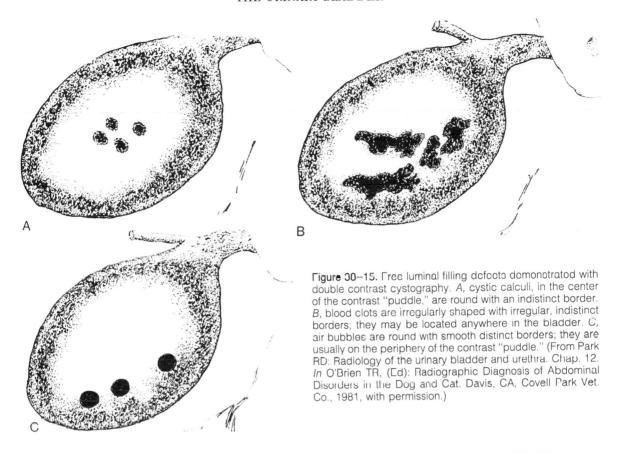

Figure 38–15. Free luminal filling defects demonstrated with double contrast cystography. A, cystic calculi, in the center of the contrast "puddle," are round with an indistinct border. B, blood clots are irregularly shaped with irregular, indistinct borders; they may be located anywhere in the bladder. C, air bubbles are round with smooth distinct borders; they are usually on the periphery of the contrast "puddle." (From Park RD: Radiology of the urinary bladder and urethra. Chap. 12. In O'Brien TR, (Ed): Radiographic Diagnosis of Abdominal Disorders in the Dog and Cat. Davis, CA, Covell Park Vet. Co., 1981, with permission.)

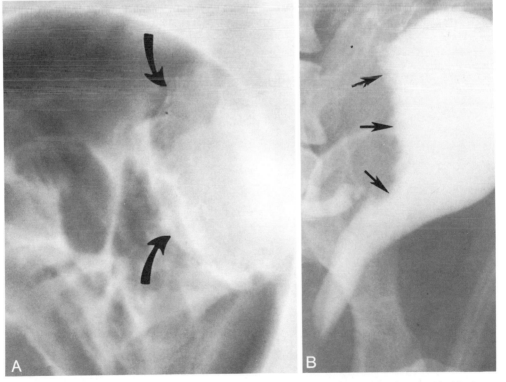

Figure 38–16. A, double-contrast cystogram. A large neoplastic mass (arrows) protrudes into the bladder lumen. There is minimal bladder wall infiltration. Contrast medium coats the ulcerated surface of the neoplasm. B, a large neoplastic lesion (transitional cell carcinoma) is on the right side of the bladder (arrows). The neoplasm causes a large filling defect with an irregular surface. Decreased bladder distensibility and asymmetry are also present.

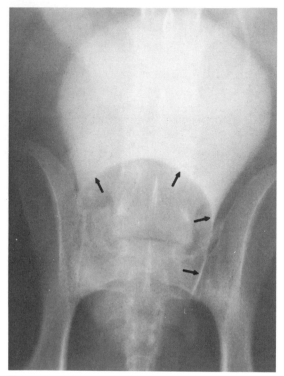

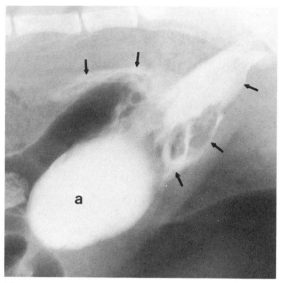

Figure 38–19. Positive-contrast cystogram in a cat. Contrast medium fills the urinary bladder (a), but extravasates into the peritoneal cavity *(arrows)*. This combination occurs most frequently with perforation or tears of the bladder neck.

Figure 38–17. Ventrodorsal radiograph of the bladder filled with contrast medium during intravenous urography. The smooth luminal filling defect *(arrows)* that projects into the bladder neck is a ureterocele.

be seen with either congenital or acquired fistulas. The most frequent organs involved are the rectum and vagina. The communicating segment is usually not outlined with contrast medium in such a way as to be detected radio-

graphically. Such fistulas are usually diagnosed in an indirect fashion on contrast cystograms, i.e., the structure that communicates with the bladder fills simultaneously or shortly after the bladder is filled with contrast medium.

Contrast extravasation into the peritoneal cavity and surrounding soft tissues has an irregular outline and usually occurs simultaneously with injection of contrast medium into the bladder (Fig. 38–19). With small bladder tears, extravasation of contrast medium may be slow,

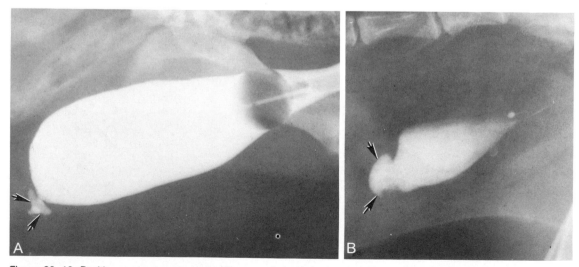

Figure 38–18. Positive-contrast cystogram with a small, irregular urachal diverticulum *(arrows)*. The air-filled balloon on the Foley catheter causes the filling defect within the bladder neck. *B,* A traumatic bladder diverticulum was identified *(arrows)*. Immediately after trauma, traumatic diverticuli must be differentiated from a bladder contusion. Contusions usually heal within 48 hours and the bladder will distend symmetrically.

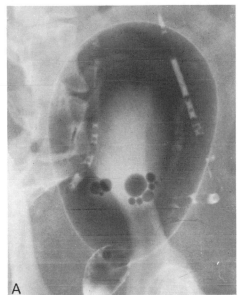

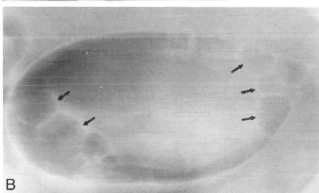

Figure 38–20. Air bubble artifacts created by cystographic procedures. *A,* small air bubbles that cause free luminal-type filling defects in the urinary bladder during double-contrast cystography. Bubbles are present in both ureters. *B,* "honeycomb" appearance created by several adjacent air bubbles *(arrows).* A large air bubble in a mostly fluid-filled bladder may produce a pseudothick bladder wall. *C,* positive contrast medium and gas may produce a similar pattern *(arrows).* The smooth borders of the pseudothick bladder wall are produced by the large air bubble border and the actual bladder wall or outer border of the contrast medium.

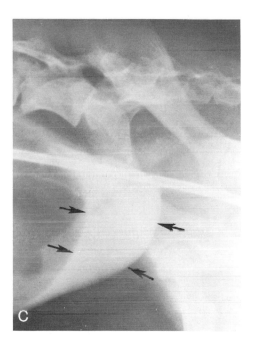

with only a small volume extravasated.[6, 35] In these instances, a second radiograph may be required 5 to 10 minutes after contrast medium injection for a positive diagnosis to be reached.

Pitfalls with Cystographic Interpretation

Interpretation pitfalls are changes noted on the radiograph that mimic actual pathologic changes. These changes are artifacts that are created during the cystographic procedure. Pitfalls commonly seen with contrast cystography are air bubble artifacts and pseudofilling defects.

There are three types of air bubble artifacts (Fig. 38–20): small air bubbles simulating calculi or other small luminal filling defects, a large air bubble simulating bladder wall thickening, and multiple air bubbles creating a honeycomb appearance. Air bubbles are radiolucent and have smooth distinct borders.

Pseudofilling defects may be mistaken for bladder neoplasia or other attached filling defects. These defects are created by inadequate bladder distension combined with external

pressure from adjacent abdominal structures. Pseudofilling defects have a smooth surface and taper on both borders (Fig. 38–21); they can be obliterated with further bladder distension.

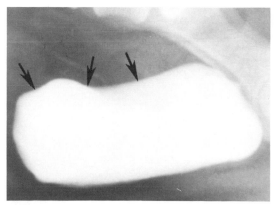

Figure 38–21. Lateral radiograph of a contrast medium-filled bladder during intravenous urography. Pseudofilling defects *(arrows)* are created by pressure on a partially distended bladder from adjacent abdominal structures.

438

References

1. Fletcher TF: Anatomy of pelvic viscera. Vet Clin North Am 4:471, 1974.
2. International Committee of Veterinary Anatomical Nomenclature: Nomina Anatomica Veterinaria. Adolf Holzhausen's successors, Vienna, 1973.
3. Miller ME, Christensen GC, and Evans HE: Anatomy of the Dog. Philadelphia, WB Saunders, 1964.
4. Nickel R, Schummer A, Seiferle E, et al: The Viscera of the Domestic Mammals. Berlin, Paul Parey, 1973.
5. Mahaffey MB, Barsanti JA, Barber DL, et al: Pelvic bladders in dogs without urinary incontinence. J Am Vet Med Assoc 184:1477, 1984.
6. Park RD: Radiology of the urinary bladder and urethra. In O'Brien TR (Ed): Radiographic Diagnosis of Abdominal Disorders in the Dog and Cat. Davis, CA, Covell Park Veterinary Co., 1981.
7. Adams WM, and DiBartola SP: Radiographic and clinical features of pelvic bladder in the dog. J Am Vet Med Assoc 182:1212, 1983.
8. Patnaik AK, and Greene RW: Intravenous leiomyoma of the bladder in a cat. J Am Vet Med Assoc 175:381, 1979.
9. Hansen JS: Persistent urachal ligament in the cat. Vet Med/Small Anim Clin 67:1090, 1972.
10. Root CR, and Scott RC: Emphysematous cystitis and other radiographic manifestations of diabetes mellitus in dogs and cats. J Am Vet Med Assoc, 158:721, 1971.
11. Ellenbogen PH, and Talner LB: Uroradiology of diabetes mellitus. Urology 8:413, 1967.
12. Middleton DJ, and Lomas GR: Emphysematous cystitis due to Clostridium perfringens in a non-diabetic dog. J Small Anim Pract 20:433, 1979.
13. Sherding RG, and Chew DJ: Nondiabetic emphysematous cystitis in two dogs. J Am Vet Med Assoc 174:1105, 1979.
14. Moreau PM, Lees GE, and Gross DR: Simultaneous cystometry and uroflowmetry (micturation study) for evaluation of the caudal part of the urinary tract in dogs: Studies of the technique. Am J Vet Res 44:1769, 1983.
15. Moreau PM, Lees GE, and Gross DR: Simultaneous cystometry and uroflowmetry (micturation study) for evaluation of the caudal part of the urinary tract function in dogs: Reference values for healthy animals sedated with xylazine. Am J Vet Res 44:1774, 1983.
16. Moreau PM, Lees GE, and Hobson HP: Simultaneous cystometry and uroflowmetry for evaluation of micturition in two dogs. J Am Vet Med Assoc 183:1083, 1983.
17. Rosin AE, and Barsanti JA: Diagnosis of urinary incontinence in dogs: Role of the urethral pressure profile. J Am Vet Med Assoc 178:814, 1981.
18. Oliver JE Jr, and Young WO: Air cystometry in dogs under xylazine-induced restraint. Am J Vet Res 34:1433, 1973.
19. Mooney JK Jr, Cox EC, and Heniman F: Vesical contamination from insertions of everting cot or catheter in inoculated canine urethra. Invest Urol 11:248, 1973.
20. Buchanan JW: Kinked catheter: A complication of pneumocystography. J Am Vet Radiol Soc 8:54, 1967.
21. Feeney DA, Johnston GR, Tomlinson MJ, et al: Effects of sterilized micropulverized barium sulfate suspension and meglumine iothalamate solution on the genitourinary tract of healthy male dogs after retrograde urethrocystography. Am J Vet Res 45:730, 1984.
22. Johnston GR, Stevens JB, Jessen CR, et al: Complications of retrograde contrast urethrography in dogs and cats. Am J Vet Res 44:1248, 1983.
23. Barsanti JA, Crowell W, Losonsky J, et al: Complications of bladder distention during retrograde urethrography. Am J Vet Res 42:819, 1981.
24. Farrow CS: Exercises in diagnostic radiology. Can Vet J 22:260, 1981.
25. Ackerman N, Wingfield WE, and Corley EA: Fatal air embolism associated with pneumourethrography and pneumocystography in a dog. J Am Vet Med Assoc 160:1616, 1972.
26. Thayer GW, Carrig CB, and Evans AT: Fatal venous air embolism associated with pneumocystography in a cat. J Am Vet Med Assoc 176:643, 1980.
27. Brodeur AE, Goyer RA, and Melick W: A potential hazard of barium cystography. Radiology 85:1080, 1965.
28. Mostofi FK: Potentialities of bladder epithelium. J Urol 71:705, 1954.
29. Stowater JL, and Springer AL: Ureterocele in a dog: A case report. Vet Med Small Anim Clin 74:1753, 1979.
30. Archibald J: Urinary system. In Archibald J (Ed): Canine Surgery, 1st Ed. Santa Barbara, American Veterinary Publications, 1965.
31. Green RW, and Bohning Jr RH: Patent persistent urachus associated with urolithiasis in a cat. J Am Vet Med Assoc 158:489, 1971.
32. Hansen JS: Patent urachus in a cat. Vet Med Small Anim Clin 67:379, 1972.
33. Osborne CA, Rhoades JD, and Hanlon GF: Patent urachus in the dog. Anim Hosp 2:245, 1966.
34. Scherzo CS: Cystic liver and persistent urachus in a cat. J Am Vet Med Assoc 151:1329, 1967.
35. Park RD: Radiographic contrast studies of the lower urinary tract. Vet Clin North Am 4:863, 1974.

CHAPTER 39

THE URETHRA

ROBERT D. PECHMAN, JR.

ANATOMY

The urethra is a sphincter and a conduit for urine from the bladder to the external environment.[1] The urethra in females is shorter in length and greater in diameter than that in males. It originates at the urinary bladder and terminates at the external urethral orifice on the ventral floor of the vagina. An external urethral sphincter is present in female dogs.[2]

The male urethra is long and thin and may be divided into three parts (Fig. 39–1). The prostatic urethra extends from the urinary bladder to the caudal border of the prostate gland. The membranous urethra extends from the caudal margin of the prostate gland to the urethral bulb of the penis in dogs and to the bulbourethral glands in cats. In both species, the distal extent of the membranous urethra is approximately at the caudal margin of the ischium. The penile urethra reaches from the caudal edge of the pelvis to the tip of the penis. The penile urethra is considerably smaller than the membranous urethra in cats; in dogs, it is partially surrounded dorsally by the os penis.[1, 2]

SURVEY RADIOGRAPHY

Radiographic evaluation of the urethra is performed most often on male dogs.[1] Radiography of the urethra of male cats may be of value in patients with feline urologic syndrome with or without urethral obstruction.[5] Radiographic examination of the urethra is not often performed in female dogs and cats.

Survey radiographs of the urethra usually yield minimal diagnostic information, but they should be carefully examined for signs of possible urethral disease. Radiopaque urethral calculi can be visible on survey radiographs. Abnormal cranial displacement of the urinary bladder may be associated with urethral rupture. Pelvic fractures, particularly in male dogs, may result in urethral injury. Contrast urethrography is indicated in all cases of suspected urethral disease.[3, 4]

CONTRAST URETHROGRAPHY

Retrograde positive-contrast urethrography is the recommended procedure to evaluate dogs and cats for suspected urethral disease;[1, 3, 4] water soluble organic iodide contrast media should be used. Oil-based contrast media, barium suspensions, and air should not be used because of the risk of urethrocavernous reflux and contrast medium embolization.[1, 4-6] Positive-contrast media should be diluted with sterile saline or sterile water to 15 per cent concentration.[1, 4]

Urethrography is performed by using a balloon-tipped catheter.[4] The catheter is inserted into the urethra and the balloon is inflated to

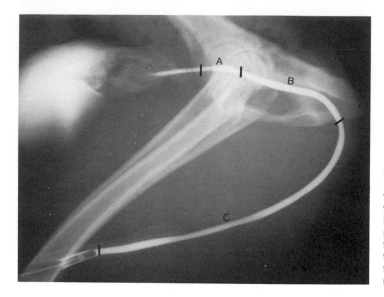

Figure 39–1. Normal positive-contrast retrograde urethrogram in a dog, lateral view. A balloon-tipped catheter is visible within the distal penile urethra. The urethra is divided into three segments: A: the prostatic urethra, B: the membranous urethra, and C: the penile urethra. The urethral mucosa is uniformly smooth and there are no filling defects in the contrast medium column.

prevent reflux of contrast medium. A 10- to 15-ml amount of contrast medium is usually required in dogs; 5 to 10 ml are adequate for cats. Radiographic exposures should be made during injection of the last 2 to 3 ml of contrast medium. A lateral view is usually adequate for diagnosis of urethral disease, but right and left ventrodorsal oblique projections are sometimes helpful. Ventrodorsal views are not often of value. It is important to position the patient with the rear legs drawn forward for the lateral radiograph to avoid superimposition of the femurs over portions of the urethra.[1, 4] Distension of the urethra, particularly the prostatic urethra, and overall quality of the contrast urethrogram may be improved if the urinary bladder is fully distended with contrast medium or sterile saline during urethrography.[5] Retro-

grade positive-contrast urethrography should be performed with care because complications can result.[7, 8] Fortunately, most of these potential complications are transient and reversible.

Urethrography should be performed in any patient with abnormal urination or hematuria that is thought to be of urethral origin. Pelvic fractures, especially in male dogs, are an indication for contrast urethrography if urinary tract injury is suspected.[4, 9–11]

RADIOGRAPHIC SIGNS OF URETHRAL DISEASE

Radiographic signs of urethral disease on contrast urethrography may be classified as filling defects in the contrast column and extravasation of contrast medium from the urethral lumen.[1]

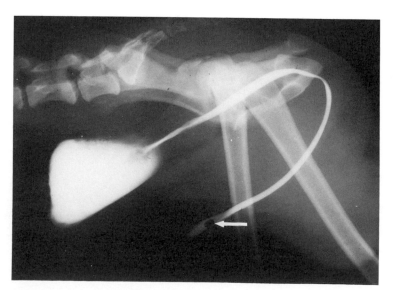

Figure 39–2. Positive-contrast retrograde urethrogram in a male dog with a solitary urethral calculus. In survey radiographs, a mineral-opacity calculus was seen near the proximal os penis. Urethrography demonstrates the calculus as a radiolucent intraluminal filling defect in the contrast medium column (arrow). The margins of the calculus are smooth and sharply defined. The remainder of the urethra is normal.

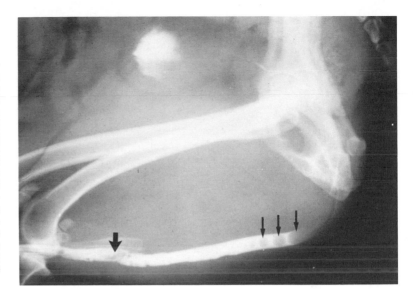

Figure 39–3. Retrograde positive-contrast urethrogram in a male dog with stranguria and a history of urethral calculi. There are intraluminal and intramural filling defects in the contrast medium column. Marked irregularity of the urethral mucosa is evident. An irregularly shaped intraluminal filling defect is present near the proximal os penis *(large arrow)* and multiple smooth, ovoid intraluminal filling defects are present in the proximal penile urethra *(small arrows)*. Surgical intervention revealed urethritis and a large blood clot within the urethra. The ovoid filling defects are intraluminal air bubbles. No urinary calculi were found.

Filling Defects. Filling defects may be intraluminal, intramural, or extramural. Intraluminal filling defects are caused by air bubbles in the contrast medium column; urethral calculi, either radiopaque or radiolucent; or blood clots (Fig. 39–2). Air bubbles are round to oval, have smooth margins, and have a distinct, sharply defined border. Urethral calculi are variable in shape, have irregular margins, and usually demonstrate a poorly defined or blurred margin. If large enough, urethral calculi may produce widening of the urethral lumen. Blood clots are irregular in shape and have poorly defined margins.

Intramural filling defects may be due to neoplasia, inflammatory diseases, or scar tissue from previous urethral surgery, or may result from careless instrumentation (Fig. 39–3). Intramural urethral lesions usually result in marked irregularity of the mucosal surface of the urethra and may cause widening or narrowing of the urethral lumen. The transitional zone from normal to abnormal urethra is usually abrupt and is sharply defined with intramural lesions.

Extramural filling defects result from compression by masses that surround the urethra (Fig. 39–4). Prostatic hyperplasia or neoplasia may result in extraluminal filling defects. The mucosal surface remains smooth and the margins of the extraluminal filling defect are smooth and tapered.[1]

Extravasation of Contrast Material. Extravasation of contrast medium indicates a disruption of the integrity of the urethra. Contrast medium accumulates in the soft tissues surrounding the site of urethral disruption (Fig. 39–5). Contrast medium may enter the perito-

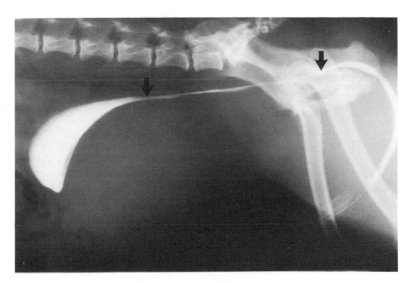

Figure 39–4. Retrograde positive-contrast urethrogram in a male dog with a large paraprostatic cyst. There is a long, extramural filling defect of the urethra *(arrows)*. The margins of the filling defect are long and tapered, indicating extramural compression of the urethra. The urethra is "stretched" and compressed by the large prostatic mass.

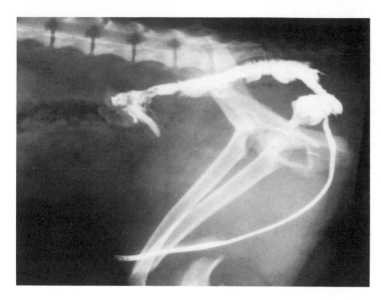

Figure 39–5. Positive-contrast retrograde urethrogram in a male dog with fractures of the pelvis and femur. There is extravasation of contrast medium into the perineal and pelvic soft tissues. Surgical exploration revealed complete transection of the membranous urethra. Urethral injuries occur frequently in male dogs with pelvic fractures.

Figure 39–6. Positive-contrast urethrogram in a male dog. There is extravasation of contrast medium through a urethral laceration into the cavernous tissues of the penis. There is opacification of the dorsal vein of the penis by contrast medium *(arrows)*. The patient was examined because of stranguria. Survey radiographs revealed a fracture of the os penis at the site of the urethral laceration. Note drainage of contrast medium into the caudal vena cava.

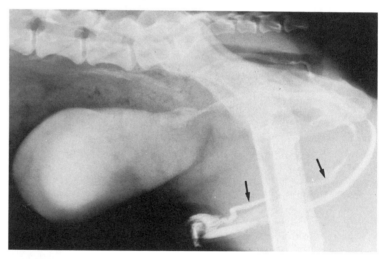

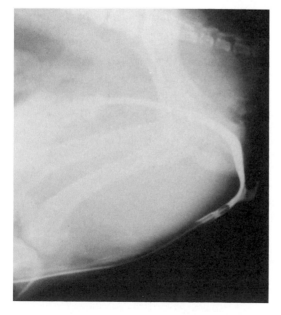

Figure 39–7. Iatrogenic urethral trauma. Urethrogram demonstrates extravasation of contrast medium from the urethra near the junction of the membranous and penile portions. This urethral laceration was the result of overzealous manipulation of a stiff, plastic urinary catheter.

neal cavity if the urethral rent is near the bladder neck, or the systemic venous circulation if urethrocavernous reflux of contrast medium occurs (Fig. 39–6).[1, 11] Pelvic fractures or fractures of the os penis may produce urethral lacerations.[9-11] Abdominal trauma may be associated with urethral rupture at the vesicourethral junction.[10, 11] Iatrogenic urethral disruptions may result from poor catheter manipulation or as a sequela to urethral surgery (Fig. 39–7).[1]

Extravasation of urethral contrast medium may also be seen when there is communication of the urethral lumen with extraurinary organs through fistulous tracts. Urethrorectal and urethrovaginal fistulae have been reported;[1, 12] these fistulae may be congenital or acquired.[1]

References

1. Park RD: Radiology of the urinary bladder and urethra. In O'Brien TR (Ed): Radiographic Diagnosis of Abdominal Disorders in the Dog and Cat. Philadelphia, WB Saunders, 1978, pp. 605–611.
2. Osborne CA, Low DG, and Finco DR: Canine and Feline Urology. Philadelphia, WB Saunders, 1972, pp. 7–8.
3. Johnston GR, Feeney DA, and Osborne CA: Urethrography and cystography in cats. Part I. Techniques, normal radiographic anatomy, and artifacts. Comp Contin Ed Pract Vet 4:823, 1982.
4. Tier JW, Spener CP, and Ackerman N: Positive contrast retrograde urethrography: A useful procedure for evaluating urethral disorders in the dog. Vet Radiol 21:2, 1980.
5. Johnston GR, Jessen CR, and Osborne CA: Effects of bladder distention on canine and feline retrograde urethrography. Vet Radiol 24:271, 1983.
6. Ackerman N, Wingfield WE, and Corley EA: Fatal air embolism associated with pneumourethrography and pneumocystography in a dog. J Am Vet Med Assoc 160:1616, 1972.
7. Johnston GR, Stevens JB, Jessen CR, et al: Complications of retrograde contrast urethrography in dogs and cats. Am J Vet Res 44:1248, 1983.
8. Johnston GR, Feeney DA, and Osborne CA: Urethrography and cystography in cats. Part II. Abnormal radiographic anatomy and complications. Comp Contin Ed Pract Vet 4:931, 1982.
9. Wingfield WE: Lower urinary tract injuries associated with pelvic trauma. Canine Pract 1:25, 1974.
10. Kleine LJ, and Thornton GW: Radiographic diagnosis of urinary tract trauma. J Am Anim Hosp Assoc 7:318, 1971.
11. Pechman RD: Urinary trauma in dogs and cats: A review. J Am Anim Hosp Assoc 18:33, 1982.
12. Osborne CA, Engen MH, Yano BL, et al: Congenital urethrorectal fistula in two dogs. J Am Vet Med Assoc 166:999, 1975.

CHAPTER 40

THE PROSTATE

JIMMY C. LATTIMER

NORMAL ANATOMY

The prostate is a small, ovoid exocrine and endocrine accessory sex gland located just caudal to the urinary bladder.[1, 5] The urethra passes through the prostate slightly dorsal to its center. The prostatic urethra is slightly dilated within the gland, but there is a slight constriction at the caudal margin. A small papilla in the dorsal wall of the midprostatic urethra, the colliculus seminalis, marks the entry point of the vas deferens. Multiple pairs of prostatic ducts enter the urethra dorsal, lateral, ventral, and caudal to the seminal hillock, providing drainage of the prostate.[3]

The prostate is located immediately ventral to the rectum and dorsal to the pubis. Because the prostate is intimately attached to the bladder and urethra, the relationship of the gland to the rectum and pubis is highly dependent on the position of the urinary bladder. If the bladder is full, it may, due to traction, pull the prostate cranially into the abdomen; if the bladder has reflexed into a perineal hernia, the prostate may be displaced into the caudal part of the pelvic canal.[3, 28] Other factors, such as the presence of disease and age, may also cause displacement of the prostate, usually in a cranial direction.

In the immature dog, the prostate usually lies completely within the pelvic canal. As the animal matures, the prostate enlarges in response to the increase in androgen levels accompanying sexual maturity.[11] By the time the animal is 3 to 4 years old, the gland has usually migrated cranially so that it is mostly, if not completely, within the peritoneal cavity.[18]

As the dog ages, the size of the normal prostate remains relatively constant until the age of 10 or 11 years; at this age the gland usually undergoes some degree of shrinkage due to atrophy.[21] The prostate may then again become intrapelvic, although this occurrence is not constant, and usually does not happen if there is any pathologic enlargement of the prostate. As previously stated, the prostate may be abnormally positioned within the pelvic canal in the mature adult dog; conditions causing this malpositioning should be considered if the prostate of the mature dog appears to be more caudal than expected.

Position and form of the prostate in the adult male cat are much the same as in the dog. The gland is much smaller than in the dog, however, and rarely, if ever, is seen on a radiograph. Reports of abnormalities of the feline prostate are rare.[18]

Although all mammals have prostate glands, prostatic disease is rare in all except dog and man. Because the dog is the only domestic animal in which the prostate is visible on radiographs, the remainder of this discussion is lim-

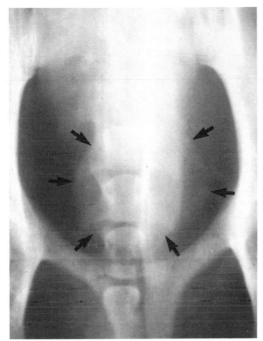

Figure 40–1. Ventrodorsal view of the pelvis illustrates a normal prostate *(arrows)*. Note that the total diameter of the prostate is only about one half that of the pelvic canal.

ited to the dog. Just as there is no average-sized dog, there is no average-sized prostate. The variation in body size between a Yorkshire terrier and a Great Dane, and all the breeds between, makes any statement regarding average absolute prostate size meaningless. It has been reported, however, that the relative weight of the prostate, defined as prostatic weight in grams divided by body weight in kilograms, is the same for all dogs except in the Scottish terrier, in which it is larger by a factor of four.[21] In the study cited, the author considered benign hyperplasia, present in 63 percent

of the dogs studied, to be normal; histologic description of the prostates from the Scottish terriers was not given.[21] Thus, the data cannot be considered evidence to support the contention that the prostate of the Scottish terrier is normally larger than that of other breeds, because Scottish terriers in the experimental group may have had prostatic hyperplasia.

A number of technical and anatomic conditions make it difficult, if not impossible, to determine the absolute size of the prostate radiographically. Therefore, knowing that the prostate of a 55-lb dog should weigh 33 g is of minimal use. The relative anatomic size of the prostate is the key indication. The normal prostate is seldom greater in diameter than one half of the width of the pelvic inlet as seen on the ventrodorsal radiograph (Fig. 40–1).

The shape of the prostate varies from almost spherical to an oval or a flattened ellipse, in which the length is approximately 1½ times the width of the gland. The normal prostate is bilobed and bilaterally symmetric on gross examination.[5, 22] It is generally not possible to differentiate lobar borders on survey radiographs; this bilobed appearance is occasionally seen, however, and should not, by itself, be considered abnormal.

The prostate is of water opacity and therefore visualization is dependent on the differential contrast with surrounding pelvic fat. If the animal is emaciated or if there is fluid in the abdomen, the prostate is obscured. When it is surrounded by pelvic fat, the prostate has a smooth well-marginated contour that may be seen on both the lateral and ventrodorsal projections. On the lateral view, the cranial and ventral borders are clearly seen where a triangular area of fat separates the prostate from the bladder and the ventral abdominal wall (Fig. 40–2).[18, 32]

Figure 40–2. Lateral view of the caudal abdomen. The position and size of a normal prostate in an adult dog can be seen. *Arrows,* the fat triangle that marks the division between the prostate and the bladder.

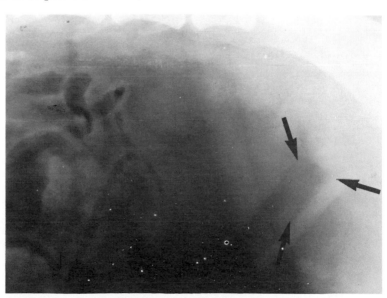

Because the prostate is usually in direct contact with the rectum, the dorsal border is often difficult to see, especially if the rectum contains feces. A full rectum may also completely obscure the prostate on the ventrodorsal view, in which the gland is seen as a circular or oval opacity centered over the pelvic inlet. Although the central portion of the prostate is usually obscured by the sacrum and caudal vertebrae, its lateral margins are often visible when the gland is completely obscured on the lateral view, especially if the gland is slightly enlarged.

The normal prostate is recognizable by its shape, opacity, and the relationship of the gland to the organs around it. If the shape or position of the gland is altered, the gland may not be recognizable other than as a nondescript opacity between the bladder, rectum, and pelvis.[6] Such an opacity does not ensure that the prostate is the cause of the mass effect, but it is the most common cause of this finding in the male dog.

Because the prostate enlarges in response to male hormones, the removal of those hormones by castration results in atrophy of the gland. Alternatively, if the animal is neutered at an early age, the prostate remains in its juvenile form. Shrinkage of the prostate almost invariably follows castration unless pre-existing diseases, such as neoplasia or severe infection with abscess formation, are present.[6, 8, 13, 21] These diseases may not be controlled by castration, but the progression of the disease may be markedly slowed. A similar effect is obtained by estrogen administration, even in an intact animal.[6] Administration of estrogen in combination with castration usually results in rapid shrinkage of the prostate, even if the diseased gland is only partially hormone-responsive. After castration or estrogen therapy, a neoplastic prostate may exhibit rapid initial shrinkage followed by tumor regrowth.[14]

In instances in which a male dog has been castrated or was given estrogen, the prostate may be so small that it is not visible radiographically. Evidence of an enlarged prostate in such animals is often a poor prognostic sign in that it indicates a disease not responsive to normal homeostatic mechanisms.[8]

DISEASES OF THE PROSTATE

Intrinsic disease of the prostate usually results in prostatic enlargement. The prostate is a compact, densely glandular organ. Therefore any proliferative, inflammatory, or traumatic insult to the gland results in enlargement. Enlargement may also occur in response to stimulation from disease processes extrinsic to the prostate. An androgen-producing testicular tumor or orchitis could result in increased prostate size due to androgen secretion or extension of disease to the prostate itself.[21]

There are several different disease processes of the prostate. The most common is benign prostatic hypertrophy in which instance the prostate enlarges due to an increase in the volume of the intercellular and ductal space rather than to an increase in intracellular volume or cell numbers. Thus, once the disease reaches a certain point, the development of dilated cystic spaces and ducts is inevitable. Solid and cystic hypertrophy are therefore different stages of the same disease, with the latter being the advanced form.[17, 21] Size of the cystic spaces varies from microscopic to large; they may become so large that they distort the shape of the entire gland. A cystic prostate usually has cysts of many different sizes, ranging from small to large.

Another common cause of prostatic enlargement is prostatitis, in which there is usually a bacterial cause for the inflammation.[2] The infection may arise within the prostate itself or it may extend to the gland from other sources, such as the bladder or testicles.[10] The prostate may also be a reservoir for reinfection or primary extension to either of these organs.[31] The degree of inflammation is dependent on the type of organism present and the condition of the prostate before infection. Obviously, a normal prostate is more resistant to infection than a hypertrophic one with many secretion-filled cystic spaces. The inflammation may vary in severity from a mild transient process that causes minimal or no clinical disease to a fulminating hemorrhagic process that rapidly destroys the entire gland.[3] The latter type of infection may easily result in rupture of the glandular capsule with extension of the infection to the peritoneal cavity, resulting in diffuse peritonitis and death.[31]

In chronic recurrent prostatitis, gradual destruction of the gland by recurrent inflammation may result in a scarred fibrotic prostate that is actually smaller than normal. A prostate such as this may not be recognized radiographically unless a urethrogram is performed to locate the gland. Chronic scarring may result in stricture of the urethra due to cicatrix formation.[14]

Prostatic abscesses may form as a result of prostatitis. As with cyst formation, the abscesses may be small or large. Large abscesses distort the shape of the gland and may eventually rupture, causing diffuse peritonitis. Abscess formation may be primary or it may be secondary to infection of a previously formed cyst. As previously stated, cysts form in advanced benign hypertrophy and are usually contained within the gland. Occasionally, cysts become so large that the shape of the gland is distorted and the predominate opacity seen on the radiograph is due to the large prostatic cyst. Such large cysts are also referred to as paraprostatic cysts, because they are no longer confined within the gland. These cysts are usually sterile but may become secondarily infected and lead to abscess formation.[30]

Occasionally, cysts form from lesions other than prostatic hypertrophy. Probably the most common cause is neoplasia.[22] Formation of functional neoplastic secretory cells without an accompanying ductal system results in a cystic structure lined with neoplastic epithelium. Osteocollagenous retention cysts are rare and of unknown origin, but they do not appear to be the direct result of cystic hypertrophy.[25]

A rare form of cyst, which is truly paraprostatic, is cystic enlargement of the wolffian ducts (uterus masculinus).[29] When this enlargement occurs, there is evidence of a bilateral tubular mass that resembles uterine enlargement. The prostate itself may or may not be enlarged and is usually not distinguishable as a separate opacity.[14]

Prostatic adenocarcinoma is relatively uncommon.[20, 27] When it occurs, this neoplastic process is often far advanced, with involvement not only of the prostate, but also of the regional lymph nodes, pelvis, and distant sites, such as the liver and lungs.[8, 9, 23] In some dogs, the prostate is massively enlarged by the tumor and in others the degree of enlargement is rather minimal. Small in situ prostatic carcinomas are unusual but do occur; they are usually manifest through the effect of their distant metastasis rather than locally, as is true for most prostatic tumors. Prostatic neoplasms are often secondarily infected or necrotic, and affected dogs may therefore have many of the signs of prostatitis. These patients are difficult to diagnose because of the tendency of the prostatitis to overshadow the neoplasia, unless signs of metastatic disease are present.[12, 15, 24] Neoplasia should always be suspected in animals that have a compatible history and signalment, especially if signs of prostatitis are present.

Trauma to the prostate may occur in instances of pelvic or abdominal injury. Perhaps the most common source of such an injury is automobile trauma. Because the prostate is encapsulated by a tough fibrous layer, it is not free to expand rapidly due to interstitial hemorrhage. The prostate therefore does not usually become enlarged due to traumatically induced bruising. Rarely, the prostate may be ruptured or avulsed. A ruptured prostate may scar and heal; if the urethra is ruptured, however, as with an avulsed prostate, surgical intervention is required to save the animal's life. Early recognition of prostatic avulsions is therefore mandatory.

Clinical Signs

The clinical signs of prostate enlargement tend to mimic the signs of other diseases. Prostatic disease usually presents with clinical signs referable to either urinary or rectal problems. Stranguria, hematuria, and pyuria are frequently seen.[3, 29, 30] Because the urethra passes through the center of the prostate, however, and prostatic disease usually progresses outward radially from the urethra, complete urethral obstruction is unusual.[4, 17] With hematuria of prostatic origin, the entire urine stream is not bloody, only the terminal portion. In fact, blood may actually appear only after all of the urine has been voided. The possibility of concurrent disease in both the bladder and prostate must also be considered. Cystitis and urethritis commonly accompany prostatitis.[10] The clinical work-up should be designed to detect such concurrent problems.

Another common complaint with prostatic disease is difficult defecation with small or ribbon-like stools.[3, 4] As the enlarging prostate displaces the colon dorsally, it compresses it against the sacrum and pelvis, resulting in a decrease in stool diameter. Extreme straining to defecate may break small mucosal blood vessels in the rectum, resulting in small amounts of fresh blood in the stool. The presence of hookworms may also be a source for small amounts of blood in the feces, and contribute to the rectal irritation, which increases the amount of straining. Severe rectal compression by the prostate may cause clinical and radiographic signs of constipation or obstipation. Such patients may not strain or even attempt to defecate. The problem is then critical and immediate, and definitive treatment must be instituted.

Another less common but important complaint is a stiff or waddling gait in the rear legs. The animal may refuse to climb stairs and jump. Owners often believe the animal has developed degenerative arthritis in the hip joint. Such animals may have severe active septic prostatitis.[3, 10] The pain caused by the prostatic infection is markedly exacerbated by walking, climbing, and jumping. Both legs are usually affected uniformly because the pain is central. These animals are also usually sensitive to palpation of the caudal abdomen. There may also be some erythema of the skin due to inflammation in this area. Gait abnormalities are seen rarely in uncomplicated benign prostatic hypertrophy.

Radiographic Changes

As previously stated, the prostate occupies the space between the pelvis, rectum, and bladder. The degree of bladder distension affects the position of the prostate. As the bladder distends, it pulls the prostate cranially into the abdomen, which may result in enhanced visualization of it. A large urinary bladder may also displace the bowel structures away from the prostate, making it more visible.

Because of its intimate relationship to the

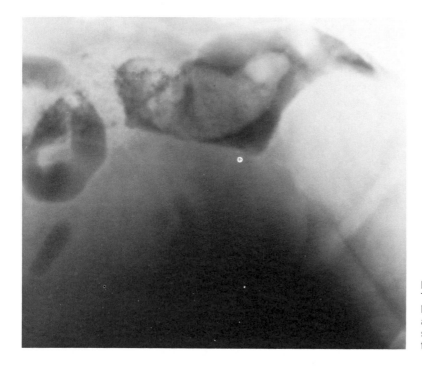

Figure 40–3. Prostatic hypertrophy. The bladder is displaced cranially. Note that the margins of the gland are still smooth, regular, and easily seen, as is the fat triangle between the prostate and the bladder.

urinary bladder, any enlargement of the prostate displaces the bladder cranially (Fig. 40–3). If the enlargement is uniform throughout the gland, displacement is in a cranial direction, along the floor of the abdomen. If, however, the enlargement is eccentric, as is often the case with cysts and abscesses, direction of bladder displacement may be somewhat different. Marked enlargement of the dorsal part of the gland by a cyst or abscess may actually extend dorsal to the bladder, compressing it against the caudal ventral floor of the abdomen (Fig. 40–4). Alternatively, if the ventral portion of

the gland is markedly enlarged, the bladder may be elevated off the floor of the abdomen (Fig. 40–5). A large prostatic cyst or abscess may extend cranially beneath the bladder, also resulting in a cranial dorsal displacement of the bladder. This latter appearance of elevation of the bladder may also be seen with severe benign prostatic hypertrophy (Fig. 40–6).

The other major radiographic sign of prostatic enlargement is dorsal displacement of the colon (Fig. 40–5). The colon normally lies in contact with the dorsal or dorsolateral surface of the bladder. As the prostatic enlargement displaces

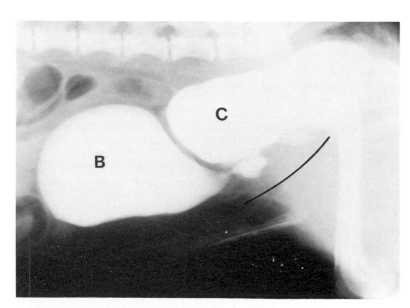

Figure 40–4. Positive-contrast cystogram. There is a large dorsally placed paraprostatic cyst (C) filled with contrast medium. Thus the cyst communicates with the urethra. The bladder is displaced cranially and ventrally. Note the relatively small size of the remainder of the prostate, as indicated by the space between the cyst and the ventral abdominal wall (line) caudal to the bladder (B).

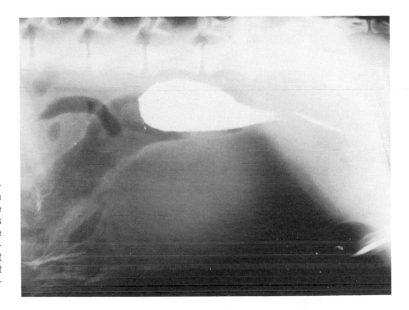

Figure 40–5. Marked dorsal displacement of the bladder (filled with positive contrast medium) by a large paraprostatic cyst (soft-tissue mass ventral to bladder). Note that the bladder and the colon are superimposed. Also note that unlike the cyst in Figure 40–4, this cyst does not appear to communicate with the urethra.

the colon dorsally, contact with the bladder is lost. Radiographically, there is separation of the ventral border of the colon and the dorsal border of the bladder. In a male dog, such a finding is virtually confirmatory of prostatic enlargement.[10] Such an appearance may also be caused by disease of the urethra, bladder, or enlarged uterus masculinis.

Prostatic enlargement may cause narrowing of the colonic lumen. Radiographically, this compression may be visible or, depending on the disease present, the colon may simply become confluent with the mass at the pelvic inlet. The latter appearance does not usually occur unless highly aggressive disease is present. The colon is often displaced to one side of the pelvic canal by a prostatic mass (Fig. 40–7).

The urethra, although not really displaced relative to the prostate, may be lifted up at the pelvic floor or displaced to one side of the pelvic canal by an enlarged prostate. This displacement of the urethra is most often seen with asymmetric prostatic disease, such as tumor growth or abscess formation. The urethra is also often elongated by its passage through a markedly enlarged prostate. The position of the urethra is impossible to ascertain unless contrast medium is used to outline it.

A tremendously enlarged prostate displaces other abdominal organs cranially. Huge prostatic lesions usually lie on the floor of the abdomen, so there is some dorsal displacement of the remainder of the abdominal contents. Prostatic and paraprostatic cysts may become

Figure 40–6. Positive-contrast cystogram. There is marked prostatic hypertrophy and the bladder is displaced cranially. Note that if the bladder were only slightly less distended, it would not reach the abdominal floor. There is reflux of contrast medium into the parenchyma of the prostate outlining dilated ducts but indicating nothing more.

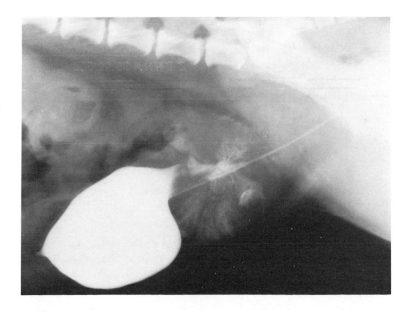

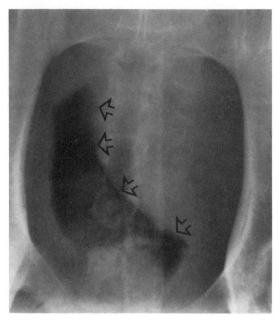

Figure 40–7. Ventrodorsal radiograph of the pelvic canal. *Arrows,* concave indentation of the colon on the left side by an enlarged prostate.

so large that they reach almost to the costal arch.[29] With masses of this magnitude, organ displacement is so severe that the actual source of the mass may be difficult to determine without the use of special radiographic procedures.

All common prostate diseases cause enlargement. As is the instance with most organs, the enlargement may be symmetric (diffuse in origin), asymmetric (focal in origin), or a combination of the two types. Combination lesions are the most common. Hypertrophy and prostatitis are examples of symmetric enlargement, whereas neoplasia and cysts are examples of asymmetric enlargement. Large prostatic and paraprostatic cysts and abscesses are generally

combination lesions that involve the entire prostate, but a single lobe predominates as the source of the radiographic lesion.[3] Because it is difficult to define the shape of the normal prostate precisely, it may be difficult to determine whether the enlarged prostate is symmetric or asymmetric when enlargement is mild. If the enlarged prostate is relatively symmetric in its relationship to the bladder, the enlargement is probably symmetric (Fig. 40–8); if not, the enlargement is asymmetric (Fig. 40–9).

The actual degree of prostatic enlargement varies tremendously for each condition. For instance, prostatic size might vary from slight enlargement to 10 times normal size for benign prostatic hypertrophy. If prostatic cysts or abscesses are present, the prostate may be as great as 20 or more times normal size, or the degree of enlargement may be minimal. Acute prostatitis and neoplasia do not usually cause the huge enlargements seen with hypertrophy and cyst formation. Some small in situ prostatic neoplasias are not recognized until the animal is examined for another problem, such as cough or lameness caused by metastasis (Fig. 40–10), or as an incidental finding at post mortem examination.

One of the most important characteristics of the prostate to evaluate is its margination. If the prostate has a smooth margin that is easily seen, the disease involving the gland is likely to be benign or is slowly progressing (Fig. 40–2), such as benign hypertrophy and low grade or chronic prostatitis. A rough or indistinct margin in the presence of adequate abdominal fat is more likely to be due to an acute or aggressive process, such as neoplasia or prostatitis (Fig. 40–11).[15, 19, 32] When the margin is indistinct or is not discernible, the impression is that of a localized peritonitis in the caudal abdomen. Except for prostatic rupture, this

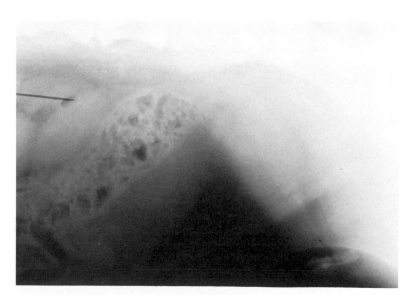

Figure 40–8. Moderate symmetric enlargement of the prostate due to hypertrophy. Note that the margins of the gland are still smooth and the fat triangle between the bladder and the prostate is still clearly visible.

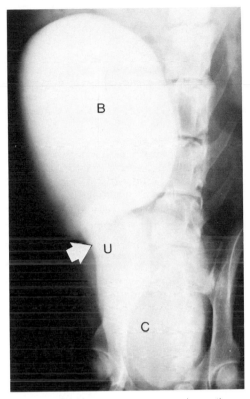

Figure 40–9. Positive-contrast retrograde urethrogram. There is an asymmetric prostatic mass. This large prostatic cyst (C) markedly displaces the urethra (U) to the right side of the pelvis. *Arrows,* the point which the urethra enters the prostate; such displacement of the urethra is typical of large cystic lesions of the prostate. B, Bladder. Some contrast medium is present in the prostatic cyst.

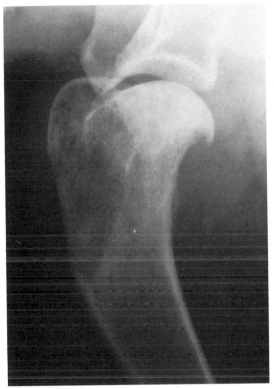

Figure 40–10. Metastatic adenocarcinoma. This large, predominantly lytic lesion in the proximal part of the humerus was the cause of lameness. The presumed radiographic diagnosis was osteosarcoma, although the histologic diagnosis at postmortem was metastatic adenocarcinoma of the prostate. The lesion in the prostate was an in situ lesion and did not grossly distort or enlarge the prostate. Multiple areas of metastasis were found throughout the body.

Figure 40–11. Prostatic adenocarcinoma. The large, irregularly shaped prostate displaces the bladder cranially along with the small bowel. The colon is displaced dorsally and the bladder is lifted off the abdominal floor. Although the tumor has not yet broken through the capsule of the gland, it distorts the outline, making its shape irregular. The margin is still smooth, probably due to the confinement of the tumor by the glandular capsule.

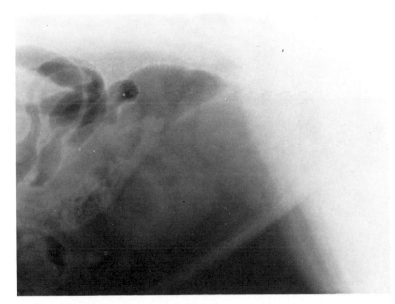

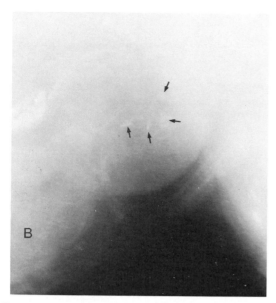

Figure 40–12. There are speckled areas of calcification *(arrows)* throughout the parenchyma of this large prostate. Calcification in association with the enlarged gland is suggestive of neoplasia. The histologic diagnosis was mucinous carcinoma of the prostate. B, urinary bladder.

assessment is probably accurate. In most aggressive prostatic diseases, even if the disease itself is confined by the glandular capsule, there is usually some secondary inflammation in the surrounding tissues. Almost all large prostatic neoplasms are infected, which accounts in part for the localized peritonitis associated with them.

Paraprostatic cysts and abscesses usually have well-defined margins that are easily seen (Fig.

40–5). An occasional abscess is poorly marginated, although this occurrence is the exception rather than the rule. Occasionally, a cyst or abscess may form in the pelvic canal; such lesions may not be readily visible on survey radiographs or produce the usual displacement of the bladder.[16] These lesions do, however, produce marked displacement and compression of the rectum, and are therefore recognized as an intrapelvic mass. The lack of regional peritonitis associated with a large abscess may be due in part to the thickness of the capsule and to the organism being of a low virulence. It is seldom possible to distinguish a cyst from an abscess on the basis of a radiographic examination alone.

Any change in the opacity of the prostate from its normal water opacity indicates severe disease. Areas of calcification within the gland are either a sign of long-standing and relatively severe prostatitis or of neoplasia (Fig. 40–12).[24, 29] Most prostate calcification is a result of neoplasia. Therefore, calcification should be considered a serious finding that warrants surgical biopsy.[28, 32]

The presence of spontaneous gas within the prostate is also an important sign. Because the prostate does not normally communicate with any air-containing organ, there is no reason for it to contain gas. The most common cause of apparent gas within the prostate is a small pocket of gas within an overlying small bowel loop. Every attempt should be made to eliminate the possibility that the gas is contained within the bowel rather than the prostate. Gas-containing small bowel loops are usually identifiable as such on one of two views; they are either seen directly or the gas bubble itself

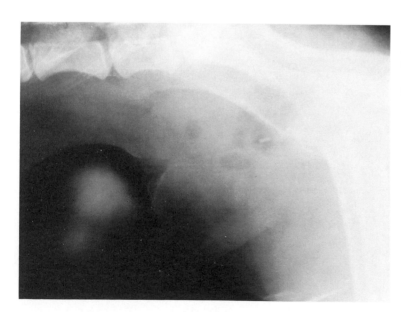

Figure 40–13. Double-contrast cystogram. There is marked enlargement of the prostate. Note the air that has refluxed into the gland. The cavities are irregular, suggestive of multiple abscesses or neoplasia.

shifts out of the prostatic silhouette. If doubt remains, gentle compression of the caudal abdomen with a paddle displaces the bowel cranially away from the prostate. Differentiation of bowel and prostate should then be possible.

A second way in which the prostate may contain air is reflux of air from the bladder during infusion of air for a negative or double-contrast cystogram (Fig. 40–13). A small amount of reflux into prostatic ducts is a normal but not consistent occurrence. Simple filling of the ducts with air does not necessarily indicate prostatic disease. Filling of air in pockets within the prostate is abnormal, however, and is most commonly associated with cyst formation secondary to benign hypertrophy. This accumulation of air within cystic areas in the prostate is probably an indication for the performance of a biopsy or aspiration of the organ, but it should not be taken as a poor prognostic sign.

The presence of intrinsic gas within the prostate indicates infection with a gas-forming organism. Coliform or clostridial prostatitis results in severe hemorrhagic necrosis of the gland. These infections rapidly destroy the gland and extend to the abdomen, resulting in a generalized peritonitis. Because of the rapidly fatal course of these infections, identification of noniatrogenic gas within the prostate should be viewed as an unfavorable prognostic sign. Even if the animal survives, severe permanent scarring of the prostate is likely. Sterility and urinary retention or incontinence may become long-term sequelae to such scarring.

Pallisade-type periosteal proliferation is sometimes seen on the ventral aspect of the caudal lumbar vertebrae and pelvis (Fig. 40–14). Such proliferation is suggestive of prostatic neoplasia.[4, 5, 7, 13, 24, 28] The proliferation may not represent bone metastasis, but rather occurs as a secondary effect of swelling of the adjacent lymph nodes, which themselves contain the actual metastatic lesions. Because the proliferation is a secondary lesion, it could conceivably occur any time there is nodal enlargement;[32] this, however, is not usually the situation. Although pallisade-type proliferation of the ventral vertebral body is occasionally seen with other diseases, it is most often seen with prostatic neoplasia. True bone metastasis of a prostatic tumor would be expected to be predominantly lytic in nature (Fig. 40–10).

Cysts and abscesses of the prostate may extend through the wall of the gland, resulting in paraprostatic cysts and abscesses. Paraprostatic cysts may also arise from outside the prostate. Occasionally, retention of secretions within the remnants of the wolffian ducts (uterus masculinus) causes them to enlarge. The disease process is self-perpetuating and results in massive enlargement. The tubules of the uterus masculinus, like the uterine horns in the female, tend to maintain their tubular shape as they enlarge. Radiographically, the appearance is identical to that of a large pyometra. There is a large tubular, soft-tissue mass in the caudal ventral abdomen. The bladder is displaced ventrally and the colon is moved dorsally. The small bowel, spleen, and perhaps even the kidneys are moved cranial and dorsal from their normal positions. This typical pattern of organ displacement seen with pyometra, if observed in a male dog, strongly suggests the possibility of a paraprostatic cyst due to enlargement of the uterus masculinus.

Special Radiographic Procedures

Few special radiographic procedures are used in the diagnosis of prostatic disease. The only technique that has been found to be uniformly useful in the evaluation of the prostate is the positive-contrast retrograde urethrogram. This procedure allows evaluation of the position of the urethra in relation to the suspected prostatic mass. Displacement of the urethra to one side,

Figure 40–14. Palisade-type periosteal reaction along the ventral aspect of L$_5$, L$_6$, L$_7$, and the sacrum. The reaction is apparently a response to enlargement and inflammation of the regional lymph nodes caused by invasion of carcinoma of the prostate. This lesion is not a constant feature with all prostate tumors, but when evident, it is suggestive of a prostatic adenocarcinoma, even if there is no gross enlargement of the prostate. (Courtesy of Dr. L. Konde, Colorado State University, Ft. Collins, CO.)

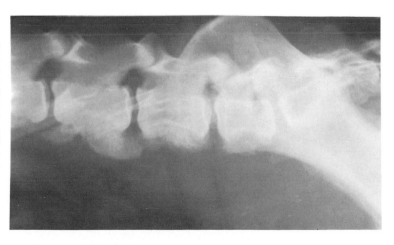

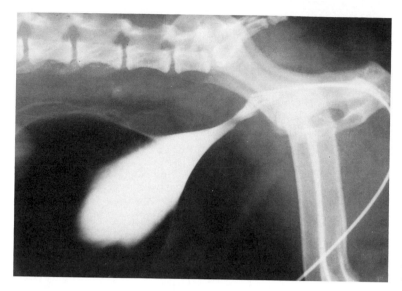

Figure 40–15. Double-contrast cystogram. The prostate is only moderately enlarged, although the urethrogram shows that the ventral portion of the gland is more enlarged than is the dorsal portion. The off-center position of the urethra suggests that the enlargement of the gland is at least in part due to either a cystic-type or a neoplastic lesion.

ventrally or dorsally, of the mass indicates that the enlargement is either extrinsic to the prostate or is occurring asymmetrically within the prostate (Fig. 40–15), the latter being the more common occurrence. The procedure also allows evaluation of the urethra itself. Invasion or stricture of the urethra in association with a prostatic mass is a poor prognostic finding, not only because of the danger that a urinary obstruction might occur, but also because it is a sign that aggressive disease is present. Evidence of either prostatic asymmetric enlargement or urethral abnormalities is a positive indication for prostatic biopsy. Such a finding also points out the difficulties likely to be encountered if resection of the disease is attempted.

A secondary benefit of the urethrogram is that it identifies the true location of the urinary bladder. In some instances, abdominal masses, such as an omental carcinoma or enlarged retained tecticle, lie just cranial to the bladder. This positioning closely mimics the appearance of an enlarged prostate that is displacing the bladder cranially. Such tumors obviously present different clinical and diagnostic problems and should be handled accordingly.

Positive identification of the bladder and its position relative to the prostate also has definite benefits when the disease process does involve the prostate. It is not always obvious from survey radiographs or palpation what is prostate and what is bladder (Fig. 40–4). This identification is necessary if a blind percutaneous aspirate or biopsy of the mass is to be attempted rather than a biopsy via laparotomy. By having identified the position of the bladder and urethra with a urethrogram, the chances of injury to the urinary tract during blind biopsy procedures are lessened.

Urethrography is easily performed in the male dog. There are at least two methods. The most common method is to insert the largest possible male urinary catheter to the point at which the tip is within the terminal portion of the pelvic urethra. The tip of the catheter can usually be felt, through the skin or rectally, as it passes over the ischial arch. Once the catheter is in place, a few milliliters of lidocaine are infused to reduce urethral spasm. After the lidocaine has been given, contrast medium is infused at a steady rate and the exposure made during infusion. The rate of contrast infusion should be sufficient to distend the urethra moderately so that any lesions within the urethra itself are easier to see.[26]

The contrast medium used is the same water-soluble iodinated contrast medium that is used for excretory urography. It should be sterile and, depending on personal preference, should have an iodine concentration of 200 to 400 mg iodine per milliliter of solution.[26]

A complete urethrogram should include at least three views: lateral and right and left ventrodorsal oblique projections, each one approximately 30 degrees from vertical. These two oblique views, in conjunction with the lateral view, allow complete visualization of the entire circumference of the urethra without interference from the overlying skeleton, as would occur if only a lateral and ventrodorsal projection were made. Much of the value of a urethrogram for diagnosis of prostatic disease is lost if only a single lateral view is acquired. The leg should not be pulled forward as is done when the penile urethra is evaluated.

An alternative and more reliable, but slightly more difficult, method of performing urethrography is to use a Foley catheter in place of a male urinary catheter. The balloon of the cath-

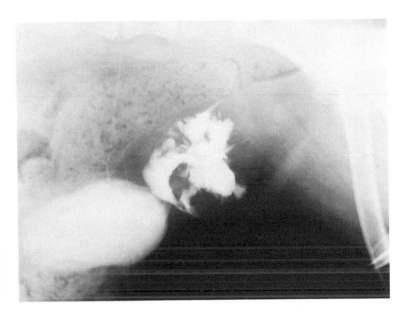

Figure 40–16. Positive retrograde urethrogram. Same dog as in Figure 40–12. There are large irregular cavities within the prostate, suggestive of neoplasia.

eter is placed within or just caudal to the proximal end of the os penis. The balloon is then inflated and the examination is performed as described.[26] The use of a Foley type catheter gives better control of contrast medium flow and prevents reflux of the contrast medium around the catheter in those instances in which there is a urethral spasm or an occlusive lesion of the urethra. Even though there may be a severe stricture of the urethra at the prostate, contrast medium can usually be forced past the obstruction to provide an accurate assessment of the degree and extent of the lesion.

Urethrography often only provides indirect evidence of disease within the prostate. If the urethra is deviated around a large mass or does not pass directly through the center of the prostate, the disease within the prostate is asymmetric, such as a cyst. If the urethra passes directly through the middle of an enlarged prostate, the disease process is more likely to be diffuse throughout the gland, such as hypertrophy or prostatitis.

Direct signs of urethral disease of prostatic origin are urethral stricturing, ulceration of the mucosa, and filling defects within the urethra itself. Ulceration or stricturing of the prostatic urethral mucosa should be regarded as highly suggestive of neoplasia of the prostate.

Extravasation of contrast medium into the prostate should not be interpreted as abnormal as long as only the prostatic ducts fill with contrast medium. This appearance is often seen in animals with a normal prostate. Only if definite pooling of contrast medium within the prostate is seen should extravasation be consid-

ered abnormal. Large, irregularly shaped cavities with rough walls that communicate with the urethra are often associated with neoplasia; biopsy is then indicated (Fig. 40–16).[16, 27] Conversely, if extravasation does not occur, the

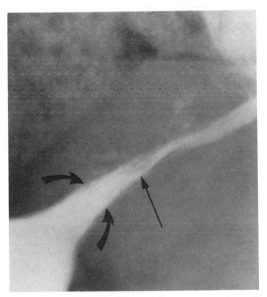

Figure 40–17. Close-up view of the prostate shows the normal appearance of the urethra when distended during positive-contrast urethrography. The small amount of contrast medium reflux into the gland is insignificant. The small filling defect (straight arrow) indicates the position of the colliculus seminalis and is a normal finding. If the prostatic urethra is not distended when radiographed, the colliculus will probably not be evident. Note that the level of the urethral sphincter (curved arrows) is well within the prostatic shadow.

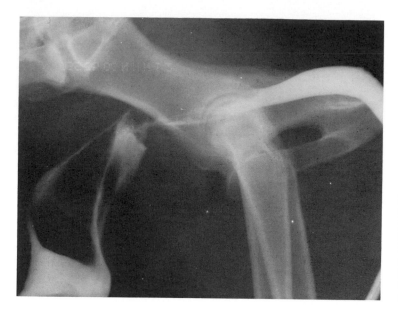

Figure 40–18. Positive-contrast ure-throgram reveals the presence of marked irregularity of the prostatic ure-thral mucosa and vesicourethral junction. Such lesions may not be visible on a double-contrast cystogram, or the true extent of the lesion may be underestimated. Diagnosis: transitional cell carcinoma.

prostate is not necessarily normal or solid. Many times, large cavitary lesions, such as cysts and abscesses, attain their size because they do not communicate with the urethra via the ductal system.[4, 29, 30] If these cavities do fill with contrast medium, they are usually ovoid, with smooth walls.

The normal prostatic urethra as seen on the urethrogram has a smooth mucosal border. The urethra is usually slightly greater in diameter near the center of the prostate and tapers slightly at the cranial and caudal borders. The degree of the central dilatation is somewhat dependent on the size of the prostate, the disease present, the degree of bladder distension, and the amount of pressure applied during injection.[3] Many examinations reveal the presence of a small filling defect in the dorsal wall of the urethra near the center of the prostate. This defect represents the colliculus seminalis and is a normal finding (Fig. 40–17). In some dogs, there may also be a normal groove in the colliculus.

The point at which the prostatic urethra joins the trigone of the bladder should be carefully evaluated. It is possible to detect small filling defects or mucosal ulcers that may be early lesions of transitional cell carcinoma (Fig. 40–18). These small lesions may be not detected on a cystogram because they are obscured by the internal urethral sphincter, which is actually encircled by the prostate.[5] By the time the

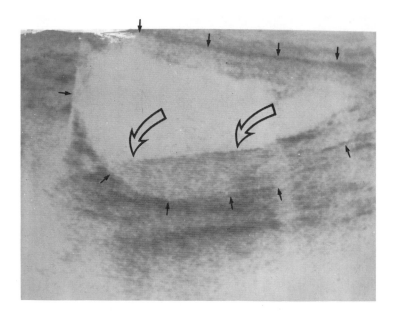

Figure 40–19. Sonogram of a large para-prostatic cyst. The large clear space indicates fluid within the cyst. *Small arrows*, capsule of the cyst. The line *(curved arrows)* of greater echodensity within the cyst is caused by a layer of sediment in the dependent portion of the cyst. The dog is in dorsal recumbency.

lesions are of sufficient size to be seen on a cystogram, the chance to fully resect them has probably been lost.

Alternative Imaging Techniques

In recent years, diagnostic ultrasound has become available for use by veterinarians. Although still principally found in university teaching hospitals, several companies now produce units specifically designed for veterinary use. Therefore, more private practices are using ultrasound for diagnosis of a variety of diseases. Evaluation of the prostate is one of the best areas to use diagnostic ultrasound as an adjunct to radiography. Unlike radiographic evaluation, which often relies on the indirect effects of prostatic disease, ultrasound provides an accurate representation of the actual internal structure of the gland. Cystic and hypercellular areas are clearly depicted and careful evaluation can reveal evidence of fibrosis and inflammation (Fig. 40–19). Although it is beyond the scope of this text to describe in detail the evaluation of sonographic images, ultrasonography is probably the easiest and most accurate noninvasive way to evaluate the prostate. Therefore, any possibly abnormal prostate should be examined sonographically if the equipment and the expertise to perform the study are available.

References

1. Aumuller G, Stofft E, and Tunn U: Fine structure of the canine prostatic complex, Anat Embryol 160:327, 1980.
2. Barsanti JA, Shotts Jr EB, Prasse K, et al: Evaluation of diagnostic techniques for canine prostate disease. J Am Vet Med Assoc 177: 160, 1980.
3. Barsanti JA, and Finco DR: Canine bacterial prostatitis. Vet Clin North Am 9:679, 1979.
4. Borthwiek R, and Mackenzie CP: The signs and results of treatment of prostatic disease in dogs. Vet Rec 89:374, 1971.
5. Christensen GC: In Evans HE and Christensen GC (Eds): Miller's Anatomy of the Dog. Philadelphia, WB Saunders, 1979, pp. 565–566.
6. Finco DR: Diseases of the prostate gland of the dog. In Morrow DA (Ed): Current Therapy in Theriogenology. Philadelphia, WB Saunders, 1980, pp. 654–661.
7. Franks LM: The spread of prostatic carcinoma to the bones. J Pathol 66:91, 1953.
8. Gill CW: Prostatic adenocarcinoma with concurrent sertoli tumor in a dog. Can Vet J 22:230, 1981.
9. Grant CA: Carcinoma of the canine prostate. Acta Pathol Microbiol Scand 40:197, 1957.
10. Griener TP, and Johnson RG: Diseases of the prostate gland. In Ettinger SJ (Ed): Textbook of Veterinary Internal Medicine, Diseases of the Dog and Cat, 2nd Ed. Philadelphia, WB Saunders, 1983, pp. 1459–1492.
11. James RW, and Heywood R: Age-related variations in the testes and prostate of beagle dogs. Toxicology 12:273, 1979.
12. Jameson RM: Prostatic abscess and carcinoma of the prostate, Br J Urol 40:288, 1968.
13. Klausner JS: Management of canine bacterial prostatitis. J Am Vet Med Assoc 182:292, 1983.
14. Kornegay J: Canine prostatic disease. SW Vet 26:257, 1973.
15. Leav I, and Ling GV: Adenocarcinoma of the canine prostate. Cancer 22:1329, 1968.
16. McClain DL: Surgical treatment of perineal prostatic abscesses. J Am Anim Hosp Assoc 18:794, 1982.
17. Metten S: A morphologic study of benign prostatic hypertrophy in the dog. Doctoral dissertation; Department of Anatomy, Colorado State University, Fort Collins, CO, 1978.
18. O'Brien, T: Normal radiographic anatomy of the abdomen. In Diagnosis of Abdominal Disorders in the Dog and Cat; Radiographic Interpretation, Clinical Signs, and Pathophysiology, Philadelphia, WB Saunders, 1978, pp. 9–47.
19. O'Brien T: Abdominal masses. In Diagnosis of Abdominal Disorders in the Dog and Cat; Radiographic Interpretation, Clinical Signs, and Pathophysiology, Philadelphia, WB Saunders 1978, pp. 85–109.
20. O'Shea JD: Studies on the canine prostate gland. II. (Prostatic neoplasms). J Comp Pathol 73:244, 1963.
21. O'Shea JD: Studies on the canine prostate gland. I. Factors influencing its size and weight. J Comp Pathol 72:321, 1962.
22. Price D: Comparative aspects of development and structure in the prostate. Natl Cancer Inst Monogr 12:1, 1962.
23. Rabut SM, and Kelch WJ: Undifferentiated carcinoma in the canine prostate. Mod Vet Pract 60:401, 1979.
24. Rendano Jr VT, and Slauson DO: Hypertrophic osteopathy in a dog with prostate adenocarcinoma and without thoracic metastasis. J Am Anim Hosp Assoc 18:905, 1982.
25. Rife J, and Thornburg LP: Osteocollagenous prostatic retention cyst in the canine. Canine Pract 7:44, 1980.
26. Root CA: Urethrography. In Ticer JW (Ed): Radiographic Techniques in Veterinary Practice, 2nd Ed. Philadelphia, WB Saunders, 1984, pp. 387–394.
27. Weaver AD: Fifteen cases of prostatic carcinoma in the dog. Vet Rec 109:71, 1981.
28. Weaver AD: Prostatic disease in the dog. Vet Annual 20:82, 1980.
29. Weaver AD: Discrete prostatic (paraprostatic) cysts in the dog. Vet Rec 102:435, 1978.
30. Zolton GM: Surgical techniques for the prostate. Vet Clin North Am [Small Anim Pract] 9:349, 1979.
31. Zolton GM, and Griener TP: Prostatic abscess—surgical approach, J Am Anim Hosp Assoc 14:698, 1978.
32. Zontine WJ: Radiographic interpretation, the prostate gland. Mod Vet Pract 56:341, 1975.

CHAPTER 41

THE UTERUS

DANIEL A. FEENEY
GARY R. JOHNSTON

The general goals of this chapter are to familiarize the reader with the radiographic techniques applicable to the uterus. Another goal is to describe the normal radiographic findings for the uterus when these techniques are applied. An additional goal is to provide a general introduction to selected abnormal findings to permit some degree of familiarity with the commonly encountered diseases as they appear radiographically. The ultimate goal is to use this information on a case by case basis to analyze the radiographic findings and to formulate a plan for definitive diagnosis, even if this is not possible using radiographic techniques alone.

IMAGING PROCEDURES

Survey radiographs are commonly used in the evaluation of the uterus. The indications and limitations of abdominal radiography as they apply to specific uterine diseases have been described in textbooks of medicine and surgery.[1-4] From a standpoint of radiographic interpretation, however, the major applications of survey radiographs to diseases of the uterus lie in confirming that the palpable abdominal mass is consistent in radiographic location with that of an enlarged uterus, or the identification of the enlarged uterus in a bitch that is difficult to palpate. Other utilizations for survey radiographs include assessment of fetal skeletons (i.e., number and degree of mineralization), assessment of progress in variations of uterine size both during pregnancy and in disease states such as pyometra, and, to a limited degree, of the assessment of fetal viability, based principally on the absence of findings consistent with fetal demise.

Two radiographic views are necessary for adequate assessment of intra-abdominal masses, including the uterus. Preparation should include the withholding of food for 24 hours and the administration of enemas to evacuate the colon at least 2 hours before radiography.[5] It is important that adequate attention be paid to technical procedures to ensure maximal radiographic contrast, because the uterus in disease states and without the presence of skeletal structures must be differentiated from bladder, colon, and other nonspecific abdominal masses. Radiographic technique is also important when the early mineralization of fetal skeletons is assessed, because in the presence of a large uterus, early fetal mineralization can be masked by poor technique.

Abdominal compression has been suggested as a possible means by which the colon, uterus, and bladder may be differentiated in the caudal abdomen.[5] The usefulness of this technique is basically limited to patients in which the uterus is not massively enlarged and can be aligned between the colon and urinary bladder by using

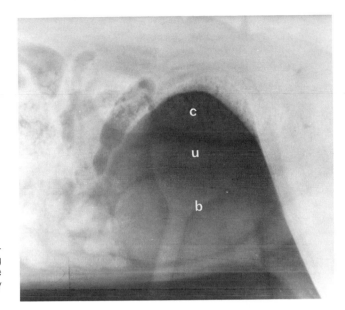

Figure 41–1. Lateral view of the caudal abdomen. Local compression was applied by using a wooden spoon during radiography. Note the separation of the colon (c), uterus (u), and urinary bladder (b).

a compression device—either a plastic paddle or a wooden kitchen spoon. An example of the type of separation that can be achieved is shown in Figure 41–1. Pneumoperitonography is a procedure that has also been suggested to aid in the definitive identification of the uterus.[5] It is our opinion, however, that pneumoperitonography is rarely indicated; usually the radiographic findings in combination with the history of the estrous cycle and results of physical examination are adequate for a diagnosis to be reached.

Hysterosalpingography is the infusion of water-soluble contrast medium through the cervix into the uterus and oviducts to outline these structures so that they can be identified when they are not of sufficient size to be seen on survey radiographs.[5–8] In our opinion, this technique is rarely indicated and should be reserved for the radiographic examination of the chronically infertile bitch or to define anomalous genital organs. An example of a ventrodorsal view of a vaginohysterosalpingogram is shown in Figure 41–2.

Ultrasonography is the use of high frequency, focused sound that can be transmitted into the tissue and reflected at tissue interfaces; the reflected sound is then detected and displayed as a two-dimensional image.[9] This technique has been advocated for the diagnosis of pregnancy in the bitch as well as confirmation of fetal viability. In our experience, it has been valuable in assessing the mildly enlarged uterus to determine whether the contents are fluid, as in pyometra; gestational sacs, indicative of pregnancy; or a mass, suggestive of neoplasia. The major shortcoming of ultrasonography is the expense of the equipment involved and the somewhat abstract appearance of the images, making interpretation without previous experi-

ence difficult. Several sonograms are shown in this chapter, but these images are paired, when possible, with survey radiographs to aid reader understanding.

NORMAL RADIOGRAPHIC FINDINGS

Non-pregnant Animal. The normal uterus has a body and two horns, and usually cannot be seen in the normal dog or cat unless the organ is enlarged by a pathologic process or pregnancy.[3] The uterus is tubular and usually is

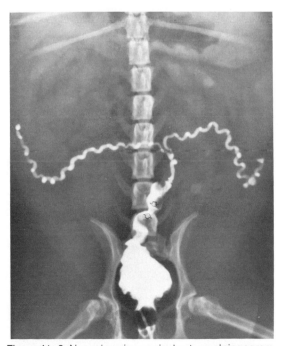

Figure 41–2. Normal canine vaginohysterosalpingogram, ventrodorsal view. The cervix can be identified (arrows).

about 1 cm in diameter.[3] The uterus is located in the mid and caudal abdomen with the uterine body between the colon and the bladder, as discussed in the preceding section concerning abdominal compression.[3] The radiopacity of the uterus is that of soft tissue and it cannot usually be differentiated from small intestine on survey radiographs.

Pregnant Animal. The size, shape, and opacity of the canine uterus during pregnancy varies with the breed, the number of feti, and the stage of gestation. The fetal development and radiographic appearance of the uterus during gestation has been described in detail elsewhere,[4, 10] but a brief summary follows. In general, uterine enlargement is detectable at approximately 30 days after ovulation.[4] The circumference of the uterine horns is then reported to be about 10 to 11 cm.[10] Spheric enlargements at the location of the gestational sacs are identifiable in the uterus between 30 and 40 days after ovulation.[4] The circumference at the spheric enlargement is then approxi-

mately 10 to 15 cm.[10] The uterus subsequently becomes smoothly tubular and has been described as sausage-shaped at about 38 to 45 days after ovulation;[4] the circumference of the uterine horns is then approximately 12 to 17 cm.[10] Early fetal mineralization is identifiable by survey radiographs at or beyond 45 days after ovulation.[4] For further specifics, including estimated crown-rump length, References 4 and 10 may be consulted. A near-term pregnancy in a normal bitch is shown as it appears radiographically in Figure 41–3.

The size, shape, and opacity of the feline uterus is similar in its variation to the dog, with major variables being number of feti and stage of gestation. The feline uterus during gestation is described, in considerable detail in Reference 11, but a brief summary follows. In the pregnant cat, detectable uterine enlargement occurs at approximately 25 to 35 days of gestation. Fetal mineralization is identified at approximately 36 to 45 days of gestation. Fetal mineralization progresses beyond this time; for crown-rump

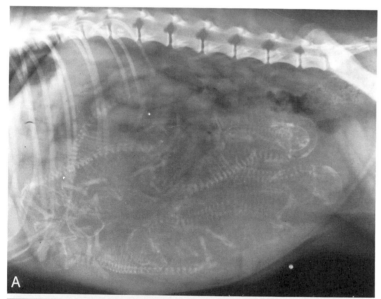

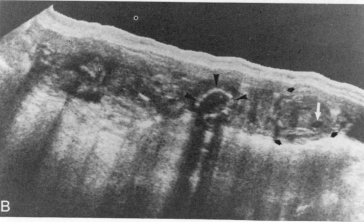

Figure 41–3. *A,* a normal pregnancy, near term, in a bitch (lateral view). Note the mineralization and alignment of the skull bones as well as the arrangement of the cervical through lumbar vertebrae and the pelvis with the appendages. *B,* sagittal sonogram with the patient in dorsal recumbency, the head to the left and the ventral abdominal wall at the top of the scan. Note the well-defined fetal head *(arrowheads)* with the shadowing phenomenon beyond it secondary to its mineralization. Also note the cross-section of another fetal torso *(black arrows)* in which echopenic areas, representing the stomach, can be identified *(white arrow).*

length estimates, the reader is referred to Reference 11.

The location of the pregnant uterus in both the dog and the cat is in the mid to caudal ventral abdomen at mid to late gestation. The enlargement of the uterus at this sight causes cranial and somewhat dorsal displacement of the small intestine, with dorsal and lateral displacement of the descending colon and some degree of ventral compression of the urinary bladder.[5]

ABNORMAL RADIOGRAPHIC FINDINGS

Number. Absence of one of the horns in a normally bicornuate uterus has been reported.[12] It is likely that there is considerable variation in the length of the uterine body versus the length of the uterine horns, especially because there is much variation in litter size with breed and body stature. Another consideration relative to the number of uterine horns or possibly the number of uterine bodies is the variable manifestation in the pseudohermaphrodite intersex anomalies. Contrast urinary and genital tract studies may be utilized to investigate intersex anomalies further, but they are often difficult to evaluate. Surgical removal and morphologic analysis is often necessary for a definitive diagnosis.

Size. Generalized uterine enlargement in the absence of fetal mineralization may be suggestive of a number of diseases in addition to the early phases of normal pregnancy before fetal mineralization. Differential diagnoses that should be considered under these circumstances include early pregnancy and possibly pseudopregnancy;[3, 4, 5, 13] pyometra, hydrometra, and mucometra;[3–5, 13, 14] uterine torsion;[3–5, 13, 15, 16] and uterine adenomyosis.[17] The radiographic manifestation of diffuse uterine enlargement is shown in Figure 41–4; unilateral pyometra was noted secondary to a sarcoma at the junction of the affected uterine horn and the uterine body. The diagnosis of an intrauterine mass was made on the basis of ultrasonographic evaluation and not on the survey radiographic evaluation, which suggested nonspecific uterine enlargement.

Generalized uterine enlargement in the presence of fetal mineralization is suggestive of pregnancy, but the possibility of torsion of the pregnant uterus should not be excluded. Clinical signs and history must then be used to differentiate these possibilities rather than radiography per se.

Localized uterine enlargement can be suggestive of a number of diseases, including neoplasia;[3, 18] cystic endometrial hyperplasia;[2, 18] localized or loculated pyometra, hydrometra, or mucometra;[14] uterine stump granuloma or abscess;[5, 19] cystic uterine remnant;[20] and uterine adenomyosis.[17] Focal uterine body enlargement confirmed as a uterine stump granuloma with urinary bladder invasion and a fistulous tract draining into the flank is shown in Figure 41–5.

Location. The normal location of the uterus in the caudal ventral mid-abdomen has been discussed, and its detection as well as location and effect on adjacent organs is highly dependent on its size.[3, 5] Herniation of the uterus through discontinuities in the abdominal wall, including the inguinal ring, can occur and may be congenital or acquired.[3] It is also possible that these herniations may occur during pregnancy. An example of uterine herniation into the subcutaneous tissues via the inguinal canal is shown in Figure 41–6. This uterus was in the early stages of gestation and contained no evidence of fetal mineralization.

Radiopacity. The normal nonpregnant and early pregnant uterus are of soft tissue or fluid radiopacity.[3–5] Other uterine conditions that also have soft-tissue radiographic characteristics are pyometra, hydrometra, mucometra, and uterine torsion.[3–5, 15, 16] As previously mentioned, history and clinical signs are necessary to differentiate among these possibilities. Gas within the uterus is generally indicative of either fetal death[3, 4] or ischemia due to uterine torsion.[2] In both instances, the gas is due to devitalization and breakdown of the tissues. An example of an emphysematous fetus is shown in Figure 41–7. A word of caution, however, lies in the fact that no attempts at catheterization of the cervix have been made when gas could have artifactually been introduced into the uterus and then been overinterpreted as evidence of intrauterine disease. The other possibility is that a gas-forming organism within an abscess of the uterine stump in the neutered patient may cause focal accumulation of air, but this is highly unlikely.[5]

Mineralization within the uterus is usually indicative of fetal skeletons, but it is imperative that the alignment of the structures, such as vertebrae, ribs, and limbs, and the shape and alignment of skull bones be assessed to differentiate a radiographically viable fetus, a dead fetus, and a mummified fetus.[3, 4] In general, radiographic evidence of axial or appendicular skeletal malalignment or collapse of the skull bones is suggestive of fetal death. Overlap and apparent compression of the structures into a smaller than expected space is more suggestive of mummification than a recent history of fetal death. An example of a mummified fetus is shown in Figure 41–8.

If the fetal skeleton appears to be tightly curled, more obvious than expected than when surrounded by uterus, or not associated with a tubular uterine radiopacity or its expected location, the possibility of ectopic pregnancies should be considered.[21, 22] Peritoneal effusion

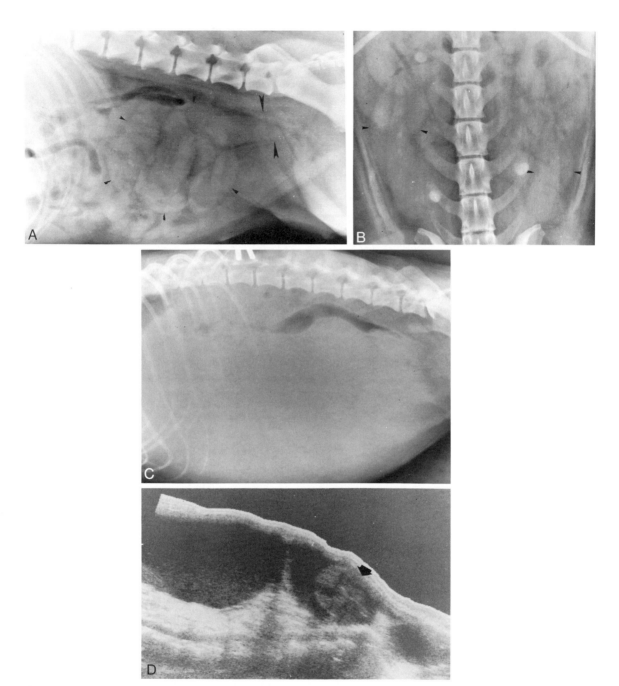

Figure 41–4. Lateral *(A)* and ventrodorsal *(B)* radiographs of a patient with a tubular, coiled, soft-tissue structure in the caudal abdomen that extends into the pelvis *(arrows)*. This structure is a moderately distended uterus, as found in pyometra. *C,* lateral view of a patient with a caudoventral abdominal mass that occupies about 60 percent of the abdominal cavity. Displacement of the viscera is consistent with uterine involvement. *D,* sagittal sonogram of the same patient (head is to the left and the ventral abdominal wall is at the top of the scan). The mass is seen to be primarily echopenic, indicating that it is fluid-filled. There is, however, an echogenic mass in the caudal portion of one of the fluid-filled subdivisions *(arrow)*. Radiologic and sonographic interpretations: a fluid-filled uterus with a mass in the region of the junction between the uterine body and the uterine horns. Surgical diagnosis: pyometra of the left uterine horn due to neoplasm (sarcoma) of the junction between the uterine horn and body.

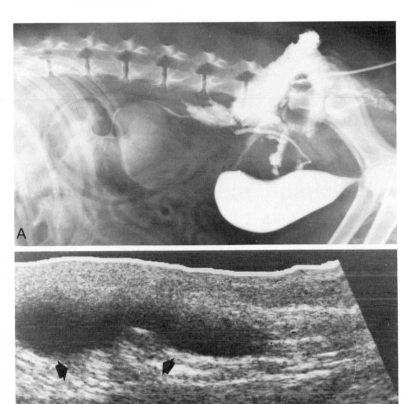

Figure 41–5. *A,* lateral view after excretory urography and left flank fistulography. Draining tract in the left flank injected with contrast medium leads to a soft-tissue mass, which displaces the urinary bladder ventrally and indents it dorsally. Only the right kidney and ureter can be identified. *B,* sagittal sonogram of the urinary bladder area (ventral abdominal wall at the top and the head to the left of the scan). An echogenic mass *(arrows)* indents into and through the wall of the urinary bladder. Radiologic diagnosis: probable uterine stump granuloma. The diagnosis was confirmed at laparotomy.

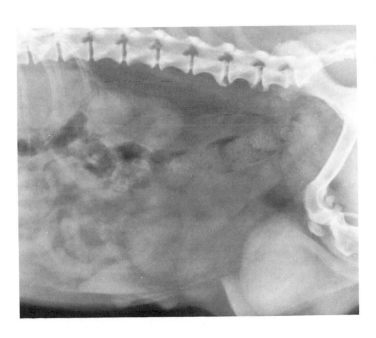

Figure 41–6. Lateral view of a bitch in midterm pregnancy with an inguinal mass. The tubular soft-tissue opacity representing the uterus extends into the subcutaneous peri-inguinal tissues. Radiologic diagnosis: inguinal hernia containing a portion of dilated uterus, probably secondary to pregnancy.

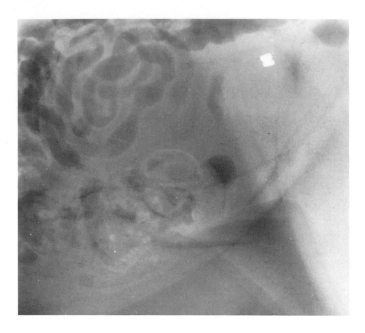

Figure 41–7. Close-up lateral view of the ventral abdomen. There is a moderately mineralized fetus within the soft-tissue uterine shadow. There is, however, gas surrounding the fetus. Radiologic diagnosis: emphysematous fetus.

may complicate the assessment of the uterine boundaries in these patients and may further confuse the diagnosis with the possibility of acute uterine rupture rather than ectopic pregnancy.[22, 23] Gentle abdominal compression and follow-up radiography may be of assistance in differentiating between these possibilities.

Function. Dystocia may be due to both maternal and fetal factors.[24] Radiographs are of minimal value in determining the maternal factors, such as uterine contractility, other than assessment of the size relationship between the fetus and the maternal pelvic canal. Radiography can be helpful in assessing one of the fetal factors, positioning relative to the maternal pelvic canal, thus providing additional evidence

for the necessity of caesarean section (Fig. 41–9). Survey radiographs can also be of value in the postpartum bitch to determine the possibility of retained fetus, but routine follow-up radiography of every pregnancy is not indicated. Abdominal palpation and clinical signs should

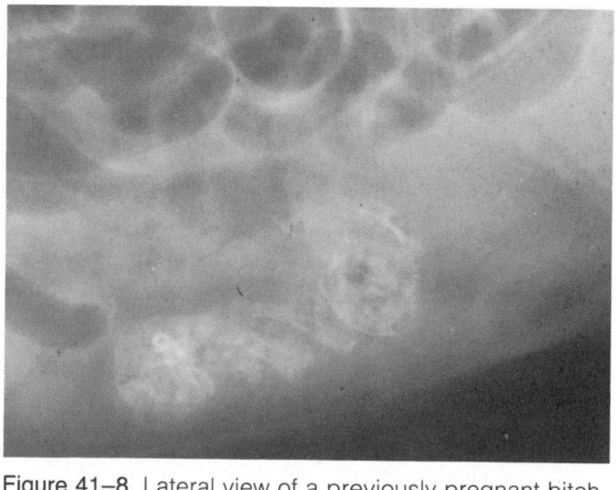

Figure 41–8. Lateral view of a previously pregnant bitch. An irregularly mineralized mass with some evidence of skull and tubular bones can be identified and is located outside the intestinal tract and in a region consistent with that of the uterus. Radiologic diagnosis: mummified fetus. The diagnosis was confirmed at surgery.

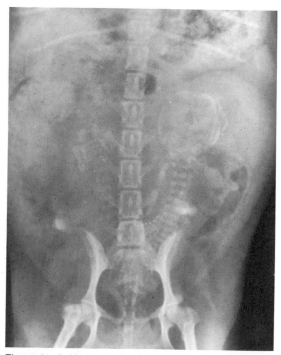

Figure 41–9. Ventrodorsal view of a small-breed bitch in dystocia. Note the transverse presentation of the enlarged, but as determined radiographically, viable fetus. Surgical diagnosis: viable single fetus, which subsequently died.

be used as major determining factors for post-partum radiography.

RELATED ABNORMAL INTRA-ABDOMINAL FINDINGS

Unexplained intra-abdominal calcific opacities may be related to previous uterine rupture or ectopic pregnancy and subsequent mummification of the involved feti. Careful radiographic scrutiny of the character of the calcified intra-abdominal masses and the possible use of serial radiographs to assess reproducibility of the location are indicated. Occasionally, ingestion of an intact body of a puppy or other small animal may complicate the differentiation of intrauterine fetal calcification or mummification, intra-abdominal ectopic pregnancy or fetal mummification, and the ingested body of a fetus or other similar-sized animal.

Variations in abdominal contrast may be somewhat nonspecific in that there are numerous causes for accumulation of abdominal fluid and free intraperitoneal air. The presence of abdominal fluid, however, especially if the patient has intestinal displacement (when intraluminal gas is present) consistent with an enlarged uterus, may be suggestive of uterine rupture with subsequent hemorrhage, ruptured pyometra, or hemorrhage from uterine torsion. Free intraperitoneal air in such patients, especially in the presence of intrauterine (perifetal) or intrafetal air, is highly suggestive of uterine rupture and fetal death.

ULTRASONOGRAPHY AND ITS APPLICATION

Ultrasonography is of greatest value in assessing the uterine contents when only soft-tissue opacity is seen radiographically. The use of ultrasonography can be of value in differentiating early pregnancy, pseudopregnancy, and pyometra when the stage of gestation is too early for fetal mineralization. Ultrasonography can also be of value in the assessment of the etiologic factors for uterine enlargement other than fluid distension, including neoplasia and adenomyosis. Fetal viability can be assessed by using real-time or M-mode ultrasonography in the identification of the fetal heart and its moving valves. The movement of the fetus as visualized on two-dimensional, real-time ultrasonography is also an indicator of fetal viability. Fetal heart and major vessels can be imaged quite readily, as demonstrated in Figure 41–10. Ultrasonography can also be helpful in confirming pregnancy in the early stage i.e., 22 to 26 days after breeding. This technique is especially useful in the obese or muscular bitch that is not amenable to manual assessment of the sacculated uterine

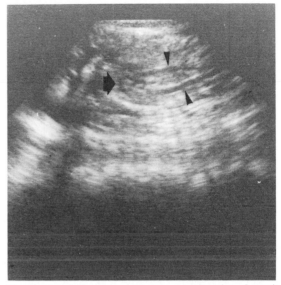

Figure 41–10. Sagittal real-time sonogram of an 8-week fetus in utero. The fetal heart *(arrow)* and the fetal caudal vena cava and fetal aorta *(arrowheads)* were functioning normally during dynamic imaging.

conformation in early pregnancy. The ultrasonic appearance of a gestational sac approximately 24 days after mating is shown in Figure 41–11.

On the basis of the previous discussion of normal and abnormal radiographic findings and the radiographic techniques that are useful to assess these findings, the gamut approach to the diagnosis of most uterine diseases should now be possible. As emphasized, it is important to assess the radiographic abnormalities in terms of the roentgen signs, especially those of opacity and geometry, and to compare the radiographic differential considerations with information obtained from the history and the

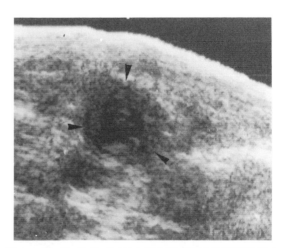

Figure 41–11. Static B-scan of a 24-day pregnancy in a normal bitch. Note the echopenic gestational sac *(arrowheads)* that contains the fetal pole.

clinical evaluation. The finding of uterine enlargement is commonly a nonspecific radiographic finding, and the differentiation of early pregnancy, uterine torsion, and pyo/hydro/mucometra necessitates careful evaluation of factors other than those identified radiographically.

Although the emphasis of this chapter has been on the radiographic findings, in particular the survey radiographic findings, it should be noted that two-dimensional, gray-scale ultrasonography may play a major role as a noninvasive diagnostic technique. When access to such techniques is afforded to the clinician, the potential usefulness of this procedure should be considered.

References

1. Buckner RG: The genital system. *In* Catcott EJ (Ed): Canine Medicine, 4th Ed. Santa Barbara, CA, American Veterinary Publishers, 1979, pp. 501–532.
2. Colby ED, and Stein BS: The reproductive system. *In* Pratt PW (Ed): Feline Medicine. Santa Barbara, CA, American Veterinary Publishers, 1983, pp. 511–534.
3. Ackerman, N: Radiographic evaluation of the uterus: A review. Vet Radiol 22:252, 1981.
4. Rendano VJ: Radiographic evaluation of fetal development in the bitch and fetal death in the bitch and the queen. *In* Kirk RW (Ed): Current Veterinary Therapy VIII. Philadelphia, WB Saunders, 1983, pp. 947–952.
5. Root CN: Interpretation of abdominal survey radiographs. Vet Clin North Am 4:763, 1974.
6. Cobb LM: Radiographic outline of the genital system of the bitch. Vet Rec 71:66, 1959.
7. Reid JS, and Frank RJ: Double contrast hysterogram in the diagnosis of retained placenta in the bitch. A case report, J Am Anim Hosp Assoc 9:367, 1973.
8. Cobb LM, and Archibald J: Radiographic appearance of certain pathological conditions of the canine uterus. J Am Vet Med Assoc 134:393, 1959.
9. Bondestam S, Alitalo I, and Karkkainen M: Real-time ultrasound pregnancy diagnosis in the bitch. J Small Anim Pract 24:145, 1983.
10. Tsutsui T: Process of development uterus, fetus, and fetal appendices during pregnancy in the dog. Bull Nippon Vet Zootech Coll 30:175, 1981.
11. Boyd JS: Radiographic identification of the various stages of pregnancy in the domestic cat. J Small Anim Pract 12:501, 1971.
12. Robinson GW: Uterus unicornis and unilateral renal agenesis in a cat. J Am Vet Med Assoc 147:516, 1965.
13. Stein BS: Obstetrics, Surgical Procedures and Anesthesia. *In* Morrow PA (Ed): Current Therapy in Theriogenology. Philadelphia, WB Saunders, 1980, pp. 865–869.
14. McAfee CT: Hydrouterus and hydroovarium in a beagle bitch. Canine Pract 4:48, 1977.
15. Shull RM, Johnston SD, Johnston GR, et al: Bilateral torsion of uterine horns in a nongrand bitch. J Am Vet Med Assoc 172:601, 1978.
16. Rendano VT, Juck FA, and Binnington AG: Hematometra associated with pseudocyesis and uterine torsion in a dog. J Am Anim Hosp Assoc 10:577, 1974.
17. Pack FD: Feline uterine adenomyosis. Feline Pract 10:45, 1980.
18. Brodey RS, and Roszel JF: Neoplasms of the Canine uterus, vagina and vulva: A clinicopathologic survey. J Am Vet Med Assoc 151:1294, 1967.
19. Spackman CJA, Caywood DD, Johnston GR, et al: Granulomas of the uterine and ovarian stumps: A case report. J Am Anim Hosp Assoc 20:449, 1984.
20. Franklin RT, and Prescott JVB: Tenesmus and stranguria from a cystic uterine remnant. Vet Radiol 24:139, 1983.
21. Carrig CB, Gourley IM, and Philbrick AL: Primary abdominal pregnancy in a cat subsequent to OHE. J Am Vet Med Assoc 160:308, 1972.
22. Tomlinson J, Jackson ML, and Pharr JW: Extrauterine pregnancy in a cat. Feline Pract 10:18, 1980.
23. DeNooy PP: Extrauterine pregnancy and severe ascites in a cat. Vet Med/Small Anim Clin 74:349, 1979.
24. Bennett D: Canine dystocia—a review of the literature. J Small Anim Pract 15:101, 1974.

CHAPTER 42

THE OVARIES AND TESTES

DANIEL A. FEENEY
GARY R. JOHNSTON

OVARIES

Imaging Procedures

Survey radiographs have limited applicability to the ovaries in their normal status. Because these organs are the basis of reproduction in the bitch, exposure to ionizing radiation should be minimized. The indications for radiography of the ovaries have been defined in textbooks of internal medicine under the applicable specific diseases.[1, 2] The major application of survey radiographs to diseases of the ovary is that of identifying a mass not palpable at physical examination or further localizing an abdominal mass to the ovary. On the basis of location, displacement of adjacent organs, and radiographic opacity, the organ of origin of the mass may be determined.[3] Survey radiographs are of considerable value in differentiating ovarian, splenic, and kidney masses. The limitations are that normal ovaries cannot be visualized and the internal architecture of ovarian masses cannot be assessed by radiography unless mineralization is present; such mineralization is uncommon.

Abdominal preparation for radiography is routine; food is withheld for 24 hours and an enema is administered, at least 2 hours before radiography.[3] As with other abdominal radiographic techniques, lateral and ventrodorsal views are indicated. It is of paramount importance that proper radiographic technique and attention to darkroom detail be emphasized because intra-abdominal contrast may be limited, even in the absence of intraperitoneal fluid. Under such circumstances, differentiation of an ovarian mass from bowel, kidney, or spleen may be difficult at best, even under ideal radiographic circumstances.

Alternative radiographic procedures that may be of assistance in assessing ovarian masses include pneumoperitonography and excretory urography. Pneumoperitonography has limited applications because the mass can usually be visualized on survey radiographs. Excretory urography provides an indirect means of assessing the ovary by assisting in identification of the kidney on the side of the mass. It may also be helpful to determine the degree of renal displacement and to separate renal parenchyma from that of the ovary if the mass has not resulted in ventral migration of the ovary into the conglomerate of small bowel away from the kidney.

Another technique that has shown promise in assessing intra-abdominal masses, including ovarian masses, is that of gray-scale ultrasonography.[4] When applicable, ultrasonographic images are provided in this chapter to complement the radiographs. Because the technique

467

involves the use of sound directed into tissue and the reconstruction of reflected echoes from variations in tissue texture, the presence of abdominal fluid and the apparent homogeneous appearance of soft-tissue masses or normal organs do not preclude assessment of internal architecture.

Normal Radiographic Findings

The normal ovaries are not seen in the normal bitch or queen. The ovaries are located just caudal to the kidneys in both species.[2, 3] The ovaries are not, however, functionally retroperitoneal as are the kidneys, and ovarian masses gravitate ventrally without extensive ventral displacement of other abdominal viscera, as is caused by a renal mass.[5]

Abnormal Radiographic Findings

Number. Usually only one, but occasionally both, ovaries may be radiographically abnormal. In our opinion, the ovary must increase in size to at least the diameter of two bowel loops to be identifiable on survey radiographs. The shape of the abnormal ovary may be variable. but ovarian masses are usually well circumscribed.[5] Depending on the specific cell type of a neoplasm, if the mass is neoplastic in origin, abdominal fluid may also be identified.

Size. A radiographically detectable mass in the appropriate anatomic region for ovary, which is usually caudal to the respective kidney and originating from the dorsal abdominal wall, should have certain differential considerations: follicular cyst,[6] luteal cyst,[6] tumors of gonadal-stromal origin,[6, 7] tumors of epithelial origin,[6, 7] germ-cell tumors (see section entitled Radiopacity),[7, 8] tumors of mesodermal origin,[7, 8] and hydrovariam.[9] An example of a well-circumscribed ovarian mass is shown in Figure 42–1, as is a sonogram from a similar patient in which both the kidney and the hypoechoic, fluid-filled ovarian cyst can be identified.

Location. The normal ovaries in both the bitch and queen lie caudal to their respective kidneys. As these structures enlarge, however, they may displace the ipsilateral kidney cra-

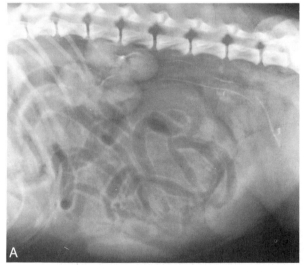

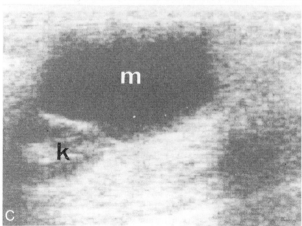

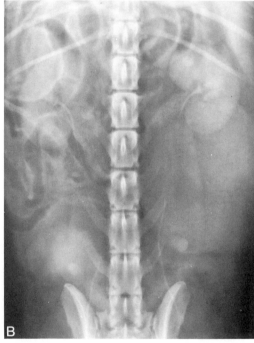

Figure 42–1. Lateral *(A)* and ventrodorsal *(B)* views of a patient with a soft-tissue abdominal mass approximately four times the size of the left kidney and located caudal and ventral to it. Kidneys are opacified secondary to the injection of contrast medium for excretory urography. Location of the soft-tissue mass is consistent with that of the ovary. *C*, real-time sonogram from a similar patient in which an echopenic (fluid-filled) mass (m) with distant enhancement associated with the caudal pole of the kidney (k) can be seen. Radiologic diagnosis: ovarian mass, sonographically consistent with simple cyst.

nially or laterally and may pull it ventrally. The degree and direction of adjacent organ displacement and extent of ovarian mass migration depend on ovarian size and the position of the patient during radiography. Abdominal viscera other than those described specifically in the previous section may be displaced. For a more extensive discussion of the evaluation of ovarian masses, the reader is directed to Reference 5.

Radiopacity. Ovarian cysts and most ovarian neoplasms are of soft-tissue or water opacity.[6, 7] Occasionally, these structures may contain mineralized areas, including those with the opacity of bone or tooth enamel. These masses are usually benign teratomas (dermoid cyst),[7, 8] but malignant teratocarcinomas have also been reported to contain calcific opacities.[10] On the basis of this assessment and the vast difference in prognosis for these two types of malignancies, it is ill-advised to base the prognosis on the presence of calcification.

Consideration. It is important to be aware of the possibility of intersex conditions, including the true and pseudohermaphrodite.[11, 12] Complex anomalies encompassing the entire genital tract and involving the urinary tract should be considered in patients with other intra-abdominal abnormalities or combined urinary and reproductive signs. Although multiple contrast radiographic procedures and ultrasonographic evaluation may be of assistance in analyzing the anomaly, it is often necessary to remove the anomalous tissue and then to evaluate it by dissection and histologic examination.

Related Abnormal Radiographic Findings

Abdominal effusion, which may occur from a wide variety of etiologies, may result from peritoneal seeding and diffuse metastasis of malignant ovarian tumors or hemorrhage due to rupture of an ovarian tumor.[13] Although ovarian tumors are less often the cause of malignant effusion, abdominal hemorrhage, or both, these lesions should at least be considered as differential possibilities in an intact bitch.

TESTES

Imaging Procedures

Survey radiographs have limited applicability to the intrascrotal testes. They are, however, of value in the assessment of abdominal masses, which include neoplastic transformation of an intra-abdominal testicle. Because of the ease of palpation of the intrascrotal testes, radiography usually provides a minimal amount of additional information. It is also important to limit all exposure to the mutagenic effects of ionizing radiation. Pneumoperitonography has limited applications for the intra-abdominal mass that may be a retained intra-abdominal testicle; the technique adds minimal specificity, and the mass is usually of sufficient size to be seen without intraperitoneal air. An additional method that does provide information on the intrascrotal and intra-abdominal testicular architecture is gray-scale ultrasonography.[14] This technique is applicable to reproductive organs because as yet no major reproductive or genetic consequences have resulted from the use of the diagnostic technique. For a more extensive discussion of the role of ultrasonography in the diagnosis of testicular disease, the reader is referred to Reference 14.

Normal Radiographic Findings

Because the testicles, epididymis, and scrotum are all soft-tissue structures, radiography is of minimal value in small animals to evaluate these organs. The accessibility of the scrotum to visual and digital inspection further minimizes the usefulness of radiography. Radiography may on occasion provide some information on the opacity (such as mineral or air) of an abnormality detected by palpation.

Ultrasonography is of assistance in noninvasively assessing the internal architecture of the testicle and epididymis as well as the nature of scrotal enlargement. Although extensive work on the ultrasonic architecture of canine and feline testicles has not been evaluated, our limited experience suggests that testicular parenchyma is usually of fairly uniform echogenicity. Increases or decreases in echogenicity and the presence of either shadowing due to mineralization or distal (far) enhancement due to intraparenchymal liquid is abnormal. For more details, Reference 14 should be consulted.

Abnormal Radiographic Findings

Detailed discussion of the embryogenesis of the testes, gubernaculum, and scrotum are beyond the scope of the current discussion; for further details, the reader should consult references 15 and 16. As with ovarian diseases, intersex anomalies must be considered. These anomalies may be evaluated by multiple contrast procedures of the lower and upper urinary tract as well as with ultrasonography, although the final diagnosis is usually determined surgically and microscopically.[11, 15] With this preface, the majority of the following discussion deals with sequelae of cryptorchidism amenable to radiographic assessment.

Intra-abdominal testicles that are of normal dimension usually cannot be identified. If the intra-abdominal testicle enlarges, however, the following considerations may apply.

Size and Shape. To be detected radiographically, the enlarged intra-abdominal testicle must be two or more times the diameter of the normal small intestine. When such a structure is identified, it must also be differentiated from other soft-tissue structures in the abdomen, such as fluid-filled cecum or bladder, spleen, and possibly prostate. In general, the radiologic consideration of the mass as an intra-abdominal testicle is either by prior sensitization to the fact that only one testicle was descended or identified at castration or by the fact that the mass cannot be associated with any other organ of origin in this male patient. The shape of the enlarged, and probably neoplastically transformed, intra-abdominal testicle is usually fairly symmetric with varying degrees of surface irregularity.

Number and Radiopacity. Usually only one of the testicles is responsible for the abdominal abnormalities in a given patient, even if both testicles are intra-abdominal. The radiographic opacity of intra-abdominal testicles is usually that of soft tissue, and no specificity can be assigned to the identification of calcific opacity within these masses; such an opacity is most likely to be dystrophic calcification rather than to suggest teratoma/teratocarcinoma, as it was in the bitch.

Location. Intra-abdominal testicles, when identified radiographically as an abdominal mass, usually lie somewhere in a parasagittal plane between the caudal pole of the ipsilateral kidney and the inguinal canal. Our experience suggests these testicles usually gravitate to the ventral abdomen as they enlarge, causing dorsal and lateral displacement of the small intestine and possible indentation or caudal displacement of the urinary bladder. An example of a neoplastically transformed intra-abdominal testicle is shown in Figure 42–2. Testicles may be identified in the inguinal canal or subcutaneous structures of the inguinal region when they succeed in exiting the abdomen during development but did not achieve the ultimate scrotal location. Subcutaneous soft-tissue masses in this region in a male dog may be identified radiographically, but differentiation from lymph

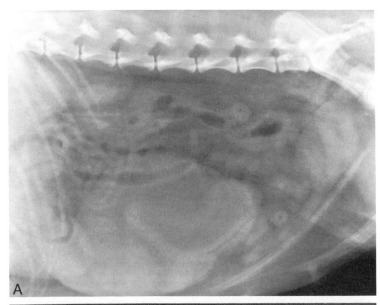
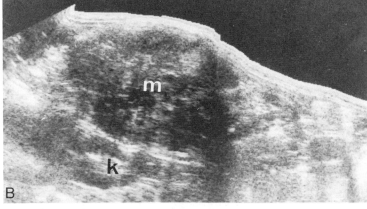

Figure 42–2. *A,* lateral radiograph of a male dog with an abdominal mass and only one palpable descended testicle. The abdominal mass in the caudal midventral abdomen is approximately four to six times the size of the kidneys. *B,* sagittal sonogram with the patient in dorsal recumbency (head to the left). There is a variably echogenic and echopenic mass (m) of similar dimensions to that seen in *A.* The right kidney (k) can be seen dorsal to the mass. Radiologic diagnosis: well-circumscribed intra-abdominal mass, probably a retained intra-abdominal testicle. The diagnosis was confirmed at laparotomy.

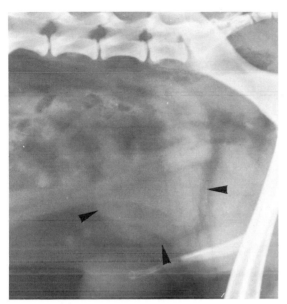

Figure 42–3. Lateral view of a male dog in which only one testicle was intrascrotal. There is an ovoid soft-tissue mass (arrowheads) in the peri-inguinal soft tissues in the region of the os penis. Surgical diagnosis: malignant transformation of an incompletely descended testicle.

node, subcutaneous tumor, or another nonspecific mass requires ultrasonographic assessment and probable microscopic examination of a fine needle aspirate. An example of an enlarged, neoplastically transformed inguinal testicle is shown in Figure 42–3.

Consideration. An intra-abdominal mass identified in a male dog fitting the size, shape, and location criteria described above must be differentiated from other intra-abdominal organs, including the spleen, bladder, cecum, and prostate; a nonspecific mesenteric mass; and a mass originating within the intestinal tract. Ultrasonography, particularly two-dimensional real-time techniques, can be valuable in this differentiation. Fine-needle aspiration biopsy and laparotomy are the alternatives worthy of consideration.

The mass, which is possibly testicle, may represent neoplastically transformed, retained testicle[7] or torsion of an intra-abdominal testicle without neoplastic transformation.[17, 18] Differentiation between these processes is based on history, abdominal palpation, and the reproductive and cutaneous manifestations of endocrine abnormalities associated with neoplastic testicular tissue.

Intrascrotal Testicle

The size and shape are the major features used to assess the intrascrotal testicle for potential abnormalities. Symmetric enlargement of the testicle or hemiscrotum is suggestive of orchitis,[19] hydrocele,[14, 19] intrascrotal testicular tor-

sion,[17, 19] and nonspecific vascular abnormalities.[19] It is worth noting that observation of the testicular mass and spermatic cord at scrotal exploratory surgery is the most definitive means of differentiation among the scrotal contents and does not carry with it the known genetic sequela of ionizing radiation to the opposite testicle. Asymmetric enlargement of the intrascrotal testicle is suggestive of neoplasia,[7] varicocele,[14] hematoma/abscess, epididymitis;[19] differentiation of these possibilities may be facilitated by information from the history and fine-needle aspiration biopsy.

As mentioned previously, an additional means of assessing the internal contents of the scrotum, including the testicle, is gray-scale ultrasonography. This method permits identification of the etiology of scrotal enlargement as to testicle, fluid retention, associated mass, and, if the testicle is the site of enlargement, the internal architecture of the offending mass. In Figure 42–4, a sagittal sonogram of a testicle containing a metastatic tumor from a primary in the lung is identified. Ultrasonography was of value in assessing the internal architecture of the mass palpated on the testicle at physical examination.

Related Intra- and Periabdominal Findings

Sublumbar (iliac or paraortic) lymphadenopathy may be identified in patients with testicular disease, and is most likely suggestive of metastasis[20, 21] or extension of an inflammatory process. Lumbar vertebral osteomyelitis and dyspondylitis have been reported in patients with inflammatory diseases of the testicle, including specifically *Brucella canis*.[22]

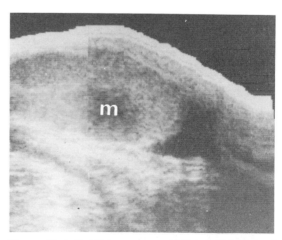

Figure 42–4. Sagittal sonogram of the right testicle. A hypoechoic mass (m) can be seen within the testicular parenchyma. A nodule was palpable at this site as well. Microscopic diagnosis: intratesticular metastatic bronchogenic carcinoma.

On the basis of the discussions of the ovary and the testes, it should now be possible to choose the appropriate method to image and assess the clinically encountered abnormality. The reader should have some perspective as to the applicability and limitations of radiography in the diagnosis of diseases involving the ovary and testes. Sufficient data and reference material have been presented to permit formulation of gamuts for radiographically encountered abnormalities. It is important to remember, however, that microscopic evaluation of neoplastic cell type, bacteriologic confirmation of inflammatory processes, or both are mandatory for definitive diagnosis.

References

1. Colby ED, and Stein BS: The reproductive system. *In* Pratt PW (Ed): Feline Medicine. Santa Barbara, CA, American Veterinary Publishers, 1983, pp. 511–554.
2. Buckner RG: The genital system. *In* Catcott EJ (Ed): Canine Medicine, 4th Ed. Santa Barbara, CA, American Veterinary Publishers, 1979, pp. 501–532.
3. Root CR: Interpretation of abdominal survey radiographs. Vet Clin North Am 4:763, 1974.
4. Gottesfeld KR: Role of ultrasound in gynecologic diagnosis. Clin Diag Ultrasound 2:207, 1979.
5. Root CR: Abdominal masses: The radiographic differential diagnosis. J Am Vet Radiol Soc 15:26, 1974.
6. Dow C: Ovarian abnormalities in the bitch. J Comp Pathol 70:59, 1960.
7. Barrett RE, and Theiler LH: Neoplasms of the canine and feline reproductive tracts. *In* Kirk RW (Ed): Current Veterinary Therapy VI. Philadelphia, WB Saunders, 1977, pp. 1263–1267.
8. Riser WH, Marcus JF, Gaibor EC, et al: Dermoid cyst of the canine ovary. J Am Vet Med Assoc 134:27, 1959.
9. McAfee LT: Hydroureters and hydrovarium in a beagle bitch. Canine Pract 4:48, 1977.
10. Patnaik AK, Schaer M, Parks JL, et al: Metastasizing ovarian teratocarcinoma in dogs. J Small Anim Pract 17:235, 1976.
11. Murti GS, Gilbert DL, and Bougmann AP: Canine intersex states. J Am Vet Med Assoc 149:1183, 1966.
12. Todoroff RJ: Canine urogenital anomalies. Comp Contin Ed Small Anim Pract 1:780, 1979.
13. Greene JA, Richardson RP, Thornhill JA, et al. Ovarian papillary cystadenoma in a bitch. J Am Anim Hosp Assoc 15:351, 1979.
14. Carroll BA, and Gross DM: High-frequency scrotal sonography. AJR 140:511, 1983.
15. Wensing CJ: Developmental anomalies, including cryptorchidism. *In* Morrow DA (Ed): Current Therapy in Theriogenology. Philadelphia, WB Saunders, 1980, pp. 583–589.
16. Bauran V, Dijkstra F, and Wensing CJ: Testicular descent in the dog. Anat Histol Embryol 10:97, 1981.
17. Pearson A, and Relly DF: Testicular torsion in the dog. A review of 13 cases. Vet Rec 97:200, 1975.
18. Naylor RW, and Thompson SMR: Intra-abdominal testicular torsion—a report of 2 cases. J Am Anim Hosp Assoc 15:763, 1979.
19. Leio DH: Canine orchitis. *In* Kirk RA (Ed): Current Veterinary Therapy VI. Philadelphia, WB Saunders, 1977, pp. 1255–1259.
20. McNeil PE, and Weaver AD: Massive scrotal swelling in two unusual cases of canine sertoli cell tumor. Vet Rec 106:144, 1980.
21. Simon J, and Rubin SB: Metastatic seminoma in a dog. Vet Med/Small Anim Clin 74:941, 1979.
22. Henderson RA, Hoerline BF, Kramer TT, et al: Disspondylitis in three dogs infected with *Brucella canis*. J Am Vet Med Assoc 165:451, 1974.

CHAPTER 43

THE STOMACH

DON L. BARBER
MARY B. MAHAFFEY

ANATOMY

The stomach is a musculoglandular organ that connects the esophagus and the duodenum. The stomach is located in the cranial abdomen, with its cranial surface in close apposition with the caudal surface of the liver. In the normal dog and cat, the empty stomach usually lies cranial to the last pair of ribs,[11, 28] but it may extend slightly caudal to the costal arch. The stomach is roughly shaped as the letter J, lying primarily in a transverse plane to the left of the median plane.

The stomach is subdivided into the cardia, fundus, body, and pyloric portions (Fig. 43–1).[11] The cardia is a small area at the esophagogastric junction. The fundus is the dome or outpouching from the left dorsal aspect of the stomach. The body is the middle portion from the fundus to the pyloric portion and is the largest portion of the stomach. The distal one third of the stomach is the pyloric portion, which is further subdivided into the pyloric antrum and the pyloric canal. The pyloric antrum is the proximal two thirds of the pyloric portion and is relatively thin-walled and slightly expanded. The pyloric canal, the distal one-third of the pyloric portion, is more muscular and contains a double sphincter.

Additional landmarks of the stomach include the greater and lesser curvatures and the angular incisure (notch).[11] The greater curvature is the convex surface of the stomach that originates at the cardia on the left and extends caudoventrally around to the pylorus. The lesser curvature is the concave surface that originates from the right of the cardia and extends cranioventrally to the pylorus. It is the shortest distance between the cardia and the pylorus. The angular notch is the point of acute angulation of the lesser curvature; it is located approximately at the junction of the body and the pyloric antrum. The mucosal surface of the stomach is thrown into numerous folds or ridges called rugal folds, rugae, or plicae. The actual ridges are due to the contour of the mucosa and submucosa.

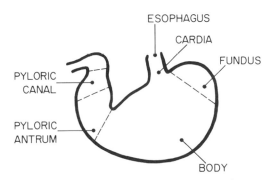

Figure 43–1. The divisions of the stomach.

473

PHYSIOLOGY

The stomach functions as a reservoir for ingested food, a digestive organ to alter food mechanically and chemically, and a propulsive organ to move ingesta along the alimentary tract. As a reservoir, the stomach can retain a large volume of ingested material. This function is facilitated by the elastic, distensible nature of the gastric wall.[28] Gastric distensibility can be documented radiographically by the size of the stomach after a meal or secondary to some gastric diseases. The body is the largest and most distensible portion of the stomach;[11] the pyloric portion, especially the pyloric canal, is the least distensible portion. As a digestive organ, mechanical actions of the stomach interrelate with gastric secretory functions. Mechanical contractions of the stomach mix ingesta with gastric secretions to convert ingested food into semiliquid chyme. As a propulsive organ, gastric contractions propel chyme through the pyloric sphincter into the duodenum.

Three types of movement have been described in the stomach: peristaltic contractions, systolic contractions of the pyloric sphincter, and diminution in size of the body of the stomach.[10] The latter type of movement is difficult to visualize radiographically. In the empty stomach, gastric walls are in close apposition and are relaxed. It was thought that with increasing distension, tension in the gastric wall increased and there was a progressive increase in strength of peristaltic contractions.[9] The relationship of gastric filling, intragastric pressure, and gastric motility, however, may not be as direct as previously thought.[39] Peristaltic contractions originate from a pacemaker near the cardia of the stomach. They are circular contractions of muscle that progress toward the pylorus as a contractile wave. Separate electrical activity occurs in the antrum, however, so that not every cycle has an antral contraction.[39] Gastric contractions are weak in the fundus and body of the stomach and are strong in the pyloric portion. As a peristaltic wave reaches the pyloric canal, increased pressure causes ejection of a small amount of luminal content into the duodenum. Systolic contraction of the pyloric sphincter, however, occurs at approximately the same time and causes closure of the sphincter and retropulsion of luminal content into the pyloric antrum to produce additional mixing.[28] Although the pyloric sphincter is open approximately two thirds of the time,[28] minimal emptying occurs during this phase due to lack of a pressure differential between the stomach and duodenum.[9] The contractile cycle of events takes approximately 12 seconds in a normal dog and occurs at a rate of approximately 5 cycles per minute.[28] Gastric motor function is affected by a wide variety of control mechanisms, which include the volume of gastric content, physical and chemical properties of gastric content, hormonal influences, and neurologic reflexes.[8, 39]

RADIOGRAPHIC EXAMINATION

Preparation. Ingesta within the stomach can obscure some lesions or simulate other lesions, and can thus create false-negative or false-positive results. Therefore, routine radiographic examination of the stomach should be performed on an animal that has been fasted for 12 to 24 hours.[34] This preparation allows for more accurate evaluation of the stomach and for continuation from survey radiography directly to contrast studies if needed. The animal may be allowed to drink water during this period as long as it does not engorge itself. Water may be withheld for 1 to 2 hours before radiography.[5] Because gastric examinations are usually part of survey radiographs of the abdomen, cleansing enemas are also usually performed to cleanse the colon of fecal material. A fecal-filled colon often hinders evaluation of the abdomen and may cause indentation of the stomach, especially by the transverse colon. Variations have been described as to the method and timing of cleansing enemas.[34] The cleansing enema should preferably be given after the fasting period to avoid the reformation of feces. The cleansing enema should be a nonirritating enema soap solution and should be given 2 to 3 hours before radiography. This interval usually allows enough time for expulsion of feces as well as gas that may have been introduced with the enema solution.

Exceptions to this standard protocol do exist. Patients with emesis or anorexia for 12 hours before radiography generally do not require fasting. In addition, the above protocol should be avoided in patients with acute abdominal disorders wherein time delays, fasting, or enemas are medically contraindicated or fluid and gas patterns in the bowel may be of diagnostic importance. Diarrhea may also preclude the need for a cleansing enema.

A consideration of medications is also an important aspect in the preparation of patients for radiographic examination of the stomach. Oral medications should be avoided. Many drugs affect gastric motility, especially anticholinergic drugs, and these preparations should be discontinued for an appropriate interval before any contrast study.[20] Drugs used for chemical restraint can also affect gastrointestinal motility and should be avoided if possible. If chemical restraint is necessary during a contrast study, acetylpromazine maleate may be the agent to use because it may have the least effect on gastrointestinal motility.[42] Triflupromazine hydrochloride may be the preferred drug if both restraint and decreased gastrointestinal motility are desired.[42] Xylazine hydrochloride may produce gastric dilatation and paralytic ileus and therefore its use should be avoided in this situation.[4]

Radiographic Techniques. Survey radiography of the stomach should always precede contrast studies of the stomach. Survey radiographs may be diagnostically adequate for some diseases of the stomach and thus preclude the need for contrast studies. In addition, survey radiography allows evaluation and subsequent adjustment of technical exposure settings in anticipation of the addition of contrast medium. A variety of contrast studies exist for evaluation of the stomach. These studies include standard gastrography with barium sulfate, low-volume gastrography, double-contrast gastrography, pneumogastrography, and gastrography with a water-soluble, organic iodide contrast medium. Standard gastrography with barium sulfate is the most commonly used technique for contrast radiography of the stomach. Low-volume gastrography may occasionally be used to document gastric displacement or in the evaluation of the stomach for certain types of foreign bodies. Double-contrast gastrography may be a more sensitive technique than single-contrast gastrography for detecting lesions of the gastric wall and mucosa,[12] but it is difficult to perform properly without fluoroscopy and chemically inducing gastric hypotonicity. In addition, sensitivity of the technique has been questioned.[18] Pneumogastrography may be of value for the diagnosis of some radiolucent foreign bodies, but the technique is infrequently used. Gastrography with an organic iodide contrast medium may be associated with many problems if used routinely.[36] This procedure should be reserved for the diagnosis of gastric perforation and is rarely used. Methods and variations of these techniques are adequately described elsewhere.[1, 5, 13, 14, 20, 25, 28]

Most radiographs in veterinary medicine are made by using conventional equipment with overhead x-ray tubes. Fluoroscopy is an extremely valuable tool in the radiographic evaluation of the stomach because it allows visualization of dynamic characteristics of the stomach; gastric motion can be observed fluoroscopically. Because the stomach frequently undergoes cyclic changes in appearance and anatomic changes characteristic of a particular disease may not be continuously present, fluoroscopy with spot filming is a valuable tool in demonstrating some diseases of the stomach. Lastly, fluoroscopy can be of value in precise positioning of some patients to best project certain gastric lesions.

Views. Most radiographs of the stomach are made with a conventional, vertically directed x-ray beam. Horizontal-beam radiography is rarely used for evaluation of the stomach. For complete evaluation of the stomach, however, four conventional views may be necessary: the ventrodorsal view with the animal in dorsal recumbency, the dorsoventral view with the animal in ventral recumbency, the right recumbent lateral view, and the left recumbent lateral view. Oblique views may occasionally be of value to isolate or project certain areas of the stomach, such as the pylorus.

NORMAL RADIOGRAPHIC FINDINGS

The radiographic appearance of the normal stomach is quite variable and depends on many factors, such as the species, breed conformation, degree of gastric distension, volume and type of gastric content, position of the patient during radiographic exposure, and the presence or absence of contrast medium within the stomach.

The stomach is located in the cranial abdomen in close apposition with the caudal surface of the liver. It is usually easy to recognize by its location, shape, and content of gas, ingesta, or both. The entire stomach may not be discernible on survey radiographs, however, if it is empty or if the gastric fluid content silhouettes with the liver and other cranial abdominal structures. As a general guide, on the lateral view, the axis of the stomach from the fundus through the body and pylorus is either perpendicular to the spine, parallel to the ribs, or somewhere between these angles (Fig. 43–2A). On the lateral view, the pylorus may be superimposed over the body or located slightly cranial to the body of the stomach. On the ventrodorsal view of the dog, the cardia, fundus, and body of the stomach are located to the left of midline and the pyloric portions are located to the right of midline. The pyloric sphincter is usually located in the right cranial abdominal quadrant at about the level of the 10th to 11th ribs, and is usually cranial to the pyloric canal.[28] The long axis of the stomach may be perpendicular to the spine with the stomach appearing to run straight across the abdomen, making the angular notch difficult to identify (Fig. 43–2B). The stomach may also have a U-shaped appearance with a more obvious angular notch and still be within its normal location, if the pyloric sphincter is not displaced (Fig. 43–2C). On the ventrodorsal view of the cat, the stomach is more acutely angled, with the pylorus located at or near the midline (Fig. 43–2D). Variations in the appearance of the stomach have been described in the dog based on the shape of the thorax and cranial abdomen and thus on breed conformation.[28] The actual shape of the stomach also varies with the degree of gastric distension, since different portions of the stomach vary in their distensibility.

One of the most important factors in the

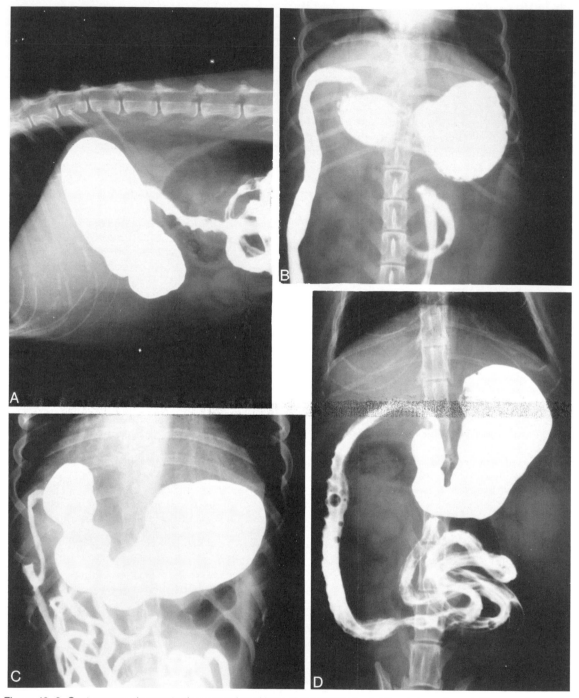

Figure 43–2. Gastrograms demonstrating normal positions of the stomach. *A,* lateral view of a cat. The gastric axis is parallel with the ribs. *B,* ventrodorsal view of a dog. The gastric axis of this dog is perpendicular to the spine. *C,* ventrodorsal view of a dog. The stomach is U-shaped and the pyloric sphincter and fundus are normally located. *D,* ventrodorsal view of a cat. The stomach is acutely angled with the pylorus located at midline.

appearance of the stomach is the position of the patient during radiographic exposure.[21] The relationship between position of the patient and radiographic appearance of the stomach is an important concept that must be understood

both for interpretation of radiographs and for the demonstration of some lesions of the stomach. Variation in appearance of the stomach with different patient positions is due to shifts in fluid and gas distribution within the lumen of the stomach. The stomach usually contains both fluid and gas within its lumen, and the fluid may either be of water opacity or positive-contrast medium opacity. This fluid and gas distribution varies with the position of the patient because fluid settles dependently due to gravity, and gas rises to the highest or uppermost portion of the lumen. Gas and positive-contrast media are relatively easy to visualize on radiographs, whereas substance of water opacity within the stomach may be more difficult to visualize due to silhouetting with other structures of similar opacity in the cranial abdomen.

To help understand the aforementioned relationship, the stomach can be described as J-shaped and positioned in a transverse plane in the cranial abdomen. Thus, as an example, with a patient positioned in dorsal recumbency for a ventrodorsal view, fluid within the lumen settles dependently to the fundus and body of the stomach. If enough fluid is present, the pyloric portion of the stomach also fills. Gas rises to the uppermost portion, which is in the pyloric antrum and body near midline. This description, or example, is illustrated in Figure 43-3. Figure 43-3 is a computed tomographic cross-sectional view of the cranial abdomen at the level of the stomach made with the dog in dorsal recumbency. Note the fluid opacity filling most of the stomach with the gas bubble floating near midline. With this image as an example, it is possible to project how the fluid and gas would be distributed if the animal were

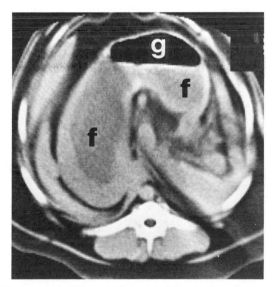

Figure 43–3. CT scan of a normal dog in dorsal recumbency at the level of the stomach. Fluid (f) fills most of the stomach, and the gas bubble (g) floats near midline. (From Baber DL: Vet Radiol 22:149, 1981 with permission.)

rotated in 90 degree increments for a left recumbent lateral view, a dorsoventral view in sternal recumbency, a right recumbent lateral view, and back to a ventrodorsal view in dorsal recumbency. These variations in appearance of the stomach are further altered by the volumes and ratios of fluid to gas within the stomach. Examples of the appearance of the stomach with various views are illustrated in Figure 43–4, which were made with a conventional, vertically directed x-ray beam.

On the ventrodorsal view (Fig. 43–4A), the gas is located in the pyloric antrum and body near midline. Fluid settles to fill the fundus, body, and pyloric portions of the stomach. A larger volume of gas would fill additional areas of the stomach. If completely empty, the fundus and body may appear as a soft-tissue nodule on the ventrodorsal view. On a dorsoventral view (Fig. 43–4B), gas rises to the cardia and fundus, and fluid settles dependently to fill the pyloric portions and part of the body. On the left recumbent lateral view (Fig. 43–4C), gas rises to the pyloric portion of the stomach, which is on the patient's right side and is thus the uppermost point of the stomach. Fluid settles dependently to the fundus and body. Occasionally, a gas pocket may be trapped in the fundic region. In this position, the fundus and body are well visualized with positive-contrast medium but are more difficult to visualize if filled with fluid of water opacity (Fig. 43–5A). On the right recumbent lateral view (Fig. 43–4D), gas rises to the fundus and body, which are on the patient's left side and thus are uppermost. With this view, the gas is often more spread out to fill the fundus and body (Fig. 43–5B) and may not stand out as discretely as on the left recumbent lateral view. In addition, fluid settles dependently to fill the pyloric portions and part of the body of the stomach. In this position, the pyloric portion is well visualized with positive-contrast medium. Occasionally, the pyloric antrum and distal part of the body may appear as a soft-tissue nodule or mass on survey radiographs if filled with fluid of water opacity and projected in the right recumbent lateral view (Fig. 43–5B).

Understanding the relationships of view, position, and findings is important in the radiographic evaluation of the stomach for several reasons. The radiographic appearance of the normal stomach is quite variable. It is thus important to recognize variations that exist in appearance of the normal stomach and to recognize how the appearance of the stomach can be altered by factors such as position of the patient and the volumes and ratios of fluid and gas within the stomach. It is also important to be able to take advantage of fluid and gas shifts

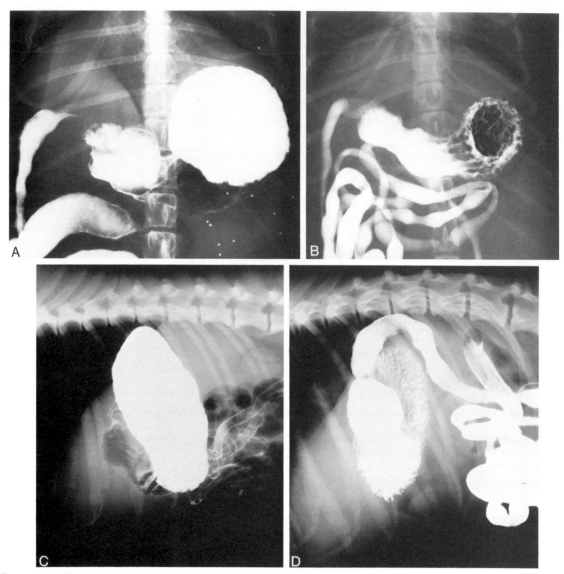

Figure 43–4. Normal variations in fluid (barium) and gas distribution within the stomach with different patient positions. *A*, ventrodorsal view, in dorsal recumbency. Gas is located in the body and pyloric antrum. Fluid settles dependently to fill the fundus, body, and pyloric portions. (Compare with Fig. 43–3.) *B*, dorsoventral view, in ventral recumbency. Gas rises to the cardia and fundus, and fluid settles dependently to fill pyloric portions and part of the body. *C*, left recumbent lateral view. Gas rises to the pyloric portion and fluid settles dependently to fill the fundus and body. *D*, right recumbent lateral view. Gas rises to the fundus and body, which are coated with barium. Fluid settles dependently to fill the pyloric portion and part of the body.

within the stomach to visualize certain portions of the stomach more clearly.

Rugal folds are not seen well on survey radiographs. With positive-contrast gastrography, rugal folds are best visualized at the peripheral portions of the stomach where they may be visualized end on as regular, small filling defects at the mucosal surface. If projected en face, rugal folds are not visible with positive-contrast gastrography unless the barium is well penetrated by the x-ray beam or the stomach

has emptied much of the original dose. Rugal folds then appear as relatively radiolucent, linear filling defects separated by barium in the interrugal spaces (Fig. 43–6). Double-contrast gastrography provides the most detailed evaluation of the gastric mucosa and rugal folds.

Radiographic evaluation of rugal folds is subjective. Rugal folds vary in size and number,[20] and the appearance of rugal folds is dependent on the degree of gastric distension. Rugal folds are more tortuous in the nondistended stomach

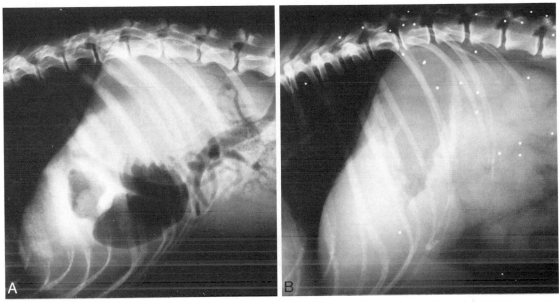

Figure 43–5. Normal variations in fluid and gas distribution within the stomach on survey radiographs. *A,* left recumbent lateral view. Gas rises to the pyloric portion and part of the body, and a gas pocket remains near the cardia. Fluid settles dependently to the fundus and body, which are difficult to visualize when filled with fluid of water opacity. (Compare with Fig. 43–4C.) *B,* right recumbent lateral view. Gas rises to fill the fundus and body. Fluid settles dependently to the pyloric portion, which appears as a soft-tissue mass.

and become more uniform and parallel to the gastric curvatures with increasing gastric distension. [14, 20] Rugal folds are smaller and more spiral in the pyloric antrum. [30] Rugal folds may not be visible if the stomach is overdistended. [13] Contractions of the stomach wall also alter the appearance of the rugal fold pattern. Size of rugal folds is difficult to quantitate, but attempts

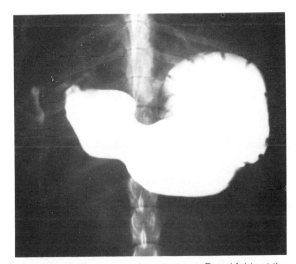

Figure 43–6. Dorsoventral gastrogram. Rugal folds at the periphery of the stomach are viewed end on and create small filling defects at the mucosal surface. Radiolucent linear filling defects are due to rugal folds projected en face.

have been made to interrelate the height of rugal folds, the width of rugal folds, and the width of interrugal spaces. [28] Rugal folds are also smaller and fewer in number in cats than in dogs. [28]

Gastric peristalsis and gastric emptying can be observed directly during fluoroscopy by using positive-contrast media. Without fluoroscopy, however, gastric peristalsis cannot be evaluated well. Although a peristaltic contraction may be seen on a conventional radiograph during gastrography, visualization of peristalsis is a chance event dependent on when the radiograph was made during the contractile cycle of the stomach. A peristaltic contraction appears as an indentation of the wall of the stomach with slight dilatation of the lumen immediately preceding the contraction. Peristaltic contractions are stronger and thus deeper and more obvious in the pyloric portion of the stomach.

Gastric emptying is evaluated on radiographs made later during a sequentially timed study. Gastric emptying should start, or be visible, within 15 minutes in most properly prepared, normal patients. [17, 19, 28] This time interval between the administration of the contrast medium and initiation of gastric emptying has been referred to as the initial gastric emptying time. [28] During gastrography with barium sulfate, the stomach generally empties within 1 to 4 hours in dogs. [17, 20] The time interval between administration of contrast medium and completion of gastric emptying has been referred to as the total gastric emptying time.[28] Minimal significance is generally applied to rapid emptying of the stomach; more significance is applied to delayed emptying. The rate of gastric emptying is a complex phenomenon, however, that is altered by a variety of factors, such as the volume of an intragastric meal, chemical and physical properties of chyme entering the duodenum, various extrinsic reflex mechanisms, and certain medications. Thus a standard approach must be used to evaluate the rate of gastric emptying radiographically. Because the stomach starts to empty faster with an increased intraluminal volume,[35] the dose of contrast medium should be standardized. Low doses of contrast medium may result in delayed gastric emptying, which in turn may lead to a false-positive diagnosis of pyloric obstruction. The type of contrast medium used, the volume of contrast medium administered, and the presence or absence of medications that can affect gastric emptying are all factors that must be considered and standardized. If these factors can be excluded as a cause of delayed gastric emptying, then such delays are most often due to psychic influences or actual disease at the pylorus. Emotional stress can inhibit gastric movement.[7] Anxiety, fear, rage, or pain induced by physical manipulation of the patient in positioning, gastric intubation, and physical restraint can contribute to delayed gastric emptying. Thus, patients with delayed gastric emp-

tying must be allowed to calm down in a quiet environment before diagnostic significance is placed on delayed gastric emptying. Also for these reasons, minimal significance is usually placed on slight or minor delays in gastric emptying if the stomach proceeds to empty in a normal manner after an initial delay.

ABNORMAL RADIOGRAPHIC FINDINGS

Displacement. The position of the stomach can be a useful indicator for the radiographic recognition or localization of some extragastric abnormalities in the cranial abdomen. Some diseases of the liver, spleen, pancreas, and diaphragm can affect the stomach. The relationship between the stomach and extragastric abnormality in the cranial abdomen may help to define the primary organ involved or to define the nature of the primary lesion.

The cranial surface of the stomach is in close apposition with the caudal surface of the liver. Thus, changes in size or position of the liver may cause a change in position of the stomach. Generalized hepatomegaly often produces caudal and dorsal displacement of the stomach.[38] This displacement may be asymmetric if the liver enlargement is asymmetric, as with a mass lesion of the liver.[28] Because the cardia of the stomach is relatively fixed in position, however, even generalized hepatomegaly produces a nonuniform displacement of the stomach. Thus, on the lateral view, generalized hepatomegaly often produces caudal and dorsal displacement

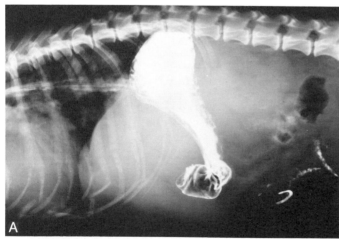
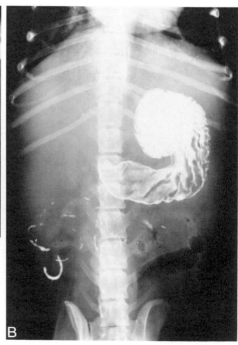

Figure 43–7. Gastric displacement due to hepatomegaly. A, lateral view. The pylorus and body are displaced caudally. B, ventrodorsal view. The pylorus and body are displaced caudally and to the left. Final diagnosis: right heart failure due to heartworm disease.

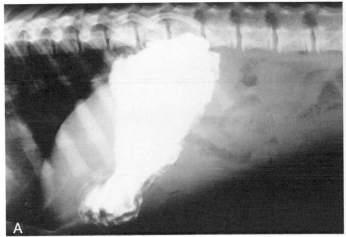

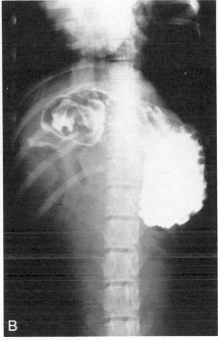

Figure 43–8. Gastric displacement due to a small liver. The pylorus and body are displaced cranially on both lateral (A) and ventrodorsal (B) views. Final diagnosis: portocaval shunt.

of the pylorus and body of the stomach. This displacement changes the axis of the stomach so that the axis is no longer parallel with the caudal ribs (Fig. 43–7A). On the ventrodorsal or dorsoventral views, generalized hepatomegaly often causes displacement of the body and pylorus of the stomach caudally and toward the left from normal (Fig. 43–7B). This displacement changes the axis of the stomach so that the axis is no longer transverse.

Because there is a minimal amount of objective, radiographic criteria of liver size, this displacement of the stomach aids in the radiographic recognition of hepatomegaly. This displacement becomes especially valuable when the liver is not visible per se on survey radiographs due to emaciation or abdominal effusion. In such patients, air within the stomach can often be used to define the axis of the stomach. A low-volume gastrogram can be readily performed if necessary to confirm the axis of the stomach.

If the diaphragm is intact, cranial displacement of the stomach relative to the diaphragm can only occur with a decrease in size of the liver. This displacement is again most obvious as a cranial displacement of the pylorus and body of the stomach, which results in an abnormal cranial angulation of the axis of the stomach on both lateral and ventrodorsal views (Fig. 43–8). A low-volume gastrogram is often of value to confirm this cranial shift in axis because many patients with small livers may also be emaciated or have abdominal effusion. Cranial

displacement of the stomach can also occur with rupture of the diaphragm and herniation of the liver, part of the liver, or the stomach into the thorax. Thus, even though the stomach may not pass through such a hernia, the axis of the stomach is important in traumatized patients suspected of having a diaphragmatic hernia. A cranial shift of the axis of the stomach may help to define whether the liver has herniated cranially through the diaphragm. A normal axis of the stomach in such cases, however, may still not completely exclude the possibility of herniation of part of the liver.

Abdominal masses that originate caudal to the stomach do not displace the stomach cranially due to the presence of the liver. Instead, such masses may distort the shape of the stomach as they press against and indent the stomach, or they may displace the stomach to the right or left. The relationship of an abdominal mass to the stomach is often of value in helping to define whether the mass originates in the liver, spleen, or pancreas (Fig. 43–9).

Gastric Foreign Bodies. Radiopaque material within the stomach is easily visualized and commonly present on survey radiographs. These opacities are most often due to ingested bone fragments and are present as an incidental finding with no clinical significance. More clinically significant foreign bodies, such as fish hooks and needles, are also readily visualized and present no diagnostic problem on survey radiographs. Occasionally, the stomach may contain a nondescript radiopaque material that

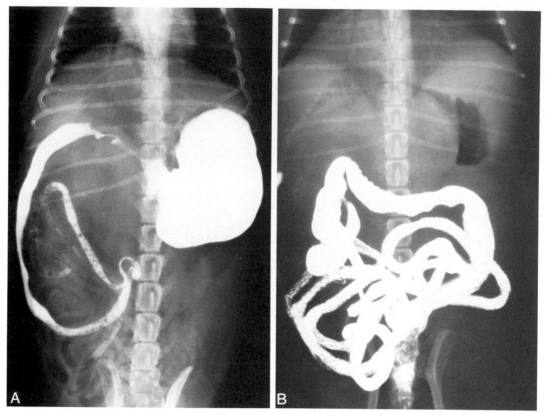

Figure 43–9. Ventrodorsal radiographs of a dog with an abdominal mass. *A,* the pylorus is displaced to the left; in addition, the cranial duodenal flexure and proximal part of the descending duodenum have a broad arc around the cranial surface of the mass, which itself is not visible. *B,* the transverse colon is displaced and curves caudally around the caudal surface of the mass. The mass is located between the proximal duodenum, pylorus, and transverse colon. Final diagnosis: pancreatic abscess.

is of questionable significance. Close correlation with clinical signs is thus important. Another factor of importance is that of persistence. If a medical or surgical emergency does not exist, repeat radiographs made 1 to 3 days later may provide valuable information (Fig. 43–10).

A greater problem exists with radiographic diagnosis of radiolucent gastric foreign bodies. Such objects are usually difficult to visualize on survey radiographs. Gastric endoscopy is valuable if equipment is available. Contrast studies may be necessary for diagnosis. Several solutions exist to aid in the radiographic demonstration of radiolucent gastric foreign bodies. The first and most simple technique is to utilize different views with different patient positioning. If the foreign body does not shift dependently with gastric fluid, then a different view may help to outline the foreign body with gas. This is most valuable if the foreign body remains in the pyloric portion of the stomach and can be outlined with gas in a left recumbent lateral view (Fig. 43–11). A low-volume gastrogram or double-contrast gastrogram may make such foreign bodies easier to visualize than a standard-

dose gastrogram with positive-contrast medium, the reason being that the larger volume of the standard gastrogram may completely obscure the foreign body and thus lead to a false-negative result. As the stomach empties during the procedure, however, the smaller amount of contrast medium within the stomach on delayed radiographs may be comparable to the low-volume gastrogram. Knowledge of patient positioning is again important because gas within the stomach during a contrast study may simulate a filling defect comparable to a foreign body. Thus, knowledge of patient positioning and fluid-air shifts within the stomach is important.

The appearance of a foreign body on a gastrogram varies depending on the type of foreign body that is present. An object such as a solid ball creates a round, discrete filling defect within the contrast medium (Fig. 43–12). If the object has a nonabsorbent surface, it may not be visible after the stomach has emptied. Conversely, a rag or sock may not create an initial filling defect because the contrast medium may permeate the object. Because of the absorption

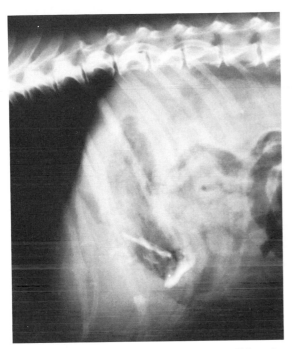

Figure 43–10. Persistent gastric foreign body. This radiopaque plastic material was also present on radiographs made 3 days previously; it was eventually removed by gastroscopy.

of contrast medium, however, the foreign body may be better visualized after the stomach has emptied due to retention of contrast medium on or within the object.

Acute Gastric Dilatation and Volvulus. Both acute gastric dilatation and gastric volvulus complex produce gas-filled enlargement of the stomach. Although both fluid and gas are present in the stomach, gaseous distension is the predominant abnormality in these acute conditions. This fact differs from chronic partial gastric outlet obstructions, in which fluid-filled gastric distension is the predominant finding.

Acute gastric dilatation is a condition that may be related to a reflex paralysis of gastric motor activity[28] and may be due to a complex variety of causes. With acute gastric dilatation, the stomach is enlarged and is filled primarily with gas, but retains its normal position and anatomic relationships. Thus, the pylorus is still located on the right and the fundus on the left. The normal position of the stomach can usually be determined on survey radiographs by using and comparing the right recumbent and left recumbent lateral views or the ventrodorsal and dorsoventral views. Recognition of the pylorus may be easier on the lateral views than on the ventrodorsal or dorsoventral views. Contrast

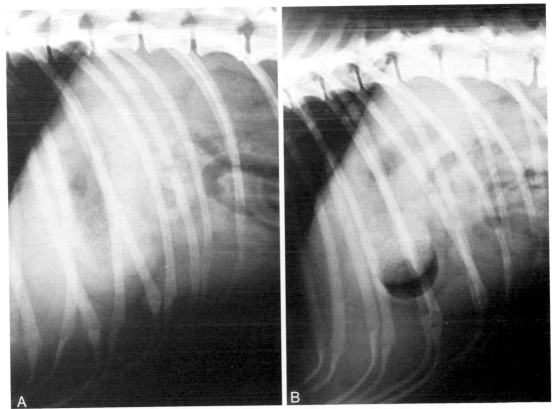

Figure 43–11. Gastric foreign body (ball) in the pyloric portion that is not well visualized on the right recumbent lateral view (A) due to fluid in the pylorus. In the left recumbent lateral view (B), gas rises to the pylorus to better outline the ball.

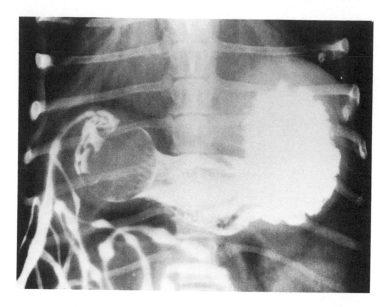

Figure 43–12. Gastric foreign body (ball) that creates a round, intraluminal filling defect on the gastrogram.

gastrography may help in this localization but is usually not necessary. It is important to avoid excessive manipulation of a patient and delays in treating a patient whose condition may be considered a medical emergency. It has been recommended that the stomach be decompressed and the patient stabilized before radiography. Gaseous distension of the stomach can also be due to aerophagia that is secondary to severe dyspnea or pain. In such cases, the gastric distension is usually less severe and other correlative findings may be present to aid in differential diagnosis.

Gastric volvulus is also associated with acute gaseous distension of the stomach. Gastric volvulus is differentiated from acute gaseous dilatation by displacement of the stomach due to its rotation. Different directions and degrees of rotation of the stomach may be present at the time of radiography, and the radiographic appearance of the stomach varies depending on the type and degree of rotation and the amount of distension.[16, 24] It appears that in most cases of gastric volvulus, as the stomach dilates, the greater curvature rotates to lie along the ventral abdominal wall. The pylorus continues to shift dorsally, cranially, and to the left, and the body of the stomach shifts toward the right.[39] The spleen follows the greater curvature toward the right.

The major radiographic feature of gastric volvulus is gas and fluid distension of the stomach with the gas being predominant, as in acute gastric dilatation. With gastric volvulus, however, the pylorus is usually displaced dorsally and to the left. Thus, radiographic determination of the location of the pylorus is the key differentiating feature. Radiographic demonstration of the location of the pylorus is best accomplished by making left and right recumbent lateral views or ventrodorsal and dorso-

ventral views. The comparative lateral views are usually of most value. When outlined by its gas content on such radiographs, the pyloric portion of the stomach appears more tubular and narrower than the rest of the stomach. Although the stomach is filled primarily with gas, it usually contains enough fluid so that the pyloric portion may fill with fluid and thus not be seen on the radiograph. Thus, both lateral views may be needed to be sure that the pylorus fills with gas and can thus be recognized. With the pylorus shifted to the left and with the patient in left recumbency, the fluid within the stomach fills the pylorus, and gas fills the rest of the stomach. With the patient in right recumbency, gas then fills the pyloric portion and fluid shifts to the fundus or body of the stomach. Thus, the radiographic finding that the pyloric portion fills with fluid on the left recumbent lateral view and fills with gas on the right recumbent lateral view indicates that the pylorus in on the left side and that the stomach has rotated (Figs. 43–13 and 43–14). Recognition of this shift is usually more difficult on the ventro-dorsal and dorsoventral views because specific recognition of the pyloric portion may be more difficult. Positive-contrast gastrography may be performed but is usually not needed. An additional variation is a volvulus of 360 degrees. In such cases, the pylorus and fundus are on their normal sides radiographically (Fig. 43–15), and diagnosis is dependent on findings at physical examination.

Gastric volvulus may also be present without severe dilatation. This situation may often exist for days or weeks after previous gastric decompression[16] or may be present at the time of initial presentation. The aforementioned radiographic principles still apply as a means to recognize rotation of the stomach (Fig. 43–16).

Compartmentalization is a term that refers to

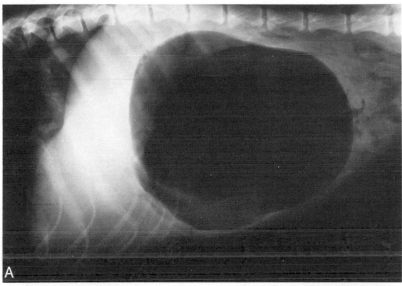

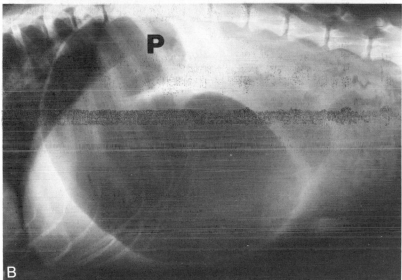

Figure 43–13. Gastric volvulus. *A,* left recumbent lateral view. The stomach is greatly distended with gas that is in the fundus and body. Fluid fills the pyloric portion, which is thus not well visualized. *B,* right recumbent lateral view. The fluid shifts into the fundic portion, and gas outlines the pyloric portion (P). These changes indicate that the pylorus is on the left and the fundus is on the right, and that there is a gastric volvulus. In this particular patient, the pylorus is directed caudally.

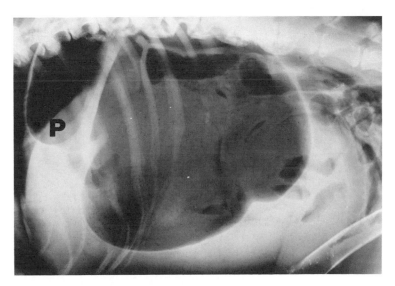

Figure 43–14. Gastric volvulus. Right recumbent lateral view. The pylorus (P) is directed cranioventrally. (Compare with Figure 43–13.)

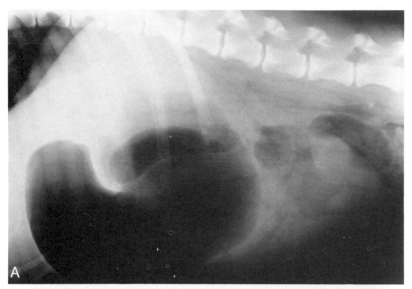

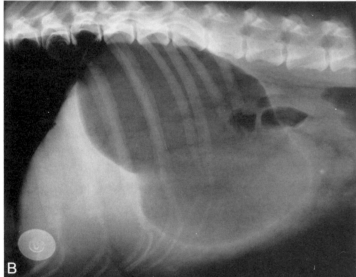

Figure 43–15. Left recumbent *(A)* and right recumbent *(B)* lateral views of a dog with acute gastric dilatation. On the basis of these radiographic findings, the pylorus and fundus are on normal sides of the abdomen. The esophagus was dilated, however, and a gastric tube could not be passed into the stomach. Final diagnosis: 360 degree gastric volvulus.

Figure 43–16. Left recumbent lateral view of a dog a few days after gastric decompression. Gastric volvulus is still present but without extreme dilatation.

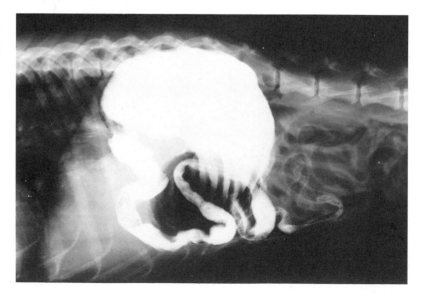

the radiographic recognition of soft-tissue bands that project into or across the gas-filled lumen of the rotated stomach. These soft-tissue bands are due to folding of the stomach on itself as the folded wall projects into the lumen and is outlined by gas within the lumen.[28] These bands may become more obvious with greater degrees of distension. With progressive distension of the stomach, the stomach wall becomes thinner. Gas within the gastric wall has also been described but is infrequent.[28]

As the stomach enlarges, other mobile structures within the abdomen are displaced caudally. With severe gastric distension, it is often difficult to visualize other abdominal organs radiographically due to crowding of these organs caudally. The spleen is also usually involved in gastric volvulus and may shift with the stomach. The spleen is usually enlarged due to impaired circulation, but its location may vary. The greater the gastric distension, the less likely the spleen is visualized radiographically due to crowding of abdominal viscera. Thus, splenomegaly and splenic displacement may be more easily visualized with less severe cases of gastric volvulus. Other changes that may be seen with volvulus include reflex paralytic ileus of the small intestine, esophageal dilatation, and cardiovascular changes within the thorax associated with shock.

Chronic Pyloric Obstruction. Obstruction of gastric emptying at the pylorus may be acute or chronic. Causes of acute obstruction include gastric volvulus as well as foreign bodies, although foreign bodies may also produce a more chronic situation. Chronic pyloric obstruction is usually due to narrowing of the pyloric orifice secondary to diseases affecting the wall or blocking the orifice, such as hypertrophic pyloric stenosis, pylorospasm, inflammation or fibrosis, neoplasia, and mucosal hypertrophy. These conditions usually cause a chronic, partial obstruction at the pylorus leading to chronic retention of gastric content. Chronic, partial obstruction of the pylorus is often manifest on survey radiographs as fluid-filled gastric distension as opposed to the acute gaseous distension of gastric volvulus (Fig. 43–17). The stomach may be quite large with chronic partial obstruction of the pylorus. The enlarged stomach may be more difficult to identify on survey radiographs, however, when it is filled with fluid than when it is filled with gas. Even when distended with fluid, the stomach still contains some gas. In these instances, however, the gas does not totally outline or fill the entire stomach. Instead, the smaller amount of gas floats as a bubble on top of the fluid and should not be mistaken as the limits of the stomach (Fig. 43–17B).

The major effect of such pyloric obstructive diseases is to restrict gastric emptying. Survey radiographic findings may vary from normal to gastric enlargement, depending on the severity and duration of the disease. With contrast studies, the major radiographic abnormality is delayed gastric emptying, especially total gastric emptying. An initial delay in gastric emptying,

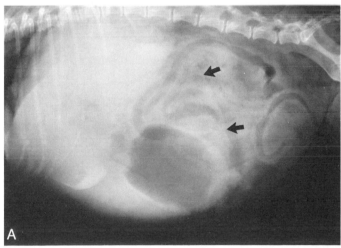
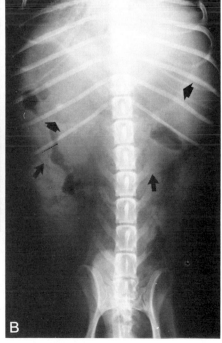

Figure 43–17. Lateral *(A)* and ventrodorsal *(B)* radiographs of two dogs with fluid-filled gastric distension due to chronic pyloric obstruction. The stomach is more difficult to identify when filled with fluid instead of gas. *Large arrows,* caudal margin of the stomach. The smaller gastric gas pocket *(small arrows* in *B)* should not be mistaken for limits of the stomach. The dog in *A* also had hepatomegaly and cholelithiasis.

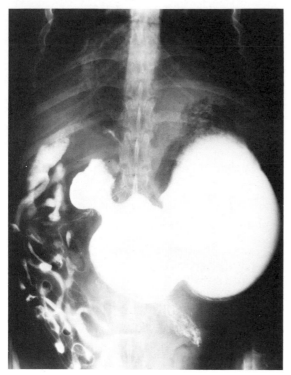

Figure 43–18. Dorsoventral radiograph 5 hours after initiation of an upper gastrointestinal tract series. There is a pronounced delay in gastric emptying, with most of the contrast medium retained within the stomach. Note the strong peristaltic contraction of the pyloric portion.

malities may be visible only during certain moments within the gastric cycle and thus are not likely to be seen on a randomly exposed radiograph. The advantage of fluoroscopy is that sequential changes of the shape of the stomach can be visualized, and thus those momentary changes that may best demonstrate certain lesions of the stomach may be documented. Even with fluoroscopy, however, it is often not possible to differentiate some pyloric obstructive diseases specifically. As an example, hypertrophic pyloric stenosis and mural inflammation or scarring can all produce an annular type of stricture of the pylorus that prevents the pylorus from opening adequately. Thus, it may be more practical to divide obstructive pyloric diseases into those that encircle the pylorus and are thus restrictive and those that obstruct the pylorus by blocking its orifice.

Restrictive diseases of the pylorus include hypertrophic pyloric stenosis, pylorospasm, inflammation or scarring, and neoplasia of the pylorus. If characteristic abnormalities are present on radiographs, they are usually those of an annular, stricture type of narrowing of the py-

however, may be of no clinical significance due to the influence of various psychic factors discussed previously. This point is especially important to remember if the stomach starts to empty normally after an initial delay or after the animal is allowed to calm down. Of more significance is a pronounced delay in gastric emptying when only a small amount of contrast medium passes from the stomach over a period of a few hours. Because the normal stomach should be empty 1 to 4 hours after administration of contrast medium, retention of most of the dose within the stomach 3 to 4 hours after administration usually indicates pyloric obstructive disease (Fig. 43–18).

It is often difficult to differentiate the pyloric obstructive diseases radiographically, especially by using conventional radiography without fluoroscopy. The stomach is a dynamic organ that rapidly changes appearance due to peristaltic waves, and a radiograph demonstrates the appearance of the stomach during only a fraction of a second. Thus, the appearance of the stomach on a radiograph depends on when the exposure was made during the cycle of change. Although some diseases may produce characteristic radiographic abnormalities, such abnor-

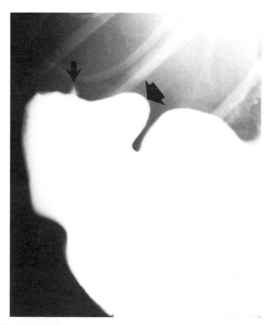

Figure 43–19. Ventrodorsal spot radiograph of the pyloric region of a dog with restrictive disease of the pylorus. The "beak" sign (small arrow) is caused by barium that fills only the entrance of the lumen of the pyloric sphincter due to an annular type of stricture. The peristaltic pouch (large arrow) is the outpouching of the pyloric antrum along the lesser curvature as a peristaltic wave pushes contrast medium up against the mass-type lesion encircling the pylorus. There was also a pronounced delay in gastric emptying. (Same dog as in Fig. 43–17B.) Final diagnosis: pyloric stenosis due to inflammation caused by an ulcer.

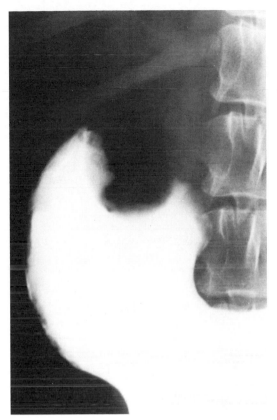

Figure 43–20. Ventrodorsal spot radiograph of the pylorus of a dog with obstructive disease of the pylorus. There is a hemispheric filling defect at the pylorus that projects into the lumen. There was pronounced delay in gastric emptying. (Same dog as in Fig. 43–18.) The filling defect was due to mucosa that was hypertrophied in a symmetric band around the pylorus. Final diagnosis: chronic plasmocytic gastritis.

pyloric sphincter (Fig. 43–20). It is again emphasized that radiographic recognition of such a lesion is usually diagnostically adequate and that specific differentiation of the underlying cause may not be possible on radiographs.

Gastric Ulcers. Gastric ulcers probably occur more often than they are recognized clinically or radiographically. The major problem in the diagnosis of gastric ulcers is the difficulty in demonstrating the ulcers on conventional radiographs. Gastric ulcers produce craters in the wall of the stomach that appear as outpouchings from the lumen (Fig. 43–21). The radiographic appearance of a gastric ulcer can be quite variable, depending on whether the ulcer is projected in profile, en face, or obliquely.[41] The appearance of the ulcer can be further altered by gastric peristalsis. Manipulation of the patient during fluoroscopy allows a more complete and continuous evaluation of the margin and contour of the stomach. Double-contrast gastrography may also be of value, because ulcers that are projected en face can be visualized with double-contrast studies but are obscured with positive-contrast gastrography.

Gastric ulcers may be benign or malignant. Benign gastric ulcers can be due to a variety of causes.[23, 33, 39] Malignant gastric ulcers occur in association with gastric neoplasia and may be

loric sphincter. If barium fills only the entrance of the lumen at the pyloric sphincter, the resultant radiographic appearance is referred to as the "beak sign."[32] If barium fills the length of the narrowed lumen through the pyloric sphincter, the resultant radiographic appearance is referred to as the "string sign."[32] A "tit sign" has been described as a relatively sharp, pointed, outpouching of the pyloric antrum along the lesser curvature as a peristaltic wave pushes contrast medium in a peristaltic pouch up against the mass-type lesion around the pylorus.[32] Variations in severity, symmetry, and radiographic projection all contribute to create variations in the radiographic appearance of pyloric restrictive lesions (Fig. 43–19).

The second group of pyloric obstructive diseases include gastric foreign bodies, mucosal inflammation or hypertrophy, and some mural lesions of the pyloric antrum. These types of lesions are more likely to produce filling defects within the lumen that occlude the orifice of the

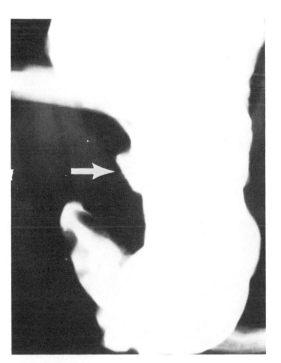

Figure 43–21. Lateral spot radiograph of the stomach of a dog with a gastric ulcer (arrow). The stomach tube is still in place. Mass lesions of the stomach are not definitive, and the ulcer is the only definitive radiographic abnormality. Final diagnosis: gastric adenocarcinoma.

due to tumor necrosis.[33] Criteria have been established for the radiographic differentiation of benign and malignant gastric ulcers in humans.[27, 31, 41] These criteria have not been well established in dogs and cats, presumably because of the lower number of recognized cases.

Radiography may provide an excellent method for the recognition of gastric ulcers. Infrequent use of gastrography, lack of fluoroscopy, insufficient views, and the infrequent use of double-contrast gastrography, however, all combine to limit the recognition of gastric ulcers in dogs and cats. In addition, experience is limited in radiographically differentiating benign and malignant gastric ulcers in dogs and cats. Ulceration is often associated with gastric carcinoma,[22, 37] and gastric ulcers in dogs that are recognized on radiographs are often due to neoplasia.[2] Thus, the radiographic recognition of a gastric ulcer should lead to strong consideration of neoplasia and further evaluation of the stomach with endoscopy and biopsy or by surgical exploration.

Gastric Neoplasia. Several types of neoplasms occur in the stomach of dogs and cats, and any region of the stomach can be involved. Adenocarcinoma is the most frequently recognized gastric tumor of dogs.[26, 37] This tumor may occur in any region of the stomach, but appears to be found most often in the pyloric portion of the stomach.[22, 30] Gastric neoplasia occurs less frequently in the cat than in the dog,[6] and lymphosarcoma is the most common type of feline gastric neoplasm.[40]

The radiographic appearance of gastric neoplasia is quite variable and depends primarily on the size, shape, and location of the tumor. The major radiographic feature is that of a mass lesion that projects into the gastric lumen, creating a filling defect within the contrast medium. The more nodular and pedunculated the lesion, the easier it is to recognize as a distinct mass-type of lesion (Fig. 43–22A). Smaller mass lesions may be totally obscured by a relatively large volume of positive contrast medium. Oblique projection, conformation of the stomach, and peristaltic contractions may all contribute to obscure some mass lesions of the stomach. Tumors that are more diffuse and less discrete are more difficult to identify. Diffuse, infiltrative lesions of the stomach wall may not produce distinct filling defects. Instead, they may alter the shape of the stomach and may produce decreased motility of the involved area. If such diffuse lesions encircle a portion of the stomach, the radiographic appearance may be that of an annular type of narrowing or one in which the stomach has decreased distensibility in the affected area (Fig. 43–22B). Because of the variations in appearance of the stomach created by patient positioning, these positions should be used to best advantage in demonstrating suspected lesions. Due to variations in appearance of the stomach created by peristalsis, persistence of a suspected abnormality on sequential radiographs is important. The radiographic recognition of a gastric ulcer should also suggest the possibility of gastric neoplasia.

Diffuse Diseases of the Stomach. The stomach can be involved diffusely by a variety of diseases that produce inflammation, hypertrophy, atrophy, or mineralization. Acute gastritis can be due to a variety of causes, infrequently

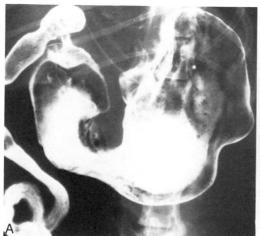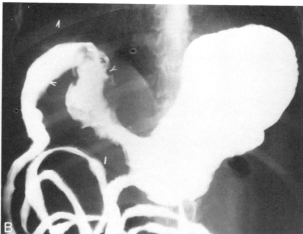

Figure 43–22. *A,* dorsoventral double contrast gastrogram of a cat. There is a nodular filling defect due to a mass lesion along the lesser curvature. Final diagnosis: lymphosarcoma. *B,* dorsoventral gastrogram of a dog. An annular mass encircles the pyloric portion and part of the body. This area failed to distend, even in sternal recumbency, and the abnormality persisted throughout the study. Final diagnosis: gastric adenocarcinoma.

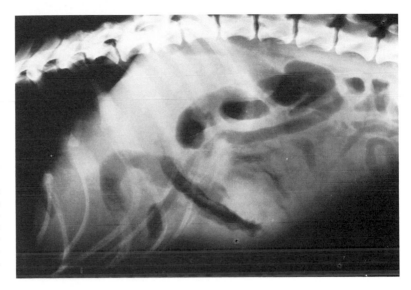

Figure 43–23. Lateral survey radiograph of the abdomen of a dog with a thick gastric wall. The thickened wall is best visualized in the ventral midabdomen, and is associated with a narrow, tubular, gas-filled lumen. Rugal folds were enlarged on a gastrogram. Final diagnosis: chronic hypertrophic gastritis.

requires radiography, and is rarely associated with radiographic abnormalities. Chronic gastritis is infrequently diagnosed clinically and can also be due to a variety of causes. Examples include diseases such as chronic atrophic gastritis, chronic hypertrophic gastritis, and eosinophilic gastritis.[39] Respectively, paucity of rugal folds, large rugal folds, and granulomatous nodules or a thickened gastric wall may be seen with these diseases (Fig. 43–23).[30] Radiographic abnormalities may be difficult to identify and may not be specific for the cause of the disease.

Soft-tissue calcification can occur in association with chronic renal failure.[29] In such patients, mineralization of the gastric wall may be visible radiographically as thin, linear, mineralized densities, (Fig. 43–24).[3] These mineralized opacities are often more easily visualized when the stomach is empty and the mineralized mucosal fold pattern is more tightly grouped.

Gastric Perforation. Perforation of the stomach is not usually recognized per se on radiographs. The major radiographic findings are usually those of abdominal effusion and free abdominal gas. These radiographic abnormalities combined with the patient's clinical signs usually lead directly to an exploratory laparotomy during which the diagnosis is made. Thus, contrast studies are rarely performed in patients with gastric perforation. If contrast gastrography is necessary, a water-soluble organic iodide contrast medium is the preferred agent, although barium sulfate may better demonstrate small tears than the iodide contrast media.[15]

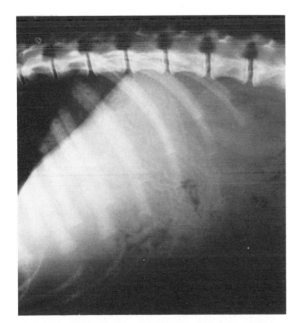

Figure 43–24. Lateral survey radiograph of the abdomen of a dog with chronic renal failure. Thin, linear, mineralized opacities that parallel the axis of the ribs are due to gastric calcification.

References

1. Allen GS, Rendano VT, Quick CB, et al: Gastrografin as a gastrointestinal contrast medium in the cat. Vet Radiol 20:110, 1979.
2. Barber DL: Radiographic aspects of gastric ulcers in dogs: A comparative review and report of 5 case histories. Vet Radiol 23:109, 1982.
3. Barber DL, and Rowland GN: Radiographically detectable soft tissue calcification in chronic renal failure. Vet Radiol 20:117, 1979.
4. Bargai U: The effect of xylazine hydrochloride on the radiographic appearance of the stomach and intestine in the dog. Vet Radiol 23:60, 1982.
5. Brawner WR, and Bartels JE: Contrast radiography of the digestive tract: Indications, techniques, and complications. Vet Clin North Am 13:599, 1983.
6. Brody RS: Alimentary tract neoplasms in the cat: A clinicopathologic survey of 46 cases. Am J Vet Res 27:74, 1966.
7. Cannon WB: The movements of the stomach studied by means of roentgen rays. Am J Physiol 1:359, 1898.

8. Cooke AR: Control of gastric emptying and motility. Gastroenterology 68:804, 1975.

9. Cornelius LM, and Wingfield WE: Diseases of the stomach. *In* Ettinger SJ (Ed): Textbook of Veterinary Internal Medicine. Vol. 2. Philadelphia, WB Saunders, 1979.

10. Davenport HW: Physiology of the Digestive Tract. 2nd Ed. Chicago, Year Book Medical Publishers, 1974.

11. Evans HE, and Christensen GC: Miller's Anatomy of the Dog. 2nd Ed. Philadelphia, WB Saunders, 1979.

12. Evans SM: Double versus single contrast gastrography in the dog and cat. Vet Radiol 24:6, 1983.

13. Evans SM, and Biery DN: Double contrast gastrography in the cat: Technique and normal radiographic appearance. Vet Radiol 24:3, 1983.

14. Evans SM, and Lauffer I: Double contrast gastrography in the normal dog. Vet Radiol 22:2, 1981.

15. Foley MJ, Ghahremani GG, and Rogers LF: Reappraisal of contrast media used to detect upper gastrointestinal perforations: Comparison of ionic water-soluble media with barium sulfate. Radiology 144:231, 1982.

16. Funkquist B: Gastric torsion in the dog. I. Radiological picture during nonsurgical treatment related to the pathological anatomy and to the future clinical course. J Small Anim Pract 20:73, 1979.

17. Funkquist B, and Garmer L: Pathogenetic and therapeutic aspects of torsion of the canine stomach. J Small Anim Pract 8:523, 1967.

18. Gelfand DW, and Ott DJ: Single- vs. double-contrast gastrointestinal studies: Critical analysis of reported statistics. AJR 137:523, 1981.

19. Gibbs C, and Pearson H: The radiological diagnosis of gastrointestinal obstruction in the dog. J Small Anim Pract 14:61, 1973.

20. Gomez JA: The gastrointestinal contrast study: Methods and interpretation. Vet Clin North Am 4:805, 1974.

21. Grandage J: The radiologic appearance of stomach gas in the dog. Aust Vet J 50:529, 1974.

22. Hayden DW, and Nielson SW: Canine alimentary neoplasia. Zentralbl Veterinarmed [A] 20:1, 1973.

23. Howard EB, Sawa TR, Nielson SW, et al: Mastocytoma and gastroduodenal ulceration. Vet Pathol 6:146, 1969.

24. Kneller SK: Radiographic interpretation of the gastric dilatation-volvulus complex in the dog. J Am Anim Hosp Assoc 12:154, 1976.

25. Morgan JP: The upper gastrointestinal examination in the cat: Normal radiographic appearance using positive contrast medium. Vet Radiol 22:159, 1982.

26. Murray M, Robinson PB, McKeating FJ, et al: Primary gastric neoplasia in the dog: A clinico-pathological study. Vet Rec 91:474, 1972.

27. Nelson SW: The discovery of gastric ulcers and the differential diagnosis between benignancy and malignancy. Radiol Clin North Am 7:5, 1969.

28. O'Brien TR: Radiographic Diagnosis of Abdominal Disorders in the Dog and Cat. Philadelphia, WB Saunders, 1978.

29. Parfitt AM: Soft tissue calcification in uremia. Arch Intern Med 124:544, 1969.

30. Patnaik AK, Hurvitz AI, and Johnson GE: Canine gastric adenocarcinoma. Vet Pathol 15:600, 1978.

31. Porcher P, and Buffard P: Malignancy of the stomach. *In* Margulis AR, and Burhenne HJ (Eds): Alimentary Tract Roentgenology. St. Louis, CV Mosby, 1967.

32. Rhodes WH, and Brodey RS: The differential diagnosis of pyloric obstructions in the dog. J Am Vet Radiol Soc 6:65, 1965.

33. Robbins SL: Pathologic Basis of Disease. Philadelphia, WB Saunders, 1974.

34. Root CR: Interpretation of abdominal survey radiographs. Vet Clin North Am 4:763, 1974.

35. Root CR, and Morgan JP: Contrast radiography of the upper gastrointestinal tract in the dog. J Small Anim Pract 10:279, 1969.

36. Rubin DL, Carroll BA, and Snow HD: The harmful effects of aqueous contrast agents on the gastrointestinal tract: A study of mechanism and means of counteraction. Invest Radiol 16:50, 1981.

37. Sautter JH, and Hanlon GF: Gastric neoplasms in the dog: A report of 20 cases. J Am Vet Med Assoc 166:691, 1975.

38. Suter PF: Radiographic diagnosis of liver disease in dogs and cats. Vet Clin North Am [Small Anim Pract] 12:153, 1982.

39. Twedt DC, and Wingfield WE: Diseases of the stomach. *In* Ettinger SJ (Ed): Textbook of Veterinary Internal Medicine. Vol. 2. 2nd Ed. Philadelphia, WB Saunders, 1983.

40. Tyler DE: Gastric neoplasia in the dog and cat. Arch Am Coll Vet Surg 6:47, 1977 (Abstract).

41. Zboralske FF: Gastric ulcer. *In* Margulis AR, and Burhenne HJ (Eds): Alimentary Tract Roentgenology. St. Louis, CV Mosby, 1967.

42. Zontine WJ: Effect of chemical restraint drugs on the passage of barium sulfate through the stomach and duodenum of dogs. J Am Vet Med Assoc 162:878, 1973.

CHAPTER 44

THE SMALL BOWEL

SANDRA V. McNEEL

Vomiting, diarrhea, weight loss, abdominal pain, and palpation of a midabdominal mass are the most frequent clinical signs of intestinal disease in small animals. Abdominal radiographs may help make a positive diagnosis or provide information that may be helpful when deciding whether medical or surgical treatment is required. Survey radiographs and intestinal contrast examinations can be useful aids to diagnosis of both acute and chronic intestinal disorders, but should not take precedence over a complete history, thorough physical examination, or pertinent laboratory tests. The animal that does not respond to symptomatic therapy for vomiting or diarrhea may also benefit from a more extensive work-up, including radiographic studies. The following information is provided as a guide to interpretation of radiographic changes that occur in the small intestinal tract. Although patients with some intestinal disorders have only one radiographic abnormality, a significant number of patients have combinations of basic roentgen signs.

ROENTGEN SIGNS IN THE NORMAL SMALL BOWEL

Table 44–1 is a summary of the roentgen signs that are most useful when interpreting intestinal radiographs. Margination, size, position, contour, and radiopacity of the bowel can often be evaluated on survey radiographs, but mucosal irregularities and abnormal peristalsis or transit time must be determined from contrast studies.

Margination. A mature dog or cat in good body condition has good definition of intestinal serosal surfaces (Fig. 44–1). The serosal margins should be smooth, and are most easily seen adjacent to the abdominal wall, where there is less superimposition of other structures. Animals less than 6 months of age or those who are emaciated have poor serosal definition due to lack of intra-abdominal fat.[28]

Size. Because of the great variation in canine body size, a specific measurement for "normal" diameter of the small bowel cannot be made. A general rule, however, is that the diameter of the normal canine small intestine may be as large as two times the width of a rib.[24] Because

TABLE 44–1. ROENTGEN SIGNS IN THE SMALL INTESTINE

Margination—Serosal surface definition
Size—Diameter of lumen
Position—Location within abdominal cavity
Shape—Contour of bowel loops
Radiopacity—Bowel wall and lumen
  contents
Architecture—Mucosa/bowel wall
  appearance

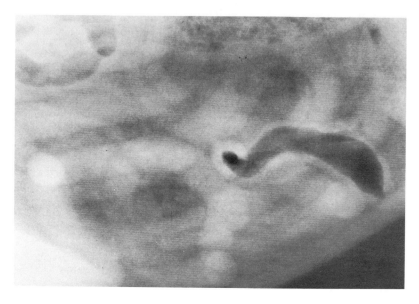

Figure 44–1. Serosal edges of small intestine are easily seen in this fat dog. Bowel segments seen end on appear as rings if the lumen contains air or as round nodules if the lumen is empty or contains a small amount of fluid.

cats tend to be similar in body size, a more specific criterion can be made: the diameter of normal feline small bowel should not exceed 12 mm.[19] Although the duodenum may be slightly wider, the jejunum and ileum should have approximately the same lumen diameter.[22] During contrast radiography, nonpersistent narrowing of the bowel lumen is due to segmental or peristaltic contractions associated with normal bowel motility. Attempting to judge the thickness of the intestinal wall on survey radiographs is hazardous; a normal empty bowel loop with a small volume of intraluminal air may be mistaken for a pathologically thickened segment. True thickening of the intestinal wall is better judged from a contrast study or, most reliably, by abdominal palpation.

Position. The small bowel should be uniformly distributed throughout the peritoneal cavity, occupying that space not taken up by distensible organs (stomach or urinary bladder) or solid organs (liver or spleen). Common variations in the position of the small bowel seen in normal dogs and cats include: (1) full stomach displaces bowel caudally; (2) distended urinary bladder displaces bowel cranially; (3) fat in the falciform ligament of obese cats displaces bowel dorsal and caudal from the ventral abdominal wall; and (4) bowel in obese dogs occupies the most ventral portion of the pendulous abdominal cavity.

In the dog, the cranial duodenal flexure is fixed along the caudal surfaces of the right liver lobes by the hepatoduodenal ligament. The descending duodenum lies along the right abdominal wall. The caudal duodenal flexure is located at midabdomen, with the ascending duodenum continuing from this point in a straight manner to the caudal portion of the stomach. Distal to this point, the loops of je-

junum may take any position not occupied by other organs.

In the cat, the cranial duodenal flexure usually creates a sharper angle with the pylorus. The descending duodenum then courses in a gently curved loop, with the caudal duodenal flexure at approximately midabdomen. As in the dog, the ascending duodenum courses in a cranial direction until it reaches the stomach; the jejunal loops are then located throughout the rest of the mesogastric area.

Shape and Contour. On survey radiographs, the small bowel may be seen as smooth, continuous, curved tubes (especially in the fat animal). In a barium study in a normal cat, distinct bead-like segments of contrast medium are seen in the duodenum (Fig. 44–2). This "string of pearls" appearance is due to the normally strong circular muscle contractions that occur during segmental intestinal peristalsis in the cat. Contrast studies are often necessary to identify abnormal shape of bowel loops.

Radiopacity. The radiopacity of the normal small intestine is quite variable due to differing opacities of material within the lumen. In the nonfasted animal any of the following contents may be seen in the lumen: air, which is radiolucent; ingesta, with a grainy or mottled appearance; fluid, which is of homogeneous fluid or soft-tissue opacity; or bone, which is radiopaque. The bowel lumen of the fasted dog or cat can be a homogeneous fluid or soft-tissue radiopacity or it may contain a small amount of ingested air. The bowel wall should also be a uniform soft-tissue opacity. This uniformity is most easily evaluated in portions of the intestine that contain air.

The opacity of the lumen during a contrast study depends upon the volume and type of contrast medium used as well as the volume of

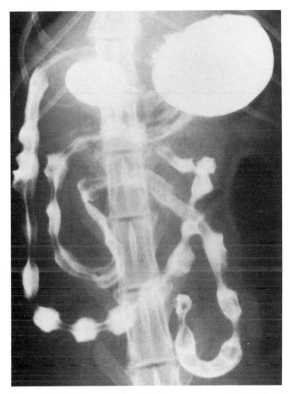

Figure 44–2. Normal feline barium upper gastrointestinal tract study. Prominent circular muscle contractions cause almost complete obliteration of the duodenal lumen during segmental peristalsis. The linear filling defect is a normal variant, attributed to a longitudinal fold of mucosa in the incompletely distended intestine.

air present. A bowel lumen filled with contrast medium appears uniformly opaque (Fig. 44–3). Bowel loops containing contrast medium and air show bubble-like radiolucent defects or contrast medium coated walls with air distension of the lumen, as seen in Figure 44–3. The

normal cat duodenum or jejunum may demonstrate a linear filling defect during a barium upper gastrointestinal tract study (Fig. 44–2). Sometimes called a pseudostring sign, this appearance is due to an indentation of a mucosal fold into the lumen. It is usually seen in those intestinal segments that are poorly distended by the contrast medium. See the description of roentgen signs of a linear foreign body to differentiate the pathologic from the normal state.

Architecture of Mucosal Surface. On survey radiographs, the mucosal surface can only be seen in air-filled segments of bowel. Barium studies are the procedures of choice to evaluate the mucosa appropriately.

During a barium upper gastrointestinal tract study, the mucosa of the normal dog may be seen as a smooth, even surface or as a finely fimbriated edge (Figs. 44–3 and 44–4, respectively). The degree of fimbriation (fringing at the barium-mucosa interface) in the normal dog is variable. This appearance has been attributed to barium dissecting between groups of aggregated villi.[36] Another variation in the normal appearance of the mucosa is the occurrence of pseudoulcers in the canine descending duodenum (Fig. 44–5). These distinct outpouchings are more commonly seen in younger dogs and indicate depressions in the bowel wall over lymphoid follicles.[22] The consistent square or conical shape without accompanying spasm and irregularity of the opposite duodenal wall helps distinguish these normal structures from true ulcers.

The cat does not have the lymphoid follicle distribution that causes pseudoulcers. The occasional finding of a radiolucent linear filling defect in the normal feline upper gastrointestinal tract has been described.

Function. Transit time of contrast medium

Figure 44–3. Normal canine barium upper gastrointestinal tract study. Bowel segments filled with barium are uniformly opaque (solid arrow). Mucosal surface is flat and smooth. Those bowel loops containing air within their lumen show a double contrast effect; barium coating the mucosa is seen as a thin opaque line, whereas intraluminal air is radiolucent (open arrow).

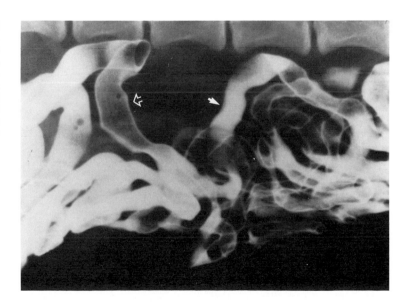

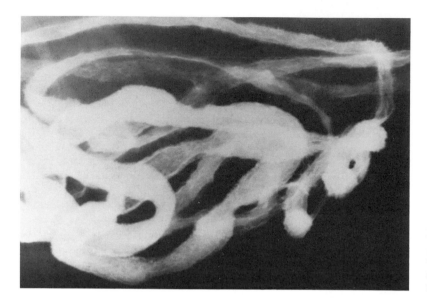

Figure 44–4. Normal canine barium upper gastrointestinal tract study demonstrates variation of the normal mucosal surface. Finely fimbriated interface between barium and mucosa is seen in some animals and is normal.

through the intestinal tract and frequency of segmental peristaltic contractions can provide some gross evidence of bowel motility. There is a wide range of normal transit times in both the cat and the dog. A guideline to those organs that usually opacify during the upper gastroin-testinal tract contrast study is given in Table 44–4. Normal peristaltic waves produce symmetric indentations along the bowel (Fig. 44–6). These indentations do not persist in the same bowel loop when serial radiographs are compared.

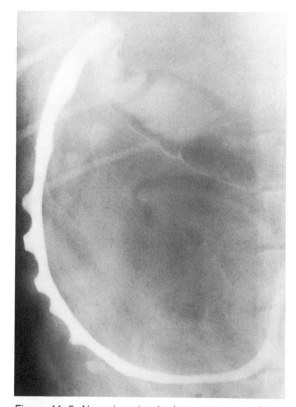

Figure 44–5. Normal canine barium upper gastrointestinal tract study demonstrates pseudoulcers in the descending duodenum. These normal outpouchings are seen only in the duodenum and more often in young animals. They are due to depressions in the mucosa at sites of lymphoid follicles.

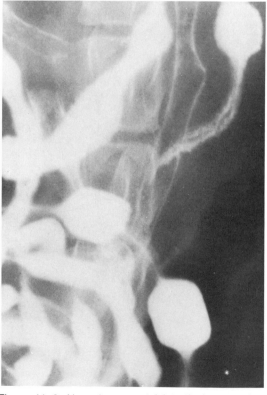

Figure 44–6. Normal segmental intestinal contractions during a canine upper gastrointestinal tract study. Normal peristalsis is indicated by symmetric indentations of the bowel wall on each side proximal and distal to the formed bolus of contrast medium.

SURVEY RADIOGRAPHY

Technique

Patient Preparation. In the patient with acute abdominal pain, acute onset of persistent vomiting, or in which enlarged fluid or air-filled bowel loops are palpable, no specific preparation for abdominal radiographs is necessary. In the elective abdominal examination, withholding food for 24 hours and administration of a cleansing warm water enema 2 to 4 hours before radiography produces the desired empty intestinal tract.

Radiographic Projections. Standard views to evaluate the small bowel are the left lateral recumbent and ventrodorsal views. Additional views that may be useful include right lateral recumbent, for changes in position of fluid or gas; standing lateral with horizontal x-ray beam, for gas-capped fluid levels seen with obstruction; and left lateral decubitus or erect ventrodorsal with horizontal x-ray beam, for free air in the peritoneal cavity (as might result from bowel perforation).

Abnormal Roentgen Signs

Margination. See Chapter 33 for a more complete description of peritoneal disorders. In summary, abnormal bowel serosal surfaces may be less distinct or more distinct than expected. Decreased or absent definition of serosal edges is found with a lack of intra-abdominal fat (abdominal walls are tucked-up in the emaciated patient) or with fluid in the peritoneal space (abdominal walls are often distended in the patient with a large volume of peritoneal fluid). The type of fluid in the peritoneal cavity cannot be determined by radiography; abdominal paracentesis with cytologic evaluation of fluid is required. Certain types of fluid, however, accumulate to the point that collection in the abdomen is radiographically detectable: peritonitis; hemorrhage (trauma, rupture of liver or spleen, coagulopathy disorders); ascites; urine (ruptured ureter or bladder); and carcinomatosis. Improved definition of serosal edges is found with free air in the peritoneal cavity, which may result from puncture of the abdominal wall, perforation of the intestine (or other hollow viscus); iatrogenic induction (recent abdominal surgery); or bacterial fermentation, and with fat deposition which may be "normal" in obese animal. Lipoma or lipomatosis is rare.

Size (Increased Lumen Diameter). The most common alteration in size is distension with air, fluid, or a combination of both. Failure of intestinal contents to pass through the tract is termed ileus. Ileus may be mechanical, caused by physical obstruction of the bowel lumen, or functional (paralytic), in which the peristaltic contractions of the bowel cease due to vascular or neuromuscular abnormalities of the intestinal wall. In functional ileus, the bowel lumen remains patent.

Evaluation of both the approximate length of bowel affected and the degree of lumen distension can aid in establishing a list of reasonable differential diagnoses. The following guidelines are presented to assist in evaluation of the radiographic sign of bowel distension. Pathologic conditions given usually show the radiographic sign being discussed. These lists are not meant to be complete, however, because a single disease process may show different radiographic appearances during its clinical course.

Focal/Mild. Less than 50 per cent of small bowel loops are distended to only three or four times the width of a rib. Possible causes for this appearance include: regional enteritis, regional peritonitis (secondary to pancreatitis), thrombosis of a segmental mesenteric artery (early, developing functional ileus), and recent or incomplete obstruction in the proximal intestinal tract (mechanical ileus).

Focal/Extensive. Less than 50 per cent of loops are greatly distended (five or six rib widths) whereas other visible portions of the small bowel may be less distended (nonuniform enlargement of lumen diameter). Possible etiologies include mechanical obstruction in the mid to distal intestine (Fig. 44–7), or volvulus of a portion of the intestine (as through a rent in the mesentery). The most common cause of extensive dilatation is mechanical obstruction, which may be caused by intraluminal occlusion (foreign body, intussusception, fecal or parasite impaction), intramural lesions (neoplasia, granulomatous infiltration as seen with histoplasmosis, strictures after trauma or previous surgery, congenital stenosis or atresia), or extraluminal pressure (adhesions, masses, hernias). As a mechanical obstruction becomes more chronic or more complete, the bowel wall becomes atonic and a functional ileus may develop. A lateral projection made with a horizontally directed x-ray beam may show gas caps (fluid levels) within the intestine that is distended as a result of mechanical ileus.[10] Severe focal bowel dilatation is a significant radiographic sign of intestinal disease. Because of the potentially life-threatening lesions that may be present, rapid surgical exploration is often warranted, especially when an abdominal mass is also palpable.

Generalized/Mild. All small bowel loops appear mildly enlarged; they may be distended with fluid or fluid/air. Possible etiologies include bacterial or viral enteritis; malabsorption; hypokalemia; the use of anticholinergic drugs, such as atropine; or mild functional ileus due to abdominal pain (Fig. 44–8).

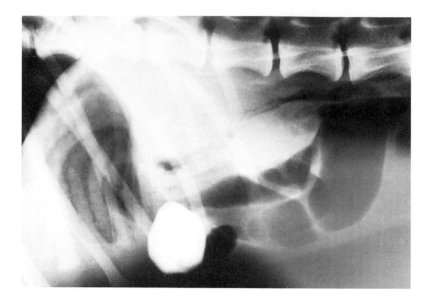

Figure 44–7. Mechanical ileus caused by a radiopaque foreign object (rock). Note the distended air-filled loops of small bowel in the ventral midabdomen are enlarged to five times the width of a rib.

Figure 44–8. Mild, generalized enlargement of small bowel lumen (four times the width of the adjacent rib). This appearance can be seen with mild, early functional ileus. This dog had a recently ruptured splenic hemangiosarcoma (not visible on this image) leading to abdominal pain and subsequent functional ileus.

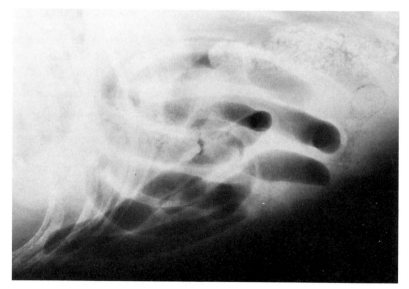

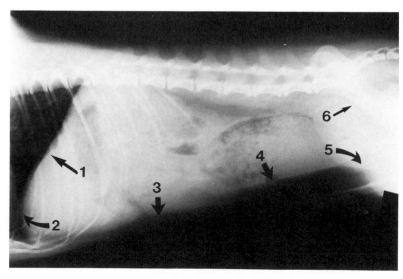

Figure 44–9. Potential locations for displacement of bowel in traumatic or congenital herniation. 1: diaphragmatic; 2: pericardial/peritoneal; 3: umbilical; 4: ventral; 5: inguinal; and 6: pelvic diaphragmatic.

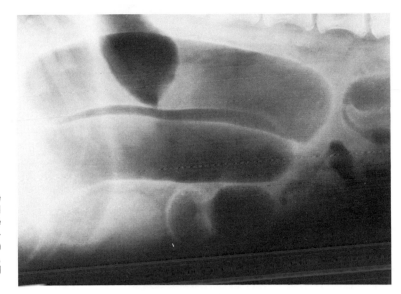

Figure 44–10. "Stacked loops" are greatly distended segments of small bowel that lie parallel and may be connected by sharp 180 degree hairpin turns. Stacking is usually seen with obstructive (mechanical) ileus, as in this dog with a corn cob jejunal obstruction.

Generalized/Extensive. If all bowel loops are uniformly distended, functional ileus is present. Possible causes of diffuse functional ileus are recent abdominal surgery with manipulation of bowel, neurologic injury (spinal trauma), and volvulus of the entire small bowel around the mesenteric root.

If bowel loops are not uniformly distended, mechanical ileus in the distal portion of the small bowel may be present, as could be seen with foreign body obstruction, tumor, stricture, or intussusception. Specific identification of the site and type of obstruction usually cannot be made on survey radiographs. Distension of the bowel lumen, however, often allows the clinician to determine the presence of obstructive ileus and to proceed directly to surgical correction.

Position. Displacement of small bowel is usually due to enlargement of adjacent organs, space-occupying mass lesions (see Chapter 32), or herniation. Potential sites for herniation of small bowel are illustrated in Figure 44–9. Contrast studies often help to define position abnormalities, especially if there is a minimal amount of air in the bowel lumen. The most common sites of small intestinal herniation are through the diaphragm, abdominal wall, inguinal canal, or pelvic diaphragm.[22]

Shape and Contour. "Stacked loops" is the term used to describe bowel segments (usually distended) that are layered closely parallel to each other. This appearance also suggests sharp hairpin turns (Fig. 44–10). Stacked loops are usually seen with mechanical ileus.

Irregular or tortuous contour may be due to

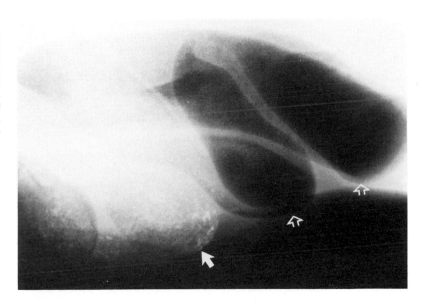

Figure 44–11. Mechanical ileus in a dog with an ileocolic intussusception. Air-distended stacked loops *(open arrows)* and small particles of radiopaque ingesta *(solid arrow)* are trapped proximal to the obstruction. The latter finding is commonly seen in cases of chronic or slowly developing partial obstruction. The intussusception itself cannot be identified.

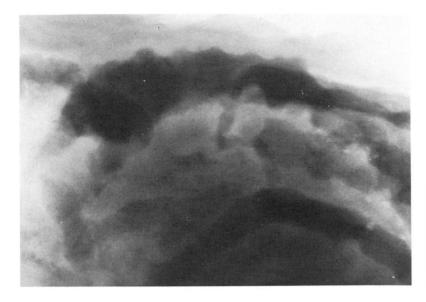

Figure 44–12. Survey radiograph suggests focal dilatation and an irregular, scalloped mucosal surface of a small bowel segment. Elevation of the length of intestine affected and the severity of changes in the mucosa require the performance of a barium study.

partial obstruction by linear foreign material or the occurrence of multiple serosal adhesions. Abnormalities in shape and contour are often easier to identify with contrast studies.

Radiopacity—Lumen Contents. Increased radiopacity occurs most commonly with radiopaque foreign objects (mineral or metallic content) (see Fig. 44–7). Small particles of radiopaque ingesta and debris may also accumulate proximal to a chronic obstruction (Fig. 44–11).

Decreased radiopacity is usually due to ingested air (aerophagia), especially if the location of the lucency changes on serial radiographs. A persistent decreased radiopacity within the bowel lumen may be a radiolucent foreign object. Fruit pits commonly contain straight geometric radiolucent defects that can be seen on survey radiographs. A contrast study is often necessary to confirm the diagnosis, however, if evidence of ileus is not present.

Radiopacity—Bowel Wall. Alterations in radiopacity of the bowel wall are unusual and may be difficult to differentiate from opacities within the lumen. Increased radiopacity occurs with dystrophic calcification within a neoplasm, granuloma, or abscess. Radiolucent defects within the intestinal wall have been seen in cases of intestinal necrosis secondary to infarction of mesenteric vessels or volvulus.

Architecture of Mucosal Surface. The mucosa cannot be adequately evaluated on survey radiographs. An irregularly scalloped appearance of the mucosa seen in air-filled segments of bowel, however, can provide an additional indication for contrast examination (Figs. 44–12 and 44–13).

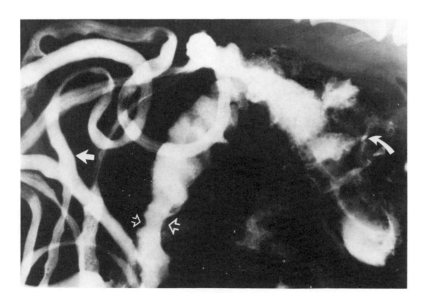

Figure 44–13. Barium upper gastrointestinal tract study (same patient as in Fig. 44–12). Normal bowel is seen proximal to the affected intestine (solid arrow). Abnormal mucosal architecture is indicated by irregular, nonsymmetric indentations of contrast medium (open arrows) and spiculated, ragged interface between barium and mucosa (curved arrow). The affected section of bowel is also moderately dilated. Histopathologic diagnosis: lymphosarcoma.

CONTRAST RADIOGRAPHY

Indications. Although the barium upper gastrointestinal study is probably the most frequently performed contrast examination in veterinary practice, the information gained is often limited. This limitation is generally due to poor patient selection and preparation or to inappropriate technique. The complete radiographic evaluation of the stomach and small bowel is time-consuming for the veterinarian and expensive for the owner (cost of an upper gastrointestinal tract study often rivals that of exploratory laparotomy). Because of the potential for a low yield of diagnostic information from this procedure, a contrast study should be reserved for the patient in which a diagnosis or approach to treatment cannot be made from clinical information and survey radiographs.

The clinical signs that most frequently warrant an intestinal contrast study[2, 12, 20, 22, 30] are: acute persistent vomiting with no changes seen on survey radiographs, recurrent vomiting (especially those animals refractory to symptomatic therapy and without other organ involvement to explain the vomiting), palpable abdominal mass without obstruction on survey radiographs, hematemesis, melena, acute abdominal pain with an unusual or unexplained abnormality seen on survey radiographs, and weight loss with intermittent or recurrent diarrhea. (Comment: contrast gastrointestinal tract studies are least informative in cases of chronic diarrhea without vomiting.) Additional information that can be gained from a contrast study includes: more thorough evaluation of mucosal abnormalities, length of intestine affected (focal, regional, or generalized), thickness of bowel wall, abnormalities in peristaltic activity and intestinal transit time, improved determination of lumen size, more complete evaluation of lumen contents, and determination of patency of lumen.

Contraindications. Contrast examination is not warranted in the patient with survey radiographic evidence of obstructive ileus.[30] Minimal additional information is to be gained, in that contrast medium passes only slowly through the atonic bowel (especially in the weakened or debilitated animal). If the clinical impression and survey radiographic findings are suggestive of mechanical obstruction, immediate surgery is indicated. Further attempts to define the specific site and type of obstructing lesion only delay and possibly complicate surgery and cause additional patient stress.

Technique. An empty gastrointestinal tract is preferred for obtaining optimal information from the contrast study. In patients with severe acute abdominal distress, however, no preparation is usually possible. In fact, the animal with an acute abdominal crisis may suffer additional injury from administration of laxatives or enemas.

For the elective upper gastrointestinal tract examination, a 24-hour fast is recommended before contrast medium administration. A thorough, flushing warm water or saline enema should be given until the returning fluid is clear. Commercial hypertonic enema preparations are not satisfactory because they do not cause evacuation of the entire colon. The enema should be given 2 to 4 hours before the contrast study to allow emptying of residual fluid and air.

TABLE 44–2. **INTESTINAL CONTRAST AGENTS**

Contrast Agent	Advantages	Disadvantages	Uses
Barium sulfate suspensions	Very radiopaque Excellent mucosal detail Remains in suspension Resists dilution Physiologically inert Low cost	Irritating if leaked into peritoneal cavity	Routine GI contrast studies
Barium sulfate, U.S.P.	Very inexpensive	Inadequate mucosal detail Tends to precipitate	Not recommended

Organic iodine solutions	Rapid transit time
	Nonirritating to serosal surfaces
	Rapidly resorbed following extraluminal leakage
		Less opaque than barium
		Poor mucosal detail
		May form precipitates
		May be absorbed across mucosa and excreted by urinary tract
		Hypertonicity causes:
		  Fluid flux into lumen
		  Dilution of contrast
		  Electrolyte imbalance ⎫
		  Dehydration ⎬ Young or debilitated patient
		Expensive
			Suspected intestinal perforation

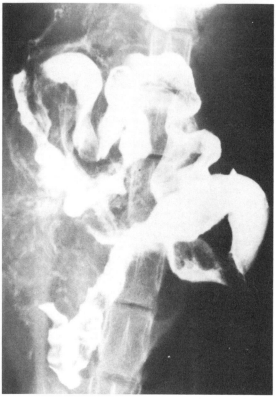

Figure 44–14. Leakage of contrast medium into the peritoneal cavity occurred due to bowel wall necrosis at multiple sites. Iodine-containing contrast media are the agents of choice when bowel perforation is suspected. After this cat vomited the iodine several times, barium was used to achieve a diagnostic study.

Because most sedative drugs used in small animal practice affect the motility of the gastrointestinal tract, their use should be avoided. General anesthetics and tranquilizers, such as promazine hydrochloride, fentanyl/droperidol, and xylazine hydrochloride, have all been shown to slow passage of barium through the intestines.[16, 39] Ketamine hydrochloride may be used in fractious cats; it has been shown to cause no apparent change in motility.[1] Medications that contain anticholinergic drugs should also be discontinued at least 24 hours (preferably 48 to 72 hours) before the contrast study.[2]

Ventrodorsal and right lateral recumbent positions are routinely used. Oblique views to highlight the pyloric sphincter or a particular abnormality may be added as needed.[6, 37]

Contrast Medium. Barium sulfate suspension is the contrast medium of choice in most situations. Micropulverized preparations are available in a dry powder form* or as a liquid suspension.† (Colibar V, Veterinary Radiographic Systems, Maitland, FL). The advantages of barium sulfate suspension are summarized in Table 44–2.[1, 2, 29, 30] If perforation of the intestinal tract is suspected, use of barium sulfate is not recommended; the combination of barium and ingesta contamination within the peritoneal cavity may cause more severe peritonitis, foreign body granulomas, or serosal adhesions.[9, 12, 23, 31] Therefore, one of the organic iodine preparations designed for the gastrointestinal tract should be used.‡ Occasionally, a small tear is missed because the iodine is reabsorbed so rapidly by the serosa. If a tear is still

*Barosperse, Mallinckrodt Pharmaceuticals, St. Louis, MO; Micropaque, Picker International, Highland Heights, OH.
†Novapaque, Picker International; Colibar V, Veterinary Radiographic Systems, Maitland, FL.
‡Gastrografin, Meglumine Diatrizoate Oral Solution, Squibb & Sons, Princeton, NJ; Oral Hypaque, Sodium Diatrizoate Liquid, Winthrop Laboratories, New York, NY.

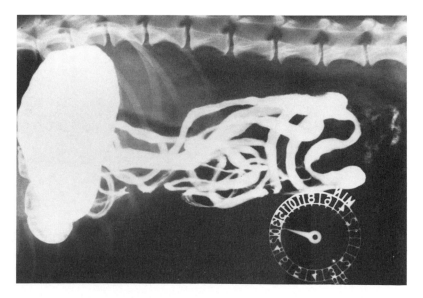

Figure 44–15. Normal canine barium upper gastrointestinal tract study, 30 minutes after contrast medium administration. Note the excellent radiopacity of the contrast medium and the sharp definition of the mucosal surface.

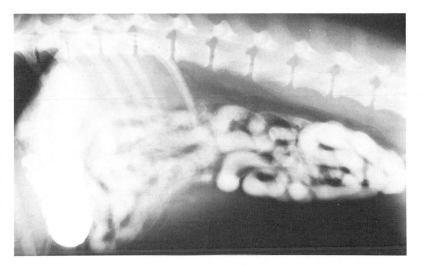

Figure 44–16. Normal canine iodine preparation upper gastrointestinal tract study, 30 minutes after contrast medium administration. Whereas contrast medium opacity is good in the bowel located in the caudal abdomen, the contrast medium is diluted (decreased opacity, poor definition of mucosa) in the cranial abdomen.

suspect after an iodine study, barium can demonstrate the leak more obviously (Fig. 44–14). Because of the rapid passage of iodine preparations through the gastrointestinal tract, these agents can also be used to determine the patency of the lumen quickly. The potentially hazardous adverse effects from the hyperosmolarity of the iodine contrast media, however, should always be kept in mind. Examples of the appearance of barium and iodine in normal small bowel are presented in Figs. 44–15 and 44–16. The advantages and disadvantages of the water-soluble contrast media are summarized in Table 44–2.

The volume of barium present within the intestinal lumen is a critical factor in the technical success or failure of an upper gastrointestinal tract study. The intestine should be distended to its reasonable physiologic maximum. Inadequate volume of contrast medium is one of the most frequent causes for nondiagnostic barium studies. The recommended dose rate for contrast medium is given in Table 44–3.

Complete descriptions of the procedure for performing an upper gastrointestinal tract study

and excellent examples of the normal appearance of the contrast-filled small bowel are available.[2, 18, 19, 20, 30] A summary of the organs usually seen at intervals after contrast medium administration is presented in Table 44–4.

Abnormal Roentgen Signs

The constant movement of the intestinal tract due to segmental and peristaltic contractions can produce some unusual appearances of the contrast medium column. Keep in mind that any single radiograph is an image of what is occurring within the gastrointestinal tract at a small fraction of a second. To avoid mistaking a contraction or a peristaltic wave for a pathologic lesion, remember that on an upper gastrointestinal tract study, the probability of a suspicious opacity being a real lesion varies directly with its frequency of occurrence; the more often the same abnormality is seen, the more likely it is to be a real lesion.

Position. Displacement of the small intestine within the confines of the peritoneal cavity is usually due to a space-occupying mass. A complete description of the direction of displacement caused by organ enlargement is available in Chapter 32. "Gathering" or crowding of bowel loops in the midabdomen is also seen with linear foreign body or adhesions from peritonitis (penetrating foreign object, pancreatitis, bite wound) or organized hemorrhage (after surgery or abdominal trauma).[34]

Herniation is another common cause of bowel displacement in small animals. Most of these herniations are in fact ruptures of one of the tissues that form the boundaries of the peritoneal cavity—diaphragm, abdominal wall, or pelvic diaphragm. Figure 44–9 is an illustration of the most common sites at which traumatic herniation occurs. Congenital hernias usually affect the diaphragm, scrotum, and umbilicus.[22]

TABLE 44–3. **RECOMMENDED DOSE RATE FOR CONTRAST MEDIUM**

Contrast Medium	Dog	Cat
Barium sulfate suspension*	6–12 ml/kg 20% (w/w)[30] or 6–10 ml/kg 60% (w/w)	12–16 ml/kg[18]
Organic iodine preparation (full strength)	2–3 ml/kg[20, 22, 30]	2 ml/kg[30]

*A large volume of relatively dilute contrast is preferred by some[30] to distend the intestinal lumen, but not to obscure radiolucent luminal filling defects. This author prefers use of the full strength barium suspension for its superior mucosal pattern definition.

TABLE 44–4. **UPPER GI FILM SEQUENCE**

	Barium	Organic Iodine	Structures Usually Opacified in Normal Animals*
Dog	Immediate	Immediate	Stomach
	15 min		Stomach, duodenum
	30 min	15 min	Stomach, duodenum, jejunum
	1 hour		Stomach, duodenum, jejunum
	2 hours	30 min	Stomach, all parts of small bowel
	4 hours	1 hour	Small bowel, colon
Cat	Immediate	Immediate	Stomach
	5 min	5 min	Stomach, duodenum
	30 min	30 min	All parts of small bowel
	60 min	60 min	Small bowel, colon

*Owing to the extreme variability of individual transit times, this list is only an approximation of the parts of the GI tract seen at these times.

Shape and Contour. Because the contour of the normal small intestinal wall is gently rounded or curved, abnormal patterns are seen as segments of bowel with persistent straight or flat walls or those that are excessively coiled or plicated. Straight contour of the wall is seen with infiltrative diseases (neoplastic lymphosarcoma, scirrhous, adenocarcinoma, granulomatous histoplasmosis) as demonstrated in Figure 44–13. Fibrosis or adhesions as might occur after trauma or focal peritonitis may also cause loss of pliability of the bowel wall.

An extensively pleated (plicated, "ribbon candy") appearance is seen when linear foreign material is trapped within the intestine.[22] In the cat, the lumen diameter is usually not greatly distended, although an increased number of bizarrely shaped gas bubbles may be present on survey radiographs.[8] If the gathering of the bowel in the midabdomen is not discernible on survey radiographs, contrast medium then allows the characteristic pleated shape to be seen (Fig. 44–17; compare with normal cat in Fig. 44–2). Although more common in cats, linear foreign material causing partial obstruction, laceration, or both, of the bowel wall with secondary peritonitis can also be seen in dogs. Common linear foreign objects include string, thread, and tinsel in the cat, and towel, carpet, string from wrapped meats, socks, or panty hose in the dog.

Radiopacity. The shape of a large radiolucent filling defect within the contrast medium column can indicate not only the presence of obstruction but also the type of lesion causing the blockage. Barium is often able to dissect between an intraluminal object and the bowel wall, allowing a more complete image of the obstruction. The following lesions may be recognized by the given shape of the intraluminal defect (see Fig. 44–18): spheric: rubber ball (common), benign tumor such as a leiomyoma (rare); elliptic: fruit pit, nut; straight edge: plastic, leather, wood splinter; hemispheric: retrograde intussusception; curved linear: ascarid

(Fig. 44–19). Other foreign objects have distinctive shapes that allow their positive identification (Fig. 44–20). If patient preparation is inadequate, particles of ingesta may appear as filling defects in the barium column (Fig. 44–21), which significantly reduces the information available from the study.

Size and Architecture. The following descriptions refer to the size of the bowel lumen, the

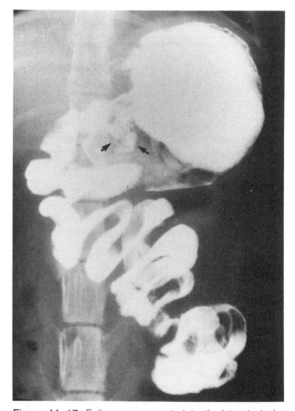

Figure 44–17. Feline upper gastrointestinal tract study, 20 minutes after administration of barium. The tightly pleated or ribbon candy appearance indicates the presence of linear foreign material. The proximal end of the foreign material is often wrapped around the base of the tongue or is caught in the pyloric antrum of the stomach (arrows).

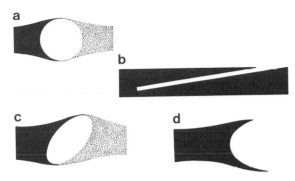

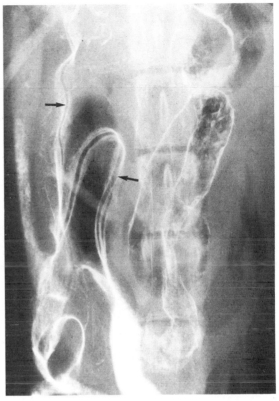

Figure 44–18. Shapes of contrast interface with an intraluminal object. The barium column (black) fills the intestine and outlines one or several surfaces of the object. Partial obstruction of the lumen allows a smaller quantity of barium (stippling) to pass. Complete obstruction shows no barium in the bowel distal to it and therefore no definition of the caudal surface of the object. a: rubber ball, spherical mass arising from the bowel mucosa (leiomyoma—rare); b: flat, straight foreign object such as hard plastic, leather, or wood splinter; c: fruit pit or nut; d: retrograde intussusception (invagination of bowel in the opposite direction of normal ingesta passage).

appearance of the mucosal surface, and the extent of the small intestine that is affected. Focal indicates one to three loops of bowel are involved, regional is used when more than three loops but less than 50 per cent of the small bowel is affected, and generalized applies to those lesions present in more than 50 per cent of the small bowel segments.

Dilated, Smooth Mucosa. This combination of roentgen signs is most frequently seen with obstruction.[10, 16a] Figures 44–20 and 44–24 show barium within the distended bowel segments proximal to a site of mechanical obstruction. With focal or regional involvement, the radiographic sign is usually seen with mechanical obstruction of recent onset or when the obstruc-

Figure 44–19. The thin, radiolucent filling defects are ascarids (arrows) Note that the defects taper at their cranial and caudal ends and that there is no evidence of abnormal size, shape, or contour of the bowel.

tion is located in the duodenum or cranial portion of the jejunum. Bowel distal to the obstruction and the unaffected bowel proximal to the obstruction are normal in size and show evidence of peristalsis. If the obstruction of the lumen is almost complete, the small volume of barium that passes the lesion may not be suffi-

Figure 44–20. Mechanical obstruction of the jejunum by a foreign object (baby bottle nipple).

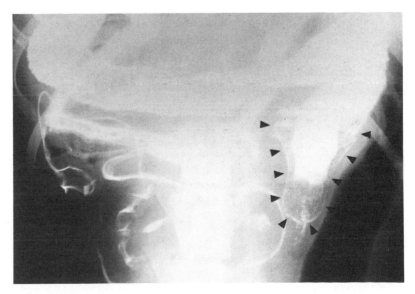

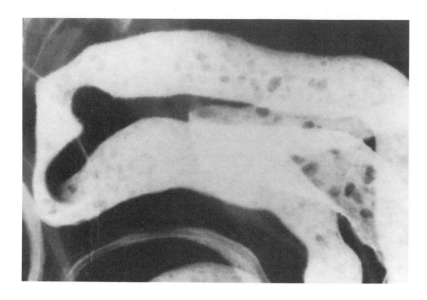

Figure 44-21. Food particles mixed with barium in a patient that had not been fasted before the contrast study. The food particles create filling defects that compromise the ability to define small intraluminal objects or nodules arising from the mucosa.

cient to distend the lumen of the remainder of the bowel (Fig. 44–20). This finding may lead to a false impression of narrowed bowel diameter distal to the obstruction.

Generalized involvement is indicated if all loops of bowel are distended uniformly, no peristaltic indentations are seen along the intestinal walls, and functional or paralytic ileus is present. Mechanical ileus may be generalized in the case of a chronic obstruction at the ileocolic junction. Mechanical ileus may also proceed to functional ileus as the bowel wall stretches, becomes atonic, and then progressively becomes ischemic. Possible etiologies of functional ileus include spinal cord trauma, peritoneal inflammation, intestinal vascular injury or thrombosis, and parasympatholytic drug administration.

Dilated, Irregular Mucosa. Usually seen as focal or regional involvement, the mucosa has an irregularly scalloped or spiculated surface; this appearance often is associated with ulceration. Regional infiltration of the jejunum by lymphosarcoma is shown in Figure 44–13. Other pathologic processes that may show similar changes in the bowel include adenocarcinoma (often produces a focal mass that is palpable, see Fig. 44–22) and histoplasmosis.[3, 25]

Narrowed, Smooth Mucosa. With focal or regional involvement, localized irritation of the bowel can cause spasm of the circular muscle component of the wall and induce hyperperistalsis. This irritation results in a radiographic appearance of numerous bead-like segments of barium on a contrast study (Fig. 44–23). A single, persistent focus of narrowed lumen can also be seen with stricture due to an intramural mass, such as a granuloma or adenocarcinoma (Fig. 44–24);[7, 27] stenosis after injury of the wall; or when barium given orally reaches an intus-

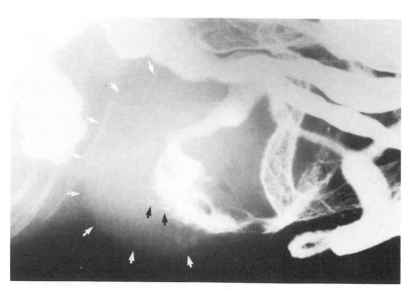

Figure 44-22. Adenocarcinoma of the jejunum during a barium upper gastrointestinal tract study. Roentgen signs include: soft-tissue mass *(white arrows),* mild focal enlargement of bowel lumen, irregular contour of mucosa, and extravasation of a small amount of contrast medium into the mass *(black arrows).*

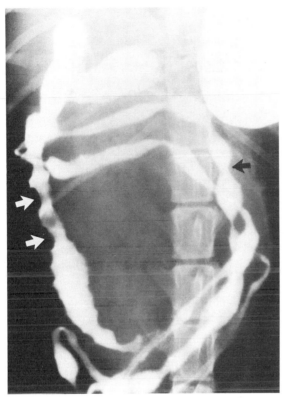

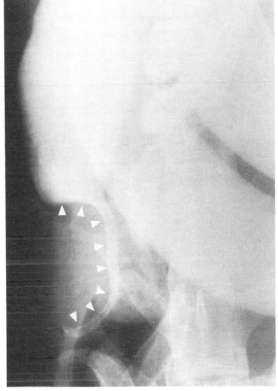

Figure 44–23. Irritation of duodenum and jejunum are indicated by irregular, serrated mucosal surface *(white arrows)* of duodenum and hypersegmentation *(black arrow).* The midcentral area, which is devoid of bowel loops, was caused by necrotic, hemorrhagic pancreatitis with abscess formation that resulted 10 days after a penetrating wound.

Figure 44–24. Eccentrically narrowed bowel lumen, smooth mucosal surface, and dilatation of bowel proximal to the narrowing characterize this focal intramural obstruction. Histopathologic diagnosis: adenocarcinoma of bowel wall. Eccentric narrowing usually occurs with a mass lesion; a post-traumatic or post-inflammatory stricture usually causes more symmetric narrowing.

susception that has occurred in the direction of normal peristalsis (forward or direct intussusception). Signs of mechanical ileus may also be present in these patients.

With more generalized involvement, hyper-

peristalsis may be seen in cases of diffuse enteritis or peritonitis, as might be caused by a variety of bacterial organisms or chemical irritants (Fig. 44–25). An insufficient volume of barium may fail to distend the bowel and may

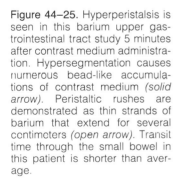

Figure 44–25. Hyperperistalsis is seen in this barium upper gastrointestinal tract study 5 minutes after contrast medium administration. Hypersegmentation causes numerous bead-like accumulations of contrast medium *(solid arrow).* Peristaltic rushes are demonstrated as thin strands of barium that extend for several centimeters *(open arrow).* Transit time through the small bowel in this patient is shorter than average.

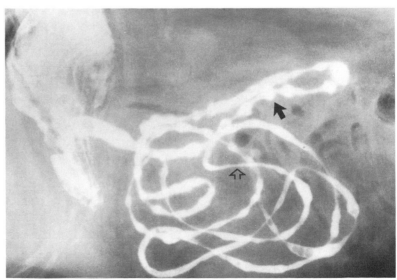

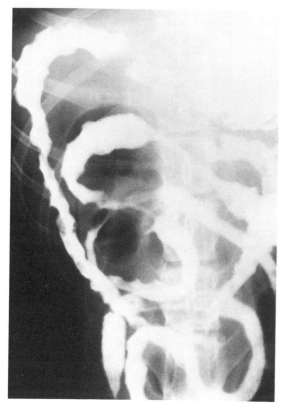

Figure 44–26. Numerous radiolucent filling defects are seen in the duodenum and less prominently in the jejunum. These defects appear as nodules or as thumbprint-like indentations of the barium column. The lumen diameter of the descending duodenum is narrowed. Possible etiologies: chronic severe inflammation or infiltrative neoplasia. Histopathologic diagnosis: lymphocytic/plasmacytic enteritis.

artifactually create an impression of bowel narrowing.

Narrowed, Irregular Mucosa. If the patient is sufficiently fat and no peritoneal fluid is present, thickening of the bowel wall may also be appreciated, especially when a mass can be palpated on physical examination. With focal involvement, ulcerative lesions most often cause this appearance. These lesions may be benign ulcers secondary to gastrin-producing pancreatic tumors (Zollinger-Ellison syndrome) or to histamine release from mast cell tumors.[13, 17, 21, 40] Ulcerated primary intestinal tumor, such as adenocarcinoma, may also have a narrowed lumen and ragged, irregular mucosa, sometimes termed "apple core" in appearance.[26, 35] Although rare, an ulcerated granuloma occurring secondary to foreign object penetration or systemic fungal spread should also be considered.

When the distribution is more regional or generalized, severe inflammatory conditions of the mucosa and bowel wall may show numerous nodular filling defects or thumbprint indentations along the mucosal surface (Figs. 44–26 and 44–27). Possible causes include lymphocytic/plasmacytic enteritis, eosinophilic enteritis, hemorrhagic gastroenteritis, or ischemia and necrosis.[4, 14, 15, 33, 38] The diameter of the bowel lumen may also vary considerably with ulcerative enteritis. Spastic contraction of circular muscles of the intestinal wall may contribute to the scalloped appearance of the barium column.

Transit Time and Peristaltic Activity. Because of the great variation in time required for

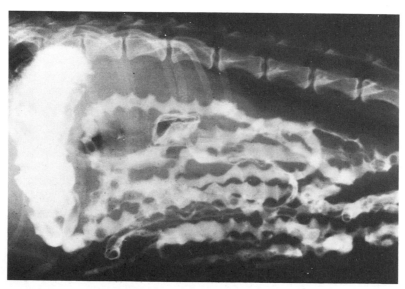

Figure 44–27. Generalized asymmetric thumbprint indentations throughout the small bowel. This pattern is unusual but suggests extensive mucosal disease, wall spasm or both. Histopathologic diagnosis: catarrhal enteritis.

barium to pass through the small bowel in the dog and cat, only those transit times that are significantly outside the normal parameters should be considered indicative of a pathologic condition. The best method for the evaluation of peristaltic activity is image-intensified fluoroscopy. Because of the limited availability of this equipment, however, those inferences concerning bowel motility that can be made from the positive-contrast radiography are mentioned.

Prolonged Transit. If barium is not cleared from the small bowel of the dog after 5 hours or of the cat after 3 hours, transit is considered abnormally slow. If lumen diameter is normal, possible causes for slow transit include anticholinergic drug administration or an inadequate volume of barium was administered (insufficient to stimulate intestinal centers of peristaltic activity).[5] If the lumen diameter is distended, atony due to mechanical or functional ileus is present.

Rapid Transit. When rapid opacification of small bowel loops occurs in combination with multiple, closely spaced peristaltic contractions, hypermotility is present. This finding is most commonly associated with acute enteritis or serosal irritation (peritonitis). Motility may be increased secondary to the increased volume and fluid nature of intestinal contents in the animal with profuse diarrhea.[18] If early opacification of many segments of the small bowel is seen without distinct peristaltic contractions, enteritis or one of the infiltrative diseases that cause malabsorption may be reducing compliance of the intestinal wall. In the latter case, segmental contractions of the wall may be obliterated and are replaced by peristaltic rushes, which move ingesta (or contrast medium) through large segments of intestine without allowing sufficient time for digestion or absorption. Peristaltic rushes may be demonstrated on a barium study as continuous loops with narrowed lumen, smooth mucosa, and decreased transit time (Fig. 44–25).

References

1. Allan GS, Rendano VT, Quick CB, et al: Gastrografin as a gastrointestinal contrast medium in the cat. Vet Radiol 20:3, 1979.
2. Brawner WR, and Bartels JE: Contrast radiography of the digestive tract: Indications, techniques and complications. Vet Clin North Am [Small Anim Pract] 13:599, 1983.
3. Brody RS: Alimentary tract neoplasms in the cat: A clinicopathologic survey of 46 cases. Am J Vet Res 27:74, 1966.
4. Burrows CF: Canine hemorrhagic gastroenteritis. J Am Anim Hosp Assoc 13:451, 1977.
5. Ehrlein H-J: A new technique for simultaneous radiography and recording of gastrointestinal motility in unanesthetized dogs. Lab Anim Sci 30:879, 1980.
6. Farrow CS, and Back RE: A modified approach: Gastrointestinal contrast examination in the cat. Feline Pract 10:20, 1980.
7. Feeney DA, Klausner JS, and Johnston GR: Chronic bowel obstruction caused by primary intestinal neoplasia: A report of five cases. J Am Anim Hosp Assoc 18:67, 1982.
8. Felts JF, Fox PP, and Burk RL: Thread and sewing needles as gastrointestinal foreign bodies in the cat: A review of 64 cases. J Am Vet Med Assoc 184:56, 1984.
9. Foley MJ, Ghahremani GG, and Rogers LF: Reappraisal of contrast media used to detect upper gastrointestinal perforations. Radiology 144:231, 1982.
10. Gibbs C, and Pearson H: The radiological diagnosis of gastrointestinal obstruction in the dog. J Small Anim Pract 14:61, 1973.
11. Goldberg HI, and Sheft DJ: Abnormalities in small intestine contour and caliber (a working classification). Radiol Clin North Am 14:461, 1976.
12. Gomez JA: The gastrointestinal contrast study. Vet Clin North Am 4:805, 1974.
13. Happe RP, van der Gaag I, Lamers CBHW, et al: Zollinger-Ellison syndrome in three dogs. Vet Pathol 17:177, 1980.
14. Hayden DW, and Van Kruiningen HJ: Lymphocytic plasmacytic enteritis in German Shepherd dogs. J Am Anim Hosp Assoc 18:89, 1982.
15. Hendrick M: A spectrum of hypereosinophilic syndromes exemplified by six cats with eosinophilic enteritis. Vet Pathol 18:188, 1981.
16. Hsu WH, and McNeel SV: Effect of yohimbine on xylazine-induced prolongation of gastrointestinal transit in dogs. J Am Vet Med Assoc 183:297, 1983.
16a. Kleine, LJ: The role of radiography in the diagnosis of intestinal obstruction in dogs and cats. Comp Contin Ed Pract Vet 1:44, 1979.
17. Middleton DJ, Watson ADJ, and Culvenor JE: Duodenal ulceration associated with gastrin-secreting pancreatic tumor in a cat. J Am Vet Med Assoc 183:461, 1983.
18. Morgan JP: The upper gastrointestinal tract in the cat: A protocol for contrast radiography. J Am Vet Radiol Soc 18:134, 1977.
19. Morgan, JP: The upper gastrointestinal examination in the cat: Normal radiographic appearance using positive contrast medium. Vet Radiol 22:159, 1981.
20. Morgan JP, and Silverman S: Radiographic evaluation of the digestive tract. In Techniques of Veterinary Radiography, 3rd Ed. Davis, CA, Veterinary Radiology Associates, 1982.
21. Murray M, McKeating FJ, Baker GJ, et al: Peptic ulceration in the dog: A clinico-pathological study. Vet Rec 91:441, 1972.
22. O'Brien TR: Small intestine. In O'Brien TR (Ed): Radiographic Diagnosis of Abdominal Disorders in the Dog and Cat. Philadelphia, WB Saunders, 1978, pp. 279–351.
23. Ott DJ, and Gelfand DW: Gastrointestinal contrast agents—indications, uses, and risks. JAMA 249:2380, 1983.
24. Owens JM: Radiographic Interpretation for the Small Animal Clinician. St. Louis, MO, Ralston Purina Co, 1982.
25. Patnaik AK, Hurvitz AI, and Johnson GF: Canine gastrointestinal neoplasms. Vet Pathol 14:547, 1977.
26. Patnaik AK, Hurvitz AI, and Johnson GF: Canine intestinal adenocarcinoma and carcinoid. Vet Pathol 17:149, 1980.
27. Patnaik AK, Liu S-K, and Johnson GF: Feline intestinal adenocarcinoma. Vet Pathol 13:1, 1976.

28. Root CR: Interpretation of abdominal survey radiographs. Vet Clin North Am 4:763, 1974.
29. Root CR, and Morgan JP: Contrast radiography of the upper gastrointestinal tract in the dog: A comparison of micropulverized barium sulfate and U.S.P. barium sulfate suspensions in clinically normal dogs. J Small Anim Pract 10:279, 1969.
30. Root CR: Contrast radiography of the alimentary tract. In Ticer JW (Ed): Radiographic Technique in Veterinary Practice. Philadelphia, WB Saunders, 1984.
31. Seltzer SE, Jones B, and McLaughlin GC: Proper choice of contrast agents in emergency gastrointestinal radiology. CRC Crit Rev Diagn Imaging 12:79, 1979.
32. Sherding RG: Diseases of the small bowel. In Ettinger SJ (Ed): Textbook of Veterinary Internal Medicine. Philadelphia, WB Saunders, 1983, pp. 1278–1345.
33. Smith SL, Tutton RH, and Ochsner SF: Roentgenographic aspects of intestinal ischemia. AJR 116:249, 1972.
34. Suter PF, and Olsson S-E: The diagnosis of injuries to the intestines, gallbladder and bile ducts in the dog. J Small Anim Pract 11:575, 1970.
35. Thielen GH, and Madewell BR: Tumors of the digestive tract. In Theilen GH and Madewell BR (Eds): Veterinary Cancer Medicine. Philadelphia, Lea & Febiger, 1979, pp. 307–331.
36. Thrall DE, and Leininger JR: Irregular intestinal mucosal margination in the dog: Normal or abnormal? J Small Anim Pract 17:305, 1976.
37. Ticer, JW: The abdomen. In Ticer JW (Ed): Radiographic Technique in Veterinary Practice. Philadelphia, WB Saunders, 1984.
38. Vest B, and Margulis AR: Experimental infarction of small bowel in dogs. AJR 92:1080, 1964.
39. Zontine WJ: Effect of chemical restraint drugs on the passage of barium sulfate through the stomach and duodenum of dogs. J Am Vet Med Assoc 162:878, 1973.
40. Zontine WJ, Meierhenry EF, and Hicks RF: Perforated duodenal ulcer associated with mastocytoma in a dog: A case report. J Am Vet Radiol Soc 18:162, 1977.

CHAPTER 45

THE LARGE BOWEL

DARRYL N. BIERY

Survey and contrast radiographic studies are diagnostic procedures that frequently enable recognition of large bowel disease. As with other diagnostic procedures, such as endoscopy and laparotomy, thorough knowledge of the anatomy of the large bowel and adjacent viscera is essential in recognizing the radiographic signs (alterations) associated with disease.

NORMAL RADIOGRAPHIC ANATOMY

The large bowel of the dog and cat is composed of the cecum, colon, rectum, and anal canal (Fig. 45–1). The cecum, a diverticulum of the proximal colon, has a different anatomic and radiographic appearance in the dog and cat (Fig. 45–2).[8] The canine cecum is semicircular ("C"- or cork-screw-shaped), compartmentalized with a cecocolic junction, and normally contains some intraluminal gas. The intraluminal gas and characteristic shape enables easy recognition of the cecum in the right midabdomen on most survey radiographs. The feline cecum, however, is usually not visible on survey radiographs. It is a short, cone-like diverticulum of the colon with no distinct cecocolic junction and no compartmentalization; it rarely contains gas. The colon of the dog and cat, the longest segment of the large bowel, is composed of a thin-walled distensible tube that is divided into ascending, transverse, and descending parts. These divisions are easily recognized on survey abdominal radiographs based on their shape, size, and location. The distal ileum enters the ascending colon from a medial direction via the ileocecal sphincter. This circular sphincter is usually not visible on survey radiographs, but it is easily identified with contrast studies, such as a barium enema. The colon has a shape similar to that of a question mark or shepherd's crook (Fig. 45–1). The junction between the ascending and transverse colon is called the hepatic or right colic flexure, and that between the transverse and descending colon is called the splenic or left colic flexure. The ascending colon and hepatic flexure are located to the right of midline. The transverse colon, which passes from right to left, lies cranial to the root of the mesentery. The splenic flexure and proximal descending colon are located to the left of midline. The distal descending colon courses to the midline and enters the pelvic canal to become the rectum. The rectum is the terminal portion of the colon, beginning at the pelvic inlet and ending at the anal canal.

The anatomic relation of the large bowel to other viscera is extremely important for the radiographic recognition of diseases of the large bowel and adjacent organs (Fig. 45–3). The

511

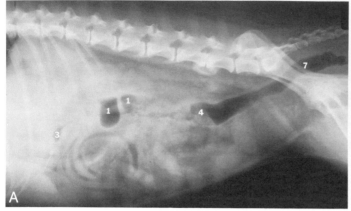

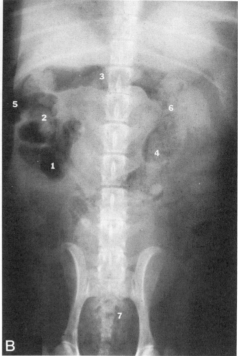

Figure 45–1. Survey lateral (*A*) and ventrodorsal *(B)* radiographs of a normal dog abdomen. The large bowel is divided into the cecum (1), ascending colon (2), transverse colon (3), descending colon (4), hepatic (5) and splenic (6) flexures, rectum (7), and anal canal. Note the admixture of gas and feces present in the cecum, colon, and rectum. In *B* the descending colon is displaced toward the right by a normal distended urinary bladder, a variation of normal.

ascending colon lies adjacent to the descending duodenum, right limb of the pancreas, right kidney, mesentery, and small bowel. The transverse colon lies adjacent to the greater curvature of the stomach, left limb of the pancreas, liver, small intestine, and root of the mesentery. The proximal descending colon lies in close proximity to the left kidney and ureter, spleen, and small bowel. The midportion of the descending colon lies adjacent to the small bowel, urinary bladder, and uterus. Because it is less

fixed, the midportion of the descending colon has a variety of normal positions in the caudal left abdomen. Normal variations are caused by various amounts of ingesta within the bowel, degree of urinary bladder distension, and amount of intra-abdominal fat. Frequently, the distended urinary bladder displaces the descending colon toward the midline or to the right of midline (Fig. 45–1). The distal portion of the descending colon and rectum are also closely associated with the urethra; sublumbar,

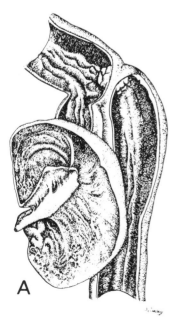

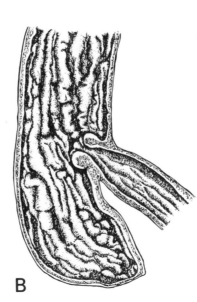

Figure 45–2. The cecum of the dog *(A)* and of the cat *(B)* are anatomically and radiographically different. The canine cecum is semicircular, compartmentalized, and normally contains some gas. The feline cecum, however, is a short, cone-like structure with no compartmentalization; it rarely contains gas. (From O'Brien TR: Radiographic Diagnosis of Abdominal Disorders in the Dog and Cat. Davis, CA, Covell Park Vet. Co., 1981, with permission.)

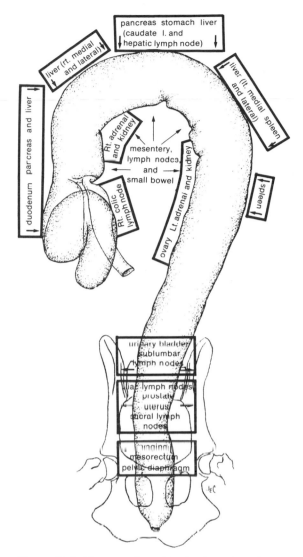

Figure 45–3. Viscera adjacent to the large bowel, on a ventrodorsal radiographic view, may cause anatomic-radiographic variations that may be alterations indicative of disease or variants of normal. *Arrows,* usual direction of large bowel position displacement when an organ enlarges. (See Fig. 45–9.) (From O'Brien TR: Radiographic Diagnosis of Abdominal Disorders in the Dog and Cat. Davis, CA, Covell Park Vet. Co., 1981, with permission.)

iliac, and sacral lymph nodes; prostate or uterus and vagina; and the pelvic diaphragm.

RADIOGRAPHIC TECHNIQUES OF LARGE BOWEL EVALUATION

Because feces and gas that produce contrasting radiographic opacities are usually present, a part or all of the large bowel is usually identifiable on survey radiographs of the abdomen. Different body positions during survey radiography distribute intraluminal gas to different parts of the large bowel, largely due to gravity.

Thus, gas is in the more nondependent portions of the colon.

When evaluating the large bowel radiographically, it is essential that the entire abdomen and pelvic area be included on two orthogonal radiographic views and that the radiographs be of diagnostic quality. The urinary bladder should be empty. Rectal examination, vigorous abdominal palpation, aerophagia from restraint and struggling, and enemas before survey radiography can increase the amount of gas or fluid present within the colon and other parts of the gastrointestinal tract. Although an abnormality in position, size, or shape of the large bowel may be seen on survey radiographs, it may not be a pathognomonic finding and a diagnosis may not be possible.

Compression radiography of the abdomen is a simple technique that may aid in further delineating the presence of a lesion. When the colon is compressed with a wooden or plastic spoon or paddle, adjacent bowel or masses are displaced or compressed, which enhances radiographic detail (Fig. 45–4). More definitive radiographic evaluation of the large bowel usually requires a contrast study via the rectal administration of barium sulfate suspension (barium enema), air (pneumocolon), or a combination of barium sulfate suspension and air (double-contrast study).

Barium enema examination is the most commonly used contrast study for examination of the large bowel. A balloon catheter is used to ensure a tight system for adequate distension of the colon. The colon must first be thoroughly cleaned by adequate preparation, a process that is frequently difficult. A microparticulate barium suspension should be used to provide a smooth coating of the mucosal surface. The colon should be filled with barium slowly, preferably with fluoroscopic observation. Because such equipment may not be available, the standard amount of barium is 10 ml per kilogram of body weight.[12] Radiographs should be made both when the colon is distended and again after evacuation. The normal colon has a smooth, contrast medium-mucosal interface and uniform diameter when the colon is distended. After evacuation of the barium, longitudinal mucosal folds are visible. If air is then infused, a double-contrast study is obtained, which provides the most detailed visualization of the mucosal surface.

A variety of radiographic appearances result from barium adhering to mucus, clumping and flocculation of barium, and filling defects of feces that is within the lumen or is adhered to the wall. The colon of the dog and cecum and colon of the cat have lymph follicles in the mucosa, which appear as spicules on a barium enema study or as pinpoint radiopacities when

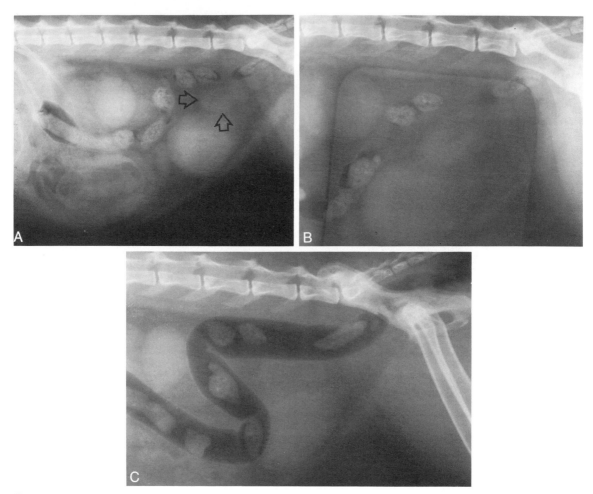

Figure 45–4. A 5-year-old female, spayed domestic shorthaired cat. *A,* survey radiograph. There is an abnormal soft-tissue mass *(arrows)* interposed between the descending colon and the urinary bladder. At surgery, the mass was a uterine stump pyometra. *B,* survey lateral recumbent radiograph of the abdomen with a compression paddle applied. The mass appears fixed and separate from the descending colon and urinary bladder. *C,* survey lateral radiograph of the abdomen after a partial pneumocolon study via retrograde introduction of gas. The soft-tissue mass (uterine stump pyometra) is visualized as an extramural mass. Feces were not removed before the contrast study was conducted.

visualized en face with a double-contrast study. These normal follicles must be differentiated from small ulcers.

The large bowel cannot be properly evaluated on an upper gastrointestinal tract study in which positive-contrast medium is administered per os. Orally administered contrast media commonly results in incomplete large bowel lumen distension as well as intraluminal filling defects due to feces. The reader is advised to consult other textbooks for more detailed information on specific techniques, procedures, complications, and limitations of large bowel radiographic techniques and contrast study procedures.[2, 8, 12] Unusual contrast studies such as rectal-colon lymphangiography and angiography are not described in this chapter.[1, 3, 11]

Complete large bowel contrast studies are time-consuming and must be done meticulously to assess the mucosa, wall, lumen, and adjacent viscera, as well as to avoid artifacts, complica-

tions, and messes, such as contrast medium on the veterinarian, equipment, and patient. Partial large bowel contrast studies, which are less thorough, quicker, and easier, can be done. These studies, performed with the introduction of small amounts of air or barium into the rectum via dose syringe, do not allow visualization of the entire large bowel or small lesions, such as mucosal irregularities. These partial studies, however, may enable visualization of large intraluminal lesions and differentiation of the colon from adjacent organs and masses (Fig. 45–4C).

Complications related to contrast studies of the colon can occur. The most serious complication is perforation and subsequent peritonitis (Fig. 45–5). Rupture can occur from a cleansing enema, improper selection or use of a barium enema catheter, overdistension of weakened or diseased bowel, or after biopsy.[10, 13] A more common complication that is of no serious con-

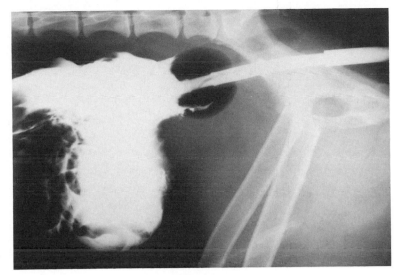

Figure 45–5. Lateral radiograph of a 5-year-old male Irish setter in which perforation of the colon occurred during a barium enema study. This complication can occur secondary to improper type and use of a closed-system catheter or to disease of the colon. The dog had a 4-month history of weight loss and straining to defecate. At necropsy, chronic prostatitis with adhesions to the colon and a localized peritonitis were evident.

sequence is retrograde filling of the distal small bowel, which obscures visualization of the colon. This complication has been reported in about one third of dogs and can occur without overdistension of the colon.[12] Spasm, which is usually transient, can also occur when the contrast medium is cold or the wall is irritated by the catheter (Fig. 45–6).

RADIOGRAPHIC FINDINGS IN LARGE BOWEL DISEASE

Disease involving or adjacent to the large bowel may produce radiographic alterations in size, shape, location, and radiopacity. Although function cannot be evaluated radiographically, the quantity or location of feces may suggest impaired motility. It must be emphasized that most radiographic descriptions and illustrations of specific large bowel diseases are not pathognomonic radiographic findings. Many different diseases have similar radiographic findings and

any one specific disease can have a spectrum of different appearances.

In the normal large bowel, the colon contains most of the feces, with small amounts or no feces in the rectum (Fig. 45–1). The diameter of the normal colon varies with the amount of feces present and defecation habits. Normally, the colon diameter should be less than the length of L_7.[8] Abnormal enlargement of the colon, certainly beyond 1½ times the length of L_7 is termed megacolon, which may be localized or generalized. Localized enlargement is usually associated with an acute disease (e.g., intussusception); generalized megacolon is usually evidence of chronic bowel dysfunction.

Generalized megacolon may be caused by pelvic trauma, with or without fracture, and narrowing of the pelvic canal; chronic partial obstruction from rectal stricture, tumor, or lymphadenopathy (Fig. 45–7); aganglionosis (e.g., Hirschsprung's disease) (Fig. 45–8); spinal anomalies (e.g., cauda equina syndrome, sac-

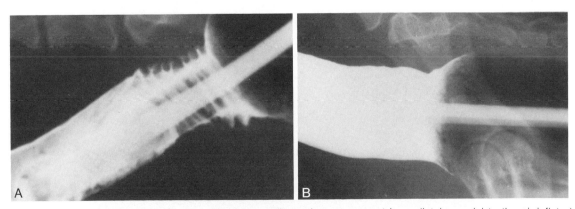

Figure 45–6. Narrowing and irregularity of the descending colon are present immediately cranial to the air-inflated Bardex catheter cuff. This was a spasm (A) and was transient as seen on a subsequent radiograph (B) made several minutes later.

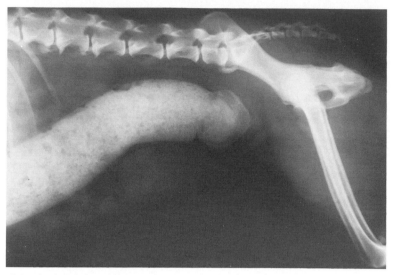

Figure 45–7. Survey lateral recumbent radiograph of the abdomen of a 9-year-old female, spayed mixed-breed dog with 5 months of progressive difficulty urinating and straining to defecate. The stools were flattened and a rectal mass was palable. The mass within the pelvis was a fibroleiomyoma causing partial colonic obstruction and megacolon. Unrelated L_7-S_1 spondylosis deformans is present.

rococcygeal agenesis in Manx cats); chronic colitis; psychogenic causes; chronic constipation (e.g., hypercalcemia and parasympathetic drugs); surgical ureterocolic diversion techniques; and anorectal congenital anomalies.[7-9]

A colon that is smaller than normal has not been reported in the dog and cat, but a congenital anomaly of duplication of the large bowel and rectum has been reported in a dog.[5]

The size and shape of the colon may be altered by congenital and acquired disease of the large bowel and adjacent viscera. These alterations can result from the chronic inflammatory disease of colitis, which may markedly shorten the bowel to a small localized lesion, such as a diverticulum or adhesion from pancreatitis.

Abnormal location of the large bowel is a common alteration consistent with large bowel disease in the dog and cat. Although there is some normal variability in the location of the large bowel, mass lesions, particularly those of organs adjacent to the colon, cause displacement of the cecum, colon, or rectum (see Chapter 32 and Figs. 45–3 and 45–9). Masses or enlargement of the uterus, prostate, and lymph

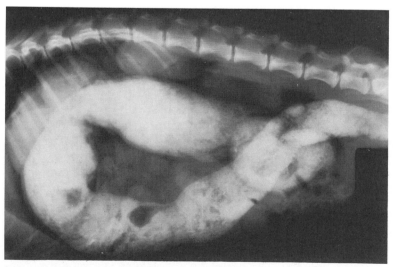

Figure 45–8. Lateral pneumoperitoneogram. Generalized megacolon is present. This 5-month-old female, mixed-breed dog had functional and histologic evidence of Hirschsprung's disease.

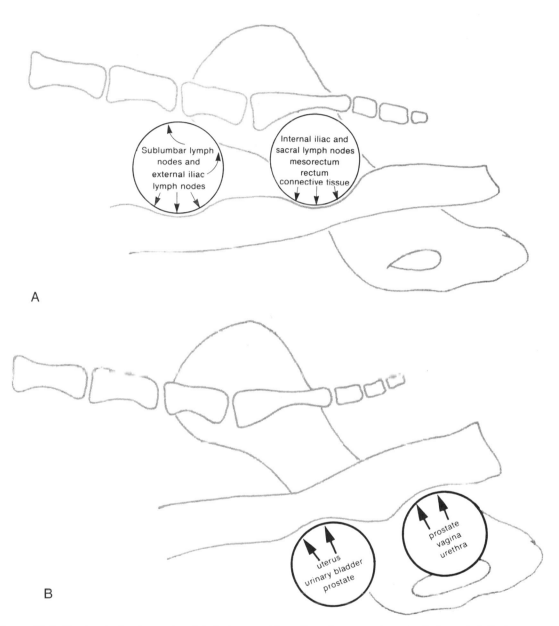

Figure 45–9. The terminal colon and rectal displacement by adjacent organ enlargement. *A,* ventral displacement of the terminal colon and rectum commonly results from sublumbar and external iliac lymph node enlargement. Although less common, a hematoma, abscess, or tumor can produce similar displacement alterations. *B,* dorsal displacement of the rectum commonly results from enlargement of the prostate, uterus, vagina, or intrapelvic urinary bladder. (From O'Brien TR: Radiographic Diagnosis of Abdominal Disorders in the Dog and Cat. Davis, CA, Covell Park Vet. Co., 1981, with permission.)

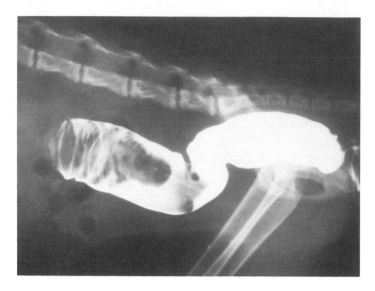

Figure 45–10. A 4½-month-old male Siamese cat with intussusception of the descending colon. Note the radiolucent filling defect and the coiled spring appearance created by the intussusceptum being outlined by barium.

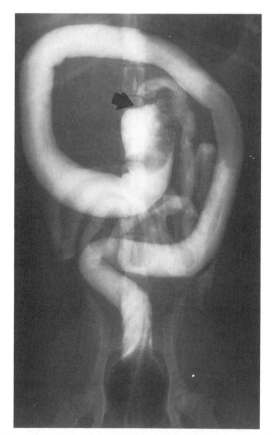

Figure 45–11. A 14-month-old male beagle had intermittent diarrhea with shreds of mucosa and blood in the stool for 5 months. On the ventrodorsal view during a barium enema examination, a cecocolic intussusception (cecal inversion) is visible as a radiolucent filling defect. Note that the remainder of the large bowel, ileocolic junction (arrow), and distal ileum are normal. The cecocolic intussusception had not been visible on two previous barium upper gastrointestinal tract studies.

nodes (mesenteric, para-aortic, and iliac) commonly alter the position and shape of the large bowel.

It is important to recognize the radiographic differences in appearance for lesions of the large bowel that are intraluminal, intramural, and extramural. These classifications as to site or origin allow differentiation of diseases such as foreign bodies, intussusception, inflammation, and benign or malignant tumors (see Chapter 44). For example, a lesion that is plaquelike is intramural and arises from the mucosal or submucosal tissues. An extramural mass usually causes extrinsic narrowing of the lumen, displacement of the bowel and adjacent viscera, or both. Some dogs appear to have an excess length of colon. Termed redundant colon, this finding seems to be a variant of normal and is not clinically significant.

The normal radiographic opacity of the colon is a variable composite of soft tissue-opaque feces, and gas. Occasionally, small pieces of bone are present. Larger pieces of bone or metallic foreign bodies, such as pins and wire and the like, are usually visible on survey radiographs. The colonic mucosal pattern cannot be evaluated on survey radiographs.

Many large bowel diseases exhibit radiographic changes in the colon that are similar to those that are often present in other parts of the gastrointestinal tract. These changes include foreign bodies; obstruction, including intussusception (Fig. 45–10) and cecal inversion (Fig. 45–11);[4, 6] inflammation (Fig. 45–12); stricture (Fig. 45–13); neoplasms (Fig. 45–14); perforation, adhesions, and diverticuli or hernia (Fig. 45–15). Most of the radiographic findings of these diseases have been discussed elsewhere

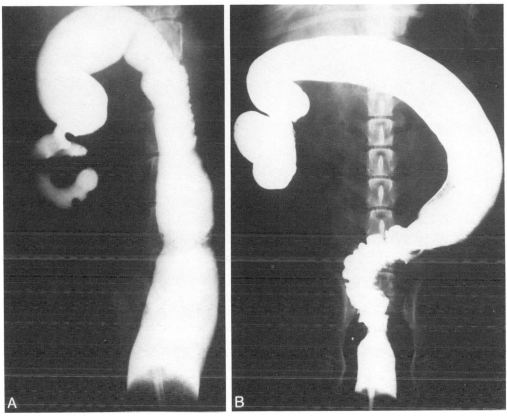

Figure 45–12. Barium enema examination revealed that two dogs were abnormal; one with generalized colitis *(A)* and the other with localized colitis *(B)*. Note the nondistensible descending colon and cecum and shortening of the colon in the more advanced and generalized disease. The localized colitis is characterized by nondistensibility and mucosal irregularity of the distal portion of the descending colon.

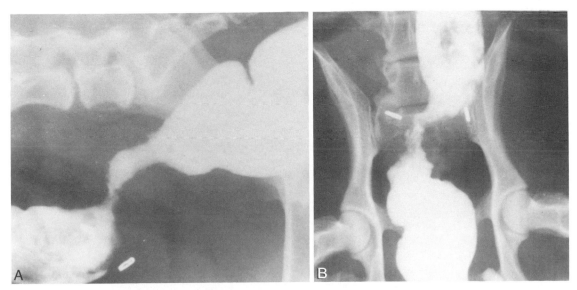

Figure 45–13. An 11-year-old female, spayed miniature Schnauzer had a 3-year history of straining to defecate with occasional soft and bloody stools. Lateral *(A)* and ventrodorsal *(B)* views of the barium enema examination demonstrate an irregular and circumferential narrowing at the junction of the descending colon and rectum. At surgery and biopsy, this narrowing was a benign stricture, presumed secondary to previous ovariohysterectomy (note surgical hemoclips).

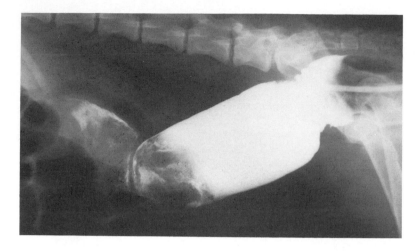

Figure 45–14. A barium enema study in a 6-year-old female German shepherd dog. An intraluminal mass is seen as a polypoid filling defect in the midportion of the descending colon. The mass was lymphoma of the colon.

in this text (Chapters 21, 32, 43, and 44), or are described in an excellent radiographic textbook of the dog and cat abdomen.[8]

In most diseases of the large bowel, particularly those that are not extramural, a contrast study is required for detection and for decision making as to the most probable diagnosis (Fig. 45–15). The radiographic findings (barium enema or double-contrast study) in large bowel disease include irregularity of the barium-mucosal interface, spasm of the bowel lumen, partial or complete occlusion of the bowel lumen, outpouching of the bowel wall due to a hernia, diverticulum, or perforation, and displacement of bowel.

As with the alterations seen on survey radiographs, the contrast study findings are also usually nonspecific. Although spasm and mucosal irregularity are commonly associated with severe local inflammation, other causes include toxicity, psychogenic factors, reflex mechanism, and idiopathic factors. Bowel inflammation (typhlitis and colitis) may have generalized or regional areas of edema, fine shallow ulceration, and increased tonus to bowel. Frequently, the acute stages of bowel inflammation have no abnormal radiographic findings.

A severe form of inflammatory disease in the dog, known as ulcerative colitis, has a spectrum of radiographic findings, which consist of mu-

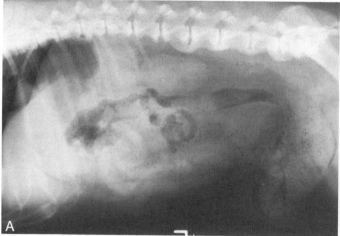

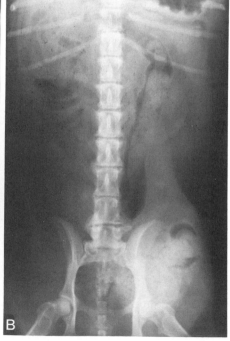

Figure 45–15. A 17-month-old mixed-breed female, spayed dog had a painful abdomen and lethargy after fighting with a larger dog. Survey lateral (A) and ventrodorsal (B) radiographs revealed a localized and dilated feces-filled segment of the descending colon, which represents a partial obstruction within a left inguinal hernia.

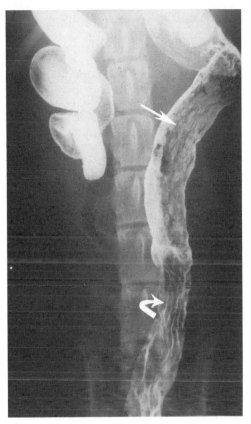

Figure 45–16 Post-evacuation ventrodorsal radiograph of a barium enema. Normal longitudinal mucosal folds of the colon *(curved arrow)* and an abnormal mucosal pattern *(straight arrow)* are visualized. The abnormal area was localized colitis and was not visible on other radiographs obtained with the colon distended with barium.

cosal and submucosal ulcers, spasticity, rigidity, and shortening of the colon (Fig. 45–12).

Narrowing of the large bowel lumen results from spasm or constriction due to neoplasia, scar tissue, or direct trauma to the bowel wall. Unlike constriction, spasm is transient and frequently is secondary to the barium enema tech-nique (Fig. 45–6). When evaluating a constriction with the use of a barium enema examination, the base and length of the defect, the mucosal surface, and mural involvement should be assessed (Fig. 45–13). Most constrictions of the large bowel are produced by neoplasms (usually carcinoma and lymphosarcoma), but benign disease, such as scar tissue, eosinophilic colitis, and ulcerative colitis, can mimic the radiographic findings of a malignant lesion.

References

1. Becker M, Adler L, and Parish JF: Rectal lymphangiography in dogs. Radiology 91:1037, 1968.
2. Brawner WB, and Bartels JE: Contrast radiography of the digestive tract: Indications, techniques, and complications. Vet Clin North Am 13:599, 1983.
3. Gomez JA, et al: Selective abdominal angiography in the dog. J Am Vet Radiol Soc 14:72, 1973.
4. Guffy MM, Wallace L, and Anderson NV: Inversion of the cecum into the colon of a dog. J Am Vet Med Assoc 156:183, 1970.
5. Jakowski RM: Duplication of colon in a labrador retriever with abnormal spinal column. Vet Pathol 14:256, 1977.
6. Kolata RJ, and Wright JH: Inflammation and inversion of the cecum in a cat. J Am Vet Med Assoc 162:958, 1976.
7. Lorenz M: Diseases of the large bowel. In Ettinger SJ (Ed): Textbook of Internal Medicine: Diseases of the Dog and Cat. 2nd Ed. Philadelphia, WB Saunders, 1983.
8. O'Brien TR: Radiographic Diagnosis of Abdominal Disorders in the Dog and Cat. Davis, CA, Covell Park Vet Co, 1981.
9. Rawlings CA, and Capps WF: Rectovaginal fistula and imperforate anus in a dog. J Am Vet Med Assoc 159:320, 1971.
10. Seaman WB, and Walls J: Complications of the barium enema. Gastroenterology 48:728, 1965.
11. Sterns EE, and Vaughan GER: The lymphatics of the dog colon. Cancer 26:218, 1970.
12. Ticer JW: Radiographic Technique in Veterinary Practice. 2nd Ed. Philadelphia, WB Saunders, 1984.
13. Toombs JP, Caywood DD, Lipowitz AJ, et al: Colonic perforation following neurosurgical procedures and corticosteroid therapy in four dogs. J Am Vet Med Assoc 177:68, 1980.

SECTION 9

MISCELLANEOUS

CHAPTER 46

AVIAN RADIOGRAPHY

SYDNEY EVANS

Interest in radiography of pet birds has increased in recent years. Birds are well suited for radiographic studies because their air sacs provide intrinsic contrast. Radiography is an inexpensive, noninvasive procedure of high diagnostic yield that is accessible to most veterinary practitioners. The small size, fragile appearance, and rapid respiratory rate of birds, however, have discouraged veterinarians from the use of radiography in their evaluation. Technically excellent radiographs can be taken with minimal patient stress. In this chapter, the technical aspects of avian radiography are briefly addressed. The reader is referred to other texts for in-depth discussions.[1, 10, 19, 27] The thrust of this chapter is on radiographic interpretation; in particular, the radiographic diagnosis of avian disease. An exhaustive discussion of avian radiographic diagnosis is not possible, but the reader is encouraged to utilize basic radiographic principles that apply to all animal species when interpreting new or unusual radiographic changes.

GROSS AND RADIOGRAPHIC ANATOMY

Several avian organ systems differ markedly from their mammalian counterparts. An excellent table of the significant anatomic differences between mammals and birds is available.[11] The purpose of the subsequent discussion is to emphasize radiographically significant aspects of avian anatomy. The emphasis is toward the budgerigar, but when possible, species variation is noted.

Skeletal System

The characteristic aspects of avian bony anatomy are pneumatic bones and the tendency toward fusion of bony parts (e.g., spine, skull, and some long bones). These features modify the avian skeleton for flight. The pneumatic nature of avian bones is often mistaken for osteoporosis.

Many bones of the avian skull have fused to lend strength and rigidity to the brain case. The skull of most birds, and parrots in particular, is kinetic; e.g., the maxillopalatal complex is articulated, allowing birds to gape. The other unique feature of the avian skull is the presence of scleral ossicles, which form a sclerotic ring around each eye. Retrobulbar mass lesions may cause displacement of the scleral ossicle.[23]

There is considerable fusion and elongation of the avian vertebral column. The only freely moving vertebrae are the cervical and caudal vertebrae. The fused thoracic region is referred to as the notarium. The last thoracic vertebrae and first caudal vertebrae fuse with the lumbosacral region to form a synsacrum. The pygostyle or coccyx represents an embryonic fusion of several caudal vertebrae.

The sternum is variable in shape and size, depending upon the frequency of flight. In flightless birds (ostrich), a keel is lacking; in strong fliers, the keel is deeper than the sternum is broad. The keel is pneumatic and communicates with the intraclavicular air sac.

The pectoral girdle comprises three bones: the scapula, blade-like and parallel to the vertebral column; the coracoid, extending from the sternum; and the clavicles, fused midventrally to form a furuncula (wishbone).

The wing is characterized by a reduction and fusion of distal elements. The humerus is pneumatic. The radius is straight and is narrower than the ulna. The carpus consists of only two bones, the radial and ulnar carpal bones. The remainder of the carpal bones fuse with the metacarpal bones to form the carpometacarpus. In the budgerigar, only three digits remain, the medial and lateral being primarily vestigial.

Because the sternum is long and supports much of the ventrum, the ventral abdominal wall and pubis are poorly developed. In most species, there is no pelvic symphysis. The pelvic limb consists of three major long bones—the femur, tibiotarsus, and tarsometatarsus—and digits I to IV.* The tibiotarsus is the largest hindlimb bone. The tarsometatarsus represents the fusion of the second, third, and fourth metatarsal bones with the tarsus.

Digestive System

The digestive tract consists of the oral cavity, pharynx, esophagus, crop, proventriculus, ventriculus (gizzard), small intestine, cecum, large intestine, and cloaca (Fig. 46–1). The crop is a dilation of the esophagus that is present in gallinaceous birds (those that nest on the ground), parrots, and a few other birds. The crop is primarily left-sided anatomically, but when filled, it may appear bilateral radiographically (Fig. 46–1A).

At the level of the heart base, the esophagus widens into the glandular stomach, the proventriculus (Fig. 46–1D and E). This structure joins the muscular gizzard (ventriculus). Because the gizzard is frequently grit-filled, it is an important radiographic landmark. The normal gizzard is left-sided, with its most cranial border at the level of the acetabulum (Fig. 46–1E). The duodenum and large intestine are not radiographically differentiable without the use of contrast medium. In general, the four

loops of ileum are packed on the right side of the gizzard. The large intestine (rectum) is short and straight, emptying into the cloaca. Ceca are of variable size, depending on species; they are small or absent in pet birds.

The avian liver is small when compared with that of the mammal, and consists of only two lobes. It lies caudal to the heart, and because the diaphragm in birds is incomplete, the liver partially surrounds the cardiac apex. This relationship gives rise to the classic hourglass shape of the heart and liver shadows in the ventrodorsal radiograph (Fig. 46–2B). The spleen is round and is located at midline dorsal to the proventriculus. It cannot always be recognized radiographically.

Respiratory and Cardiovascular Systems

The avian respiratory system is a complex interrelationship between lung and air sacs; the latter communicate with the medullary cavity of some of the bones. The lungs are small and compact, fitting against the dorsum of the thorax (Fig. 46–2A). In simplistic terms, interconnecting tubes, or parabronchi, constitute the lung. The parabronchi are radiographically identifiable as a honeycomb appearance. The air sacs lack blood vessels, are thin walled, and are homogeneously black radiographically. There are four paired and one unpaired air sacs extending from the thoracic inlet to the most caudal aspect of the coelom (Fig. 46–2).* These sacs function as bellows to receive and deliver air through the lungs. The syrinx, or voicebox, is an expansion of tracheal cartilage near the tracheal bifurcation and is peculiar to avian species. In ducks and geese, the syrinx is greatly expanded and resembles an "osseous bulla" radiographically. In most pet birds, however, the syrinx is small and is not radiographically visible as a structure separate from the trachea.

The avian heart is comparatively larger and longer than that of a mammal. It has four chambers and is located at midline, just caudal to the syrinx (Fig. 46–2). The apex is nestled into the lobes of the liver.

Genitourinary Tract

The kidneys are elongated and trilobed as a result of their location in three depressions of the synsacrum (Fig. 46–2A). They extend from the sixth rib caudally to the sacral region. Most

---

*No bird has more than four digits. The ostrich has two, some species have three, and most birds have four digits.

*Birds do not have a complete diaphragm and the body cavity is a coelom. The coelom is divided into thoracic and abdominal areas.

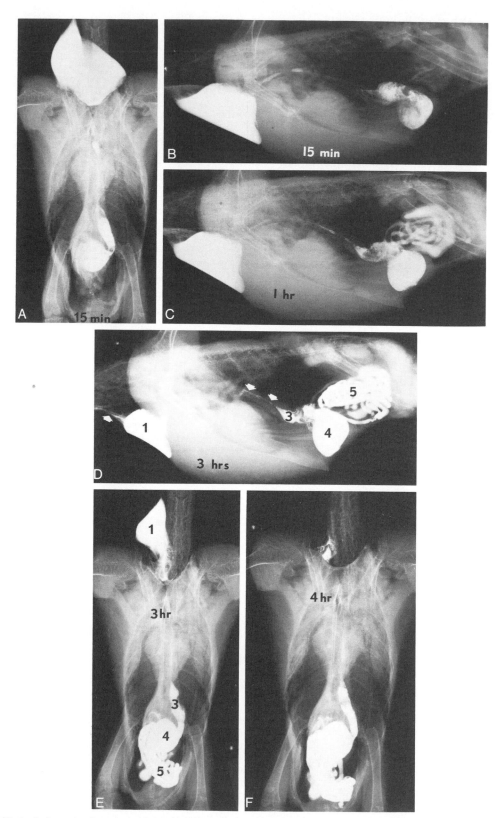

Figure 46–1. *A–F,* ventrodorsal and lateral projections from a gastrointestinal tract examination of an adult Amazon parrot. Only selective radiographs are shown. The 3-hour radiographs are labeled for organ identification. 1: crop; 3: proventriculus; 4: ventriculus (gizzard); 5: intestines; 6: esophagus *(arrows).*

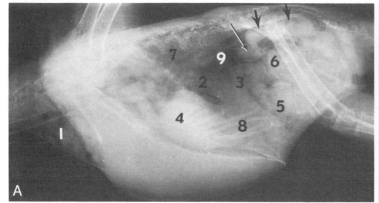

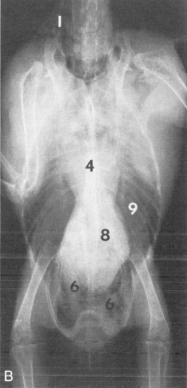

Figure 46–2. Lateral *(A)* and ventrodorsal *(B)* radiographs of a normal 8-year-old male African grey parrot. 1: crop; 2: distal esophagus; 3: proventriculus; 4: heart; 5: area of gizzard; 6: area of intestines; 7: lung; 8: liver; 9: air sac; 10: kidney *(black arrows)*; 11: gonad *(black and white arrow)*.

birds do not have a urinary bladder and the ureters enter the cloaca.

The gonads and adrenals are located at the cranial tip of the kidneys (Fig. 46–2A). The testes are paired and are not normally visible radiographically. They may enlarge in some species during the breeding cycle. Extreme physiologic enlargement of the testes is not usually seen in the male budgerigar. The left ovary is unpaired and is not seen radiographically unless it is diseased or undergoes physiologic enlargement. The left oviduct and uterus (shell gland) are not visible unless an egg or disease process is present.

RADIOGRAPHIC TECHNIQUE

Handling and Positioning. For details of handling and positioning, the reader is referred to the reference list.[10, 14, 19, 27, 28] Only certain important points are subsequently reviewed.

It is an exceptional circumstance for which sedation or anesthesia is necessary to take excellent quality, well-positioned avian radiographs. Many methods and apparatus for physical restraint are available, and their use is dictated by available help, state radioprotection laws, and personal preference. The author has been most successful when one or two persons restrain the patient. Tape* may be used for the wings. Care should be taken that personnel are properly protected against radiation exposure.

Excellent positioning is of paramount importance. A minor degree of rotation in these small patients can obscure abnormalities or mimic displacement of viscera. The keel and vertebrae are superimposed in a satisfactorily positioned ventrodorsal radiograph (Fig. 46–2B). The legs and wings are extended away from the body to preclude superimposition of extremity musculature over the coelom. The right and left acetabulae and scapulohumeral joints are superimposed in a symmetric lateral radiograph (Fig. 46–2A).

As in mammals, the respiratory phase affects the radiographic appearance of the organs. The air sacs, wings, heart, and liver can vary in size and radiopacity with respiration. This factor is difficult to control in birds, and must be taken into account during interpretation.

Film Screen Combinations and Technical Factors. There are many film screen combinations and radiographic techniques that are available for avian radiography; several are listed in Table 46–1). For additional technical factors,

---

*Dermicel paper first aid tape, Johnson & Johnson, New Brunswick, NY 08103.

TABLE 46–1. **TECHNIQUES FOR AVIAN RADIOGRAPHY**

Screen	Film	Body Part	mAs	kVp	Other
Par speed[1]*	Par speed[2]†	Whole body	5.0	42 = lateral 50 = ventrodorsal (parakeet)	— —
Par speed*	Par speed[2]‡	Extremity	5.0	42	—
High detail‡	Par speed[2]†	Whole body	6.7	40 kVp for first 2 cm. Add 2 kVp for each additional 1 cm	36-in film-tube distance. Remove filter.
High detail§ (rare earth)	Single emulsion[5]‖	Whole body	6.7	< 40 gr: 48–52 40–60 gr: 53–56 > 60 gr: 56–64	36-in film-tube distance. Remove filter.

*Dupont par speed screens.
†Kodak XRP-1 par speed film.
‡Kodak X-omatic fine intensifying screen in X-omatic cassette.
§Kodak Lanex fine screen in Kodak X-omatic cassette (extremity system).
‖Kodak NMB-1 film.

the reader is referred to the reference list.[1, 10, 14, 19, 27]

SPECIAL PROCEDURES

The most commonly performed special procedure is the upper gastrointestinal tract examination (Fig. 46–1). The indications for such a study include diarrhea, regurgitation, vomition, abnormal palpation, as well as use of positive-contrast medium to determine organ location.[15]

Barium is always administered via a stomach tube. The dose of barium administered depends on patient size, from 0.5 ml for a canary to 15 ml for large parrots. Ventrodorsal and lateral radiographs are taken at 0 and then 30 minutes, 60 minutes, 2 hours, and 4 hours later. In normal studies, the crop is filled immediately; the proventriculus and gizzard are filled after 30 minutes (Fig. 46–1A-C). After 1 hour, barium has filled the small intestine (Fig. 46–1C). By 2 to 4 hours, the crop should be completely empty (Fig. 46–1F) although varying amounts of barium may remain in the proventriculus, gizzard, small and large intestine, and cloaca. If indicated, a radiograph may be taken at 24 hours.

Excretory Urography. Avian urography has been described.[16] A dose of 1.5 mg iodine per gram of body weight of water-soluble iodinated contrast medium (sodium diatrozoate) is injected into the brachial vein while the bird is immobilized with chemical or mechanical restraint. Radiographs are taken at 10 seconds, 60 seconds, and 2 minutes and the contrast medium is excreted within 5 to 7 minutes. The kidneys, ureters, and cloaca can be visualized in a normal study. Other special studies, such as celiography (positive-contrast peritoneography), have been described.[14]

BODY SYSTEMS, DISEASES, AND RADIOGRAPHIC DIFFERENTIAL DIAGNOSES

Musculoskeletal System

The most common musculoskeletal abnormalities are fractures. Fracture types and diagnoses

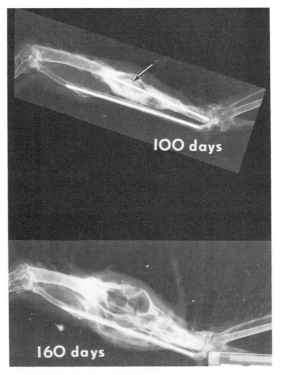

Figure 46–3. Follow-up radiographs of a simple transverse fracture of the radius and ulna. At 100 days after fracture, a sequestrum is present (arrow). The sequestrum and the pin were removed and further expansion of the cavity occurred by 160 days. At that time, extensive purulent material was removed by curettage.

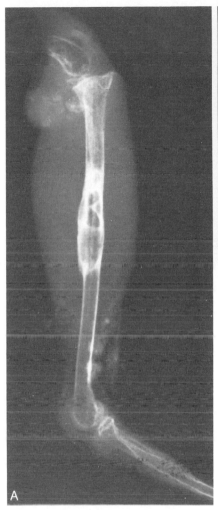
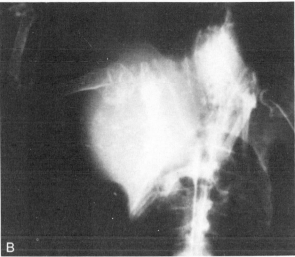

Figure 46–4. *A*, post-mortem radiograph of the tibiotarsus of a duck. The nonaggressive midshaft lesion was confirmed to be avian tuberculosis. *B*, the scapula of a parakeet in which a highly aggressive bony lesion can be seen. A neoplasm was confirmed by aspirate analysis.

are similar to those in mammals, as is fracture healing when viewed radiographically.[7, 20] Local sequestration, however, may be more common in birds than in mammals (Fig. 46–3). Because some of the medullary cavities and air sacs communicate, air sac infection may be a complication of open fractures.

Bony neoplasms[13, 22] and infections[2, 18] have been reported in birds. There are no controlled studies as to whether avian bone responds to disease in a manner similar to that of mammals. It is the author's experience, however, that criteria for aggressive (Fig. 46–4*B*) and nonaggressive (Fig. 46–4*A*) bone lesions can be applied to the bird (see Chapter 2).

Because some avian bones are pneumatic, it is easy to mistake their apparent decreased radiopacity for osteoporosis. True osteoporosis is characterized by decreased contrast between bone cortex and soft tissue. Pathologic fractures are common in birds fed an improper diet.[24]

Bony hyperostoses and increased medullary radiopacity have been described in female budgerigars with disturbances of estrogen production.[26] Heavy egg layers on simple seed diets are likely to exhibit skeletal changes associated with massive calcium utilization in producing egg shell. A number of these patients also have some body wall herniation (Fig. 46–5).

Digestive System

Abnormalities of the gastrointestinal tract are frequently the basis for avian whole body radiographs. The liver is best evaluated on the ventrodorsal radiograph, in which it normally forms an hourglass shape with the heart. The relative size of the "waist" of the hourglass depends upon the avian species and body condition (Fig. 46–6). Hepatomegaly of any etiology can cause changes in this shadow. Differential diagnosis of hepatomegaly includes lipid hepatopathy, neoplastic invasion, hepatitis, and infection. It should be noted that a large intra-abdominal mass may mimic hepatomegaly. As well, poor positioning, e.g., legs not fully ex-

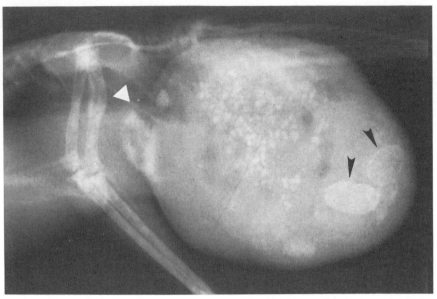

Figure 46–5. Lateral radiograph of a female parakeet. A large body wall hernia contains bowel, gastrointestinal content, and collapsed calcified eggs *(black arrowheads)*. There is increased medullary radiopacity in the long bones, referred to as polyostotic hyperostosis. The combination of polyostotic hyperostosis and body wall hernias in obese female parakeets is due to hyperestrogenism. A healed fracture of one femur is also seen *(white arrowhead)*.

tended, may cause the appearance of hepatomegaly.

The spleen is best seen in the lateral radiograph as a round, well-circumscribed opacity

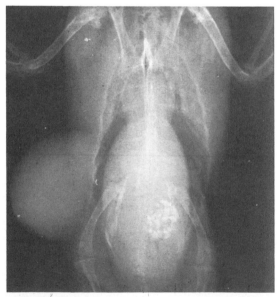

Figure 46–6. An obese female parakeet was examined for a mass on the right body wall. At surgery, the mass was found to be a lipoma. Loss of the normal cardiohepatic hourglass shape and caudal gizzard displacement can be seen. Hepatomegaly due to lipid deposition was suspected; the hepatomegaly resolved with treatment.

dorsal to the proventriculus. It is only seen well in medium to large-sized birds. Splenic tumors and infectious splenic enlargement often occur. Splenic tumors may appear as irregular coelomic masses and may cause organ displacement. Smooth and generalized splenic enlargement is usually associated with a systemic infection, such as Chlamydia psittaci (psittacosis) or tuberculosis[21] (Fig. 46–7).

Radiographic changes in the tubular gastrointestinal tract are similar to those in mammals and the same tenets of diagnosis should be applied (see Chapter 44). The avian gastrointestinal tract rarely contains air and its presence should signal aerophagia or disease of the intestine itself.

Disease of the esophagus is best identified in the lateral radiograph. Air in the esophagus may be caused by aerophagia or obstruction. The crop, a diverticulum of the esophagus, may become impacted[6] or inflamed, and clinical signs of regurgitation occur (Fig. 46–8). A small amount of barium, air, or a combination should be given to evaluate the crop. It may be necessary to lavage the crop first so that food materials are not misinterpreted as mucosal abnormalities.

The most common abnormalities of the proventriculus and ventriculus are impactions, although inflammation due to parasites, yeast, and bacteria have been reported.[17] Intussusception, although rare, has been diagnosed post mortem in a budgerigar and a parrot.[3]

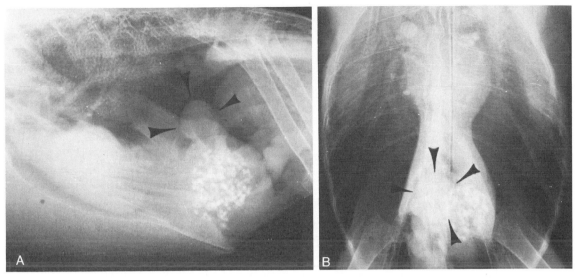

Figure 46–7. *A* and *B*, radiographs of a 2-year-old male macaw. A well-circumscribed, round shaft-tissue mass dorsal to the gizzard on the midline *(arrowheads)* is an enlarged spleen. An elevated titer to *Chlamydia psittaci* (psitticosis) was confirmed.

Changes in the intestine are interpreted as they are in mammals (see Chapter 44). Paralytic obstruction associated with systemic disease can occur (Fig. 46–9), as does mechanical obstruction due to intra- or extraluminal disease (Fig. 46–10). Enteritis is common in all pet bird species and has been reported in association with systemic infection, bowel infection, lead poisoning, viral infections, and parasites (Fig. 46–11).

Figure 46–8. An adult male cockatoo. Lateral radiograph *(A)* reveals a large soft-tissue mass *(arrows)* at the thoracic area inlet. A technetium pertechnetate thyroid scan *(B)* was performed on a normal dove (left) and on the patient (right). Note the bilateral enlargement of the patient's thyroid and the lack of background activity. The patient–pinhole collimator distance was approximately equal in both scans. (Courtesy of Dr. Jeff Wortman, University of Pennsylvania.)

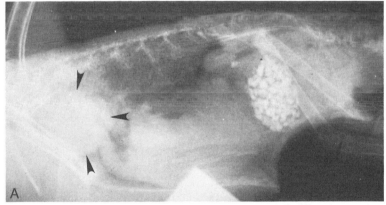

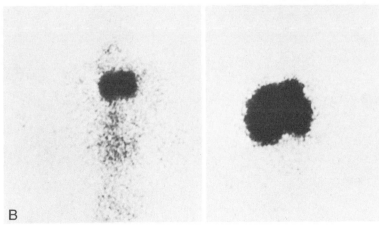

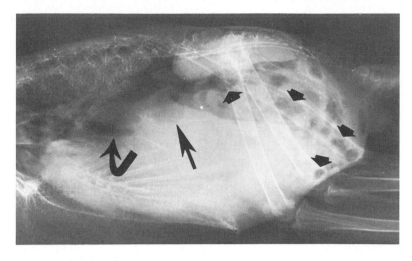

Figure 46–9. A 3-year-old Amazon parrot. The esophagus *(curved arrow)*, proventriculus *(large arrow)*, and multiple loops of small bowel *(small arrows)* contain air. Diagnosis: paralytic ileus secondary to generalized systemic bacterial infection.

Diseases of the intracoelomic space, like the peritoneal cavity in mammals, may cause radiographic changes. The tenets of diagnosis and list of differentials are identical to those in mammals. In addition, peritonitis due to escape of egg yolk material is a comparatively common condition in caged birds. Ascitic fluid in the coelomic spaces has been seen in several mynah birds associated with iron-storage hepatopathy.[25] Ascites due to hepatic neoplasms, hepatitis, and nephritis have also been reported.

Genitourinary Tract

Abnormalities of the genitourinary tract are common, especially in budgerigars. Although avian intravenous urography has been described,[16] the genitourinary tract is usually evaluated on survey radiographs.

Most reports of urinary tract disease detail post-mortem changes. Knowledge of the clinical signs associated with avian urinary tract disease is scant. Acute and chronic renal inflammation, renal tumors, cysts and parasitic invasion, and uric acid deposition have been described.[12] Changes in size associated with renal masses (cysts, tumors, and parasites) and radiopacity (calcifications) have personally been seen. Renal masses or generalized enlargement are best seen in the lateral radiograph and must be differentiated from pathologic or physiologic gonadal enlargement. Occasionally, renal abnormalities (nephritis) are associated with ascites and a specific mass cannot be demonstrated. In patients in which the gizzard is grit-filled, caudal and ventral displacement may be identified.

Physiologic gonadal enlargement must be dif-

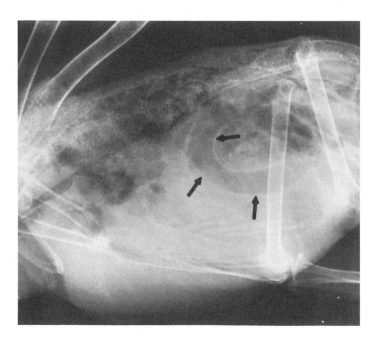

Figure 46–10. An adult cockatoo. A single, severely gas-distended loop of small bowel can be seen *(arrows)*. Post mortem, adhesions of the small bowel to the liver were present, resulting in a mechanical bowel obstruction.

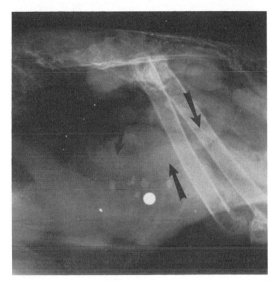

Figure 46–11. A 3-year-old cockatoo. There is a metallic foreign body within the gizzard. Fluid distension of bowel (enteritis) is also present *(arrows)*. Blood lead levels were elevated.

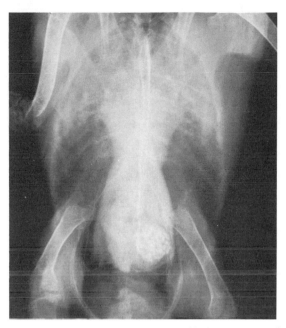

Figure 46–12. A 3-year-old parrot with acute onset of dyspnea. There is an abnormal, increased radiopacity of the air sacs, especially when these structures are compared to the surrounding air. Extensive hemorrhage of the air sacs and lung was diagnosed post mortem.

ferentiated from pathologic processes (usually by behavioral means). Mass enlargement (neoplasia and cysts) of the testes and ovary are common in psittacine birds, particularly budgerigars. Masses in this area, as with the kidney, cause ventral and usually caudal displacement of the gizzard. This displacement is variable, however, and ovarian masses have been seen to displace the gizzard cranially or caudally. Abnormalities of the oviduct are less common, with the exception of egg binding. Chronic oviduct impaction, oviduct prolapse, and oviduct rupture resulting in yolk peritonitis have been described.[9] The former two conditions result in midcoelomic masses and organ displacement, the latter condition in loss of coelomic detail.

Respiratory and Cardiovascular Systems

Changes in the avian lower respiratory tract are difficult to identify unless they are gross or asymmetric. Inspiratory-expiratory variation makes subtle increased air sac radiopacity difficult to identify.

Air sacculitis, either inflammatory, nutritional (hypovitaminosis A), or parasitic all result in a homogeneous increased air sac radiopacity. One guideline to identify increased sac radiopacity is to compare the opacity of the air sacs with that of the surrounding air; they should be quite close (Fig. 46–12). Mycotic air sac infections result in patchy increases in radiopacity (Fig. 46–13).

The lungs should resemble a honeycomb on the lateral radiograph. This pattern results from

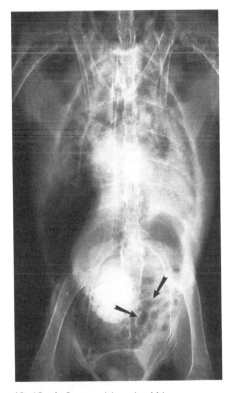

Figure 46–13. A 2-year-old male African grey parrot. There is extensive radiopacity that involves the right thoracic air sac and lung. A silhouette sign with the heart is evident. The intestines contain a large amount of air *(arrows)*, probably due to aerophagia. Bacterial air sacculitis and pneumonia were found post mortem.

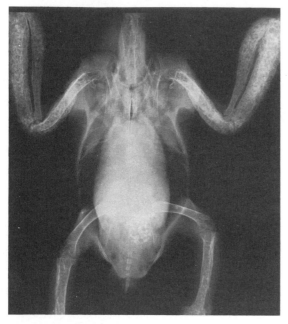

Figure 46–14. A 3-year-old Amazon parrot. The normal cardiohepatic hourglass shape is absent. There is an extensive lacy periosteal proliferative change that involves the diaphyses of most of the long bones. Post mortem, extensive pericardial effusion was present. The bony changes are hypertrophic osteopathy.

the masses of parabronchi seen end on. Lung masses may result from infection,[21] edema, and metabolic abnormalities. Neoplastic lung masses are rare in birds in contrast to mammals. End-on views of large pulmonary vessels, however, may mimic the interstitial neoplastic masses commonly seen in mammals.

Although abnormalities of the upper respiratory tract are frequently noted in birds, radiography is often not helpful because of the intricate detail and small size of the avian skull.

Congestive heart failure is rare, but has been reported in a mynah bird and a Pukeko. Cardiac enlargement[4, 9] results in loss of the normal cardiohepatic hourglass shape (Fig. 46–14). Other cardiovascular abnormalities reported in birds are atherosclerosis, pericarditis, myocarditis, parasitism, and neoplasia.[8, 29] Although the author has not radiographed these conditions, it is expected that the changes mimic those seen in mammalian hearts.

References

1. Altman RB: Radiography. Vet Clin North Am [Small Anim Pract] 3:165, 1973.
2. Altman RB: Disorders of the skeletal system. In Petrak ML (Ed): Diseases of Cage and Aviary Birds. Philadelphia, Lea & Febiger, 1982.
3. Beach JE: Diseases of budgerigars and other caged birds. A survey of post mortem findings. Vet Rec 74:10, 1962.
4. Beehler BA, Montali RJ, and Bush M: Mitral valve insufficiency with congestive heart failure in a Pukeko. J Am Vet Med Assoc 177:934, 1980.
5. Blackmore DK: Diseases of the reproductive system. In Petrak ML (Ed): Diseases of Cage and Aviary Birds. Philadelphia, Lea & Febiger, 1982.
6. Bowen S: What is your diagnosis? J Am Vet Med Assoc 173:1258, 1978.
7. Bush M, Montali RJ, Novak GR, and Everett A Jr: The healing of avian fractures. A histological xeroradiographic study. J Am Anim Hosp Assoc 12:768, 1976.
8. Cooper JE, and Pomerance A: Cardiac lesions in birds of prey. J Comp Pathol 92:161, 1982.
9. Ensley PK, Hatkin J, and Silverman S: Congestive heart failure in a greater mynah. J Am Vet Med Assoc 175:1010, 1979.
10. Evans SM: Avian radiographic diagnosis. Comp Contin Ed Pract Vet 3:7, 1981.
11. Evans JE: Anatomy of the budgerigar. In Petrak ML (Ed): Diseases of Cage and Aviary Birds. Philadelphia, Lea & Febiger, 1982.
12. Hasholt J, and Petrak ML: Diseases of the urinary tract. In Petrak ML (Ed): Diseases of Cage and Aviary Birds. Philadelphia, Lea & Febiger, 1982.
13. Liu S, Dolenszk EP, and Tappe JP: Osteosarcoma with multiple metastases in a Panama boat-billed heron. J Am Vet Med Assoc 181:1396, 1982.
14. McMillan MC: Avian radiology. In Petrak ML (Ed): Diseases of Cage and Aviary Birds. Philadelphia, Lea & Febiger, 1982.
15. McMillan MC: Avian gastrointestinal radiography. Comp Contin Ed Pract Vet 5:273, 1983.
16. McNeel SV, and Zenoble RD: Avian urography. J Am Vet Med Assoc 178:366, 1981.
17. Minsky L, and Petrak ML: Diseases of the digestive system. In Petrak ML (Ed): Diseases of Cage and Aviary Birds. Philadelphia, Lea & Febiger, 1982.
18. Montali RJ, Bush M, Thoen CO, and Smith E: Tuberculosis in captive exotic birds. J Am Vet Med Assoc 169:920, 1967.
19. Morgan JP, and Silverman S: Techniques of Veterinary Radiography. Davis, CA, Veterinary Radiology Associates, 1982, pp. 241–244.
20. Newton CD, and Zeitlin S: Avian fracture healing. J Am Vet Med Assoc 170:620, 1977.
21. Peavey GM, Silverman S, Howard EB, Cooper RS, et al: Pulmonary tuberculosis in a sulfur crested cockatoo. J Am Vet Med Assoc 169:915, 1976.
22. Petrak ML, and Gilmore CE: Neoplasms. In Petrak ML (Ed): Diseases of Cage and Aviary Birds. Philadelphia, Lea & Febiger, 1982.
23. Rambow VJ, Murphy JC, and Fox JG: Malignant lymphoma in a pigeon. J Am Vet Med Assoc 179:1266, 1981.
24. Randell MG: Nutritionally induced hypocalcemic tetany in an Amazon parrot. J Am Vet Med Assoc 179:1277, 1981.
25. Randell MG, Patnaik AK, and Gould J: Hepatopathy associated with excessive iron storage in mynah birds. J Am Vet Med Assoc 179:1214, 1981.
26. Schlumberger HG: Polyostotic hyperostosis in the female parakeet. Am J Pathol 35:1, 1959.
27. Silverman S: Avian radiographic technique and interpretation. In Kirk RW (Ed): Current veterinary therapy V. Philadelphia, WB Saunders, 1974.
28. Stone RM: Clinical examination and methods of treatment. In Petrak ML (Ed): Diseases of Cage and Aviary Birds. Philadelphia, Lea & Febiger, 1982.
29. T-W-Fiennes RN: Diseases of the cardiovascular system, blood and lymphatic system. In Petrak ML (Ed): Diseases of Cage and Aviary Birds. Philadelphia, Lea & Febiger, 1982.

CHAPTER 47

ALTERNATE IMAGING

JEFFREY A. WORTMAN
NORMAN W. RANTANEN

There has been a virtual explosion in imaging technology as a result of the ongoing search for better, safer, and noninvasive diagnostic procedures. Conventional radiographic imaging has been improved by rare-earth intensifying screen and film technology. Nuclear medicine imaging, ultrasound, and computer-based imaging procedures, such as x-ray computed tomography (X-CT) and magnetic resonance imaging (MRI) have been developed and refined. In general, the incorporation of these newer imaging methods into veterinary medicine has been slow, due in part to the high costs of purchasing and maintaining the necessary equipment and facilities and the economics of veterinary practice. These imaging procedures are in greater use in veterinary medicine, however, as equipment costs decrease, used equipment becomes available, and there is access to human clinical or research facilities. These alternative imaging methods are available at many veterinary teaching institutions.

This chapter is a discussion of the principles of some of these imaging technologies with examples of applications in veterinary medicine. Of necessity, these imaging methods are discussed briefly; there are, however, many texts devoted to detailing their clinical applications.

X-RAY COMPUTED TOMOGRAPHY (X-CT)

In 1972, at the Annual Congress of the British Institute of Radiology, Godfrey Hounsfield introduced computed tomography to the medical community with the EMI Mark I brain scanner. He called this revolutionary new imaging technique computerized axial transverse scanning. There have since been many names for this imaging technique, the most commonly used names or acronyms being computed or computerized tomography (CT) and computerized axial tomography (CAT). Since the advent of another computer-reconstructed imaging method, magnetic resonance imaging (MRI), x-ray CT (X-CT) is now used for added specificity.

In conventional radiography, the x-ray film records the results of an x-ray beam passing through a patient. In X-CT, an axial or cross-sectional image is reconstructed by computer analysis of transmitted x-ray intensity recorded by sensitive detectors. The resultant picture is called an image or slice.

The original EMI scanner was designed specifically for the head. It was capable of producing a pair of cross-sectional images after a 4 to 5-minute scan time. Significant technical improvements have occurred such that newer equipment can produce higher resolution im-

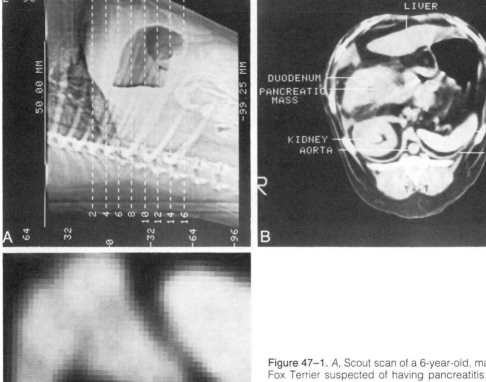

Figure 47–1. *A*, Scout scan of a 6-year-old, male Wire-haired Fox Terrier suspected of having pancreatitis. The dog was in dorsal recumbency. Locations of alternate transverse slices are indicated by dashed lines and slice numbers. Barium is in the colon from an upper gastrointestinal tract study performed the previous day. *B*, Slice 14 demonstrates a poorly delineated mass adjacent to the descending duodenum that was thought to represent inflammatory reaction of pancreatitis. *C*, a magnified portion of slice 14 that includes the aorta, diaphragm, and a portion of the spleen demonstrates the concept of the digital matrix of the image. The shade of each square block (pixel) is determined by the x-ray attenuation (CT number) of the tissue volume (voxel) represented by the square. The dog was clinically normal after a 2-week course of symptomatic treatment for pancreatitis.

ages in seconds. These extremely short scan times now permit the imaging of virtually all organs without deleterious image degradation from motion.

With the exception of infants, human patients rarely require sedation for X-CT studies. Dogs and cats, however, usually require heavy sedation or anesthesia to prevent patient motion during the study. The animal is usually placed in dorsal or ventral recumbency on a movable table, and the body part of interest is carefully positioned and centered to the x-ray tube and detector housing (gantry) by using external laser alignment lights. An initial image, called a scout scan (Fig. 47–1A), which appears similar to a survey radiographic image, is obtained by moving the patient through the gantry while the x-ray tube and detectors remain stationary. The scout view is used to verify correct patient positioning, as a guide to the operator to determine the number and location of subsequent slices that are to be obtained, and in interpretation to assess slice location.

During the studies, sequential slices through the area of interest are obtained. For each slice, the x-ray tube emits a finely collimated x-ray beam in multiple exposures, e.g., 300 to 600, as it rotates around the patient. The intensity of the x-ray beam emerging from the patient is quantitated by an array of detectors that, depending on equipment design, either can be stationary around the circumference of the rotation ring or can rotate in conjunction with the x-ray tube. This information passes from the

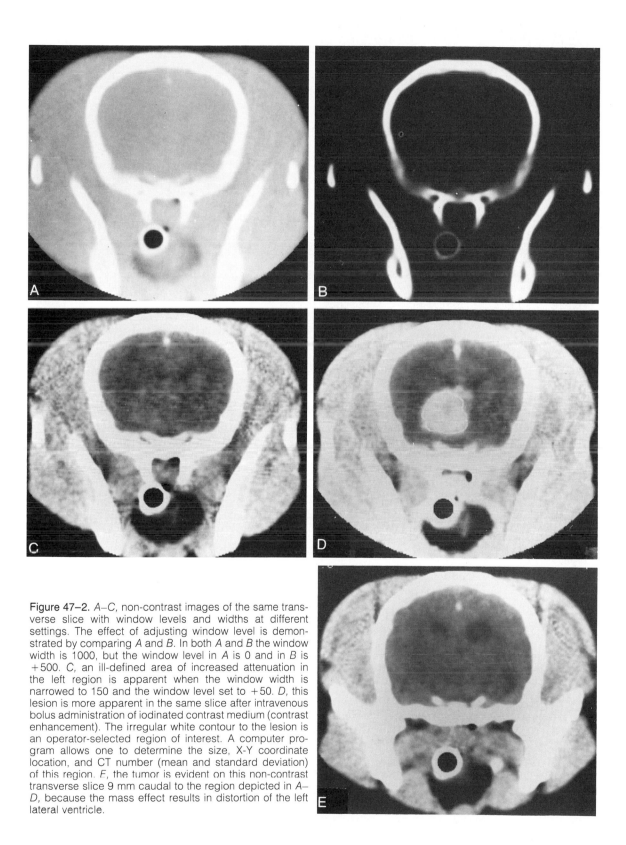

Figure 47–2. *A–C,* non-contrast images of the same transverse slice with window levels and widths at different settings. The effect of adjusting window level is demonstrated by comparing *A* and *B.* In both *A* and *B* the window width is 1000, but the window level in *A* is 0 and in *B* is +500. *C,* an ill-defined area of increased attenuation in the left region is apparent when the window width is narrowed to 150 and the window level set to +50. *D,* this lesion is more apparent in the same slice after intravenous bolus administration of iodinated contrast medium (contrast enhancement). The irregular white contour to the lesion is an operator-selected region of interest. A computer program allows one to determine the size, X-Y coordinate location, and CT number (mean and standard deviation) of this region. *F,* the tumor is evident on this non-contrast transverse slice 9 mm caudal to the region depicted in *A–D,* because the mass effect results in distortion of the left lateral ventricle.

data acquisition system to the computer, which evaluates, computes, and reconstructs the results into a picture displayed on a television screen (Fig. 47–1B). The cross-sectional image of the body part is displayed in a digital matrix, which is divided into tiny two-dimensional square blocks called pixels (picture elements), with each block assigned a CT number proportional to the degree that the volume represented by that block, called a voxel (volume element), attenuated the x-ray beam (Fig. 47–1C). The original EMI scanner used an 80 × 80 matrix (6400 pixels), which is a relatively coarse matrix size when compared with the 160 × 160 (25,600 pixels) or 320 × 320 (102,400 pixels) matrices of newer generation equipment. The scale of CT numbers is arbitrary, but it commonly ranges from minus 1000 (for air) to plus 1000 (for compact bone). In this scale, fat has a CT number of about minus 50 and soft tissues about plus 35. The gray scale on an X-CT scan is similar to conventional radiographs in that tissue physical density and atomic number are directly proportional to opacity (whiteness).

With conventional radiography, one cannot usually perceive visible differences between tissues with only slight differing physical properties. One of the real strengths of X-CT is the capability of adjusting the contrast on the gray scale image to show slight differences in x-ray attenuation, even as small a percentage as 0.5; it is customary to view X-CT images at extremely high contrast when compared with conventional radiographs, which makes these relatively small differences visible. There are two basic adjustments that affect the appearance of the image, a brightness and a contrast control. Adjustment in the brightness control, usually called the window level, determines the CT number that will be the mid-gray level of the image (Fig. 47–2A and B). Adjustment of the contrast control, usually called the window width, determines the range of CT numbers that will be shown from black to white in the image (Fig. 47–2A and C). For example, the CT numbers for intracranial soft tissues range from approximately plus 5 for cerebrospinal fluid to plus 25 for gray matter. Therefore, there is a difference of 20 CT numbers between the least dense and the most dense of the intracranial tissues. If a narrow window width, e.g., 150, is selected at a window level of plus 50, any structure with a CT number of minus 25 or lower would be black and any structure with a CT number of plus 125 or greater would be white. All structures with CT numbers in between minus 25 and plus 125 would be displayed in the gray scale of the image. The difference between the least dense and most

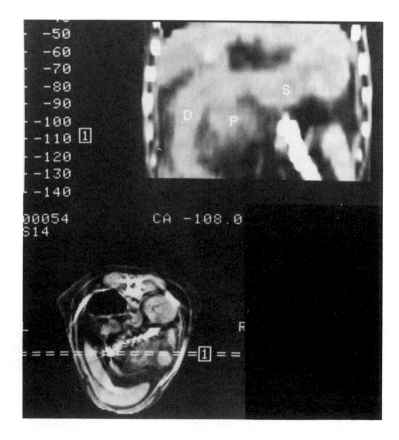

Figure 47–3. At lower left is a transverse slice of the same dog as in Figure 47–1 but in ventral recumbency. The upper midportion of the figure is a computer-reformatted image in the dorsal plane indicated by dashed lines on the transverse image. S: stomach; D: descending duodenum; P: pancreatic mass. Barium is seen in the descending colon.

dense intracranial tissue in this example is about 13 percent of the full scale (20/150), which results in sufficient difference to be seen (Fig. 47–2C).

In addition to viewing X-CT images at relatively high contrast settings at the appropriate window level, contrast agents are also often utilized to improve image contrast. Intravenously administered urographic agents are commonly used to identify vasculature or to demonstrate differences between normal and diseased tissue blood supply. For example, many brain tumors have a higher CT number after intravenous administration of contrast medium (contrast enhancement) than without contrast medium (Fig. 47–2C and D). This difference is due to increased vascularity, increased capillary permeability from disruption of the blood brain barrier, or both. Orally adminis-

tered organic iodides or barium sulfate are sometimes used to identify bowel loops in abdominal X-CT studies. Subarachnoid injections of metrizamide are used in X-CT studies of spinal disease to delineate the spinal cord and subarachnoid space. Some lesions are recognized by disruption of normal anatomy (mass effect) (Fig. 47–2E).

Another diagnostic advantage of X-CT technology is the ability to reformat the study images into a new plane of interest, e.g., to reconstruct data from a transverse scan into dorsal-plane images (Fig. 47–3). Computer software programs also enable the operator to measure distances or to outline a region of interest and then to determine its mean CT number, size, and location in the X, Y, Z coordinate system (Fig. 47–2D).

MAGNETIC RESONANCE IMAGING (MRI)

MRI is one of the newest diagnostic imaging techniques. Preliminary results with prototype equipment suggest that MRI will have a significant impact on medical imaging. The MRI technique is based on the physical effect of nuclear magnetic resonance discovered independently by Bloch and Purcell in 1946. As with X-CT images, MRI images are computer

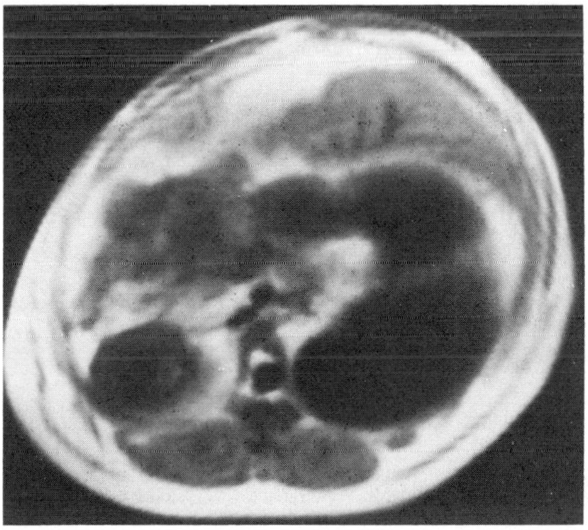

Figure 47–4. Magnetic resonance image. This axial slice is of the same dog as in Figures 47–1 and 47–3, at a similar plane to that displayed in Figures 47–1B or 47–3. Bone and flowing blood in the major vessels produce a low-intensity signal and are therefore black. Fat produces a high-intensity signal and is white. The pancreatitic mass is again an ill-defined region ventral and medial to the right kidney, and medial and adjacent to the descending duodenum. (Compare with Fig. 47–1B.)

reconstructed in a digital matrix and are reproduced as gray tones or color gradations (Fig. 47–4).

A major advantage of MRI is the absence of ionizing radiation. The basis of imaging is a strong magnetic field on the order of hundreds to thousands of times the strength of the earth's magnetic field, and a finely tuned radiofrequency transmitter and receiver. Nuclei with an odd number of particles, protons, neutrons, or both, possess angular momentum and behave like magnets spinning in random directions. When the patient is placed in the magnetic field, these nuclei with angular momentum (hydrogen nuclei being of particular interest) tend to align in the direction of the magnetic field. Finely tuned radiofrequency pulses in a precise sequence are used to disturb the nuclear alignment. The protons absorb energy from the radiofrequency waves, change the direction of their spins, and align themselves against the magnetic field. The absorbed energy is quickly radiated away as electromagnetic energy of the same frequency as the radiofrequency source, and protons tend to realign their spins with the external magnetic field in between radiofrequency pulses. This signal is picked up by a radiofrequency coil (antenna) and is then analyzed and processed by a computer to reconstruct the image. The MRI signal intensity is a synthesis of the hydrogen concentration (proton density), the T_1 (longitudinal or spin lattice) and T_2 (transverse or spin-spin) relaxation times of the tissue, and blood movement. The relative weight of these components in the signal is dependent on the pulsing sequence used.

The T_1 and T_2 relaxation times play an important role in providing contrast between different soft tissues. The T_1 and T_2 times can vary over a range of 500 percent, whereas the hydrogen content of most soft tissue varies over a range of approximately 20 percent. Dramatically different images of the same tissue slice can be obtained depending on the imaging method and pulsing sequence selected. Data are now being accumulated to determine optimal imaging methods and pulsing sequences for various body parts and disease states.

MRI equipment is only now commercially available. The equipment is expensive, in the range of 1 to 2 million dollars. The impact on veterinary medicine will therefore be through access to the equipment in human facilities.

NUCLEAR MEDICINE IMAGING

Nuclear medicine imaging (scintigraphy) involves the administration of a radiopharmaceutical followed by immediate or delayed imaging of the distribution of the radioactivity as it is present within the body. The basis for imaging then is the differential localization of the radiopharmaceutical among or within various tissues and organs, as well as differences between healthy and diseased tissues. Radiopharmaceutical distribution can be categorized into several underlying physiologic mechanisms (Table 47–1). Most of the radiopharmaceuticals and studies tend to be organ-specific rather than disease-specific. Radiopharmaceuticals have been developed to evaluate many organs and tissues satisfactorily.

Two important considerations for a radiopharmaceutical are the radioactive properties, which relate primarily to the radionuclide used, and the distribution properties, which relate to its chemical form. Because of its nearly ideal radionuclidic properties, technetium 99m (^{99m}Tc) is the radionuclide incorporated into most of the radiopharmaceuticals suitable for clinical use in veterinary medicine. ^{99m}Tc is a transitional metal with chemical properties that allow it to be incorporated into a variety of drugs with different localizing properties suitable to image most of the major organ systems (Table 47–1). ^{99m}Tc has a 6-hour half-life and decays with almost 100 percent gamma ray emission of 140 keV energy. Much of the radiation hazard to personnel, patient, and environment is minimized by these properties. General precautions are similar to those required for handling an infectious animal or agent. Radioactive waste is held for decay and is then disposed of as ordinary waste. ^{99m}Tc is the decay product of molybdenum 99, a common by-product of nuclear reactors. A shielded source of molybdenum 99 (technetium generator) can be purchased each week, which will provide the daily clinical needs for ^{99m}Tc.

The imaging system most commonly used is known as a gamma camera. It consists of a stationary detector that contains a single 11 to 16-in diameter sodium iodide crystal that is activated with thallium. The crystal is collimated to allow localization of the source of radioactive decay within the patient. When an incident gamma photon enters the crystal, its energy is converted to light. An array of photomultiplier tubes that are optically connected to the crystal convert the light to electrical energy and amplify the electrical signal. After further modification and processing, the electrical pulse carries information on positioning and pulse height. This information is displayed on a persistence scope for immediate viewing and also on a cathode-ray tube screen for Polaroid photography to produce a hard copy image. The image can also be recorded on x-ray film in any of several optional formats, e.g., 1, 4, or 16 images on an 8 × 10-in x-ray film. The data can also be stored on magnetic tape or disc for later image processing or computer analysis.

Decay events in the entire field of view are processed simultaneously. Rapidly dynamic events, such as a flow of a bolus of radioactivity through the cardiac chambers, can be recorded

TABLE 47–1. MECHANISMS OF RADIOPHARMACEUTICAL LOCALIZATION

Mechanism	Organ	Agent
Active transport	Thyroid	^{123}I, ^{131}I, ^{99m}TcO$_4^-$
Simple or exchange diffusion	Bone	^{18}F, ^{99m}Tc-phosphates
	Brain	^{99m}Tc-glucoheptonate
Compartmental localization	Heart	^{99m}Tc-red blood cells
Capillary blockade	Lung	^{99m}Tc-macroaggregated albumin
Cell sequestration	Spleen	Heat-damaged ^{51}Cr-red blood cells
Phagocytosis	Liver/spleen	^{99m}Tc-sulfur colloid
Metabolic function precursor	Pancreas	^{75}Se-selenomethionine
Antigen-antibody reaction	Tumor	^{131}I-antitumor antibodies

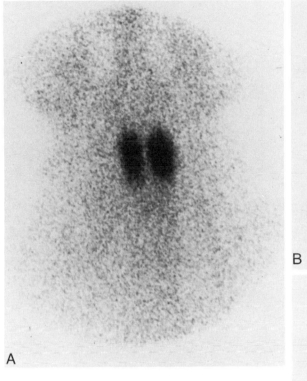

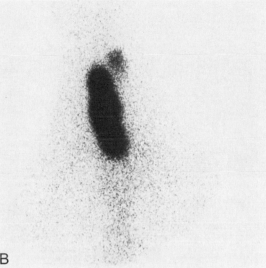

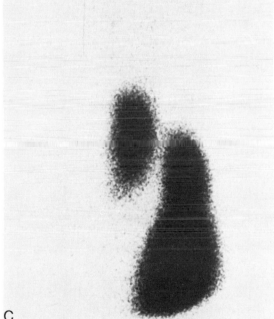

Figure 47–5. Normal *(A)* and abnormal *(B* and *C)* thyroid scans (ventral images of the neck region) in a cat. The head is at the top of the image and the animal's right side is to the viewer's left. These studies were obtained about 15 minutes after intravenous injection of 1 to 2 mCi sodium ⁹⁹ᵐTc-pertechnetate. A pinhole collimator was used. *A,* note the bilateral symmetry of the thyroid lobes and the relatively high soft-tissue background activity. *B* and *C,* toxic nodular goiter. In *B,* note the multilobulated appearance of the enlarged right thyroid lobe and the nodular involvement at the cranial aspect of the left thyroid lobe. In *C,* note the extensive bilateral involvement with caudal intrathoracic extension of the multilobulated left thyroid lobe.

by taking several sequential images during the first pass of the bolus through the heart.

The imaging protocol is dependent on the study performed. The radiopharmaceutical is usually administered intravenously. For most procedures involving the use of technetium radiopharmaceuticals in dogs and cats, 1 to 10 mCi of activity are used. Horses receive a proportionally larger injected dose. With these doses, each static image takes from less than 1 minute to approximately 3 minutes to generate. Resolution is greatest at the surface of the detector and activity distributed at a distance from the surface is more poorly resolved. Con-

sequently, multiple views are usually obtained for complete evaluation. The views are named for the part closest to the detector.

In veterinary medicine, most scans are performed by using ⁹⁹ᵐTc either in ionic form as ⁹⁹ᵐTc O₄⁻, the form in which it is obtained from the generator, or is chemically bound to another pharmaceutical. Most ⁹⁹ᵐTc radiopharmaceuticals can be easily prepared on an as-needed basis from commercially available kits.

Although some animals cooperate fully, sedation is often necessary to facilitate restraint and positioning of the patient for imaging. If the patient is not anesthetized, one or two

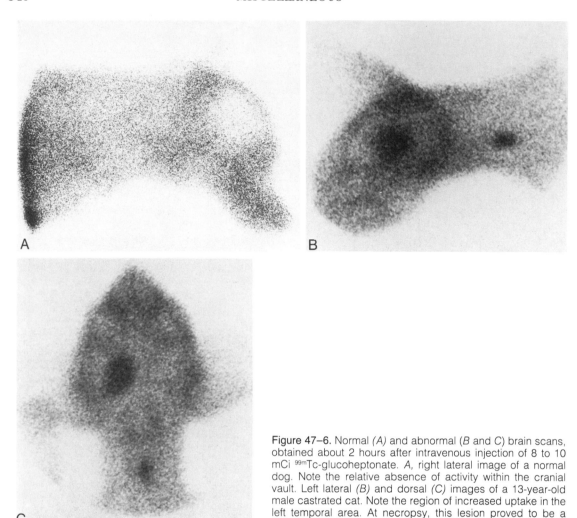

Figure 47–6. Normal *(A)* and abnormal *(B* and *C)* brain scans, obtained about 2 hours after intravenous injection of 8 to 10 mCi ^{99m}Tc-glucoheptonate. *A,* right lateral image of a normal dog. Note the relative absence of activity within the cranial vault. Left lateral *(B)* and dorsal *(C)* images of a 13-year-old male castrated cat. Note the region of increased uptake in the left temporal area. At necropsy, this lesion proved to be a meningioma.

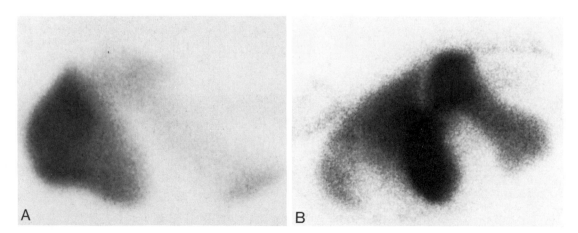

Figure 47–7. Normal *(A)* and abnormal *(B)* liver-spleen scans obtained about 20 minutes after intravenous injection of 3 to 6 mCi ^{99m}Tc-sulfur colloid. *A,* left lateral image of a normal beagle. *B,* left lateral image of a 3-year-old female boxer with a portosystemic shunt. Note the small liver and increased splenic, pulmonary, and skeletal uptake of the radiopharmaceutical.

people are required to hold the animal in position. After the imaging procedure, the patient is housed in relative isolation for 24 to 48 hours during which time the body burden of radioactivity is reduced to a negligible level and the animal is then handled as a nonradioactive patient. Radioactive wastes are stored for decay to background activity levels and then are disposed of routinely. For ^{99m}Tc radioactive waste, such decay occurs in 2 to 3 days.

Examples of normal and abnormal thyroid scans (Fig. 47–5), brain scans (Fig. 47–6), and liver scans (Fig. 47–7) are presented. There have been many reports of the clinical use of nuclear medicine imaging procedures in veterinary medicine.

DIAGNOSTIC ULTRASOUND

EQUIPMENT

Two basic types of portable diagnostic ultrasound instruments have gained popularity in veterinary imaging. It should be noted that the instruments in current use were designed for use in people; only the shape of the scanheads have been modified by some manufacturers for use in animals. The most popular type of ultrasonic equipment is the low-cost linear array scanner, which is used primarily in obstetrical examination of the mare. The second most popular type is the mechanical sector scanner, which can perform a larger variety of examinations in animals. A smaller number of static B-mode scanners are in use, primarily in veterinary schools. A definition of the basic "modes" of ultrasound and the methods of display is warranted before discussion of the instrumentation.

Amplitude modulation or A-mode ultrasound displays information as distance versus amplitude of the returning echoes. The height of the peaks is proportional to the amplitude of the returning echoes (Fig. 47–8). Brightness modulation or B-mode ultrasound displays the returning echoes as dots, the brightness of which are proportional to their amplitudes (Fig. 47–9). One can imagine viewing the tips of the peaks of the A-mode display on end as if they have been turned 90 degrees toward the reader. Some ultrasound instruments display both A- and B-mode. M-mode or TM-mode (motion or time motion), which are popular for use in cardiac studies, is the same B-mode principle, although the display is different. An actual two-dimensional image is not displayed, rather a tracing is made on light-sensitive paper or is displayed on a monitor. The various levels of

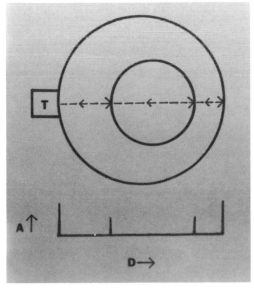

Figure 47–8. A-mode or amplitude modulation. The sound beam originates from the transducer (T) and encounters interfaces within tissue. At each interface of differing acoustic impedance, a portion of the sound is reflected back to the transducer. The returning echo is displayed as a peak, the height of which is proportional to its amplitude (A). The depth of the interfaces can be determined from the horizontal scale (D).

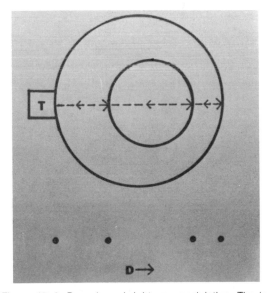

Figure 47–9. B-mode or brightness modulation. The interfaces are seen as dots, with their amplitude proportional to their intensity on the display screen. In this diagram, the transducer (T) is held in one position without movement for graphic purposes. When the transducer is moved (static B-mode), the image is formed by the operator. With real-time (sector) scanning, the crystals rotate or wobble through an arc of 60 to 100 degrees to form a pie-wedge image (see Fig. 47–11).

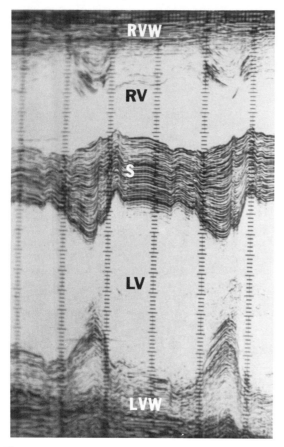

Figure 47–10. M-mode or motion mode is a form of B-mode in which the tracing is made on light-sensitive paper. The transducer is held as in Fig. 47–9. The dot display would move if the heart were the internal structure of the graph. No image is formed per se, but graphic movement of cardiac walls and other structures is recorded. RVW: right ventricular wall; RV: right ventricle; S: septum; LV: left ventricle; LVW: left ventricular wall.

cardiac muscle correspond to the undulant lines (Fig. 47–10).

Currently, the bulk of the imaging performed in veterinary medicine is B-mode imaging in real time. For several years, B-mode imaging in human medicine was performed with "static" scanners; the operator actually "painted" the image on the display screen while physically moving the crystal over the patient's skin surface. This type of imaging, although useful in examining disease states, is losing favor to real-time scanning techniques. With real-time imaging, multiple crystals or single oscillating crystals are used and information is continuously upgraded and displayed on a nonstorage monitor. The transducer containing the crystals is held on the skin over the area of interest and a moving image is obtained. Because the crystals of a mechanical sector scanner obtain information through an arc, the image is wedge-shaped, varying from 60 to 100 degrees depending on the instrument (Fig. 47–11). With linear array scanheads, the crystals are continually fired and a rectangular image is formed on the monitor. Each crystal forms a scan line on the monitor (Fig. 47–12).

Real-time scanning instruments, mechanical sector or linear array, are most effective for animal scanning. One advantage of the sector scanner is the small contact area needed to couple the sound beam to the body surface. Linear array scanheads have long, narrow contact surfaces, which can be difficult to couple to the irregular body contours, especially in small animals or when tissue deep to the ribs is scanned. With real-time imaging, the patient can be less cooperative as far as movement and the study can still be performed. With static imaging, patient motion often compromises the study because the crystal must be physically

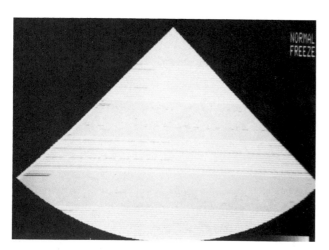

Figure 47–11. Shape of the 90-degree sector image seen on the display screen. One crystal that wobbles or three to four crystals that rotate through a sector of 60 to 100 degrees are commonly used in sector scanning. The contact surface of the transducer is always displayed at the top of the sector image.

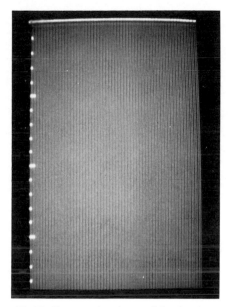

Figure 47–12. Rectangular shape of the image seen on the display screen of a linear array instrument. Each crystal forms a scan line on the monitor. The transducer contact surface is always displayed at the top of the rectangular image.

moved over the area to form the image. Static scanners are effective, although chemical restraint is often required, the instrument is large and cumbersome, more time is needed for each examination, and the scanners are more expensive than the portable real-time instruments.

METHODOLOGY

Ultrasound at the frequencies used (2.25 to 10 MHz) does not penetrate bone (mineral) or air (gas), because they are near-perfect reflectors. Thus, areas of the body surface covered with thick hair pose a problem with trapped air, and this hair should be removed. The best image quality in small animals is obtained when the hair is clipped with a #40 clipper; in large animals the area should be clipped and shaved. Some studies, however, can be performed without hair removal. If the hair is not too thick and is free of debris, and a copius amount of aqueous coupling gel is used, the hair need not be removed, especially if only size, shape, and position of the underlying organs need be determined or if the possibility of fluid within a body cavity is to be ruled out. Cardiac examinations can usually be performed with a sector scanner from a single site or from a few sites without clipping the hair.

The depth of penetration of ultrasound is frequency-dependent and is based on an atten-uation rate of approximately 1 dB/cm/MHz. For example, a 3.0-MHz ultrasound beam would be attenuated at a rate of 3.0 dB/cm. A 7.5-MHz beam would be attenuated at 7.5 dB/cm. Therefore, the lower frequency sound beam would penetrate further than the higher frequency beam. It follows then that superficial tissues should be examined with higher frequency sound than that used for deeper structures.

Two considerations must be made for the resolving power of the transducer with ultrasound. The ability of the sound to differentiate two objects along the axis of the beam is termed axial resolution and can be thought of as depending on the frequency. The ability of the sound to differentiate two objects side by side is termed lateral resolution. Lateral resolution is determined by the physical size of the transducer crystal. Therefore, larger crystals, which are needed to produce low frequency sound, have poorer resolving power, but they penetrate further into tissue. Conversely, smaller crystals, which produce higher frequency sound, have better resolving power, but they do not penetrate as great a distance.

Crystals used in mechanical sector scanners can be tightly focused in all planes; linear array crystals can only be focused in one plane. Therefore, mechanical sector scanners have inherently better resolution than do linear arrays.

Diagnostic ultrasound can be used to examine virtually any soft tissue in large and small animals. Most of the techniques performed in human imaging are possible in animals. Knowledge of anatomy, ultrasound physics, and sound-tissue interaction are necessary to achieve diagnostic images and to allow accurate interpretation. The reader is referred to several excellent texts dedicated to the physics of ultrasound and sound-tissue interaction.

The goal of the ultrasonographer is to image accurately the acoustical interfaces of the tissue or organ of interest. The size, shape, position, texture, and dynamics of the anatomy in question may then be determined. The set-up of the various instruments necessary to produce high quality images is not addressed in this discussion. It should be stressed, however, that like tissues should appear the same throughout the image. This will preclude introducing artifacts in the image and will allow tissues to be examined within the scanning plane. Tissues should be scanned in more than one plane and any abnormalities should be documented in different planes.

As with any diagnostic imaging technique, permanent record of the images is essential. There are a number of recording options available for the sonographer, including videotape,

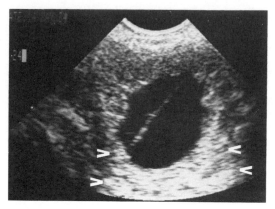

Figure 47–13. Transrectal scan of a cystic structure (equine twin pregnancy). There is acoustic enhancement of the deeper tissues *(arrows)* due to lack of attentuation of the sound beam as it passes though fluid. Note the darkness of the tissue adjacent to the enhanced area.

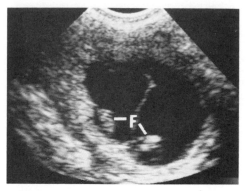

Figure 47–14. Transrectal scan of equine twins (F) made at 26 days gestational age. During the examination, both fetal hearts could be seen beating. The thin white line is the division between the gestational sacs.

Polaroid film, and multiformat cameras. Some of the commercially available systems interface with a video cassette recorder. Videotape is the best way to capture dynamic studies, such as cardiac examinations. Polaroid filming is the most popular method in private practice today; it is convenient and most portable systems have a polaroid camera as an option. Multiformat cameras, which place a number of images on imaging film, are limited to institutions because of their high cost and lack of portability. These cameras do produce the best "hard copy" of the studies, however. With the real-time scanners, the image is "frozen" on the screen and photographs can be taken.

The most important feature of ultrasound is its ability to distinguish solid versus cystic lesions. Cysts have few, if any, acoustic interfaces and should be anechoic (echo-free). The leading edge of the cyst should be well defined and acoustic enhancement of the far wall should be apparent (Fig. 47–13). Fluids within lesions or body cavities may be homogeneous with no acoustic interfaces, as with a cyst, or there may be echoes that originate from within the fluid that correspond to cellular or inflammatory debris (composite fluid).

CLINICAL USE

Large Animals. Diagnostic ultrasound has been used most often in the horse, although A-mode ultrasound has been used in sheep and swine for several years. Transrectal imaging of the reproductive tract of the mare has become a commonly accepted technique. The most popular instrument used is the linear array scanner, usually with a 3.0-MHz scanhead; scanheads with 5.0 MHz are also available for the linear

array. It is possible to image the pregnant mare 14 days after breeding (or earlier) and to detect twins (Fig. 47–14). Fetal viability can be determined as early as 22 to 23 days with the use of sector scanners.

Intracardiac lesions in horses can be imaged with diagnostic ultrasound. Vegetative lesions can be documented (Fig. 47–15). It is possible to utilize microbubble injection techniques in young horses to diagnose definitively suspected septal defects. A great amount of information concerning cardiac chamber size, presence of pericardial fluid, and valve excursion can be obtained.

Pleural effusion can be a diagnostic challenge, although it is possible to detect minimal amounts of fluid within the thoracic cavity. Fluid can be classified as clear or composite,

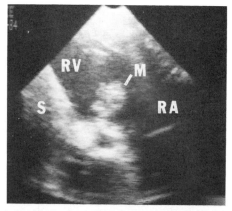

Figure 47–15. From a videotape of a cardiac examination of a 3-year-old colt with clinical evidence of vegetative endocarditis. The heart base is to the right and the apex is to the left. The heart is in diastole. RV: right ventricle; RA: right atrium; S: interventricular septum; M: vegetative mass attached to the right atrial wall dorsal to the tricuspid valve.

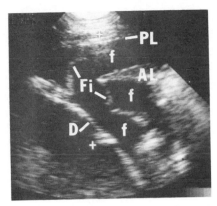

Figure 47–16. Pleural effusion between the costal margins of the left side of the thorax of a 2-year-old Standardbred filly. Dorsal is to the right, ventral is to the left, and the skin surface is at the top of the image. PL: parietal pleural surface; f: thoracic fluid, Fi: fibrin loosely attached to diaphragm (D); AL: atelectatic ventral lung border.

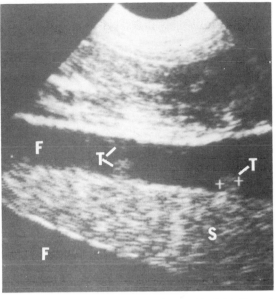

Figure 47–18. Scan of a horse with ascitic fluid (F) and implantation metastases of squamous cell carcinoma (T) on the peritoneum and serosal surface of the spleen (S).

and areas of atelectasis and necrosis or abscess formation of the lung can be found (Fig. 47–16). Ultrasound is extremely useful to monitor fluid removal or recurrence on a daily basis because of its noninvasive properties.

Renal ultrasound examinations not only allow determination of size, shape, and position of the kidneys, but also hydronephrosis and the presence or absence of mineral within the kidney may be detected. Transrectal examination of the ureters and urinary bladder as well as the left kidney can be performed (Fig. 47–17).

Examination of the liver can be performed from the right or left sides to determine if hepatomegaly exists. Neoplastic enlargement of

the liver can also be diagnosed by the change in textural quality or the presence of abnormal masses within the liver parenchyma.

Ascites can be readily determined and tumor growth within the abdominal cavity can be documented. Tumors can be seen within the wall of the gut and can also be seen growing as implants on serosal surfaces (Fig. 47–18).

Structural damage (fiber tearing) within the tendons and ligaments of the extremities can be imaged with high frequency sound (7.5 MHz or higher). Figure 47–19 illustrates a cross-

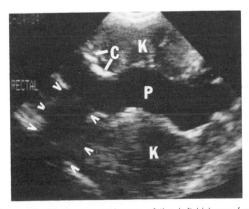

Figure 47–17. Transrectal scan of the left kidney of a 3-year-old filly with hydronephrosis secondary to renal and ureteral calculi. The transducer–rectal wall interface is at the top of the scan. K: left kidney; P: dilated renal pelvis; C: renal calculi producing acoustic shadowing of the deeper structures (arrows). Mineral is a near-perfect reflector that blocks the sound that produces the shadow.

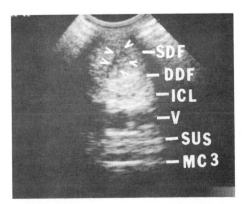

Figure 47–19. Cross-sectional image of the middle of the metacarpus of a 3-year-old colt. There is an area of fiber tearing (arrows) and hemorrhage within the superficial digital flexor. SDF: superficial digital flexor; DDF: deep digital flexor; ICL: inferior check ligament; V: vessels; SUS: suspensory ligament; MC3: palmar surface of the third metacarpal bone.

sectional scan of acute fiber tearing and hemorrhage within the superficial flexor tendon. Virtually any superficial connective tissue or muscle can be imaged. Knowledge of sound-tissue interaction is needed to interpret subtle changes within connective tissue structures.

These examples are but a few of the applications of ultrasound in the evaluation of the horse. Guided biopsy techniques can be used to sample any abnormal fluid accumulation or body tissue, because needles can be accurately placed within the tissues under ultrasonic guidance.

Small Animals. Because ultrasound instruments are designed for people, they work extremely well for small animal imaging. Usually, higher frequencies (5.0 and 7.5 MHz) are used because of the smaller size. Larger dogs may require 3.0 MHz, however, especially if they are obese. Sector scanners, because of their small contact area, work better for small animals than do linear array scanners. Static B-mode scanners can be used, although patient motion is a factor.

Pregnancy can be diagnosed at less than 20 days gestation in the bitch and queen (Fig. 47–20). The fetal pulse can often be detected at 17 days of gestation or less with high frequency sound (7.5 MHz).

Thoracic scanning techniques for detection of neoplasia can often add additional information to the radiographic examination. Intrathoracic, extracardiac tumors have been documented with ultrasound.

Ultrasound has offered a new dimension to cardiac imaging in dogs and cats. Both real-time and M-mode studies can offer significant diagnostic and prognostic information in the evaluation of the heart. Valvular lesions, pericardial effusion, cardiomyopathy, and cardiac neoplasia can be diagnosed ultrasonically.

Abdominal tumors that have been palpated

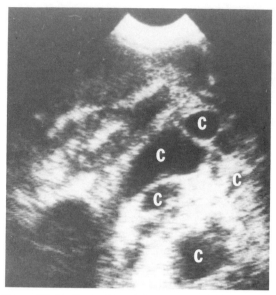

Figure 47–21. Scan of an abdominal mass proved to be hemangiosarcoma of the spleen of an aged dog. Note the multicystic (C) appearance of the mass with homogeneous (anechoic) areas within a more dense stroma.

or seen on conventional radiographs can often be characterized with ultrasound. Hemangiosarcoma, for instance, has a characteristic ultrasonic appearance (Fig. 47–21). It is also often possible to detect metastatic disease, which obviates exploratory laparotomy in abdominal neoplasia. Prostatic imaging is valuable in the older male dog. Neoplasia can often be detected on an ultrasound examination, and guided biopsy techniques can be performed safely.

The urinary tract is well-evaluated with diagnostic ultrasound techniques. The urinary bladder appears as a cystic structure, and growths within the bladder wall can be imaged noninvasively. Ultrasound-guided centesis of the bladder or renal pelvis for culture can be performed.

FUTURE DIRECTION

Diagnostic ultrasound, because it is a noninvasive means of imaging, will find its place in animal imaging. For the horse, it often provides information that cannot be obtained with more invasive methods without difficulty. Cardiac studies in all animal species have enhanced our ability to diagnose and understand cardiac disease, especially in the horse. No longer will disease of the abdominal organs of horses be only suspected. Because of the ease of adapting the technology to the body size of the smaller animals, ultrasound will become an alternative to more invasive methods of diagnosis.

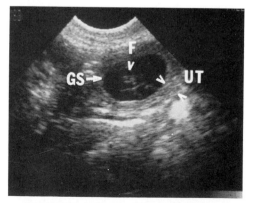

Figure 47–20. Scan of a canine pregnancy at 28 days gestational age. F: fetus; GS: gestational sac; UT: uterine wall. The skin surface is at the top of the scan.

References

X-CT

Texts

Christensen EE, Curry III TS, and Dowdey JE: An Introduction to the Physics of Diagnostic Radiology, 2nd Ed. Philadelphia, Lea & Febiger, 1978.

Greenberg M, Greenberg BM, and Greenberg IM: Essentials of Body Computed Tomography. Philadelphia, WB Saunders, 1983.

Haaga JR, and Alfidi RJ: Computed Tomography of the Whole Body. St. Louis, CV Mosby, 1983.

Moss AA, Gamsu G, and Genant HK: Computed Tomography of the Body. Philadelphia, WB Saunders, 1983.

Newton TH: Advanced imaging techniques. In Modern Neuroradiology, Vol. 2, San Anselmo, CA, Clavadel Press, 1984.

Journal Articles

Barber DL: Imaging: Radiography II. Vet Radiol 22:149, 1981.

Fike JR, and Cann CE: Contrast medium accumulation and washout in canine brain tumors and irradiated normal brain: A CT study of kinetics. Radiology 151:115, 1984.

Fike JR, and Cann CE: Radiation effects in the canine brain quantified by CT. J Comput Assist Tomogr 7:565, 1983.

Fike JR, LeCouteur RA, and Cann CE: Anatomy of the canine brain using high resolution computed tomography. Vet Radiol 22:236, 1981.

Fike JR, Druy EM, Zook BC, et al: Canine anatomy assessed by computerized tomography. Am J Vet Res 41:1823, 1980.

Fike JR, Le Couteur RA, Cann CE, et al: Computerized tomography of brain tumors of the rostral and middle fossas in the dog. Am J Vet Res 42:275, 1981.

Fike JR, Cann CE, Davis RL, et al: Radiation effects in the canine brain evaluated by quantitative computed tomography. Radiology 144:603, 1982.

LeCouteur RA, Fike JR, Cann CE, et al: Computed tomography of brain tumors in the caudal fossa of the dog. Vet Radiol 22:244, 1981.

LeCouteur RA, Fike JR, Cann CE, et al: X-ray computed tomography of brain tumors in cats. J Am Vet Med Assoc 183:301, 1983.

LeCouteur RA, Fike JR, Scagliotti RH, et al: Computed tomography of orbital tumors in the dog. J Am Vet Med Assoc 180:910, 1982.

Marincek B, and Young SW: Computed tomography of spontaneous canine neoplasms. Vet Radiol 21:181, 1980.

Smallwood JE, and Healey WV: Computed tomography of the thorax of the adult nubian goat. Vet Radiol 23:135, 1982.

Turrel JM, Fike JR, and LeCouteur RA: Radiotherapy of brain tumors in dogs. J Am Vet Med Assoc 184:82, 1984.

Magnetic Resonance Imaging

Texts

Mansfield P, and Morris PG: NMR Imaging in Biomedicine. New York, Academic Press, 1982.

Margulis AR, Higgins CB, Kaufman L, et al: Clinical Magnetic Resonance Imaging. San Francisco, University of California, 1984.

Partain CL: Nuclear Magnetic Resonance and Correlative Imaging Modalities. New York, The Society of Nuclear Medicine, 1984.

Partain CL, James AE, Rollo FD, et al: Nuclear Magnetic Resonance (NMR) Imaging. Philadelphia, WB Saunders, 1984.

Wolf GL, and Popp CA: NMR: A Primer for Medical Imaging. Thorofare, NJ, Slack, Inc., 1983.

Young SW: Nuclear Magnetic Resonance Imaging: Basic Principles. New York, Raven Press, 1984.

Journal Articles

Bloch F: Nuclear induction. Physiol Rev 70:460, 1946.

Koutcher JA, and Burt CT: Principles of nuclear magnetic resonance. J Nucl Med 25:101, 1984.

Koutcher JA, and Burt CT: Principles of imaging by nuclear magnetic resonance. J Nucl Med 25:371, 1984.

Lauterbur PC: Image formation by induced local interactions: Examples employing NMR. Nature 242:190, 1973.

Purcell EM: Resonance absorption by nuclear magnetic moments in a solid. Physiol Rev 69:37, 1946.

Pykett IL: NMR imaging in medicine. Sci Am 246:78, 1982.

Pykett IL, Newhouse JH, Buonanno FS, et al: Principles of nuclear magnetic resonance imaging. Radiology 143:157, 1982.

Nuclear Medicine Imaging

Texts

Baum S, Vincent NR, Lyons KP, et al: Atlas of Nuclear Medicine Imaging. New York, Appleton-Century-Crofts, 1981.

Freeman LM: Clinical Radionuclide Imaging, 3rd Ed. Orlando, FL, Grune & Stratton, 1984.

Maisey MN, Britton KE, Gilday DL: Clinical Nuclear Medicine. London, Chapman & Hall, 1983.

Matin P: Clinical Nuclear Medicine. Garden City, NY, Medical Examination Publishing, 1981.

Mettler FA, and Guiberteau MM: Essentials of Nuclear Medicine Imaging. Orlando, FL, Grune & Stratton, 1983.

Rocha AF, and Harbert JC: Textbook of Nuclear Medicine: Clinical Applications. Philadelphia, Lea & Febiger, 1979.

Journal Articles

Allhands RV, Kallfelz FA, and Lust G: Radionuclide joint imaging. An ancillary technique in the diagnosis of canine hip dysplasia. Am J Vet Res 41:230, 1980.

Barber DL, and Roberts RE: Imaging: Nuclear. Vet Radiol 24:50, 1983.

Devous Sr MD, and Twardock AR: Techniques and applications of nuclear medicine in the diagnosis of equine lameness. J Am Vet Med Assoc 184:318, 1984.

Koblik PD, Hornof WJ, and Breznock EM: Quantitative hepatic scintigraphy in the dog. Vet Radiol 24:226, 1983.

Koblik PD, Hornof WJ, and Breznock EM: Use of quantitative hepatic scintigraphy to evaluate spontaneous portosystemic shunts in 12 dogs. Vet Radiol 24:232, 1983.

Peterson ME, and Becker DV: Radionuclide thyroid imaging in 135 cats with hyperthyroidism. Vet Radiol 25:23, 1984.

Selcer BA: Imaging: Bone. Vet Radiol 24:243, 1983.

Turrel JM, Feldman EC, Hays M, et al: Radioactive iodine therapy in cats with hyperthyroidism. J Am Vet Med Assoc 184:554, 1984.

Ueltshi G: Bone and joint imaging with Tc99m-labeled phosphates as a new diagnostic aid in veterinary orthopedics. J Am Vet Radiol Soc 18:80, 1977.

Wolff RK, Merickel PS, Rebar AH, et al: Comparison of bone scans and radiography for detecting bone neoplasms in dogs exposed to 238PuO$_2$. Am J Vet Res 41:1804, 1980.

Wortman JA: Veterinary nuclear medicine imaging. Acta Med Vet 28:331, 1982.

Diagnostic Ultrasound

Texts

Feigenbaum H: Echocardiography, 3rd Ed. Philadelphia, Lea & Febiger, 1981.

Goldberg BB: Abdominal Ultrasonography, 2nd Ed. John Wiley & Sons, 1984.

Hagen-Ansert SL: Textbook of Diagnostic Ultrasonography. St. Louis, CV Mosby, 1983.

Kremkau FW: Diagnostic Ultrasound, Physical Principles and Exercises, New York, Grune & Stratton, 1980.

Powis RL, and Powis WF: A Thinkers Guide to Ultrasonic Imaging. Baltimore and Munich, Urban & Schwarzenberg, 1984.

Powis RL: Ultrasound Physics for the Fun of It. Cleveland, OH, Technicare Corporation, 1980.

Skolnick ML: Real-Time Ultrasound Imaging in the Abdomen. New York, Springer, 1981.

Journal Articles

Allen DG: Echocardiographic study of the anesthetized cat. Can J Comp Med 46:115, 1982.

Baylen BG, Garner DJ, Laks MM, et al: Improved echocardiographic evaluation of the closed-chest canine: Methods and anatomic observations. JCU 8:335, 1980.

Bonagura JD, and Pipers FS: Diagnosis of cardiac lesions by contrast echocardiography. J Am Vet Med Assoc 182:396, 1983.

Boon J, Wingfield WE, and Miller CW: Echocardiographic indices in the normal dog. Vet Radiol 24:214, 1983.

Cartee RE: Diagnostic real time ultrasonography of the liver of the dog and cat. J Am Anim Hosp Assoc 17:731, 1981.

Cartee RE: Ultrasonography—a new diagnostic technique for veterinary medicine. Vet Med/Small Anim Clin 75:1523, 1980.

Cartee RE, Selcer BA, and Patton CS: Ultrasonographic diagnosis of renal disease in small animals. J Am Vet Med Assoc 176:426, 1980.

Chevalier F, and Palmer E: Ultrasonic echography in the mare. J Reprod Fertil [Suppl] 32:423, 1982.

Dennis MO, Healeigh RC, Pyle RL, et al: Echocardiographic assessment of normal and abnormal valvular function in beagle dogs. Am J Vet Res 39:1591, 1978.

Feeney DA, Johnston GR, and Hardy RM: Two-dimensional, gray scale ultrasonography for assessment of hepatic and splenic neoplasia in the dog and cat. J Am Vet Med Assoc 184:68, 1984.

Ginther OJ: Effect of reproductive status on twinning and on side of ovulation and embryo attachment in mares. Theriogenology 20:383, 1983.

Ginther OJ: Mobility of the early equine conceptus. Theriogenology 19:603, 1983.

Ginther OJ: Intrauterine movement of the early conceptus in barren and postpartum mares. Theriogenology 21:633, 1984.

Ginther OJ: Fixation and orientation of the early equine conceptus. Theriogenology 19:613, 1983.

Ginther OJ, and Pierson RA: Ultrasonic anatomy and pathology of the equine uterus. Theriogenology 21:505, 1984.

Ginther OJ, and Pierson RA: Ultrasonic evaluation of the mare reproduction tract: Principles, equipment and technique. J Equine Vet Sci 3:195, 1983.

Ginther OJ, and Pierson RA: Ultrasonic evaluation of the mare reproductive tract: Ovaries. J Equine Vet Sci 4:11, 1984.

Hauser ML, Rantanen NW, and Modransky PD: Ultrasonic examination of the distal interphalangeal joint, navicular bursa, navicular bone and deep digital flexor tendon. J Equine Vet Sci 2:95, 1982.

Hauser ML, and Rantanen NW: Ultrasound appearance of the palmar metacarpal soft tissues of the horse. J Equine Vet Sci 3:19, 1983.

James EA, Osterman FO, Bush RM, et al: The use of compound B-mode ultrasound in abdominal disease of animals. J Am Vet Radiol Soc 17:106, 1976.

Konde LJ, Wrigley RH, Park RD, et al: Ultrasonographic anatomy of the normal canine kidney. Vet Radiol 25:173, 1984.

Modransky PD, Rantanen NW, Hauser ML, et al: Diagnostic ultrasound examination of the dorsal aspect of the equine metacarpophalangeal joint. J Equine Vet Sci 3:56, 1983.

Nyland TG, Park RD, Lattimer JC, et al: Ultrasonic patterns of canine hepatic lymphosarcoma. Vet Radiol 25:167, 1984.

Nyland TG, Park RD, Lattimer JC, et al: Gray-scale ultrasonography of the canine abdomen. Vet Radiol 22:220, 1981.

Nyland TG, and Benard WV: Application of ultrasound in veterinary medicine. Cal Vet 36:21, 1982.

Nyland TG, Mulvany MH, and Strombeck DR: Ultrasonic features of experimentally induced, acute pancreatitis in the dog. Vet Radiol 24:260, 1983.

Nyland TG, and Park RD: Hepatic ultrasonography in the dog. Vet Radiol 24:74, 1983.

Palmer E, and Draincourt MA: Use of ultrasound echography in equine gynecology. Theriogenology 13:203, 1980.

Park RD, Nyland TG, Lattimer JC, et al: B-mode gray-scale ultrasound: Imaging artifacts and interpretation principles. Vet Radiol 22:204, 1981.

Pipers FS, Bonagura JD, Hamlin RL, et al: Echocardiographic abnormalities of the mitral valve associated with left-side heart diseases in the dog. J Am Vet Med Assoc 179:580, 1981.

Pipers FS, Zent W, Holder R, et al: Ultrasonography as an adjunct to pregnancy assessments in the mare. J Am Vet Med Assoc 183:328, 1984.

Pipers FS, and Hamlin RL: Echocardiography in the horse. J Am Vet Med Assoc 170:815, 1977.

Pipers FS, and Hamlin RL: Clinical use of echocardiography in the domestic cat. J Am Vet Med Assoc 176:47, 1980.

Pipers FS, Muir WW, and Hamlin RF: Echocardiography in swine. Am J Vet Res 39:707, 1978.

Pipers FS, Reef V, and Hamlin RL: Echocardiography in the domestic cat. Am J Vet Res 40:882, 1979.

Rantanen NW: The use of diagnostic ultrasound in limb disorders of the horse: A preliminary report. J Equine Vet Sci 2:62, 1982.

Rantanen NW: Ultrasound appearance of normal lung borders and adjacent viscera in the horse. Vet Radiol 22:217, 1981.

Rantanen NW, and Ewing III RL: Principles of ultrasound and application in animals. Vet Radiol 22:196, 1981.

Rantanen NW, Gage L, and Paradis MR: Ultrasonography as a diagnostic aid in pleural effusion of horses. Vet Radiol 22:211, 1981.

Rantanen NW, Torbeck RL, and DuMond SS: Early pregnancy diagnosis in the mare using transrectal ultrasound scanning techniques: A preliminary report. J Equine Vet Sci 2:27, 1982.

Soderberg SF, Boon JA, Wingfield WE, et al: M-mode echocardiography as a diagnostic aid for feline cardiomyopathy. Vet Radiol 24:66, 1983.

Spaulding K: Ultrasonic anatomy of the tendons and ligaments in the distal metacarpal-metatarsal region of the equine limb. Vet Radiol 25:155, 1984.

Thomas WP: Two-dimensional, real-time echocardiography in the dog: Technique and anatomic validation. Vet Radiol 25:50, 1984.

Thomas WP, Sisson D, Bauer TG, et al: Detection of cardiac masses by two-dimensional echocardiography. Vet Radiol 25:65, 1984.

Torbeck RL, and Rantanen NW: Early pregnancy detection in the mare with ultrasonography. J Equine Vet Sci 2:204, 1982.

Traub JL, Rantanen NW, Reed S, et al: Cholelithiasis in four horses. J Am Vet Med Assoc 181:59, 1982.

INDEX

Note: Page numbers in *italics* refer to illustrations; page numbers followed by (t) refer to tables.

Hemarthrosis, in dogs, 127–128

Hematoma, in companion animals, calcification of, 17, *119*
    subpleural, *242*
    in equidae, ethmoid, 73, *74*

Hemivertebra(e), in companion animals, 44, 45(t), *46*

Hemophilia, in dogs, hemarthrosis due to, 127–128

Hemorrhage, pulmonary, in race horses, 347–348

Hepatomegaly, in companion animals, 393, *393*
    displacement of abdominal viscera by, *360–361*, 361–363
    displacement of stomach by, 480, *480*

Hernia (companion animals), diaphragmatic, 250–251
    barium sulfate examination for, 250, *251*
    causes of, 250
    clinical signs of, 250
    congenital predisposition to, 254–257
    hiatal, *230*, 255–257
        clinical signs of, 255
        paraesophageal, 255, *256*
        radiographic signs of, 255–256, 256(t)
        sliding, 255, *256*
        types of, 255
    inguinal, *389*
        due to pregnancy, 463
    peritoneopericardial, 244, 254–255, 393, *394*
        radiographic signs of, 254(t), 255
    pleural fluid as sign of, 253
    traumatic, 251–253
        radiographic signs of, 250(t), 251, *252, 253*

Hiatal hernia. See under *Hernia*.

Hip, joint mice in, in companion animals, 122
    causes of, 123(t)

Hip dysplasia (dogs), 123–126
    coxofemoral subluxation as sign of, 124–125, *125*
    development of, 124
    early changes in, 124–125
    heritability of, 123
    pathologic joint changes in, 125
    radiographic diagnosis of, accuracy of, 124, 125(t)

Hirschsprung's disease, in companion animals, 515, *516*

Histoplasmosis, hepatic involvement in, in companion animals, 395

Horses, amyloblastic odontoma in, 59
    alveolar periostitis in, 59, *61*
    bone tumors in, 59–60
    head of, normal anatomy of, 65–70. See also specific structures and disorders.
        radiographic evaluation of, 64–81
    hyoid-temporal bone function in, 58–59, *60*
    infraorbital canal of, *66, 68, 69*
    intermaxillary septum of, *66, 68, 68*

Horses (*Continued*)
    interphalangeal joint abnormalities in, 187–192. See also *Interphalangeal joints.*
    mandibular fractures in, 57–58, *57–58*
    mandibular osteoma in, 59, *61*
    skull fractures in, 57–59, *57–59*
        normal suture vs., 58, *58, 59*

Humeral condyle, osteochondritis dissecans of, in companion animals, *90*

Humeral fractures, in companion animals, healing of, 102, *103*
    non-union of, 109, *110*

Hydrarthrosis, intermittent, in equidae, 173

Hydrocephalus (in companion animals), degree of calvarial distortion due to, 22–23
    radiographic signs of, 22, *23*

Hydronephrosis (companion animals), 372, *372*, 412
    pyelographic appearance of, 416(t), *417*
    ureteral obstruction with, *415*

Hydronephrosis (equidae), ultrasound diagnosis of, *545*

Hydrothorax (equidae), 334

Hyoid bone, radiographic identification of, in companion animals, 211

Hyoid-temporal bone fusion, in horses, 58–59, *60*

Hyperparathyroidism (companion animals), alveolar bone loss in, 25, 30
    loss of radiographic opacity due to, 25
    primary, 25, *26*
    secondary, 25, *25*
        nutritional, *94–95*, 95
    skull signs of, 25
    spinal changes due to, 49

Hyperthyroidism (companion animals), osteopenia due to, 49

Hypertrophic osteopathy, in companion animals, 132, *132*

Hypervitaminosis A, in cats, vertebral body proliferation with, 47

Hypoadrenocorticism, microcardia due to, in companion animals, 291, *292*

Hypodermoclysis, 237

Hypoglossal defect, in dogs, 227

Hypovolemia, in companion animals, microcardia due to, 291
    pulmonary changes in, 313
    vena cava in, 284

Hysterosalpingography, in companion animals, 459, *459*

Ileocolic intussusception, in companion animals, *499*

Ileum, anatomy in companion animals, 511

Ileus, functional, in companion animals, 498, *499*

Ileus (*Continued*)
    paralytic, in birds, *530*

Image formation, principles of, 1–4

Infectious arthritis, of proximal interphalangeal joint, in equidae, *191*

Infraorbital canal, of horse, *66, 68, 69*

Inguinal hernia, in companion animals, *389*
    due to pregnancy, 463

Injury, bone responses to, 13–17

Interlobar fissures, 270–271, *270–272*

Intermaxillary septum, of horse, visualization of, *66, 68, 68*

Interosseous ligaments, metacarpal, lesions in equidae, 162, *163*

Interphalangeal joints (equidae), abnormalities of, 187–192
    alignment of, 187–189
    decreased width of, *185*
    distal, luxation of, *190*
    flexural deformities of, 187–188, *189*
    periarticular bone margins in, 191–192, *192*
    visualization of, 178, *179*
    proximal, degenerative arthritis of, 185
        dorsal subluxation of, 188, *189*
        radiographic appearance of, 190, *191*
        width and subchondral bone opacity in, 190, *191*
    soft tissue lesions of, 189, *190*

Intervertebral disc (companion animals), 51–56
    calcification of, 53, *53, 54,* 55
    disease of, incidence and pathophysiology of, 52–53
        spondylosis vs., *53,* 55, *55*
    herniation of, 52–55, *54*
    mineralization of, 53

Intervertebral disc space, collapse of, 54

Intervertebral foramen, enlargement of, in companion animals, 48

Intranasal cysts, in horses, 73

Intrapatellar fat pad sign, in companion animals, 121

Intravenous urography, in companion animals, 409–410, 409(t)

Intussusception (companion animals), cecocolic, *518*
    colonic, *518*
    gastroesophageal, *223, 233*
    ileocolic, *499*

Involucrum, complicating bone healing, 112, *112*

Iodides, organic, for contrast bladder cystography, 430(t)

Jaw locking, open mouth, in companion animals, 31

Jejunum (companion animals), adenocarcinoma of, in companion animals, *506*
    foreign object in, *505*
    obstruction of, *499*